ADVANCES IN

Immunology

VOLUME 47

ADVANCES IN
Immunology

EDITED BY

FRANK J. DIXON

*Scripps Clinic and Research Foundation
La Jolla, California*

ASSOCIATE EDITORS

K. Frank Austen
Leroy E. Hood
Jonathan W. Uhr

VOLUME 47

ACADEMIC PRESS, INC.
Harcourt Brace Jovanovich, Publishers

San Diego   New York   Berkeley   Boston
London   Sydney   Tokyo   Toronto

COPYRIGHT © 1989 BY ACADEMIC PRESS, INC.
All Rights Reserved.
No part of this publication may be reproduced or transmitted in any form or
by any means, electronic or mechanical, including photocopy, recording, or
any information storage and retrieval system, without permission in writing
from the publisher.

ACADEMIC PRESS, INC.
San Diego, California 92101

United Kingdom Edition published by
ACADEMIC PRESS LIMITED
24-28 Oval Road, London NW1 7DX

LIBRARY OF CONGRESS CATALOG CARD NUMBER: 61-17057

ISBN 0-12-022447-X (alk. paper)

PRINTED IN THE UNITED STATES OF AMERICA
89 90 91 92   9 8 7 6 5 4 3 2 1

CONTENTS

Regulation of Immunoglobulin E Biosynthesis
KIMISHIGE ISHIZAKA

I.	Introduction	1
II.	Mechanisms for the IgE Antibody Response	1
III.	Isotype-Specific Regulation by IgE-Binding Factors (IgE-BFs)	12
IV.	Immunological Approaches for Suppression of the IgE Antibody Response	28
	References	40

Control of the Immune Response at the Level of Antigen-Presenting Cells: A Comparison of the Function of Dendritic Cells and B Lymphocytes
JOSHUA P. METLAY, ELLEN PURÉ, AND RALPH M. STEINMAN

I.	Introduction	45
II.	Tissue Distribution of Dendritic Cells and B Lymphocytes	47
III.	The Cell Surface of Dendritic Cells and B Lymphocytes	57
IV.	Antigen Presentation	64
V.	APC Requirements during T Cell-Dependent Antibody Responses	81
VI.	Discussion—Four Components of APC Function	87
VII.	Conclusion—Consequences of Having Two Different Types of APCs	101
	References	105

The CD5 B Cell
THOMAS J. KIPPS

I.	Introduction	117
II.	CD5 B Cells Defined	118
III.	Anatomic Localization of CD5 B Cells	120
IV.	CD5 B Cells in Ontogeny	121
V.	CD5 B Cells in Aging	122
VI.	CD5 B Cell Malignancies	123
VII.	CD5 as a Marker for B Cell Activation	125
VIII.	CD5 B Cells Define a Distinct B Cell Lineage	128
IX.	CD5 B Cells after Human Bone Marrow Transplantation	129
X.	CD5 B Cell Physiology	130
XI.	Physiology of the CD5 Surface Antigen	143
XII.	Genetic Influence on the Relative Numbers of CD5 B Cells	147
XIII.	CD5 B Cells in Human Autoimmune Diseases	148
XIV.	Immunoglobulin Gene Expression in Murine CD5 B Cell Lymphomas	150

XV.	Immunoglobulin Gene Expression in Human CD5 B Cell Malignancies	152
XVI.	CD5 B Cells and the Primordial Immune Network	159
XVII.	Conclusion	161
	References	162

Biology of Natural Killer Cells

GIORGIO TRINCHIERI

I.	Introduction	187
II.	Measurement of NK Cell-Mediated Cytotoxicity	189
III.	Phenotypic and Genotypic Characteristics of NK Cells	196
IV.	Origin and Differentiation of NK Cells	219
V.	Activation and Effector Mechanisms of NK Cells	234
VI.	Interaction between NK Cells and the Central Nervous System	266
VII.	NK Cells and Reproduction	269
VIII.	NK Cells and Hematopoiesis	272
IX.	Antimicrobial Activity of NK Cells	282
X.	NK Cells and Adaptive Immunity	291
XI.	Anti-Tumor Activity of NK Cells	295
XII.	Alterations of Human NK Cell Number and Function in Other Pathological Conditions	300
	References	303

The Immunopathogenesis of HIV Infection

ZEDA F. ROSENBERG AND ANTHONY S. FAUCI

I.	Introduction	377
II.	The Etiological Agent	378
III.	Immunopathogenic Mechanisms	385
IV.	Neuropsychiatric Manifestations	403
V.	Immune Response to HIV	405
VI.	Summary and Conclusions	411
	References	414

The Obese Strain of Chickens: An Animal Model with Spontaneous Autoimmune Thyroiditis

GEORGE WICK, HANS PETER BREZINSCHEK, KAREL HÁLA, HERMANN DIETRICH, HUGO WOLF, AND GUIDO KROEMER

I.	Introduction	433
II.	Development of the Strain—Breeding Requirements	435
III.	Clinical and Histopathological Characteristics	438
IV.	Humoral and Cellular Immune Reactions	444
V.	Altered Thyroid Function—Target Organ Defect	456
VI.	Potential Effector Mechanisms	465
VII.	Disturbed Immunoregulation	469

VIII.	Genetics	481
IX.	Conclusion	491
	References	494

INDEX   501

CONTENTS OF RECENT VOLUMES   525

Regulation of Immunoglobulin E Biosynthesis

KIMISHIGE ISHIZAKA

*The Johns Hopkins University,
School of Medicine at Good Samaritan Hospital,
Baltimore, Maryland 21239*

I. Introduction

It has been established that immunoglobulin E (IgE) antibodies against allergen cause hay fever and are involved in the other allergic diseases. A crucial role of IgE antibodies in reaginic (Type I) hypersensitivity immediately raised a question as to whether the antibody response can be suppressed. To achieve this goal, however, one has to learn cellular mechanisms involved in the IgE antibody response. Extensive studies in rodent systems in the past 18 years indicated that the IgE antibody response to protein antigens shares common mechanisms with the IgM and IgG antibody responses to T cell-dependent antigens. However, the IgE antibody response in experimental animals has several characteristics not easily demonstrated in the IgG antibody response. The purpose of this review is to summarize some unique features for the antibody response of the IgE isotype and to discuss possible approaches to controlling the IgE antibody response.

II. Mechanisms for the IgE Antibody Response

A. Dissociation between the IgE and IgG Antibody Responses *in Vivo*

Many years ago Sherman *et al.* (1940) determined reaginic antibody titers in the sera of hay fever patients by Prausnitz–Küstner reactions, and observed that the antibody titers in the sera of ragweed-sensitive patients were persistent. This observation was confirmed by radioimmunoassay. Quantitative measurements of serum IgE antibodies in ragweed-sensitive patients who had not received immunotherapy showed that the antibody level persists throughout the year and that most patients showed secondary IgE antibody response after the ragweed season (Ishizaka and Ishizaka, 1973). Because an average half-life of IgE in the serum is 2.3 days in humans (Waldman, 1969), it appears that IgE antibodies are being formed continuously in hay fever patients.

A persistent IgE antibody formation observed in atopic patients was difficult to reproduce in experimental animals. When mice and rats were immunized with a protein antigen adequate for the maximal IgG antibody response, the IgE antibody response was transient and the antibodies disappeared within 3–4 weeks after the priming immunization (Revoltella and Ovary, 1969). In these animals a booster injection of the same antigen failed to induce the secondary IgE antibody response. Such difficulties were overcome by Levine and Vaz (1970), who immunized several strains of inbred mice with a minute dose of various antigens incorporated into aluminum hydroxide gel (alum). When certain inbred strains were immunized with an appropriate immunogen, repeated immunization at 4-week intervals induced the secondary IgE antibody response. Subsequently, E. M. Vaz et al. (1971) succeeded in obtaining a persistent IgE antibody response by immunization of SW-55 mice with a minute dose (0.1 μg) of alum-absorbed ovalbumin (OVA). The IgE antibody titer persisted for several months without any booster immunization.

Systematic studies by N. M. Vaz et al. (1971) as well as those by others showed that the IgE antibody response is controlled by immune response genes which are linked to the major histocompatibility complex (MHC). When minute doses of alum-absorbed immunogen were used for immunization, only high-responder strains gave IgE and IgG_1 antibody responses. Even in these strains, the magnitude of the IgE antibody response did not parallel the IgE antibody response to the same antigen when different adjuvants were employed for immunization. *Bordetella pertussis* vaccine and alum are effective adjuvants for the IgE antibody response, while complete Freund's adjuvant (CFA) is less effective (Ishizaka, 1976). Furthermore, when high-responder mice were immunized with a potent immunogen, together with an appropriate adjuvant, an increase in the dose of immunogen made the IgE antibody transient and caused a dissociation between the IgG and IgE antibody responses (Ishizaka and Okudaira, 1973).

An entirely different type of genetic control was found in the mouse, which uniquely controls the IgE isotype. For example, SJL mice as well as AKR mice showed a poor IgE antibody response to various protein antigens in spite of a substantial IgG antibody response (Levine, 1971). Under certain conditions, such as nematode infection, SJL mice could form IgE; however, the SJA/9 strain, which was derived from BALB/c and SJL, could not synthesize IgE (Yaoita et al., 1982). Breeding experiments showed that this genetic control is not linked to the MHC. It appears that not only immune response genes but also this genetic control operate in determining whether a given mouse strain will produce

IgE antibody to a given antigen. These findings collectively indicate that the persistent IgE antibody response to a given antigen is obtained in the mouse only when a high-responding, high-IgE-producing strain is immunized with a minute dose of a potent immunogen together with an appropriate adjuvant.

Dissociation between the IgE and IgG antibody responses can be obtained under various conditions. For example, the IgE antibody response is selectively enhanced by low-dose X-rays of rodents or by treatment of the animals with cyclophosphamide (Chiorazzi *et al.*, 1976; Tada *et al.*, 1971). Even low-responder mouse strains such as SJL produced IgE antibodies if they were irradiated prior to immunization with an alum-absorbed potent immunogen. On the other hand, repeated injections of CFA prior to immunization with alum-absorbed protein antigen selectively suppressed the IgE antibody response to the antigen without affecting the IgG antibody response (Tung *et al.*, 1978).

In both humans and experimental animals, infections with some nematodes enhance IgE synthesis (Johansson *et al.*, 1968; Rousseaux-Provost *et al.*, 1977). If one primes rats with an appropriate antigen for an IgE antibody response and then infects the animals with the nematode *Nippostrongylus brasiliensis* (Nb), IgE antibody formation against the priming antigen is selectively enhanced (Jarrett and Steward, 1972). Augmentation of the antibody response, after the nematode infection, is directed to the IgE isotype; neither IgG_1 nor IgG_2 antibody response to the same antigen was affected by the infection (Block *et al.*, 1973). These findings collectively suggest that the IgE antibody response is controlled not only by antigen-specific mechanisms but also by some additional mechanisms selective for the IgE isotype.

B. IgE Synthesis *in Vitro*

1. IgE Antibody Response by Rabbit Lymphocytes

In order to analyze the mechanisms involved in IgE synthesis, *in vitro* systems for IgE antibody response are quite useful. The first successful studies for the elicitation of the secondary IgE antibody production *in vitro* were carried out by Ishizaka and Kishimoto (1972). They immunized outbred rabbits with dinitrophenyl derivatives of *Ascaris* extract (DNP-Asc) in alum for the IgE antibody response. After a booster immunization with alum-absorbed DNP-Asc, animals giving the secondary IgE antibody response were selected, and their mesenteric lymph node (MLN) cells were obtained 2 weeks after the booster immunization. The primed MLN cells were incubated with homologous antigen for 24 hours, and after being washed the cells were cultured in Marbrook chambers for 6 days. The basic findings obtained in these studies were that rabbits which had developed good primary and secondary IgE antibody responses *in vivo* provided MLN cells that were capable of being stimulated *in vitro* to develop IgE as well as IgG and IgM antibody responses. Because the rabbits used in the experiments were outbred, the limitation of this system was that lymphocytes from two different animals could not be mixed in the culture. Nevertheless, Kishimoto and Ishizaka (1973) were able to dissect the respective roles of carrier-specific helper cells and hapten-specific B memory cells in the development of anti-DNP IgE antibody response. Rabbits were immunized with alum-absorbed DNP-Asc for the IgE antibody response and then were supplementally immunized with ragweed antigen (Rag) in alum or CFA. Their MLN cells were stimulated with either DNP-Asc or DNP-Rag for the antibody response. The MLN cells from the animals that received a supplemental immunization of alum-absorbed Rag formed both IgE and IgG anti-DNP antibodies upon stimulation with either DNP-Asc or DNP-Rag. On the other hand, MLN cells of rabbits that received a supplemental immunization of Rag included in CFA formed IgG anti-hapten antibodies, but not IgE antibody, upon stimulation with DNP-Rag, while the same cells formed both IgE and IgG antibodies when stimulated by DNP-Asc. These findings indicate that carrier-specific T cell populations developed by supplemental immunization differ depending on the adjuvant employed, and suggest that the differences in the T cell population are responsible for the dissociation between the IgE and IgG antibody responses.

2. *IgE-Forming Cell Response of Rat Lymphocytes*

In order to carry out the analysis of cellular regulatory mechanisms on the IgE production in the rat, Suemura *et al.* (1978) established a system to quantitate the development of plasma cells containing cytoplasmic IgE. Thus, MLN cells of rats infected with Nb were obtained 4 weeks after the infection, and such cells were cultured for 5 days in the presence or absence of an appropriate concentration of Nb antigen. The cells were fixed and stained by indirect immunofluorescence for cytoplasmic content of IgE, IgM, or IgG. Under these conditions stimulation of MLN cells from infected rats with Nb antigen resulted in the development of a substantial number of plasma cells that can be stained for IgE, IgM, or IgG. The Ig-forming cell response was T cell dependent. It was also found that depletion of IgE-bearing cells in the MLN cells followed by stimulation with Nb antigen resulted in a marked decrease in IgE-containing cells without affecting the development of IgM- or IgG-containing plasma cells. The same method was employed to observe Ig-forming cell responses to DNP derivatives of OVA (DNP-OVA) (Suemura and Ishizaka, 1979). Rats were immunized with DNP-OVA included in CFA. After a booster immunization, their MLN cells were cultured with 1 μg/ml of DNP-OVA for 5 days, and plasma cells containing IgE or IgG were enumerated. As expected, a substantial number of IgG-containing plasma cells but very few IgE-containing plasma cells developed in the cultures. As described in Section III, this system was useful for demonstrating IgE-potentiating factor (IgE-PF), which selectively enhanced IgE-forming cell response without affecting the IgG-forming cell response.

3. In Vitro Synthesis of IgE by Cultured Mouse Lymphocytes

The IgE antibody response in inbred mouse strains provided most useful information on the mechanisms of IgE synthesis. However, *in vitro* IgE antibody responses by murine lymphoid cells have been most difficult to reproduce. When mice of a good IgE producer strain were immunized with alum-absorbed antigen for the persistent IgE antibody response, their spleen cells spontaneously released a substantial amount of IgE antibodies. Incubation of their spleen cells with homologous antigen for 24 hours, followed by culture of the antigen-stimulated cells, resulted in a decrease of IgE antibody formation, while IgG antibodies in culture supernatant increased upon antigenic stimulation (Danneman and Michael, 1977).

Successful demonstration of the stimulation of murine IgE synthesis *in vitro* was reported by Kimoto *et al.* (1977). These investigators immunized BALB/c mice with three injections of alum-absorbed DNP-OVA or DNP-Asc at 4-week intervals and stimulated their spleen cells with homologous antigen for 24 hours. The cells were recovered, washed to remove the antigen and cultured for 6 days using the Marbrook system. The IgE and IgG_1 antibodies were detected in culture supernatants. The antibody responses required T cells and depended on carrier-specific helper T cells. Kimoto *et al.* (1977) confirmed the findings of Kishimoto and Ishizaka (1973). Thus, they primed BALB/c mice with alum-absorbed Asc for priming carrier-specific helper cells and proved that Asc-specific helper cells generated by this priming collaborated with DNP-specific B cells raised by immunization with alum-absorbed DNP-OVA; mixture of the two cell populations responded to DNP-Asc for the IgE and IgG anti-DNP antibody responses. However, the carrier-specific T cells obtained by priming with Asc included in CFA provided helper activity only for the IgG antibody response.

Subsequently, Suemura *et al.* (1981) modified the method. They immunized BALB/c mice by injecting alum-absorbed DNP derivatives of keyhole limpet hemocyanin (DNP-KLH) twice, and stimulated the spleen cells with homologous antigen for IgE-forming cell responses. Since the quantity of antihapten antibody response was limited, they evaluated the immune response by enumerating IgE- and IgG-forming cells by the reversed-plaque technique. Nevertheless, *in vitro* development of IgE-forming cell response or IgE antibody response in antigen-stimulated cultures is not consistent. Although the other investigators frequently employed similar methods, success of the response is highly dependent on the immunization regimen for priming the donor of B cells.

Recently, however, a consistent method was developed based on the participation of interleukin (IL)-4-producing helper T cells in the IgE synthesis. As will be described below, stimulation of B cells with lipopolysaccharide (LPS) in the presence of 300–1000 U/ml of IL-4 induced not only IgM and IgG formation but also IgE synthesis (Coffman *et al.*, 1986). It was also found that cognate interaction of B cells with an antigen-primed, IL-4-producing T cell clone resulted in the differentiation of B cells into plasma cells that form either IgG_1 or IgE.

4. IgE Synthesis by Human Lymphocytes

Numerous investigators have reported that peripheral blood mononuclear cells (PBMCs) from patients with elevated serum IgE levels synthesized substantial amounts of IgE in culture, whereas PBMCs from nonatopic donors failed to synthesize a detectable amount of IgE (Fisher and Buckley, 1979; Romagnani *et al.*, 1980; Saxon *et al.*, 1980). Since the concentration of IgE detected in culture supernatants was low, the possibility was raised that PBMC cells contained preformed IgE, or bore IgE on their surface, and the protein was released into culture supernatants during the culture. Indeed, several investigators claimed that nearly one half of IgE released into culture supernatants may represent IgE preformed *in vivo* (Sampson and Buckley, 1981; Turner *et al.*, 1983). However, if partially purified B cells from atopic individuals were cultured, the percentage of preformed IgE by the B cells of hyper-IgE individuals was less than 10–20% of the final IgE synthesized in 7 days' culture (Leung and Geha, 1986). It appears that B cells of atopic donors synthesize substantially more IgE than do normal B cells *in vitro*. The cell source of IgE synthesized in cultures appears to be light-density-activated B cells (Saxon *et al.*, 1980).

For understanding of the mechanisms controlling the IgE response of human lymphocytes, several laboratories have studied the ability of pokeweed mitogen (PWM) to induce human PBMCs to synthesize IgE, with conflicting results. Although the attempts were successful in some laboratories by selecting culture conditions and the dose of PWM (Saxon and Stevens, 1979; Zuraw *et al.*, 1981), PWM failed to stimulate IgE synthesis by normal PBMCs in most studies and inhibited spontaneous formation of IgE by PBMCs from atopic patients (Fisher and Buckley, 1979; Saryan *et al.*, 1983). Similarly, *Staphylococcus aureus* Cowan I strain and Epstein–Barr virus consistently stimulated normal PBMCs for IgG formation, but gave conflicting results on IgE synthesis (Deguchi *et al.*, 1983; Saryan *et al.*, 1983). Failure of IgE synthesis in these systems was not due to suppressor T cells, because depletion of OKT8$^+$ (CD8$^+$) T cells in normal PBMCs did not enhance the IgE synthesis (Saryan *et al.*, 1983).

Differentiation of human B cells for IgE synthesis was achieved by using alloreactive T cells. Lanzavecchia (1984) has reported that human alloreactive T cell clones can induce IgE secretion by B cells. The finding suggested that cognate interaction through HLA-DR determinants expressed on the relevant B cells could activate IgE synthesis by normal B cells. Indeed, the results were confirmed by Umetsu *et al.* (1985). B cells from both normal and allergic donors could be induced to synthesize Igs of all isotypes, including IgE, when they were cocultured with some alloreactive T cell clones. The results indicated that resting B cells can be activated for IgE synthesis under conditions of cognate interaction with helper T cells. Obviously, not all alloreactive T cell clones can induce the formation of IgE. From the findings described below, the T cell clones that form IL-4 would be essential for the production of IgE.

On the other hand, IgE synthesis by B cells of atopic individuals can be stimulated through bystander effects as well. When B cells lacking the stimulatory alloantigens are cultured in the presence of alloreactive T cell clones stimulated by third-party monocytes bearing the appropriate alloantigens, IgE was detected in culture supernatants (Umetsu *et al.*, 1985). Under the same culture conditions, B cells from nonatopic donors failed to synthesize IgE, although increased amounts of IgG, IgM, and IgA were produced by B cells from both atopic and nonatopic individuals. It appears that both resting and preactivated precursor B cells are present in the peripheral blood of atopic individuals and that only the latter B cell population responded to lymphokines released from alloreactive T cells.

C. T Cells and B Cells Involved in the IgE Antibody Response

1. Precursors of IgE-Forming Cells

Extensive studies of the surface Ig (sIg) on mouse B cells by many investigators showed that resting B cells bear IgM and IgD, and that the B cells bearing the other isotypes are derived from the virgin B cells

(Warner, 1974). It is generally accepted that lymphocytes bearing IgG or IgA are already committed to the synthesis of the respective isotypes after differentiation. The same principle may apply for the precursors of IgE-forming cells. Although the number of sIgE$^+$ B cells is low, sIgE$^+$ B cells were demonstrated in rodent lymphoid tissues, under certain conditions (Uede et al., 1984). However, early demonstration of IgE-bearing B cells may largely be due to binding of external IgE to FcεRII on B cells. Katona et al. (1983) reported that the proportion of IgE-bearing B cells in BALB/c spleen cells increased after infection with Nb, but the majority of IgE on the cells was passively bound through the receptors for IgE (FcεRII). IgE on these B cells could be removed by exposure of the cells to acid pH. Furthermore, the majority of B cells in a normal, unprimed mouse formed rosettes with IgE-coated erythrocytes (Vander-Mallie et al., 1982), and the majority of sIgM$^+$ sIgD$^+$ B cells in normal human peripheral blood could be stained with monoclonal anti-FcεRII antibodies in immunofluorescence (Kikutani et al., 1986b). Nevertheless, B cells with intrinsic sIgE can be demonstrated under certain circumstances. As described above, a persistent IgE antibody response can be obtained by immunization of a high-IgE-producing (BDF$_1$) mouse strain with alum-absorbed OVA. Transfer of their spleen cells into irradiated syngeneic mice followed by a booster immunization of the recipients with alum-absorbed OVA, results in an extremely high IgE antibody response. A substantial portion of B cells in the spleen of the recipients bears IgE, which cannot be removed by exposure of the cells to acid pH (Uede et al., 1984). It was also found that some IgE-producing hybridomas bear sIgE on their surface (Suemura et al., 1983). Thus, the precursors of IgE-forming cells appear to express sIgE at certain stages of differentiation.

2. Role of IL-4 and IL-4-Producing Helper T Cells

The IgE antibody response is highly T cell dependent, and nude mice failed to respond to alum-absorbed antigen for the IgE antibody response. These findings suggest that T cell-derived lymphokines are involved in the differentiation of B cells to IgE-forming cells. Recently, evidence was presented that IL-4 from helper T cells is involved in the differentiation of B cells to IgE-forming cells. It is well known that stimulation of mouse B cells with LPS results in the differentiation of B cells and the formation of a variety of Ig isotypes, except IgE (Parkhouse and Cooper, 1977). However, culture of the same B cells for 5 days with LPS together with 300–1000 units/ml of recombinant IL-4 resulted in the formation of IgE and selective enhancement of IgG$_1$ formation (Coffman et al., 1986), which was accompanied by decreases in IgG$_{2b}$

and IgG$_3$ formation. For this effect, it is not necessary that IL-4 be present from the start of the cultures but it must be added by day 2 for maximum IgE and IgG$_1$ enhancement (Coffman and Carty, 1986). It was also found that culture of pure B cells with LPS and IL-4 resulted in the appearance of sIgE- and sIgG$_1$-bearing B cells (Snapper et al., 1988b) and that depletion of sIgE$^+$ B cells developed in the culture abolished LPS plus IL-4-induced IgE formation. Since neither IL-4 itself nor anti-IgM plus IL-4 induced the differentiation of B cells for IgE synthesis, the major effect of IL-4 in the system appears to be switching of sIgM$^+$ sIgD$^+$ B cells for the expression of sIgG$_1$ and/or sIgE (Snapper et al., 1988a). It is known that IL-4 enhances the biosynthesis of Ia molecules and FcεRII in B cells (Conrad et al., 1987; Noelle et al., 1984). A relatively low concentration (3–5 units/ml) of IL-4 is sufficient for this effect. The concentration of IL-4 required for switching of B cells for IgE synthesis is much higher than the physiological concentration of IL-4. However, Coffman et al. (1988) demonstrated that the presence of IL-5 together with IL-4 diminished the minimum concentration of IL-4 for IgE synthesis to 5–10 U/ml.

The effect of IL-4 on the IgE synthesis was also demonstrated in human PBMCs. Recently, Péne et al. (1988a,b) have shown that culture of normal human PBMC cells with 100 U/ml of human IL-4 resulted in the formation of IgE. In this system, however, both T cells and monocytes are required for the induction of IgE synthesis by normal B cells. The same observations were made by Prete et al. (1988).

It has been shown that the effect of IL-4 on B cells is counteracted by γ-interferon (IFNγ). This lymphokine inhibits not only the IL-4-induced increase in Ia expression (Mond et al., 1986) and FcεRII (Conrad et al., 1987) on resting B cells, but also the formation of IgE and IgG$_1$ by B cells stimulated with LPS plus IL-4 (Coffman and Carty, 1986). Only 1–10 antiviral U/ml IFNγ totally inhibits IL-4 plus LPS-induced IgE and IgG$_1$ production. Although IFNγ could be inhibitory to the production of other isotypes by LPS-stimulated B cells, inhibition of IgG and IgM production by this concentration of IFNγ was less than 50%. The IL-4-induced formation of IgE by human PBMCs was also suppressed by IFNγ and IFNα (Péne et al., 1988b). These findings suggest that the proportion among various lymphokines in the environment of B cells may affect the distribution of antibodies among various isotypes.

As described in Section II,A, the IgE antibody response is obtained by immunization of high-responder mice with a minute dose of alum-absorbed antigen. This finding suggests that differentiation of B cells to IgE-forming plasma cells is triggered by cognate interaction between antigen-specific helper T cells and B cells, rather than by lymphokines released from helper T cells. Mosmann et al. (1986) described that mouse helper T cell clones can be classified into two subtypes, i.e., TH_1 and TH_2, which produce different ILs upon antigenic stimulation. Both subsets express Lyt-1 and L3T4; however, TH_1 produces IL-2, IFNγ, and lymphotoxin, while TH_2 produces IL-4 and IL-5. The other lymphokines, such as IL-3 and granulocyte–macrophage colony-stimulating factor, are produced by both subsets. It is not clear whether these two subsets exist as distinct lineages or whether a single helper T cell can give different patterns of lymphokine production, depending on the nature of the stimulus or the environment of the cells. Nevertheless, the lymphokine secretion phenotypes of TH_1 and TH_2 clones are quite stable, suggesting that individual stimulated helper T cells may express only one phenotype. Coffman et al. (1988) found that both TH_1 and TH_2 clones can provide help to B cells under appropriate conditions; however, there are important differences in the Ig isotypes produced by B cells in response to the different subsets. Thus, these investigators employed rabbit IgG-specific TH_1 and TH_2 clones established by Tony and Parker (1985) and induced polyclonal activation of normal B cells by culture of the cells with rabbit anti-mouse Ig antibodies and the helper T cell clone. As shown in Table I, TH_2 clones gave much better help than did TH_1 clones for the production of Ig. The majority of the Ig produced by the polyclonal activation of B cells by the TH_2 clone was IgM and IgG_1 but a substantial quantity of IgE was also produced in the system. When the same B cells were cultured with a rabbit IgG-specific TH_1 clone and rabbit anti-mouse Ig, only

TABLE I
ISOTYPE DISTRIBUTION OF POLYCLONAL RESPONSE OF NORMAL B CELLS TO RGG-SPECIFIC HELPER T CELL CLONES[a]

Isotype	TH_2 (ng/ml)	TH_1 (ng/ml)	TH_1 + IL-2 + anti-IFNγ (ng/ml)
IgM	98,000	248	65,000
IgE	187	<1	<1
IgA	484	<1	825
IgG_1	21,600	<8	5280
IgG_{2a}	39	14	2760
IgG_{2b}	189	<8	135
IgG_3	354	<8	474

[a] Coffman et al. (1988).

IgM was detected in culture supernatants. The results shown in Table I indicate that helper T cells for Ig production are TH_2 cells rather than TH_1 cells. Since IFNγ could be suppressive for the production of Ig, these investigators supplemented the TH_1 system with anti-IFNγ and IL-2. As shown in Table I, addition of anti-IFNγ antibodies and IL-2 to the system enhanced the formation of IgM, IgG_1, and IgG_{2a} but did not give the formation of IgE. However, the addition of IL-4 to the TH_1 system resulted in the formation of IgE. These results indicate that TH_2 cells are essential for IgE synthesis and suggest that the distribution of antibodies among various isotypes differ depending on the proportion between the two subsets of helper T cells.

Requirement of TH_2 cells and IL-4 for IgE synthesis may partly explain the dissociation between the IgE and IgG antibody responses. It is not known whether different types of adjuvant may affect the distribution of helper T cells between the two subsets. However, it became clear that spleen cells of mice infected with the nematode Nb formed IL-4 (Finkelman et al., 1986b). This lymphokine is almost undetectable in culture supernatants when mice were primed with a protein antigen and their spleen cells were stimulated by homologous antigen. Detection of IL-4 in the culture supernatant of lymphoid cells of Nb-infected animals indicates that the nematode infection enhances the production of IL-4 through unknown mechanisms and suggested that IL-4 enhanced the IgE synthesis. IL-4 may also explain the strain differences in IgE synthesis. As described, nude mice as well as those of the SJA/9 strain failed to form IgE even after *Nippostrongylus* infection. However, stimulation of B cells from SJA/9 and nude mice with LPS together with recombinant IL-4 induced the formation of IgE (Azuma et al., 1987). The results suggest that this strain may have deficiencies in the production of IL-4 but not in the precursor B cells of IgE-forming cells.

Series of experiments indicating the essential role of IL-4 or IL-4-producing T helper cells for IgE synthesis provided *in vitro* systems for the production of IgE. It has been shown that the presentation of conalbumin to the conalbumin-specific TH_2 clones D10.G4 cells by unprimed B cells results in the differentiation of B cells for Ig-forming cells (Keegan et al., 1989). In this system conalbumin-primed B cells are not required. Indeed, coculture of B cells from CBA or C3H strains with mitomycin-treated D10.G4 cells in the presence of conalbumin for 6 days resulted in the production of both IgG_1 and IgE. Since normal B cells can process conalbumin, these cells present antigen to D10 cells, which in turn stimulate B cells for differentiation to IgE-forming cells. The same principle may apply for human lymphocyte systems. Prete et al. (1988) have shown that many human $CD4^+$ T cell clones produce both IL-4 and IFNγ and indicated that TH_1 and TH_2 phenotypes do not apply for human T cells. However, they demonstrated that the ability of the helper T cell clones to induce *in vitro* IgE synthesis in human B cells correlated with their ability to release IL-4 and inversely related to their ability to release IFNγ. Ohehir *et al.* (1988) established helper T cell clones specific for *Dermatophagoides farinae* from PBMCs of house dust-sensitive patients. Culture of an IL-4-producing T cell clone and autologous B cells in the presence of the antigen resulted in the formation of IgE.

III. Isotype-Specific Regulation by IgE-Binding Factors (IgE-BFs)

A. Biological Activities of IgE-BFs

Dissociation between the IgE and IgG antibody responses raised the possibility that the IgE antibody response may be regulated not only by antigen-specific helper and suppressor T cells but also by a mechanism selective for this isotype. Since the infection of antigen-primed rats with Nb selectively potentiated the IgE antibody response (Jarrett and Steward, 1972) and the IgE-specific potentiation is dependent on T cells (Jarrett and Ferguson, 1974), it was anticipated that T cells of Nb-infected rats would selectively enhance the differentiation of IgE B cells to IgE-forming cells. Indeed, T cells obtained 2 weeks after Nb infection, as well as soluble factors from the T cells, selectively enhanced the *in vitro* IgE-forming cell response of DNP-OVA-primed rat MLN cells to homologous antigen (Suemura *et al.*, 1980). The T cell factors responsible for the selective potentiation of IgE response had affinity for IgE and could be purified by absorption with IgE-coupled Sepharose, followed by elution at acid pH (Suemura *et al.*, 1980; Yodoi *et al.*, 1980). The factors could be detected by their ability to inhibit rosette formation of $FcεR^+$ lymphocytes with IgE-coated erythrocytes.

Subsequent experiments revealed that T-cell factors having affinity for IgE, i.e., IgE-BFs, exhibit heterologous biological activities and physicochemical properties. Normal MLN cells did not release IgE-BFs, but incubation of the cells with homologous IgE resulted in the formation of IgE-BFs. When MLN cells obtained from rats 8 days after Nb infection were incubated with IgE, cells produced IgE-BFs, which selectively suppressed, rather than enhanced, the *in vitro* IgE response (Hirashima *et al.*, 1980a). The major cell source of IgE-PFs and IgE-suppressive factors (IgE-SFs) appeared to be T cells.

Formation of IgE-BFs is not confined to rodent lymphocytes. Human lymphocytes activated by mixed-lymphocyte cultures produced IgE-BFs upon incubation with homologous IgE (Ishizaka and Sandberg, 1981). Saryan *et al.* (1983) reported that peripheral T cells of patients with hyper-IgE syndrome or atopic dermatitis produced soluble factors that have affinity for IgE and selectively enhance the IgE synthesis by the peripheral blood lymphocytes of allergic individuals. On the other hand, Leung *et al.* (1984) reported that sera of nonatopic individuals who have extremely low serum IgE levels contained IgE-BFs, which selectively suppressed the IgE formation by the peripheral blood lymphocytes of atopic patients.

The targets of IgE-BFs appear to be sIgE$^+$ B cells, which are already committed for IgE synthesis. Incubation of splenic B cells and plasma cells from IgE-producing BDF$_1$ mice with affinity-purified rodent IgE-SFs resulted in a marked decrease in the number of sIgE$^+$ B cells, IgE plaque-forming cells, and IgE-containing plasma cells (Uede *et al.*, 1984). The same IgE-SFs also suppressed IgE formation by IgE-producing hybridomas that bear sIgE (Suemura *et al.*, 1983; Uede *et al.*, 1984). The same principle will apply for human lymphocyte systems. IgE-PFs from an FcϵR$^+$ human T cell clone (Young *et al.*, 1984) and those from a human T cell hybridoma (Kisaki *et al.*, 1988) enhanced spontaneous formation of IgE by the B cells of allergic patients, and enhanced IgE formation by the B cells induced by alloreactive T cells under bystander conditions. Young *et al.* (1984) have shown that the targets of IgE-PFs are low-density sIgE$^+$ B cells circulating in patients with symptomatic allergic rhinitis. B cells from normal nonatopic individuals or patients with asymptomatic seasonal allergic rhinitis, whose cell cultures had no detectable levels of *de novo* spontaneous IgE synthesis, did not respond to IgE-PFs. However, stimulation of normal B cells with certain allogeneic T cell clones renders them responsive to IgE-PFs (Leung *et al.*, 1986). These observations suggest that IgE-PFs act primarily as differentiation signals on preactivated sIgE$^+$ B cells. It should be noted that the major effect of IL-4 in the IgE synthesis is switching of resting B cells to sIgE$^+$ B cells. On the other hand, IgE-PFs and IgE-SFs appear to regulate the differentiation of sIgE$^+$ B cells to IgE-forming cells. Since IgE-BFs bind to sIgE$^+$ B cells but not to B cells bearing the other isotype(s), the effect of IgE-BFs is selective for this isotype.

B. Correlation between the IgE Response and the Biological Activities of IgE-BFs

It was found that IgE-BFs are formed under various experimental conditions, including incubation of normal rodent lymphocytes with homologous IgE (Yodoi and Ishizaka, 1980). Important findings obtained in a series of experiments were that selective enhancement of the IgE response by various immunological maneuvers was accompanied by the formation of IgE-PFs, while procedures for suppressing the IgE response induced the formation of IgE-SFs. Thus, a single injection of *Bordetella pertussis* vaccine, which is the best adjuvant for the IgE response, induces the formation of IgE-PFs (Hirashima *et al.*, 1981a). In contrast, repeated injections of CFA, which is known to selectively suppress the IgE response to an unrelated antigen, induce the formation of IgE-SFs (Hirashima *et al.*, 1980b). It was also found that the formation of IgE-BFs is associated with the immune response. Immunization of Lewis rats with KLH absorbed to alum resulted in the formation of IgE antibodies, and their spleen cells formed IgE-PFs upon antigenic stimulation. However, when the same strain was immunized with KLH included in CFA, no IgE antibody response was obtained, and their spleen cells formed IgE-SFs upon antigenic stimulation (Uede *et al.*, 1982).

Similar findings were observed in the mouse as well. When high-IgE-producer BDF_1 mice were immunized with a minimum dose of alum-absorbed OVA for persistent IgE antibody formation, their spleen cells formed IgE-PFs upon antigenic stimulation (Uede and Ishizaka, 1984). In contrast, intravenous injections of OVA into the same strain, which suppress the IgE antibody response to alum-absorbed OVA, primed their spleen cells for the formation of IgE-SFs (Jardieu *et al.*, 1984). Kishimoto *et al.* (1976) described that priming of BALB/c mice with DNP derivatives of mycobacteria (DNP-Myc) suppressed the IgE antibody response to alum-absorbed DNP-OVA, and that spleen cells of DNP-Myc-primed mice released IgE-specific suppressive factor (IgE-TsF) upon incubation with DNP-bovine serum albumin (BSA) (Suemura *et al.*, 1977). Their subsequent experiments showed that IgE-TsF had affinity for IgE, and belonged to IgE-BFs (Suemura *et al.*, 1981).

Strain differences in the IgE response also have correlation with biological activities of IgE-BFs formed. In contrast to BDF_1 mice immunization of SJL mice with alum-absorbed antigen and incubation of their spleen cells with the antigen resulted in the formation of IgE-SFs (Uede and Ishizaka, 1984). Such a strain difference in the nature of IgE-BFs was observed even without immunization. It was found that incubation of normal mouse spleen cells or rat MLN cells with homologous IgE resulted in the formation of IgE-BFs (Uede *et al.*, 1983a; Yodoi and Ishizaka, 1980). When normal lymphocytes from Lewis rats or BALB/c mice were incubated with homologous IgE, IgE-BFs formed by the cells were a mixture of IgE-PFs and IgE-SFs. Incubation of spleen cells of a high IgE producer, BDF_1 mice, with mouse IgE resulted in the formation of IgE-PFs. In contrast, normal SJL mouse spleen cells formed IgE-SFs upon incubation with IgE (Uede and Ishizaka, 1984). However,

SJL mice produced IgE antibodies if they received low-dose X-rays or cyclophosphamide prior to immunization, and the spleen cells of the treated mice formed IgE-PFs upon incubation with the homologous antigen (Akasaki and Ishizaki, 1987). These findings collectively indicate that IgE-PFs are formed whenever IgE synthesis is enhanced and/or IgE antibody response is induced, while IgE-SFs are formed in various conditions in which the IgE response is suppressed.

The same principles may be applied to human IgE-BFs. As described, T cells of patients with hyper-IgE syndrome, such as atopic dermatitis, constitutively secrete IgE-PFs (Saryan et al., 1983) while sera of nonatopic individuals, who have extremely low serum IgE levels, contained IgE-SFs (Leung et al., 1984). The correlations between an enhancement of the IgE response and the formation of IgE-PFs and between suppression of the IgE response and the formation of IgE-SFs strongly suggest that IgE-BFs are involved in the regulation of the IgE response *in vivo*.

C. Physicochemical Properties and Structure of IgE-BFs

The T cell-derived IgE-BFs are glycopeptides and are heterogeneous with respect to their molecular mass. When spleen cells of antigen-primed rats or mice were stimulated by homologous antigen or IgE, the IgE-BFs formed by the cells consisted of the 60-, 30-, and 15-kDa species (Uede et al., 1983a). Rodent T cell hybridomas, i.e., 23B6 and 231 F_1 (Huff et al., 1982; Jardieu et al., 1985a), as well as human T cell hybridoma 166A2 (Huff et al., 1986), formed the three species when they were incubated with homologous IgE. Another rodent hybridoma, 23A4 (Huff et al., 1982), and two human T cell hybridomas, 166G11 and 400G2 (Huff et al., 1986), formed the 60- and 30-kDa IgE-BFs upon incubation with IgE. An $Fc\epsilon R^+$ human T cell clone, which was established from the peripheral blood of an atopic dermatitis patient, constitutively secreted the 60- and 15-kDa IgE-PFs (Young et al., 1986).

The major differences between the 15-kDa IgE-PFs and the 15-kDa IgE-SFs appear to be carbohydrate moieties. The 15-kDa IgE-PFs from both rodent T cells and human T cell hybridomas have affinity for lentil lectin and concanavalin A (Con A) (Huff et al., 1986; Yodoi et al., 1980). The 15-kDa IgE-SFs from both species failed to bind to the lectins, but have affinity for peanut agglutinin (PNA) (Hirashima et al., 1980a; Huff et al., 1986). Although the 60-kDa IgE-SFs do not necessarily bind to PNA, the 60-kDa IgE-PFs from both species have affinity for lentil lectin (Jardieu et al., 1985b).

The amino acid sequence of the rodent IgE-BF peptide was revealed by gene cloning. Martens et al. (1985) incubated the rodent T cell hybridoma 23B6 with rat IgE to induce the formation of IgE-SFs, and obtained mRNA from the cells. They constructed cDNA libraries from the mRNA and isolated four cDNA clones encoding IgE-BFs. Transfection of COS 7 monkey kidney cells with the cDNA clone in mammalian cell expression vector pcD resulted in the formation of IgE-BFs. None of the IgE-BFs derived from the four cDNA clones suppressed the *in vitro* IgE-forming cell response, but the products of two cDNA clones selectively potentiated the IgE response. The IgE-BFs derived from one of the cDNA clones, i.e., clone 8.3, consisted of two species of about 60 and 11 kDa. Both species of the IgE-BFs had affinity for lentil lectin and selectively potentiated the IgE response of rat MLN cells.

The nucleotide sequence of cDNA clone 8.3 revealed a putative protein coding region of 556 amino acids (Fig. 1). The peptide contained two potential sites for N-linked glycosylation (CHO site) and several potential sites for posttranslational proteolytic cleavage (shown by arrows in Fig. 1). The molecular weight of the peptide calculated from the predicted amino acid sequence was approximately 62,000 and corresponded to the 60-kDa IgE-BFs formed by transfection with the cDNA clone. Thus, the 11-kDa IgE-PFs must be a cleavage product of the 60-kDa peptide. The 11-kDa IgE-PFs have affinity for lentil lectin, indicating that the molecules contain one of the two sites for *N*-glycosylation. Martens *et al.* (1987) constructed a carbohydrate attachment site mutant of clone 8.3, so that the product of the mutant would lack the amino-terminal proximal carbohydrate attachment site (CHO_1). The mutation changed the asparagine residue of the Asn-Trp-Ser sequence at CHO_1 site to a glutamine residue. However, transfection of COS 7 cells with the mutant resulted in the formation of both the 60- and 11-kDa IgE-PFs, which had affinity for lentil lectin, indicating that the 11-kDa IgE-PFs contain the amino-terminal distal glycosylation (CHO_2) site. These investigators found that antigenic determinant, recognized by the monoclonal antibody OX-3, is oligosaccharide attached to the CHO_1

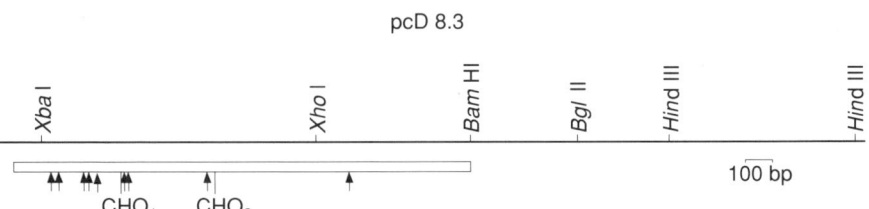

FIG. 1. Restriction map of pcD clone 8.3 encoding rodent IgE-BF. Bottom bar indicates the putative protein coding region. Potential *N*-linked glycosylation sites (CHO) and proteolytic cleavage sites (arrows) are shown.

site and/or the conformational determinant, expression of which requires glycosylation at the CHO_1 site. Failure of the 11-kDa IgE-PFs to bind to the antibody indicates that the factors do not contain the CHO_1 site (Martens et al., 1987). However, the 11-kDa factors bound to antibodies against a synthetic peptide corresponding to a segment between the two CHO sites, indicating that the 11-kDa factors contain this segment.

It was found that a DNA segment near the carboxy terminus of clone 8.3 has a striking homology with a highly conserved region of the reverse transcriptases of several retroviruses (Martens et al., 1985). Indeed, the cDNA clone hybridized with a cloned mouse intracisternal A particle (IAP) gene but not with DNA from several other cloned retroviruses (Moore et al., 1986). A comparison of the DNA sequence of clone 8.3 and a partial sequence of the genomic IAP clone showed that these sequences share extensive homology throughout the region of the cDNA clone from which the 11-kd IgE-BFs are derived. Furthermore, rabbit antiserum against electrophoretically isolated IAP structural protein gp73 absorbed not only IgE-BFs derived from cDNA clone 8.3 but also those produced by either the hybridoma 23B6 or the MLN cells of Nb-infected rats. However, neither IAP nor gp73 is released from the cells. Many cells transcribe IAP genes abundantly but do not express detectable IgE-BFs or FcεR. It was also found that only a small number (four of 70) of the cross-hybridizing cDNA clones from the 23B6 library express IgE-BF activity. It is apparent the IgE-BF gene and IAP genes belong to the same family. However, this does not necessarily mean that IgE-BFs are IAPs.

Gene cloning of rodent IgE-BFs suggested possible relationships among the 60-, 30- and 15-kDa IgE-BFs from the T cell hybridoma 23B6 and those from murine T cells (Jerdieu et al., 1985b). Since the 60-kDa IgE-BF molecule is composed of a single polypeptide chain, the 30- and 15-kDa IgE-BFs should be posttranslational cleavage products of the 60-kDa precursor molecules. A fraction of the 60-kDa IgE-BF was cleaved by reduction and alkylation treatment to yield the 30-, 15-, and 10-kDa IgE-BFs and the same treatment of the 30-kDa IgE-BF yielded the 15- and 10-kDa fragments. Reduction and alkylation of the recombinant 60-kDa IgE-PF also yielded the 11-kDa IgE-PF. It appears that a fraction of the 60-kDa peptide was already cleaved by proteolytic enzyme(s), but the fragments were held together by intrachain disulfide bonds. Since the predicted amino acid sequence of the recombinant 60-kDa peptide contains nine cysteine residues (Martens et al., 1985), it was anticipated that some of these residues were involved in intrachain disulfide bonds.

Differences between 15-kDa IgE-PF and IgE-SF and their affinities for various lectins suggested a possible role of carbohydrate moieties in their biological activities. The hypothesis was supported by the fact that rat T cells activated by 10 μg/ml of Con A, which produced IgE-PFs upon incubation with IgE, produced IgE-BFs with suppressive activity when they were incubated with IgE in the presence of tunicamycin, which inhibits the assembly of N-linked oligosaccharides (Yodoi et al., 1981a). Pretreatment of the same Con A-activated cells with glucocorticoids, followed by incubation with IgE or with IgE in the presence of lipocortin, a phospholipase-inhibitory protein, induced the formation of IgE-SFs, which had affinity for PNA (Uede et al., 1983b; Yodoi et al., 1981b). Furthermore, the T cell hybridoma clone 23B6, which produces IgE-SFs upon incubation with IgE, formed IgE-PFs when incubated with IgE in the presence of monoclonal antilipocortin antibody, which activated phospholipase (Huff et al., 1983). Such a switching of the biological activities of IgE-BFs was observed in a human T cell hybridoma as well (Huff et al., 1986). When the hybridoma 166A2 were incubated with homologous IgE, essentially all IgE-BFs formed by the cells had affinity for Con A. However, only a small fraction of the factors had affinity for lentil lectin, and the factors exerted only weak potentiating activity on the IgE response. If the same cells were incubated with IgE in the presence of bradykinin, which activates phospholipase A_2, essentially all IgE-BFs formed by the cells had affinity for lentil lectin, and the factors had much higher potentiating activity than those formed in the absence of bradykinin. In contrast, incubation of the hybridoma cells with IgE in the presence of lipocortin resulted in the formation of IgE-BFs having affinity for PNA (but not for Con A), and these factors selectively suppressed the IgE response.

The capacity of a T cell clone to form either IgE-PFs or IgE-SFs under different conditions suggested that IgE-PFs and IgE-SFs are structurally related. The hypothesis was supported by transfection of COS 7 cells with a single cDNA clone. The transfection of the cells with cDNA clone 8.3 resulted in the formation of both the 60- and 11-kDa IgE-PFs. However, when the transfection was carried out in the presence of tunicamycin, IgE-BFs formed by the cells lacked affinity for lentil lectin and Con A, and the factors suppressed the IgE response (Martens et al., 1987). The results suggest that IgE-PFs and IgE-SFs may share a common structural gene, therefore a common polypeptide chain, and that biological activities of IgE-BFs are determined by a posttranslational glycosylational process.

The effect of tunicamycin on the biological activities of IgE-BFs indicates that N-linked, mannose-rich oligosaccharide(s) in the IgE-PF molecules is essential for their biological activities. As described above, the recombinant 60-kDa IgE-BF of the carbohydrate attachment site mutant of cDNA clone 8.3 lacks an N-linked oligosaccharide attached to the CHO_1 site but contains an N-linked oligosaccharide attached to the CHO_2 site and exerted potentiating activity on the IgE response (Martens *et al.*, 1987). This result suggests that N-linked oligosaccharide(s) attached to the CHO_2 site is essential for IgE-potentiating activity.

Structures of oligosaccharides in IgE-PF and IgE-SF molecules are unknown. However, evidence was obtained that the 15-kDa rat IgE-PF has both N-linked oligosaccharide and O-linked oligosaccharide(s) and their terminal residues are sialic acids (Yodoi *et al.*, 1982). The biological activities of the 15-kDa IgE-PF were lost by treatment of the factors with neuraminidase (Yodoi *et al.*, 1980), indicating that the terminal sialic acid residues are essential for potentiating activity. On the other hand, the 15-kDa IgE-SF appears to contain O-linked oligosaccharides whose terminal residues are galactose → N-acetylgalactosamine (Yodoi *et al.*, 1982). Although this factor does not have affinity for either Con A or lentil lectin, it is not clear whether the factor contains an N-linked oligosaccharide having no affinity for the lectins or lacks such an oligosaccharide. Nevertheless, N-linked oligosaccharide does not appear to be involved in the function of IgE-SFs, because the presence of tunicamycin does not affect the biological activities of IgE-SFs formed by T cells (Yodoi *et al.*, 1982).

D. Structure of FcεRII on B Lymphocytes and B Cell-Derived IgE-BFs

Since IgE-BFs have affinity for IgE, it was originally anticipated that the factors were derived from FcεRII on lymphocytes (Yodoi *et al.*, 1980). It was well established that the majority of $FcεR^+$ cells are B cells in both humans and rodents (Fritche and Spiegelberg, 1978; Gonzalez-Molina and Spiegelberg, 1977), and that lymphoblastoid cells transformed by Epstein–Barr virus bear a high density of FcεR (Gonzalez-Molina and Spiegelberg, 1976). Kikutani *et al.* (1986b) reported that essentially all mature $μ^+δ^+$ human B lymphocytes bear FcεR, as determined by immunofluorescence with monoclonal anti-FcεRII antibody, while other subsets of B cells bearing surface IgG, IgA, or IgE do not express FcεRII. The FcεRs on mouse B cells and human lymphoblastoid RPMI 8866 cells represent a single polypeptide chain of 49 and 47 kDa, respectively (Conrad and Petersen, 1984). Sarfati *et al.* (1984) acually have shown that culture supernatants of human B lymphoblastoid RPMI 8866 cells contain soluble substances which inhibit rosette formation of $FcεR^+$ with IgE-coated erythrocytes. The major component of this factor was 25–29 kDa, was bound to monoclonal antibody against FcεRII and was proved to be a fragment of the receptors (Ikuta *et al.*, 1987; Sarfati *et al.*, 1987a).

Structures of FcεRIIs on RPMI 8866 cells and IgE-BFs derived from the cells became clear by cloning of genes for the receptors by three groups of investigators (Ikuta *et al.*, 1987; Kikutani *et al.*, 1986a; Ludin *et al.*, 1987). The receptor molecule is a single glycopeptide chain consisting of 321 amino acids. The hydrophilicity plot of the peptide indicates the lack of an amino-terminal signal sequence and the presence of a putative transmembrane portion near the amino-terminal end (amino acid residues 35–45). The findings suggest that the carboxy terminus is exposed to the cell exterior and the amino terminus is cytoplasmic. The sequence of the peptide has homology with animal lectins such as chicken hepatic lectin, human and rat asialoglycoprotein receptor, and rat mannose-binding protein C, of which the amino terminus is located on cytoplasmic slide (Ikuta *et al.*, 1987; Kikutani *et al.*, 1986a). The nucleotide sequence of the FcεRII gene shares no homology with that of rodent T cell-derived IgE-BFs described above nor FcγR on lymphocytes (Raretch *et al.*, 1987) or α chain of FcεRI on rat basophilic leukemia cells (Kinet *et al.*, 1987). Partial amino acid sequence of the 25-kDa soluble fragment indicates that the fragment with affinity for IgE represents the carboxy-terminal half, i.e., amino acids 148–321, of the receptor peptide (Ikuta *et al.*, 1987; Kikutani *et al.*, 1986a). Thus, the fragment appears to be a proteolytic cleavage product of FcεRII.

The predicted amino acid sequence of FcεRII peptide also indicated that the receptors on human B cells have only one N-linked glycosylation site, and that the 25-kDa IgE-binding fragment does not contain any N-linked glycosylation site (Ikuta *et al.*, 1987). The fragment was detected in the sera of both normal individuals and atopic patients by radioimmunoassay using monoclonal anti-FcεRII antibody (Sarfati *et al.*, 1986). However, lack of an N-glycosylation site in the 25-kDa fragment indicates that the soluble fragment of the FcεRII is distinct from T cell-derived IgE-PFs, which have affinity for both Con A and lentil lectin.

It is well known that FcεRIIs on mouse B cells also degrade at the cell surface by proteolytic enzyme into a 38-kDa soluble fragment and a 10-kDa fragment, the latter of which remains associated with the cell membrane (Lee *et al.*, 1987). The soluble fragment from mouse B cells bound to monoclonal anti-FcεRII antibody. However, in contrast to the human FcεRII fragment, soluble fragments from mouse FcεRII do not have affinity for IgE (Lee *et al.*, 1987). Thus, in rodent systems, FcεRIIs on B cells cannot be the source of IgE-BFs. This finding is in agreement with previous observations that rodent IgE-BFs are derived from T cells, rather than B cells (Yodoi and Ishizaka, 1980).

FcεRIIs are expressed not only on B cells but also on macrophages (Melewitz and Spiegelberg, 1980), platelets (Joseph *et al.*, 1983), and activated eosinophils (Capron et al., 1984). However, Kikutani et al. (1986a) could not detect FcεR mRNA in human T cell lines nor in normal T lymphocytes by Northern blot analysis. The mRNA was detected only in the human T lymphotropic virus (HTLV)-I-transformed T cell line (Kawabe et al., 1988). Indeed, Sarfati et al. (1987b) identified FcεRII and its fragments from HTLV-I-transformed cell line cells by sodium dodecyl sulfate–polyacrylamide gel electrophoresis. Immunofluorescence staining of peripheral blood lymphocytes with monoclonal anti-FcεRs failed to demonstrate FcεRIIs on normal T cells. However, Young et al. (1984) established a human T cell clone bearing FcεR from peripheral blood lymphocytes of atopic dermatitis patients. Furthermore, both rodent T cell hybridomas (Huff et al., 1984) and human T cell hybridomas (Kisaki et al., 1987) responded to homologous IgE and to antibodies reacting to FcεRIIs for the formation of IgE-BFs. These findings suggest that a subset of T cells from both humans and rodents probably bears a minimum number of cell surface receptors for IgE, which is not sufficient for detection either by rosetting or by immunofluorescence. Since a monoclonal antibody against human IgE-BFs, which did not cross-react with FcεRIIs on B cells, also stimulated the human T cell hybridoma for the production of IgE-BFs (Kisaki et al., 1987), it is possible that the receptors on T cells may be structurally different from FcεRIIs on B cells.

A relationship between FcεRIIs on B cells and those on activated eosinophils and macrophages was revealed. Yokota et al. (1988) reported two species of human FcεRIIs, i.e., FcεRIIa and FcεRIIb. Sequence analysis of the cloned cDNA of the two forms showed that they differ only at the amino-terminal cytoplasmic region and that the two forms are generated through the utilization of different transcriptional initiation sites and alternative RNA splicing. FcεRIIa was found constitutively in normal human B cells, while FcεRIIb was found in eosinophils, macrophages, B cells and HTLV-1-transformed T cell lines. Normal human B cells and monocytes express FcεRIIb only after stimulation by IL-4.

The biological role of FcεRII on B cells is unknown. Sarfati et al. (1984) reported that the soluble fragments of FcεRII on RPMI 8866 cells enhanced the IgE synthesis of human lymphocytes. Péne et al. (1988b) found that IL-4-induced IgE synthesis by normal human PBMCs was suppressed by anti-FcεRII antibody, suggesting that either FcεRII or its fragments are involved in the differentiation of B cells to IgE-forming cells. However, soluble fragments of recombinant FcεRII failed to enhance the IgE synthesis. An interesting finding on FcεRII is that this molecule is identical to a B cell differentiation antigen, known as CD23, or Blast-2 (Bonnefoy et al., 1987; Yukawa et al., 1987), which is especially prominent after Epstein-Barr virus infection of B cells (Thorley-Lawson et al., 1985). Gordon et al. (1986a) found that in the presence of phorbol ester, a monoclonal antibody against CD23 induces the progression of B cells through the G_1 phase of the cell cycle. The antibody also enhances the release of the CD23 fragment, i.e., the 25-kDa FcεRII fragment, from B cells (Guy and Gordon, 1987). Since the monoclonal anti-CD23 has proliferative effects on B cells, similar to low-molecular-weight B cell growth factor, it was speculated that CD23 is a receptor for low-molecular-weight B cell growth factor (Gordon et al., 1987b). It is quite possible that FcεRIIs on B cells and/or on the 25-kDa soluble fragments of the receptor molecules are involved in B cell transformation.

E. MECHANISMS FOR THE FORMATION OF IgE-BFs

1. Lymphokines for the Induction of IgE-BF Formation

Analysis of the cellular mechanisms for the selective formation of either IgE-PFs or IgE-SFs by rodent lymphocytes under various experimental conditions showed that the major cell sources of IgE-BFs are Lyt-1$^+$ T cells that bear either FcεR or Fcγ R or both. When rats and mice were treated with CFA or *Bordetella* pertussis vaccine, their macrophages and/or monocytes were activated and released Type I interferon, which in turn stimulated FcR$^+$ T cells to form IgE-BFs (Hirashima et al., 1981b,c). Purified mouse IFNβ induced normal lymphocytes for the formation of IgE-BFs (Uede et al., 1983a). When animals were primed with a protein antigen and their spleen cells were stimulated with the homologous antigen, Lyt-1$^+$, antigen-primed helper T cells released T cell factor(s) which stimulated unprimed FcR$^+$ T cells to form IgE-BFs (Uede and Ishizaka, 1982). Recombinant mouse IFNγ, but none of the IL-1, IL-2, IL-3, and IL-4, induced normal BALB/c splenocyte formation of IgE-BFs (Adachi et al., 1988). Recently, Carini et al. (1988) demonstrated that peripheral blood T cells of human immunodeficiency virus (HIV)-1-infected patients formed IgE-BFs and that formation of the factors by the cells was enhanced by incubation of the cells with homologous IgE. In some HIV-1-infected patients FcεRIIs were demonstrated on both CD4$^+$ and CD8$^+$ T cells. It was also found that PBMCs of some HIV-1-infected patients release soluble factor(s) which induces normal T cells to form IgE-BFs. This cytokine does not appear to be IFNγ, because neither IFNγ (25-50 U/ml) nor recombinant IL-4 (5-10 U/ml) induced the same normal T cells to form IgE-BFs. It is not known why recombinant mouse IFNγ induces normal mouse spleen cells to form IgE-BFs, whereas recombinant human IFNγ failed to induce peripheral blood human T cells to form IgE-BFs. It is quite possible that activation of T cells is required for them to respond to IFNγ for the production of the factors.

It was shown that IL-4 induced biosynthesis of FcεRIIs in B cells and enhanced the expression of the receptors on their surface (Conrad et al., 1987; Defrance et al., 1987). In the rodent systems incubation of B cells with 3-5 U/ml of IL-4 increased the density of FcεRIIs on the majority of B cells and enhanced the release of the 38-kDa fragments of the receptors which lacked affinity for IgE. However, culture of normal mouse spleen cells or B cells with IL-4 did not contain a detectable amount of IgE-BFs, as determined by rosette inhibition (Adachi et al., 1988). Human IL-4 also induced an increase in FcεRIIs on human peripheral blood B cells, particularly if the cells had been activated by anti-μ chain antibodies (Defrance et al., 1987), and enhanced the release of the 25-kDa fragments of FcεRII which had affinity for IgE. It was also noted that the effect of IL-4 on B cells to enhance the expression of both Ia molecules and FcεRII was prevented by IFNγ in both human and rodent systems (Conrad et al., 1987; Defrance et al., 1987).

2. Lymphokines Controlling the Biological Activities of IgE-PFs or IgE-SFs

When BDF_1 mouse spleen cells were stimulated with the T cell-derived "inducer" of IgE-BFs, i.e., IFNγ, IgE-PFs were formed. Stimulation of SJL mouse spleen cells with the same inducer resulted in the formation of IgE-SFs (Vede and Ishizaka, 1984). Thus, IFNs do not determine the biological activities of IgE-BFs. Under physiological conditions biological activities of the factors formed by FcR^+ T cells are controlled by two T cell factors, i.e., glycosylation-enhancing factor (GEF) and glycosylation-inhibiting factor (GIF), which regulate the posttranslational glycosylation processes of the IgE-BF peptide (Ishizaka, 1984). GEF is derived from a subset of $Lyt-1^+$ T cells. When animals are treated with pertussis vaccine for the selective formation of IgE-PFs, pertussis toxin stimulates $Lyt-1^+$ T cells to form GEF (Hirashima et al., 1981b; Iwata et al., 1983a). Immunization of Lewis rats or BDF_1 mice with alum-absorbed antigen results in priming of not only helper T cells but also $Lyt-1^+$, FcR^+ T cells, and this latter subset releases GEF upon antigenic stimulation (Vede and Ishizaka, 1982). Thus, when unprimed FcR^+ T cells are stimulated by inducers (IFNs) in the presence of GEF, these cells selectively form IgE-BFs having a "proper" N-linked oligosaccharide, which potentiate the IgE response (cf. Fig. 2). Recent experiments showed that IL-4 induces normal T cells for the formation of GEF. Thus, it appears that IL-4 not only facilitates the switching of resting B cells to $sIgE^+$ B cells but also enhances the differentiation of $sIgE^+$ B cells to IgE-forming cells through the selective formation of IgE-PFs.

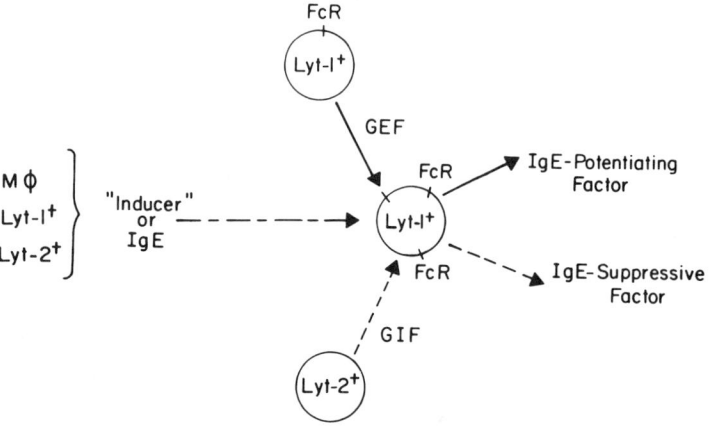

FIG. 2. Schematic models for the selective formation of IgE-PFs or IgE-SFs. FcR$^+$ T cells form IgE-potentiating factor in the presence of GEF, but the same cells form IgE-suppressive factor in the presence of GIF. MΦ, Macrophage.

On the other hand, the same FcR$^+$ T cells selectively form IgE-SFs, when the cells are stimulated by inducers (IFNs) or IgE in the presence of GIF (Fig. 2). When Lewis rats are primed with a protein antigen included in CFA, not only Lyt-1$^+$ helper T cells but also Lyt-2$^+$ T cells are primed. Thus, antigenic stimulation of spleen cells results in the formation of IFNγ from TH$_1$ cells and GIF from Lyt-2$^+$ T cells, and these two factors in combination stimulate FcR$^+$ T cells to form IgE-SFs (Uede and Ishizaka, 1982). Repeated injections of CFA also stimulate Lyt-2$^+$ T cells to form GIF (Uede et al., 1983b). It was found in the mouse that Lyt-2$^+$ I-J$^+$ antigen-specific suppressor T cells are the major source of GIF (Jardieu et al., 1984).

GIF from lymphocytes of CFA-treated rats had a molecular weight of 13,000–15,000 and bound to monoclonal antibody against lipocortin (lipomodulin), a phospholipase-inhibitory protein (Uede et al., 1983b). The lymphokine did not exert phospholipase-inhibitory activity by itself, but inhibited phospholipase A$_2$ after treatment with alkaline phosphatase. Thus, it appears that GIF is a phosphorylated derivative of phospholipase-inhibitory protein. Purified lipocortin from rabbit neutrophils (Uede et al., 1983b) as well as recombinant human lipocortin I, at the level of 0.1 μg/ml, could switch normal mouse lymphocytes for the selective formation of IgE-SFs. It was also found that treatment of normal mouse splenic lymphocytes with glucocorticoids induced Lyt-2$^+$ T cells for the formation of GIF (Jardieu et al., 1986). An

TABLE II
Correlation Among the IgE Response, Nature of IgE-BFs, and Modulators of Glycosylation

imental edures	IgE response	IgE-BFs	Modulators of glycosylation
n (2 weeks)	Enhancement	Potentiating	GEF
pertussis BP) treatment	Enhancement	Potentiating	GEF
im priming[a]	IgE antibody response	Potentiating	GEF
priming[b]	IgE antibody response	Potentiating	GEF
idoma 12H5	IgE antibody response	Potentiating	GEF
ient	Suppression	Suppressive	GIF
A priming[a]	No IgE antibody response	Suppressive	GIF
riming[b]	No IgE antibody response	Suppressive	GIF
domas 23B6,	—	Suppressive	GIF

rain rats were immunized with KLH.
SJL mice were immunized with alum-absorbed OVA.

The Lyt-1$^+$ T cells of BDF$_1$ mice constitutively form GEF, se of SJL mice form GIF. Therefore, upon antigenic stimula- en cells of antigen-primed BDF$_1$ mice form IgE-PFs, whereas SJL mice form IgE-SFs (Vede and Ishizaka, 1984). One may that the balance between GEF and GIF determines the nature iological activities of IgE-BFs formed, and these factors in turn he IgE response.

t known why GEF and GIF compete with each other in terms osylation of IgE-BFs. Biochemical analysis of the effect of GEF cell hybridoma, 23A4 cells, revealed that GEF activated e-associated enzymes such as methyltransferases and phos- C and induced Ca^{2+} influx and the formation of diacylglycerol, turn activated Ca^{2+}-activated, phospholipid-dependent nase (protein kinase C) (Akasaki et al., 1985). GEF also induced of arachidonate from the cells (Iwata et al., 1984b). It appears induces the activation of phospholipase A$_2$ and phospholipase T cells. Since GIF is a derivative of phospholipase-inhibitory ntagonistic effects between GEF and GIF with respect to the ion of IgE-BFs may be related to activation versus inactiva- ospholipase A$_2$ in the cells by the two lymphokines.

interesting observation was that GIF from
I-J determinant(s); GIF from H-2^b strains
and a monoclonal anti 1-J^b, while GIF fro
I-J^k antibodies (Jardieu et al., 1986). It i
a fragment of lipocortin. However, GIF
properties and an antigenic determinan
speculate that the phospholipase inhibito
is important in its immunological functic
by recent findings that a synthetic inh
2(p-amylcennamoyl)-amino-4-chlorobenz
hybridoma from the formation of IgE-PF
while neomycin, a well-known phospholi

It was found that GEF was inactivate
tease, bound to p-aminobenzamidine aga
by elution with benzamidine (Iwata et a
inhibitors of trypsinlike enzymes on GE
kallikreinlike enzyme. This speculation w
trypsin and kallikrein, as well as brady
kininogen by kallikrein, have GEF activi
selective formation of IgE-PFs. However,
and binds to acid-treated Sepharose (Iw
of GEF to switch the nature of IgE-BFs
d-lactose and N-acetylgalactosamine, indic
tion by binding to d-galactose on the cel
species, of 45–55 and 25 kDa, as estimated
1988). One of the unique properties of m
kine binds to alloantibodies against MHC
H-2^k mice bound to anti-Ia^k alloantibodi
bound to anti-Ia^b alloantibodies (Iwata

GIF and GEF compete with each othe
tion process of IgE-binding peptide(s).
interact with each other, but a mixture o
the nature of IgE-BFs formed by T cell
physiological conditions, the balance bet
determine the nature of the IgE-BFs form
systems in which the IgE antibody respo
pressed. IgE-PFs are always detected whe
(Iwata et al., 1984a). It should be note
in culture supernatants of splenic lymph
produced. On the other hand, formatic
panied by the formation of GIF (Ishizak
even to genetic differences between a hig

3. Formation of IgE-BFs by Antigen-Specific T Cells

Induction of IgE-PF or IgE-SF formation by lymphokines, described above (cf. Fig. 2), does not exclude the possibility that some of the antigen-specific T cells may form IgE-BFs. Indeed, we have obtained an antigen-specific mouse T cell clone and antigen-specific T cell hybridomas which produce IgE-BFs upon incubation with OVA-pulsed syngeneic macrophages. It was found that some of the antigen-specific T cell hybridomas such as $231F_1$, constitutively formed GIF, and produced both IgE-SFs and IgG-suppressive factors upon incubation with OVA-pulsed macrophages (Jardieu et al., 1985a). We have also obtained the mouse T cell hybridoma 12H5, which produced IgE-PFs and IgG-potentiating factors upon antigenic stimulation (Iwata et al., 1988). As expected, this type of hybridoma constitutively secretes GEF.

The response of this T cell hybridoma to the antigen is MHC restricted. T cell hybridoma $231F_1$ cells respond to OVA-pulsed macrophages of BDF_1 or BALB/c mice for the production of IgE-SFs, but not to OVA-pulsed macrophages of $H-2^k$ or $H-2^b$ strains nor to free OVA. Hybridoma 12H5 cells respond to OVA-pulsed macrophages of BDF_1 or $H-2^b$ strain for the production of IgE-PFs, but not to OVA-pulsed macrophages of $H-2^d$ or $H-2^k$ strains (Iwata et al., 1988). It was also found that pretreatment of antigen-presenting cells with monoclonal anti-IA^d antibody prevented antigen presentation to $231F_1$ cells for IgE-BF production. Similarly, treatment of antigen-presenting cells with anti-IA^b, but not with anti-IA^k, alloantibodies prevented antigen presentation to the 12H5 cells for the formation of IgE-BFs (Iwata et al., 1988). Furthermore, the antigen recognized by these hybridomas does not appear to be the native molecules. BDF_1 macrophages that were pulsed with urea-denatured OVA or tryptic digests of the protein stimulated $231F_1$ cells and 12H5 cells for the formation of IgE-BFs. Recent experiments in collaboration with A. Kubo of the National Jewish Hospital have shown that treatment of the 12H5 cells or $231F_1$ cells with monoclonal anti-T cell receptor (α, β) antibody or anti-CD3 antibody, followed by incubation of the cells in protein A-coated wells, resulted in the formation of IgE-BFs. The results collectively indicate that these antigen-specific T cell hybridomas bear T cell receptors, which are probably composed of α and β chains and CD3 complex, and recognize a "processed" antigen in the context of Ia molecules on the antigen-presenting cells. Since the same hybridomas respond to mouse IgE for the formation of IgE-BFs, these T cells should bear a minimum number of FcϵR (and FcγR) as well.

When a suspension of antigen-primed spleen cells was incubated *in vitro* with homologous antigen, unprimed FcR^+ T cells stimulated by lymphokines (Fig. 2) may be the major source of IgE-PFs or IgE-SFs. However, antigen-specific T cells may well be the major source of IgE-BFs *in vivo*. It is conceivable that cognate interaction between the antigen-specific regulatory T cells with antigen-presenting cells in lymphoid tissues results in the formation of IgE-BFs, and the factors in turn play an important role in the regulation of the IgE antibody formation in the tissues.

IV. Immunological Approaches for Suppression of the IgE Antibody Response

Immunotherapy of hay fever has been one of the most popular treatments of the disease. Although the clinical effects of the treatment are appreciated, it is obvious that they are not due to the suppression of the IgE antibody formation. Nevertheless, long-term treatment of ragweed-sensitive hay fever patients by specific allergens frequently prevented the secondary IgE antibody response after the pollen season (Ishizaka and Ishizaka, 1973). These classical findings suggest the possibility that IgE antibody formation against specific antigens in hay fever patients may be manipulated by immunological procedures.

A. Regulation of the IgE Antibody Response by Antigens

Regulation of the IgE antibody response by means of antigen-specific mechanisms has been attempted either through (1) tolerization of B cells or (2) manipulation of the population of T cells that regulate the differentiation of B cells to IgE-forming cells. Katz et al. (1973) induced B cell tolerance by injecting hapten coupled with a nonimmunogenic carrier, d-glutamic acid d-lysine copolymer (dGL). Injections of DNP-dGL before immunization with DNP-OVA completely suppressed the primary and secondary antihapten IgE antibody responses, and an injection of the dGL conjugates into immunized animals terminated the ongoing antihapten antibody formation. The effect of the treatment was persistent and specific for the haptenic group. Suppression is due to inactivation of hapten-specific B cells and applies to all immunoglobulin isotypes, including IgE. Subsequently, Lee and Sehon (1981) employed DNP conjugates of polyvinyl alcohol (PVA) to terminate the anti-DNP IgE antibody response. Like DNP-dGL, DNP-polyvinyl alcohol conjugate inactivates hapten-specific B cells. However, this approach cannot be applied for clinical purposes, because the antigen-conjugate will cause anaphylactic reactions in patients before tolerizing B cells.

Another approach to regulating the antihapten IgE antibody response is to induce antiidiotypic antibodies. If the antihapten antibodies are restricted to certain idiotypes, idiotype-specific regulation may be applied. Blaser et al. (1980) reported that antiidiotypic antibody suppressed primary IgE antibody response and ongoing antibody formation against the benzyl penicilloyl group. They also demonstrated in BALB/c mice that the production of antiidiotypic antibodies against syngeneic anti-OVA antibodies resulted in depression of both antihapten and anticarrier IgE antibody formation against DNP-OVA (Blaser et al., 1981).

The third approach is to regulate the IgE antibody response by inducing antigen-specific suppressor T cells. It has been shown that intravenous injections of a soluble antigen without adjuvant into naive mice facilitate the generation of antigen-specific suppressor T cells. Since allergic patients are already sensitive to allergen, an injection of native allergen will cause allergic symptoms. To avoid such a side effect, chemically modified antigens that lost the major antigenic determinant in the native antigen were employed to modulate the antibody response. Indeed, neither urea-denatured OVA (UD-OVA) nor urea-denatured ragweed antigen E reacts with the antibodies against the native antigens, but could prime helper T cells for the antigen (Ishizaka et al., 1975; Takatsu and Ishizaka, 1975). It was also found that intravenous injections of OVA or UD-OVA into OVA-primed BDF_1 mice induced the generation of antigen-specific suppressor T cells, and this treatment suppressed the primary antibody responses of mice to alum-absorbed OVA or DNP-OVA. Suppressor T cells generated by UD-OVA treatment were specific for OVA. Transfer of the splenic T cells of the UD-OVA-treated mice into naive syngeneic mice suppressed the antihapten antibody response of the recipient to DNP-OVA, but the same splenic T cells failed to suppress the antibody response of the recipients to DNP-KLH (Takatsu and Ishizaka, 1976a). Suppressor T cells induced by the UD antigen can suppress the IgE antibody response better than IgG antibody response. Nevertheless, regulation of antibody response by their cells is not restricted to the IgE isotype.

Evidence was obtained that antigen-specific suppressor T cells, which were obtained by the treatment of OVA-primed mice with UD-OVA, could suppress even the ongoing IgE antibody formation (Takatsu and Ishizaka, 1976b). When such a suppressor T cell population was transferred into OVA plus alum-immunized, syngeneic mice, after the IgE antibody titer of the recipients reached maximum, the IgE antibody titer declined. The results suggested that the generation of antigen-specific suppressor T cells might be an effective method to suppress the IgE antibody formation against a specific allergen.

Generation of antigen-specific suppressor T cells by repeated injections of UD-OVA suggested that the treatment might be effective for suppressing the ongoing IgE antibody formation. Indeed, the IgE antibody titer in the serum of OVA- or DNP-OVA-primed mice declined to one quarter to one eighth after three intravenous injections of 100 μg of UD-OVA. However, the antibody titer became stable after the treatment, and repeated treatment did not show a significant effect (Takatsu and Ishizaka, 1976b). A question arises as to why UD-OVA treatment suppressed the primary antibody response almost completely but has only marginal suppressive effects on the ongoing antibody formation. Since UD-OVA-pulsed macrophages stimulate helper T cells (Takatsu and Ishizaka, 1975), one may speculate that the effect of the UD-OVA treatment may differ, depending on the size of helper T cell populations in the primed mice. When the animals are immunized for the persistent IgE antibody response, their lymphoid tissues contain a relatively large population of antigen-specific helper T cells. In this situation, UD-OVA will not only induce antigen-specific suppressor T cells but will also expand the population of antigen-primed helper T cells. Under certain conditions, UD-OVA treatment may rather enhance the antibody response. When BDF_1 mice were primed with a suboptimal dose (10 ng) of alum-absorbed OVA, the IgE antibody was not detected in their serum. However, the IgE antibodies against OVA became detectable after repeated injections of UD-OVA into the OVA-primed animals. These findings suggested that UD-OVA cannot be applied for the treatment of allergic patients.

Chemically modified antigens were developed through other approaches. Lee and Sehon (1978) prepared conjugates of OVA with polyethylene glycol (PEG) and tried to use the conjugates for the suppression of the IgE antibody response. Immunological properties of OVA-PEG conjugates appear to be similar to those of UD-OVA. Both modified antigens lack the major antigenic determinants in the native antigen molecules. Injections of OVA-PEG conjugates to naive animals induced the generation of antigen-specific suppressor T cells and suppressed the primary antibody response to native OVA or DNP-OVA (Lee et al., 1981). However, OVA-PEG has marginal effects on the ongoing IgE antibody formation (Sehon, 1982). Series of experiments with modified antigens indicate that the generation of antigen-specific suppressor T cells would be an effective maneuver to suppress the IgE antibody formation against allergens. However, a modified antigen may not be appropriate for the treatment, unless one can prepare a tolerogen that selectively generates suppressor T cells without stimulating helper T cells.

B. Selective Suppression of IgE Synthesis by Anti-IL-4 and IFNγ

In view of an essential role of IL-4 for the development of IgE-forming cells and IgG$_1$-forming cells, Finkelman et al. (1986a) determined the effect of a monoclonal anti-IL-4 on the IgE and IgG$_1$ production *in vivo*. They used Nb infection and an injection of goat anti-mouse IgD antibodies to induce an enhanced IgE synthesis, and injected monoclonal anti-IL-4 antibody prior to the infection or injection of anti-IgD. The results clearly showed that an intraperitoneal injection of ascitic fluid, which contained approximately 20 mg of anti-IL-4, markedly suppressed the IgE production in both systems, but failed to affect the IgG$_1$ production. Subsequently, the same investigators determined possible effects of anti-IL-4 on the IgE antibody response to a protein antigen. They primed BALB/c mice with alum-absorbed DNP-KLH for the IgE antibody response and injected 20 mg of a highly purified anti-IL-4 into antigen-primed mice at the same time as a booster immunization with homologous antigen. The antibody completely blocked the secondary IgE antibody response, but neither IgG$_1$ nor IgG$_{2a}$ antibody response was affected by the treatment (Finkelman et al., 1988b). They have also shown that injections of anti-IL-4 antibody suppressed the ongoing IgE antibody formation. These results supported the concept that IL-4 is required for the IgE response. However, surprising results in the experiments were that an injection of 1-2 mg of anti-IL-4 into mice failed to affect the IgE synthesis and that even 20 mg of the antibody failed to affect IgG$_1$ synthesis (Finkelman et al., 1986a).

Finkelman et al. (1988a) also tried to suppress the *in vivo* IgE synthesis by IFNγ, which counteracts with IL-4. Enhanced IgE and IgG$_1$ formation was induced by injecting goat anti-mouse IgD antibodies. The anti-IgD-treated mice received intraperitoneal injections of 12,500-50,000 U of IFNγ twice daily for 3 days (days 2-4) and serum Ig levels were determined on days 8 and 9. Their results showed that the treatment with 25,000 U of IFNγ per injection reduced both IgE and IgG$_1$ levels to one fifth to one tenth, and the treatment with 12,500 U of IFNγ per injection diminished both IgE and IgG$_1$ levels to about one half. The decrease in IgE and IgG$_1$ synthesis by IFNγ was accompanied by a slight increase in IgG$_{2a}$ synthesis. However, 6250 U of IFNγ per injection did not give a significant effect on IgE and IgG$_1$ syntheses. The results indicate that IFNγ can regulate IgE and IgG$_1$ synthesis *in vivo*. However, the quantities of IFNγ to regulate the IgE synthesis were too much for clinical purposes. Preliminary experiments also suggested that the ongoing IgE antibody formation against protein antigens was difficult to suppress by treatment with IFNγ.

C. Suppression of IgE Antibody Response by GIF

Isotype-specific enhancement and suppression of *in vitro* IgE synthesis by IgE-PFs and IgE-SFs, respectively, suggest that these lymphokines are actually involved in the selective regulation of IgE synthesis. It is quite reasonable to speculate that IgE-SFs may suppress the IgE synthesis *in vivo*. However, effects of IgE-SFs in the *in vivo* IgE antibody response have never been studied, because of anticipation that IgE-BFs administered intravenously may be bound by IgE before reaching lymphoid tissue.

Analysis of the mechanisms for the selective formation of IgE-PFs or IgE-SFs indicated that the balance between GEF and GIF in the environment of FcR^+ T cells determines the nature and the biological activities of IgE-BFs formed by the T cells, and the latter factors in turn regulate IgE synthesis (Ishizaka, 1984) (cf. Fig. 2). If this is the case, one can speculate that the treatment of OVA plus alum-immunized BDF_1 mice with GIF may switch FcR^+ T cells from the formation of IgE-PFs to the formation of IgE-SFs, and thereby may suppress the IgE antibody response. To test this possibility, BDF_1 mice were immunized with alum-absorbed DNP-OVA for the persistent IgE antibody response, and a group of the mice was treated by repeated intravenous injections of GIF from a hybridoma (Akasaki *et al.*, 1986). The preparation of GIF was obtained by affinity purification of the factor with antilipocortin-Sepharose, and affinity-purified GIF was injected every 2 days either intravenously or intraperitoneally into the DNP-OVA-primed mice for 3 weeks. The GIF treatment completely suppressed not only the IgE antibody response but also the IgG antibody response. The same treatment suppressed the ongoing IgE antibody formation as well. If one immunizes BDF_1 mice with alum-absorbed DNP-OVA for persistent IgE antibody formation and then begins to treat the animals after the IgE antibody titer reaches maximum, IgE antibody titer markedly declines and the IgG antibody titer significantly diminishes (Akasaki *et al.*, 1986).

To analyze the cellular mechanisms of immunosuppression, two groups of BDF_1 mice were immunized with alum-absorbed OVA, and one group was treated by intravenous injections of GIF every 2 days. Two weeks after the priming, when the IgE antibody titers of untreated mice reached maximum, their spleen cells were incubated with OVA. Spleen cells of untreated mice produced IgE-PFs and GEF, while those of GIF-treated mice formed IgE-SFs and GIF upon antigenic stimulation. Thus, GIF treatment of OVA-primed mice switched their spleen cells from the formation of IgE-PFs to the formation of IgE-SFs. GIF in culture supernatants of spleen cells does not represent a carryover of the injected lymphokine. GIF employed for the treatment failed to bind to OVA–Sepharose, while the majority of GIF in the culture supernatant of BDF_1 spleen cells bound to OVA–Sepharose and was recovered by elution at acid pH. Furthermore, GIF in the supernatant bound to anti-I-J^b alloantibodies, whereas GIF injected into the animals bound to anti-I-J^k antibodies. Thus, it appears that splenic lymphocytes of GIF-treated mice formed their own GIF. The cell source of OVA-binding GIF was Lyt-2^+ T cells, suggesting that GIF treatment of OVA-primed mice facilitated the generation of antigen-specific Lyt-2^+ suppressor T cells, which form OVA-binding GIF upon antigenic stimulation (Akasaki et al., 1986). Indeed, antigen-specific suppressor T cells were detected in the spleen cells of OVA-primed, GIF-treated mice. Transfer of their splenic T cells suppressed the antihapten antibody response of syngeneic recipients to DNP-OVA but did not affect the antibody response of another group of recipients to DNP-KLH. The results suggested that the GIF treatment of OVA-primed mice facilitated the generation of antigen-specific suppressor T cells and that these cells were responsible for immunosuppression (Akasaki et al., 1986).

Since the antigen-binding GIF is derived from I-J^+, Lyt-2^+ T cells (Jardieu et al., 1984), it was anticipated that this lymphokine may have an immunosuppressive effect. Thus, OVA-specific suppressor T cells were induced by repeated intravenous injections of OVA into BDF_1 mice, and antigen-specific T cell clones were established from their spleen cells. The T cell clone was then fused with BW5147 cells. Some of the hybridomas constitutively secreted GIF that lacked affinity for OVA. Upon incubation with OVA-pulsed syngeneic macrophages, the same hybridomas formed not only GIF with affinity for OVA but also IgE-SFs (Jardieu et al., 1987). Recognition of antigen by the hybridomas was MHC restricted. A representative hybridoma, $231F_1$, produced OVA-binding GIF and IgE-SFs when the cells were incubated with OVA-pulsed macrophages of H-2^d mice or A20.3 cells of BALB/c origin. However, the same hybridoma cells constitutively secreted nonspecific GIF and failed to form IgE-BFs when they were incubated with OVA-pulsed macrophages of H-2^b or H-2^k mice. It was also found that the formation of IgE-BFs by antigenic stimulation of the $231F_1$ cells was inhibited by pretreatment of the antigen-presenting cells with monoclonal anti-I-A^d antibody but not with anti-I-E antibody. Recent experiments showed that incubation of the same cells with syngeneic antigen-presenting cells together with UD-OVA or tryptic digests of UD-OVA resulted in the formation of IgE-BFs and OVA-binding GIF. Treatment of the $231F_1$ cells with either monoclonal antibody against T cell receptor α, β, or anti-CD3 (145-2C11) antibody, followed by culture of the antibody-treated cells in protein A-coated wells, also induced the formation of both IgE-BFs and OVA-binding GIF. It appears that the hybridoma expresses T cell receptors that recognize a fragment of OVA associated with Ia molecules.

The OVA-binding GIF from the $231F_1$ cells bound to OVA-Sepharose and antilipocortin–Sepharose and were recovered from the column by elution at acid pH, but the factor did not bind to either KLH–Sepharose or BSA–Sepharose. The OVA-binding GIF consisted of the 80- and 40-kDa molecules as estimated by gel filtration, while nonspecific GIF from the same cells were 50 and 13–15 kDa (Jardieu et al., 1987). Reduction and alkylation treatment of the 40-kDa OVA-binding GIF resulted in the formation of the 15-kDa, nonspecific GIF, suggesting that the OVA-binding GIF consists of an antigen-binding polypeptide chain and a nonspecific GIF (Jardieu and Ishizaka, 1987). It was also found that OVA-binding GIF suppressed the antibody response of BDF_1 mice in a carrier (OVA)-specific manner (Jardieu et al., 1987). In the experiments shown in Fig. 3, OVA-binding GIF from the $231F_1$ cells were purified by affinity chromatography on OVA-coupled Sepharose or antilipocortin–Sepharose. Nonspecific GIF from unstimulated $231F_1$ cells was purified by using antilipocortin–Sepharose. The GIF activities of the three preparations were comparable in terms of the ability to switch BALB/c spleen cells for the formation of IgE-SFs. Groups of BDF_1 mice were immunized with either alum-absorbed DNP-OVA or DNP-KLH, and each group received three intravenous injections of a GIF preparation. The results shown in Fig. 3 indicate that OVA-binding GIF was much more effective than was nonspecific GIF for suppressing the antihapten IgE antibody response to DNP-OVA. It was also noted that OVA-binding GIF recovered from antilipocortin–Sepharose was as effective as the eluates from OVA-Sepharose with respect to their ability to suppress the antibody response. In this schedule of treatment, OVA-binding GIF and nonspecific GIF exerted only marginal and comparable suppressive effects on the antibody response to DNP-KLH. Carrier-specific suppression of OVA-binding GIF was also observed in the IgG_1 antihapten antibody response. The results imply that the antigen-binding GIF is a TsF.

Another common property shared by the antigen-binding GIF and antigen-specific TsF is association of I-J determinants with the molecules. Both the antigen-binding and nonspecific GIFs bound to alloantibodies specific for I-J determinant(s). It appears that antigen-binding GIF is composed of an antigen-binding chain and an I-J$^+$ chain, the latter of

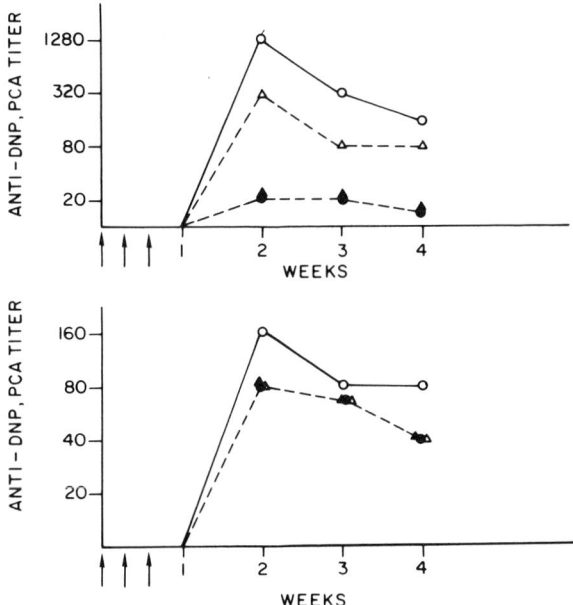

FIG. 3. Suppression of antihapten IgE antibody response to alum-absorbed DNP-OVA (top) or alum-absorbed DNP-KLH (bottom) by OVA binding (●--●, ▲--▲) or nonspecific GIF (△--△). OVA-binding GIF was purified by using either OVA–Sepharose (●--●) or antilipocortin Sepharose (▲--▲), injected intravenously into animals, as shown by the arrows. ○—○, Saline.

which also reacts with monoclonal antilipocortin (Jardieu and Ishizaka, 1987). Recent experiments also showed that the antigen-specific GIF, but not the nonspecific GIF, from the $231F_1$ cells bound to monoclonal antibody 14-12 (Ferguson et al., 1985), which reacts with effector suppressor factor. On the other hand, collaboration with the group of M. Dorf at Harvard University indicated that the monoclonal antilipocortin (141B9) bound not only GIF but also 4 hydroxy-3-nitrophenyl acetyl hapten-specific TsF_1 (Okuda et al., 1981) and TsF_3 (Furusawa et al., 1984) from CKB strain-derived Ts hybridomas (Steele et al., 1989). It appears that OVA-binding GIF from the $231F_1$ cells is similar to glutamic acid–alanine–tyrosine-specific TsF_2 (Turck et al., 1986), KLH-specific TsF (Saito and Taniguchi, 1984) and NP-specific TsF_3 (Furusawa et al., 1984) in terms of their immunosuppressive effects and antigenic structures. The findings collectively suggest that GIF treatment facilitates the generation of antigen-specific supressor T cells, which produces antigen-specific TsF upon antigenic stimulation.

D. Construction of Antigen-Specific Suppressor T Cell Hybridomas from Antigen-Primed T Cell Populations

Since the *in vivo* treatment of OVA-primed mice with nonspecific GIF facilitated the generation of suppressor T cells which produce their own GIF, attempts were made to reproduce the effects of GIF *in vitro*. The protocol of the experiments is shown in Fig. 4. BDF_1 mice were immunized with alum-absorbed OVA for the IgE antibody response, and their spleen cells were obtained 2 weeks after the immunization, when the IgE antibody titer had reached maximum. The spleen cells were cultured with OVA to activate antigen-primed T cells, and the activated T cells were propagated by IL-2 in the presence or absence of GIF for 4 days. Since antigen-specific T cells should have selectively proliferated during the culture, the cells recovered from the cultures were stimulated with OVA-pulsed syngeneic macrophages. Upon antigenic stimulation, the original spleen cells, as well as T cells, propagated in the absence of GIF produced IgE-PFs and GEF. In contrast, the same T cells propagated in the presence of GIF produced IgE-SFs and GIF (Fig. 4). The GIF detected in the culture supernatant bound to OVA-coupled Sepharose and was recovered by elution at acid pH. Since GIF added to T cells together with IL-2 during their propagation did not have affinity for OVA, GIF in culture supernatant of antigen-stimulated T cells does not appear to be a carryover of the GIF added in previous cultures. The results indicated that the addition of nonspecific GIF during the propagation of antigen-specific T cells facilitated the generation of antigen-specific T cells that produce their own GIF (Iwata and Ishizaka, 1988).

In order to determine whether the antigen-binding GIF from the T cells has immunosuppressive effects, OVA-primed T cells were propagated by IL-2 in the presence of nonspecific GIF and such T cells were fused with BW5147 cells to construct hybridomas. GIF-producing hybridomas

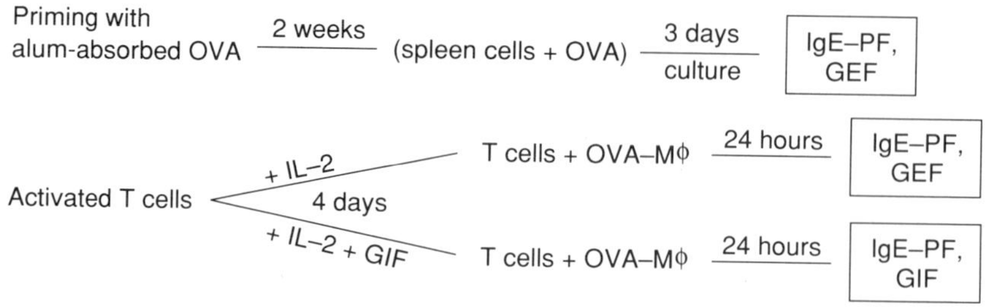

FIG. 4. Protocol of experiments for the generation of suppressor T cells *in vitro* by GIF. Mφ, Macrophage.

were selected and stimulated with OVA-pulsed syngeneic macrophages. One representative hybridoma, which produces OVA-binding GIF upon antigenic stimulation, was cultured with OVA-pulsed antigen-presenting cells, and OVA-binding GIF in culture supernatants were purified using OVA–Sepharose. In the experiments shown in Fig. 5, groups of BDF_1 mice were immunized with either alum-absorbed DNP-OVA or DNP-KLH, and they were treated with four intravenous injections of OVA-binding GIF from the hybridoma. It is evident that OVA-binding GIF suppressed the antihapten IgE antibody response to DNP-OVA without affecting the antibody response to DNP-KLH (Iwata and Ishizaka, 1988).

This series of experiments provides a maneuver for obtaining antigen-specific suppressor factor from antigen-primed T cell populations. One may anticipate that the protocol described above for mouse spleen cells

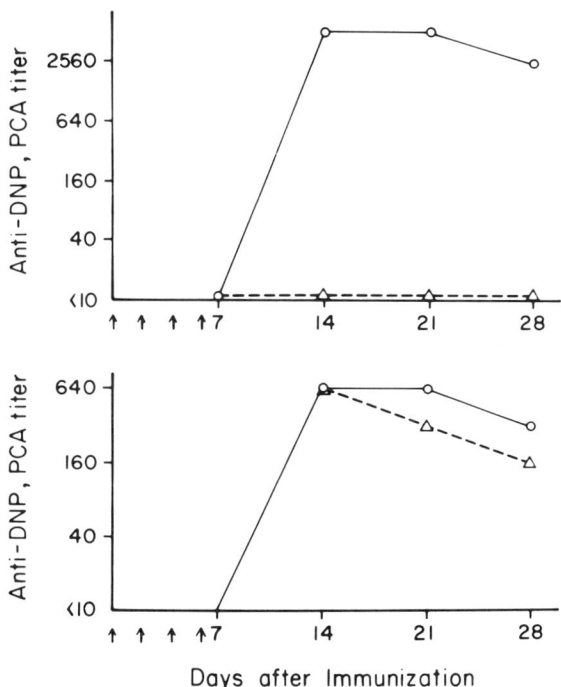

FIG. 5. Suppression of antihapten IgE antibody response to DNP-OVA (top) or DNP-KLH (bottom) by OVA-binding GIF (△--△) from a hybridoma which was constructed by the protocol shown in Fig. 4. OVA-binding GIF was given intravenously into the immunized animals. ○——○, Saline.

might be applied to generate antigen-specific suppressor T cells from the lymphocytes of allergic patients. As an experimental model we chose patients allergic to honey bee venom. Since the major allergen in honey bee venom is phospholipase A_2 (King et al., 1976), PBMCs from allergic patients were cultured with bee venom phospholipase A_2 which had been denatured by treatment with guanidine hydrochloride in the presence of reducing reagent. This treatment completely inactivated enzymatic activity of the allergen (King et al., 1976), but the denatured antigen should maintain the sequence of a peptide that would stimulate antigen-specific T cells. Since human GIF was not available, T cells activated by the denatured antigen were propagated by IL-2, in the presence or absence of recombinant human lipocortin (Wallner et al., 1986) (cf. Fig. 4). T cells propagated under these conditions were recovered and incubated with autologous monocytes in the presence of the denatured bee venom phospholipase A_2. As expected, T cells propagated by IL-2 alone produced IgE-PFs and GEF, while those propagated in the presence of lipocortin produced IgE-SFs and GIF. It became apparent also that the latter T cells constitutively released nonspecific GIF lacking affinity for bee venom phospholipase A_2, but stimulation of the same cells with phospholipase A_2-pulsed syngeneic monocytes resulted in the formation of GIF that had affinity for bee venom phospholipase A_2. As the stimulation of the T cells by antigen should go through T cell receptors, we anticipated that stimulation of the same T cells with anti-CD3 (OKT3) may induce the formation of antigen-binding GIF. Indeed, the T cells cultured in OKT3-coated wells formed IgE-BFs and GIF that had affinity for bee venom phospholipase A_2. Thus, we succeeded in generating antigen-specific T cells that can form antigen-binding GIF.

Attempts were made to construct human T cell hybridomas that produce GIF. PBMCs of a bee venom-sensitive patient were stimulated with denatured bee venom phospholipase A_2, and the cells were propagated by IL-2 in the presence of human lipocortin. The cells were then fused with a hypoxanthine guanine phosphoribosyl transferase-deficient mutant of T cell line CEM (BUC cells). One of the hybridomas that constitutively secrete GIF was expanded and cultured on OKT3-coated wells. GIF produced by the hybridoma had affinity for phospholipase A_2-Sepharose. As we do not have an appropriate system for demonstrating the antibody response of human peripheral blood lymphocytes to bee venom phospholipase A_2, we cannot evaluate immunosuppressive activity of antigen-specific GIF. However, considering the fact that antigen-binding GIF from mouse T cells suppresses the *in vivo* antibody response of syngeneic mice in a carrier-specific manner, we suspect that allergen-binding GIF from human T cell hybridomas may suppress the antibody response of the donor of parent T cells to specific antigen.

Many problems with antigen-binding GIF remain to be solved. It is not known how this lymphokine or antigen-specific TsF suppresses the antibody response. Although the target of effector TsF is believed to be antigen-primed helper T cells (Lopez et al., 1986), the mechanism for the suppression has to be explored. If antigen-binding GIF is identical to one of the antigen-specific TsFs, what is the role of phospholipase-inhibitory activity of GIF in the immunosuppression? Recent studies on antigen-specific suppressor T cells indicated that suppressor T cells possess T cell receptors (Kuchroo et al., 1988; Weiner et al., 1988). The results are in agreement with our findings that GIF-producing T cell hybridomas bear the CD3 complex. If the GIF (TsF)-producing suppressor T cells actually bear T cell receptors, a possible relationship between the factors and T cell receptors has to be elucidated. Zheng et al. (1988) indicated that TsF from a cloned T cell hybridoma, which is specific for a synthetic polypeptide, has the same fine specificity as that of T cell receptors on the cells. This principle probably applies to protein antigen systems. Our recent experiments in collaboration with H. Grey (Cytel Corporation, La Jolla, California) demonstrated that the $23IF_1$ cells responded to a truncated peptide, corresponding to amino acids 307–317 in the OVA molecule, in the context of an MHC product on antigen-presenting cells. Furthermore, the binding of OVA-binding GIF from the cells to OVA-coupled Sepharose was inhibited by the same peptide, suggesting that T cell receptors and antigen-binding T cell factors may share common specificity. It is well established that T cell receptors recognize "processed antigen" associated with the MHC product, but the T cells do not respond to nominal antigen. If antigen-binding GIF and T cell receptors share a common structural gene, how do the factors bind to the nominal antigen? All of these questions should be resolved. Nevertheless, construction of antigen-specific suppressor T cell hybridomas from the peripheral blood lymphocytes of atopic patients and preparation of antigen-binding TsF from such hybridomas may provide a new approach to suppressing the IgE antibody response to allergens.

Acknowledgments

Research in our laboratory on the regulation of the IgE antibody response was supported by U.S. Health and Human Services Grants AI-11202 and 14784 and by National Science Foundation Grant DCB-8519489. The author expresses great appreciation to his colleagues who have worked on the subject for the past 18 years.

References

Adachi, M., Arai, N., and Ishizaka, K. (1988). *J. Immunol.* **141**, 2358.
Akasaki, M., and Ishizaka, K. (1987). *Int. Arch. Allergy Appl. Immunol.* **82**, 417.
Akasaki, M., Iwata, M., and Ishizaka, K. (1985). *J. Immunol.* **135**, 4069.
Akasaki, M., Jardieu, P., and Ishizaka, K. (1986). *J. Immunol.* **136**, 3172.
Azuma, M., Hirano, T., Miyajima, H., Watanabe, N., Yagita, H., Enomoto, S., Furusawa, S., Ovary, Z., Kinashi, T., Honjo, T., and Okumura, K. (1987). *J. Immunol.* **139**, 2538.
Blaser, K., Nakagawa, T., and deWeck, A. L. (1980). *J. Immunol.* **125**, 24.
Blaser, K., Nakagawa, T., and deWeck, A. L. (1981). *J. Immunol.* **126**, 1180.
Block, M. K., Ohman, J. L., Waltin, J., and Cygan, R. W. (1973). *J. Immunol.* **110**, 197.
Bonnefoy, J.-Y., Aubry, J.-P., Peronne, C., Wijdenes, J., and Banchereau, J. (1987). *J. Immunol.* **138**, 2970.
Capron, M., Spiegelberg, H. L., Prin, L., Bennich, H., Butterworth, A. E., Pierce, R. J., Quaissi, M. A., and Capron, A. (1984). *J. Immunol.* **132**, 462.
Carini, C., Margolick, J., Yodoi, J., and Ishizaka, K. (1988). *Proc. Natl. Acad. Sci. U.S.A.* **85**, 9214.
Chiorazzi, N., Fox, D. A., and Katz, D. H. (1976). *J. Immunol.* **117**, 1629.
Coffman, R. L., and Carty, J. (1986). *J. Immunol.* **136**, 949.
Coffman, R. L., Seymour, B. W. P., Lebman, D. A., Hiraki, D. D., Christiansen, J. A., Shrader, B., Cherwinski, H. M., Savelkoul, H. F., Finkelman, F. D., Bond, M. W., and Mosmann, T. T. (1988). *Immunol. Rev.* **102**, 5.
Coffman, T., Ohara, J., Bond, M., Carty, J., Zlotnik, A., and Paul, W. E. (1986). *J. Immunol.* **136**, 4538.
Conrad, D. H., and Peterson, L. H. (1984). *J. Immunol.* **132**, 796.
Conrad, D. H., Waldschmidt, T. J., Lee, W. T., Rao, M., Keegan, A. D., Noelle, R. J., Lynch, R. G., and Kehry, M. R. (1987). *J. Immunol.* **139**, 2290.
Danneman, P. J., and Michael, G. (1977). *J. Exp. Med.* **146**, 1534.
Defrance, T., Aubry, J. P., Rousette, F., Vanherviliet, B., Bonnefoy, J. Y., Arai, N., Takabe, Y., Yokota, T., Lee, F., Arai, K., DeVries, J., and Banchereau, J. (1987). *J. Exp. Med.* **165**, 1459.
Deguchi, H., Suemura, M., Ishizaka, A., Ozaki, Y., Kishimoto, S., Yamamura, Y., and Kishimoto, T. (1983). *J. Immunol.* **131**, 2751.
Ferguson, T. A., Beaman, K. D., and Iverson, M. (1985). *J. Immunol.* **134**, 3163.
Finkelman, F. D., Katona, L. M., Urban, J. F., Jr., Snapper, G. M., Ohara, J., and Paul, W. E. (1986a). *Proc. Natl. Acad. Sci. U.S.A.* **83**, 9675.
Finkelman, F. D., Ohara, J., Goroff, D. K., Smith, J., Villacreases, N., Mond, J. J., and Paul, W. E. (1986b). *J. Immunol.* **137**, 2878.
Finkelman, F. D., Katona, I. M., Mossman, T. R., and Coffman, R. L. (1988a). *J. Immunol.* **140**, 1022.
Finkelman, F. D., Katona, I. M., Urban, J. F., Holmes, J., Ohara, J., Tung, A. S., Sample, J. G., and Paul, W. E. (1988b). *J. Immunol.* **141**, 2335.
Fisher, P. M., and Buckley, R. H. (1979). *J. Immunol.* **123**, 1788.
Fritche, R., and Spiegelberg, H. L. (1978). *J. Immunol.* **121**, 471.
Furusawa, S., Minami, M., Sherr, D. H., and Dorf, M. E. (1984). *In* "Cell Fusion Gene Transfer and Transformation" (R. F. Beers, Jr. and E. G. Bassett, eds.), p. 299. Raven Press, New York.
Gonzalez-Molina, A., and Spiegelberg, H. L. (1976). *J. Immunol.* **117**, 1838.
Gonzalez-Molina, A., and Spiegelberg, H. L. (1977). *J. Clin. Invest.* **59**, 616.

Gordon, J., Rowe, M., Walker, L., and Guy, G. R. (1986a). *Eur. J. Immunol.* **15**, 1075.
Gordon, J., Webb, A. J., Walker, L., Guy, G. R., and Row, M. (1986b). *Eur. J. Immunol.* **16**, 1627.
Guy, G. R., and Gordon, J. (1987). *Proc. Natl. Acad. Sci. U.S.A.* **84**, 6239.
Hirashima, M., Yodoi, J., and Ishizaka, K. (1980a). *J. Immunol.* **125**, 1442.
Hirashima, M., Yodoi, J., and Ishizaka, K. (1980b). *J. Immunol.* **125**, 2154.
Hirashima, M., Yodoi, J., and Ishizaka, K. (1981a). *J. Immunol.* **126**, 838.
Hirashima, M., Yodoi, J., and Ishizaka, K. (1981b). *J. Immunol.* **127**, 1804.
Hirashima, M., Yodoi, J., Huff, T. F., and Ishizaka, K. (1981c). *J. Immunol.* **127**, 1810.
Huff, T. F., Uede, T., and Ishizaka, K. (1982). *J. Immunol.* **129**, 509.
Huff, T. F., Uede, T., Iwata, M., and Ishizaka, K. (1983). *J. Immunol.* **131**, 1090.
Huff, T. F., Yodoi, J., Uede, T., and Ishizaka, K. (1984). *J. Immunol.* **132**, 406.
Huff, T. F., Jardieu, P., and Ishizaka, K. (1986). *J. Immunol.* **136**, 955.
Ikuta, K., Takami, M., Kim, L. W., Honjo, T., Miyoshi, T., Tagaya, Y., Kawabe, T., and Yodoi, J. (1987). *Proc. Natl. Acad. Sci. U.S.A.* **84**, 819.
Ishizaka, K. (1976). *Adv. Immunol.* **23**, 1.
Ishizaka, K. (1984). *Annu. Rev. Immunol.* **6**, 513.
Ishizaka, K., and Ishizaka, T. (1973). In "Asthma: Physiology, Immunopharmacology, and Treatment" (K. F. Austen and L. M. Lichtenstein, eds.), p. 55. Academic Press, New York.
Ishizaka, K., and Kishimoto, T. (1972). *J. Immunol.* **109**, 65.
Ishizaka, K., and Okudaira, H. (1973). *J. Immunol.* **110**, 1067.
Ishizaka, K., and Sandberg, K. (1981). *J. Immunol.* **126**, 1692.
Ishizaka, K., Okudaira, H., and King, T. P. (1975). *J. Immunol.* **114**, 110.
Isata, M., and Ishizaka, K. (1988). *J. Immunol.* **141**, 3270.
Iwata, M., Huff, T. F., Uede, T., Munoz, J. J., and Ishizaka, K. (1983a). *J. Immunol.* **130**, 1802.
Iwata, M., Munoz, J. J., and Ishizaka, K. (1983b). *J. Immunol.* **131**, 1954.
Iwata, M., Huff, T. F., and Ishizaka, K. (1984a). *J. Immunol.* **132**, 1286.
Iwata, M., Akasaki, M., and Ishizaka, K. (1984b). *J. Immunol.* **133**, 1505.
Iwata, M., Fukutomi, Y., Hashimoto, T., Sato, Y., Sato, H., and Ishizaka, K. (1987). *J. Immunol.* **138**, 2561.
Iwata, M., Adachi, M., and Ishizaka, K. (1988). *J. Immunol.* **140**, 2534.
Jardieu, P., and Ishizaka, K. (1987). In "Immune Regulation of Characterized Peptide" (G. Goldstein, J. F. Bach, and H. Witzell, eds.), UCLA Symp., p. 595. Liss, New York.
Jardieu, P., Uede, T., and Ishizaka, K. (1984). *J. Immunol.* **133**, 3266.
Jardieu, P., Uede, T., and Ishizaka, K. (1985a). *J. Immunol.* **135**, 922.
Jardieu, P., Moore, K., Martens, C., and Ishizaka, K. (1985b). *J. Immunol.* **135**, 2727.
Jardieu, P., Akasaki, M., and Ishizaka, K. (1986). *Proc. Natl. Acad. Sci. U.S.A.* **83**, 160.
Jarrett, E. E. E., and Ferguson, A. (1974). *Nature (London)* **250**, 420.
Jarrett, E. E. E., and Steward, D. D. (1972). *Immunology* **23**, 749.
Johansson, S. G. O., Melbin, T., and Vahlquist, B. (1968). *Lancet* **1**, 1118.
Joseph, M., Auriault, C., Capron, A., Vrong, H., and Viens, P. (1983). *Nature (London)* **303**, 819.
Katona, I. M., Urban, J. F., Sherr, J. I., Kannellopoulos-Langevin, C., and Finkelman, F. D. (1983). *J. Immunol.* **130**, 350.
Katz, D. H., Hamaoka, T., and Benacerraf, B. (1973). *Proc. Natl. Acad. Sci. U.S.A.* **7**, 2776.
Kawabe, T., Takami, M., Maeda, Y., Saito, S., Mayumi, M., Mikawa, H., Arai, K., and Yodoi, J. (1988). *J. Immunol.* **141**, 1376.

Keegan, A. D., Snapper, C. M., Dusen, R. V., Paul, W. E., and Conrad, D. H. (1989). *J. Immunol.* **142**, 3868.
Kikutani, H., Inui, S., Sato, R., Barsumian, E. L., Owaki, H., Yamasaki, K., Kaisho, T., Uchibayashi, N., Hardy, R. F., Hirano, T., Tsumasawa, S., Sakiyama, F., Suemura, M., and Kishimoto, T. (1986a). *Cell (Cambridge, Mass.)* **47**, 657.
Kikutani, H., Suemura, N., Owaki, H., Nakamura, H., Sato, R., Yamasaki, K., Barsumian, E. I., Hardy, R. R., and Kishimoto, T. (1986b). *J. Exp. Med.* **164**, 1455.
Kimoto, M., Kishimoto, T., Noguchi, S., Watanabe, T., and Yamamura, Y. (1977). *J. Immunol.* **118**, 840.
Kinet, J. P., Metzger, H., and Kochan, J. (1987). *Biochemistry* **26**, 4605.
King, T. P., Sobotka, A. K., Kochunmain, L., and Lichtenstein, L. (1976). *Arch. Biochem. Biophys.* **172**, 661.
Kisaki, T., Huff, T. F., Conrad, D. H., Yodoi, J., and Ishizaka, K. (1987). *J. Immunol.* **138**, 3345.
Kisaki, T., Leung, D. Y., Jardieu, P., Geha, R. S., and Ishizaka, K. (1988). *Eur. J. Immunol.* **18**, 1663.
Kishimoto, T., and Ishizaka, K. (1973). *J. Immunol.* **111**, 720.
Kishimoto, T., Hirai, Y., Suemura, M., and Yamamura, Y. (1976). *J. Immunol.* **117**, 394.
Kuchroo, V. K., Steele, J. K., Billings, P. R., Selvaraj, P., and Dorf, M. E. (1988). *Proc. Natl. Acad. Sci. U.S.A.* **85**, 9209.
Lanzavecchia, A. (1984). *Eur. J. Immunol.* **13**, 820.
Lee, W. T., Rao, M., and Conrad, D. H. (1987). *J. Immunol.* **139**, 1191.
Lee, W. Y., and Sehon, A. H. (1978). *Int. Arch. Allergy Appl. Immunol.* **56**, 159.
Lee, W. Y., and Sehon, A. H. (1981). *J. Immunol.* **126**, 414.
Lee, W. Y., Sehon, A. H., and Akebloom, E. (1981). *Int. Arch. Allergy Appl. Immunol.* **64**, 110.
Leung, D. Y. M., and Geha, R. (1986). *J. Clin. Immunol.* **6**, 273.
Leung, D. Y. M., Young, M., Wood, N. L., and Geha, R. S. (1986). *J. Exp. Med.* **163**, 713.
Leung, D. Y. M., Biozek, C., Frankel, R., and Geha, R. S. (1984). *Clin. Immunol. Immunopathol.* **32**, 339.
Levine, B. B. (1971). In "Biochemistry of the Acute Allergic Reactions" (K. F. Austen and E. L. Becker, eds.), p. 1. Blackwell, Oxford.
Levine, B. B., and Vaz, N. M. (1970). *Int. Arch. Allergy Appl. Immunol.* **39**, 156.
Lopez, M. T., Soresen, C. M., and Kapp, J. A. (1986). *J. Immunol.* **136**, 798.
Ludin, C., Hofstetter, H., Sarafati, M., Levy, C., Sutter, U., Alaimo, D., Kelchkerr, E., Frost, H., and Delespesse, G. (1987). *EMBO J.* **6**, 109.
Martens, C. L., Huff, T. F., Jardieu, P., Trounstein, M. L., Coffman, R. L., Ishizaka, K., and Moore, J. W. (1985). *Proc. Natl. Acad. Sci. U.S.A.* **82**, 2460.
Martens, C. L., Jardieu, P., Trounstein, M. L., Sturat, S. G., Ishizaka, K., and Moore, K. W. (1987). *Proc. Natl. Acad. Sci. U.S.A.* **84**, 809.
Melewitz, F. M., and Spiegelberg, H. L. (1980). *J. Immunol.* **125**, 1026.
Mond, J. J., Carmen, J., Sarina, C., Ohara, J., and Finkelman, F. D. (1986). *J. Immunol.* **137**, 3534.
Moore, K. W., Jardieu, P., Mietz, J. A., Trounstine, M. L., Kuff, E. L., Ishizaka, K., and Martens, C. L. (1986). *J. Immunol.* **131**, 4283.
Mosmann, T. R., Cherwinski, H., Bond, M. W., Giedlin, M. A., and Coffman, R. L. (1986). *J. Immunol.* **236**, 2348.
Noelle, R., Krammer, P. H., Ohara, J., Uhr, J., and Vitetta, E. S. (1984). *Proc. Natl. Acad. Sci. U.S.A.* **81**, 6149.
Ohehir, R. E., Bal, V., Quint, D., Mogel, R., Kay, A. B., Zanders, E., and Lamb, J. (1988). *FASEB J.* **2**, A-1442 (abstr.).

Okuda, K., Minami, M., Furusawa, S., and Dorf, M. E. (1981). *J. Exp. Med.* **154**, 1838.
Parkhouse, R. E. M., and Cooper, M. D. (1977). *Immunol. Rev.* **7**, 105.
Péne, J., Rousset, F., Briere, F., Chrétien, I., Paliard, X., Banchereau, J., Spits, H., and DeVries, J. E. (1988a). *J. Immunol.* **141**, 1212.
Péne, J., Rousset, F., Briere, F., Chrétien, I., Bonnefoy, J.-Y., Spits, H., Yokota, T., Arai, N., Arai, K., Banchereau, J., and DeVries, J. E. (1988b). *Proc. Natl. Acad. Sci. U.S.A.* **85**, 6880.
Prete, G. D., Maggi, E., Parronchi, P., Chrétien, I., Tiri, A., Macchia, D., Ricci, M., Banchereau, J., DeVries, J., and Romagmani, S. (1988). *J. Immunol.* **140**, 4193.
Ravetch, J. V., Luster, A. D., Weinshank, K., Kochar, J., Pavlorec, A., Portony, D. A., Hulmes, J., Pan, Y. E., and Unkeless, J. C. (1987). *Science* **234**, 718.
Revoltella, R., and Ovary, Z. (1969). *Immunology* **17**, 45.
Romagnani, S., Del Prete, G. G., Maggi, E., Troncone, R., Giudizi, M. G., Almerigogna, F., and Ricci, M. (1980). *Clin. Exp. Immunol.* **42**, 571.
Rousseaux-Provost, T., Bazin, H., and Capron, A. (1977). *Immunology* **33**, 501.
Saito, T., and Taniguchi, M. (1984). *J. Mol. Cell. Immunol.* **1**, 137.
Sampson, H. A., and Buckley, R. H. (1981). *J. Immunol.* **127**, 829.
Sarfati, M., Rector, E., Wong, K., Rubio-Trujilo, M., Sehon, A., and Delespesse, G. (1984). *Immunology* **53**, 197.
Sarfati, M., Nutman, T., Fonteya, C., and Delespesse, G. (1986). *Immunology* **59**, 569.
Sarfati, M., Nakajima, T., Frost, H., Kilcher, E., and Delespesse, G. (1987a). *Immunology* **60**, 539.
Sarfati, M., Nutman, T. B., Suter, U., Hofstetter, H., and Delespesse, G. (1987b). *J. Immunol.* **139**, 4055.
Saryan, J. A., Leung, D. Y. M., and Geha, R. (1983). *J. Immunol.* **130**, 242.
Saxon, A., and Stevens, R. H. (1979). *Clin. Immunol. Immunopathol.* **14**, 474.
Saxon, A., Morrow, L., and Stevens, R. H. (1980). *J. Clin. Invest.* **65**, 1457.
Sehon, A. H. (1982). *Prog. Allergy* **32**, 161.
Sherman, W. B., Stull, A., and Cook, R. A. (1940). *J. Allergy* **11**, 225.
Snapper, C. M., Finkelman, F. D., and Paul, W. E. (1988a). *Immunol. Rev.* **102**, 51.
Snapper, C. M., Finkelman, F. D., Steoany, D., Conrad, D. H., and Paul, W. E. (1988b). *J. Immunol.* **141**, 489.
Steele, J. K., Kuchroo, V. K., Kawasaki, H., Jayaraman, S., Iwata, M., Ishizaka, K., and Dorf, M. E. (1989). *J. Immunol.* **142**, 2213.
Suemura, M., and Ishizaka, K. (1979). *J. Immunol.* **123**, 918.
Suemura, M., Kishimoto, T., Hirai, Y., and Yamamura, Y. (1977). *J. Immunol.* **119**, 159.
Suemura, M., Urban, J. F., Jr., and Ishizaka, K. (1978). *J. Immunol.* **121**, 2413.
Suemura, M., Yodoi, J., Hirashima, M., and Ishizaka, K. (1980). *J. Immunol.* **125**, 148.
Suemura, M., Shiho, O., Deguchi, H., Yamamura, Y., Böttcher, I., and Kishimot, T. (1981). *J. Immunol.* **127**, 465.
Suemura, M., Ishizaka, A., Kobatake, S., Sugimura, K., Maeda, K., Nakanishi, K., Kishimoto, S., Yamamura, Y., and Kishimoto, T. (1983). *J. Immunol.* **130**, 1056.
Tada, T., Tanuguchi, M., and Okumura, K. (1971). *J. Immunol.* **106**, 1012.
Takatsu, K., and Ishizaka, K. (1975). *Cell. Immunol.* **20**, 276.
Takatsu, K., and Ishizaka, K. (1976a). *J. Immunol.* **116**, 1257.
Takatsu, K., and Ishizaka, K. (1976b). *J. Immunol.* **117**, 1211.
Thorley-Lawson, D. A., Nadler, L. M., Bhan, H. K., and Schooley, R. T. (1985). *J. Immunol.* **134**, 3007.
Tony, H.-P., and Parker, D. C. (1985). *J. Exp. Med.* **161**, 223.
Tung, A. S., Chiorazzi, N., and Katz, D. H. (1978). *J. Immunol.* **120**, 2050.
Turck, C. W., Kapp, J. A., and Webb, D. R. (1986). *J. Immunol.* **137**, 1904.

Turner, K. J., Holt, P. G., Holt, B. J., and Cameron, K. J. (1983). *Clin. Exp. Immunol.* **51**, 387.
Uede, T., and Ishizaka, K. (1982). *J. Immunol.* **129**, 3191.
Uede, T., and Ishizaka, K. (1984). *J. Immunol.* **133**, 359.
Uede, T., Huff, T. F., and Ishizaka, K. (1982). *J. Immunol.* **129**, 1384.
Uede, T., Sandberg, K., Bloom, B. R., and Ishizaka, K. (1983a). *J. Immunol.* **130**, 649.
Uede, T., Hirata, F., Hirashima, M., and Ishizaka, K. (1983b). *J. Immunol.* **130**, 878.
Uede, T., Huff, T. F., and Ishizaka, K. (1984). *J. Immunol.* **133**, 803.
Umetsu, D. T., Leung, D. Y. M., Siraganian, R., Jabara, H. H., and Geha, R. S. (1985). *J. Exp. Med.* **162**, 202.
Vander-Mallie, R., Ishizaka, T., and Ishizaka, K. (1982). *J. Immunol.* **128**, 2306.
Vaz, E. M., Vaz, N. M., and Levine, B. B. (1971). *Immunology* **21**, 11.
Vaz, N. M., Phillips-Quadriata, J. M., Levine, B. G., and Vaz, E. M. (1971). *J. Exp. Med.* **134**, 1335.
Waldman, T. A. (1969). *N. Engl. J. Med.* **28**, 1170.
Wallner, B. P., Mattalicano, R. J., Hession, C., and Cate, R. L. (1986). *Nature (London)* **320**, 77.
Warner, N. L. (1974). *Adv. Immunol.* **19**, 67.
Weiner, D. B., Liu, J., Hanna, N., Bluestone, J. A., Caligan, J. E., William, W. V., and Greene, M. I. (1988). *Proc. Natl. Acad. Sci. U.S.A.* **85**, 6077.
Yaoita, Y., Kumagai, Y., Okumura, K., and Honja, T. (1982). *Nature (London)* **297**, 697.
Yodoi, J., and Ishizaka, K. (1980). *J. Immunol.* **124**, 1322.
Yodoi, J., Hirashima, M., and Ishizaka, K. (1980). *J. Immunol.* **125**, 1436.
Yodoi, J., Hirashima, M., and Ishizaka, K. (1981a). *J. Immunol.* **126**, 877.
Yodoi, J., Hirashima, M., and Ishizaka, K. (1981b). *J. Immunol.* **127**, 471.
Yodoi, J., Hirashima, M., and Ishizaka, K. (1982). *J. Immunol.* **128**, 289.
Yokota, A., Kikutani, H., Tanaka, T., Sato, R., Barsumian, E. L., Suemura, M., and Kishimoto, T. (1988). *Cell (Cambridge, Mass.)* **55**, 611.
Young, M. C., Leung, C. Y. M., and Geha, R. S. (1984). *Eur. J. Immunol.* **14**, 871.
Young, M. C., Geha, R. S., Maksad, K. N., and Leung, D. Y. M. (1986). *Eur. J. Immunol.* **16**, 985.
Yukawa, K., Kikutani, H., Owaki, H., Yamasaki, K., Yokota, A., Nakamura, H., Barsumian, E. L., Hardy, R. R., Suemura, M., and Kishimoto, T. (1987). *J. Immunol.* **138**, 2576.
Zheng, H., Boyer, M., Fotedar, A., Singh, B., and Green, D. R. (1988). *J. Immunol.* **140**, 1351.
Zuraw, B. L., Nonaka, M., O'Hair, C., and Katz, D. H. (1981). *J. Immunol.* **127**, 1169.

This article was accepted for publication on 27 February 1989.

Control of the Immune Response at the Level of Antigen-Presenting Cells: A Comparison of the Function of Dendritic Cells and B Lymphocytes

JOSHUA P. METLAY, ELLEN PURÉ, AND RALPH M. STEINMAN

Rockefeller University and Irvington Institute of Medical Research, New York, New York 10021

I. Introduction

Dendritic cells represent a family of bone marrow-derived cells which are found in small numbers in most lymphoid and nonlymphoid tissues (Table I). The Langerhans cells of the skin, the veiled cells of the afferent lymph, the interdigitating cells of the thymic medulla and T cells areas of peripheral lymphoid organs, and the lymphoid dendritic cells isolated from lymphoid tissues are all members of this distinct lineage of leukocytes. As is detailed in this review, the dendritic cell family begins with a bone marrow precursor that likely seeds most nonlymphoid tissues. Following deposition of antigen, nonlymphoid dendritic cells may be mobilized to present antigen locally or to migrate with that antigen via the blood and lymph to the T cell areas of lymphoid organs. Except for the bone marrow precursor, dendritic cells in all tissues from which they have been isolated are potent antigen-presenting cells (APCs) for a variety of T cell-dependent immune responses.

In an analogous sense B lymphocytes also encompass a diverse array of developmental stages, each with distinct functional properties. Even within one antigen-specific B cell clone virgin B cells, B cell blasts, "memory" B cells, and plasma cells each have distinct properties, including the capacity to function as APCs.

Thus, the immune system contains two diverse groups of cells, both of which can present antigens to T cells. There have been recent reviews on the APC function of dendritic cells (Austyn, 1987; Austyn and Steinman, 1988; Steinman and Inaba, 1989) and B cells (Chesnut and Grey, 1986). Both function as APCs in the sense that under appropriate experimental conditions, these cells can form a major histocompatibility complex (MHC)–antigen complex that can be recognized by the antigen receptor on T cells (TCR) and stimulate those T cells to respond. While we review data on the capacity of dendritic cells and B cells to present antigens, our emphasis is on the different physiological features of these APCs, including their relative contributions *in vivo*.

TABLE I
TISSUES FROM WHICH DENDRITIC CELLS HAVE BEEN ISOLATED

Site	Reference
Peripheral lymphoid organs	
Mouse spleen	Steinman and Cohn (1973), Steinman et al. (1979), Nussenzweig et al. (1981)
Rat lymph node	Klinkert et al. (1978, 1982)
Mouse Peyer's patch	Spalding et al. (1983)
Human tonsil	Hart and McKenzie (1988)
Central lymphoid organs	
Murine thymus	Kyewski et al. (1986), Inaba et al. (1988), Crowley et al. (1989)
Chicken thymus	Oliver and LeDourain (1984)
Human thymus	Pelletier et al. (1986)
Nonlymphoid organs	
Rat skin, liver	Klinkert et al. (1982)
Mouse skin	Schuler and Steinman (1985), Witmer-Pack et al. (1987)
Mouse lung	Sertl et al. (1986)
Rat lung	Holt et al. (1987)
Human skin	Romani et al. (1989b)
Afferent lymph	
Rat	Mayrhofer et al. (1986), Fossum (1984), Pugh et al. (1983), Mason et al. (1981)
Mouse	Rhodes and Agger (1987)
Rabbit	Kelly et al. (1978), Knight et al. (1982)
Pig	Drexhage et al. (1979)
Sheep	Bujdoso et al. (1989)
Human	Spry et al. (1980)
Blood, human	Van Voorhis et al. (1982), Kuntz-Crow and Kunkel (1982), Santiago-Schwartz et al. (1985), Gaudernack and Bjercke (1985), Knight et al. (1986), Young and Steinman (1988), Vakkila et al. (1987)
Exudates	
Rat peritoneal cavity	Klinkert et al. (1982)
Human synovial fluid	Zvaifler et al. (1985)

We develop in this chapter three areas where there have been recent advances. The first is that dendritic cells and B lymphocytes differ considerably in terms of their tissue distribution *in situ* and their surface properties. The relevance of these differences to APC function will be considered. The second is that each cell has distinct effects when tested for APC function *in vitro* and *in situ*. Presentation of soluble proteins,

MHC and Mls antigens, viral antigens, and T cell-dependent antigens for antibody formation is each dealt with separately. The evidence that both B cells and dendritic cells regulate their APC function depending on their tissue localization and exposure to antigen and cytokines will be stressed. The third area relates to the mechanism of APC function, which includes how each APC processes antigen, acquires antigen *in vivo*, and forms stable contacts with responsive T cells.

II. Tissue Distribution of Dendritic Cells and B Lymphocytes

The histories of dendritic cells and B lymphocytes—their origin, movements, and turnover *in situ*—are distinct (Table II). In considering B cells, we refer only to the major population of conventional B cells that are surface immunoglobulin positive (Ig^+) and $CD5^-$, not smaller subpopulations such as the $CD5^+$ B cells in peritoneal exudates (Herzenberg et al., 1986) and thymus (Miyama-Inaba et al., 1988) or the IgD^{poor} B cell in the splenic marginal zone (MacLennan et al., 1982). The functions of these latter populations vis-à-vis antigen presentation, have not been analyzed extensively.

A. Origin

B cells and dendritic cells both originate from bone marrow progenitors. The events whereby progenitor B cells, termed pro-B cells, develop into monoclonal mature B cells, with a single or clonotypic receptor for antigen, have been defined. The pro-B cell has Ig genes in germline configuration and is represented by cell lines such as LyD9 (Kinashi et al., 1988). The next stage, the pre-B cell, has rearranged the Ig

TABLE II
Tissue Distribution and Movements of Dendritic Cells and B Lymphocytes[a]

Compartment	B lymphocyte	Dendritic cell
Bone marrow	Pro-B → Pre-B → B	Ia^- precursor
Circulation	Blood ($t_{1/2}$ weeks/months)	Afferent lymph ($t_{1/2}$ hours)
Lymphoid organs	B cell areas Antigen ↓	T cell areas Antigen ↑
Nonlymphoid organs	Plasmablasts to eliminate antigen	Sentinel cells to present antigen

[a]A more detailed review of the history of dendritic cells has appeared recently (Fossum, 1989).

heavy-chain locus and contains cytoplasmic μ. These cells can be identified in marrow. In μ transgenic mice the introduction of membrane μ genes suppresses rearrangement at the heavy-chain locus in most cells (Nussenzweig et al., 1987), thereby ensuring monoclonality. The pre-B cell then differentiates further into the B cell by rearrangements at the λ and/or $\varkappa$ light-chain locus and expression of membrane IgM. The vast majority of cells express IgM and IgD that share the same V_H and are produced by a common precursor transcript. As will be emphasized in Section IV,A, the fact that B cells are clonal and capable of relatively high-affinity and specific interactions with one versus many antigens is a salient distinction from dendritic cells, which lack antigen specificity.

Mature B cells are a major component of isolated marrow suspensions, some 50% of the leukocytes in mouse marrow being B cells. Possibly, although we are not aware of direct evidence, the mature marrow B cell is capable of presenting antigen, since it is not overtly different from mature B cells in other organs.

Dendritic cells in mouse spleen (Steinman et al., 1974b), rat lymph (Pugh et al., 1983), and mouse epidermis (Katz et al., 1979; Frelinger et al., 1979) are bone marrow derived, i.e., in irradiation chimeras the vast majority of dendritic cells in the chimera are of donor bone marrow origin. However, the precursor has not been isolated. A single study has shown that Ia^- bone marrow cells in the rat can develop into typical Ia^+ dendritic cells (Bowers and Berkowitz, 1986), but the factors controlling this development and the identification of discrete dendritic cell colonies remain elusive. One cannot identify mature dendritic cells in the marrow by morphology (Steinman and Cohn, 1973), expression of the 33D1 antigen (Nussenzweig et al., 1982), or mixed-leukocyte reaction (MLR)-stimulating activity (Steinman and Witmer, 1978). In unpublished experiments we also have been unable to induce the formation of typical dendritic cells from mouse bone marrow cultures even in the presence of factors that stimulate myeloid [granulocyte-macrophage (GM)] growth and differentiation, i.e., interleukin-3 (IL-3), GM colony-stimulating factor (GM-CSF), G-CSF, or M-CSF. Therefore, it would seem that dendritic cell development is under controls distinct from phagocyte development. There is no evidence that mature functioning dendritic cells are normally formed in the marrow. This situation is much like the T lymphocyte lineage, which derives from the marrow but differentiates elsewhere, especially in the thymus.

In summary, a good deal is known about the development of B cells in the marrow. Monoclonal, immunocompetent cells are produced there in the apparent absence of any antigenic stimulus. Rather little is known about dendritic cells in the marrow, except that they originate there but cannot be identified as mature cells, i.e., dendritic, Ia-rich, and MLR-stimulatory cells.

B. LIFE SPAN AND TURNOVER

Detailed reviews are available for B cells in Volume 91 of the *Immunological Reviews* series and for dendritic cells in an article by Fossum (1989). The rate of formation of new B cells in mouse marrow is extensive. When a mouse is given radiolabeled thymidine, 50% of the marrow surface Ig^+ cells have incorporated [^{3}H]thymidine in 32-38 hours (Osmond and Nossal, 1974). Since the turnover of B cells in the periphery is likely to be much slower (see below), most of the newly formed cells in the marrow must die there.

Only one series of studies concludes that the turnover of B cells in the periphery is rapid. By looking at the life span of lipopolysaccharide (LPS)-responsive B cells in unresponsive, histocompatible recipients, Freitas and Coutinho (1981) obtained evidence for very rapid turnover, i.e., most cells were lost in 1-2 days. However, Ron and Sprent (1985) found a life span of weeks to months when trinitrophenyl (TNP)-Ficoll-responsive B cells were followed in recipients that had the *xid* deficiency. The latter data are more consistent with the life spans of several weeks that were noted using labeling with [^{3}H]uridine and [^{3}H]thymidine (Howard, 1972; Sprent, 1973).

Upon antigenic stimulation, B cells expand clonally. The extent of clonal expansion during an antibody response *in situ* seems limited for antibody-secreting cells, since their levels typically peak within 4-7 days of the administration of antigen. Additional clonal expansion occurs during the formation of the memory B cell pool. This expansion likely occurs in the germinal centers of lymphoid organs (Fleidner *et al.*, 1964; Sordat *et al.*, 1970). These are collections of proliferating B cells that are evident for at least 1-2 weeks after the administration of antigens and whose formation is T cell dependent (Jacobson *et al.*, 1974). B cell proliferation in germinal centers is thought to be driven by antigen-antibody complexes which are retained on the surface of follicular dendritic cells (Nossal *et al.*, 1968; Szakal and Hanna, 1968; Chen *et al.*, 1978b). Germinal center or follicular dendritic cells are distinct from the dendritic cells under discussion in this review. The two cell types exhibit morphological differences, and isolated lymphoid dendritic cells do not carry detectable immune complexes (Steinman and Cohn, 1974; Tew *et al.*, 1982). Recent studies reveal that the surface phenotypes of follicular dendritic cells and lymphoid dendritic cells are entirely distinct in human tonsil (Schriever *et al.*, 1989; Hart and McKenzie, 1988) and mouse lymphoid tissues (Humphrey *et al.*, 1984; Schnizlein *et al.*, 1985).

Dendritic cell turnover varies markedly, depending on the compartment under study. In mouse spleen and rat lymph, turnover is rapid, with half-times of less than 1 week (Steinman et al., 1974b; Pugh et al., 1983; Fossum, 1989). Thus, if one administers [^{3}H]thymidine repeatedly, the percentage of labeled dendritic cells increases at a steady rate, corresponding to 5–10% of the total pool per day. The site in which dendritic cells are proliferating (incorporating [^{3}H]thymidine) is not known. Dendritic cells, once in the lymph or lymphoid tissue, do not seem to be proliferating, since they do not label with a 1-hour pulse of [^{3}H]thymidine.

The turnover of dendritic cells in nonlymphoid tissues may be very slow, as illustrated by some of the findings with epidermal Langerhans cells (LCs). In bone marrow chimera experiments the influx of donor-derived LCs into the epidermis occurs with half-times on the order of weeks to months (Katz et al., 1979), and some host LCs can persist for close to 1 year. In guinea pig epidermis the [^{3}H]thymidine labeling index of LCs is about 0.3%, but this can approach 3% with application of a contact allergen (Gschnait and Brenner, 1979). Our preliminary findings are that it is not possible to label even 0.1% of the LCs in mouse ear epidermis following repeated daily injections of [^{3}H]thymidine in the steady state (unpublished observations), confirming the report by MacKenzie (1975). Another study has reported that substantial numbers of LCs can be labeled following the administration of bromodeoxyuridine (BrDU), and then epidermis can be double labeled with anti-Ia and anti-BrDU antibodies (Caernielewski et al., 1985). Thus, more data are required to assess the turnover rates of Ia$^+$ tissue dendritic cells.

C. LOCALIZATION IN LYMPHOID ORGANS

B cells in lymphoid organs are primarily found in regions called follicles, or B cell areas. Useful diagrams and typical results using immunolabeling of tissue sections with anti-B cell Mabs, are available for lymph node and spleen (MacLennan and Gray, 1986). B cell follicles are the site in which germinal centers develop during a T cell-dependent immune response. Small numbers of CD4$^+$ T cells also are found in germinal centers (Bhan et al., 1981).

It has long been suspected that the primary localization of dendritic cells is the T cell, rather than the B cell area. This is because a cell with many similarities to isolated dendritic cells, the interdigitating cell (IDC) is found in the T cell area of lymphoid organs (periarteriolar sheath of spleen, paracortex and deep cortex of lymph node, the interfollicular cortex of Peyer's patch, and the thymic medulla) (Scollay et al., 1980; Heusermann et al., 1974; Veerman, 1974; Veerman and Van Ewijk,

1974; Kaiserling et al., 1974; Duijvestijn et al., 1983; Veldman and Kaiserling, 1980; Fossum et al., 1980). IDCs have irregularly shaped nuclei and abundant pale cytoplasm by light microscopy, and by electron microscopy, they have a shape most consistent with the presence of abundant long processes. Thus, the plasma membrane shows deep but closely spaced indentations which would occur if pseudopods or veils were compressed upon one another. There is little evidence of secretory function (rough endoplasmic reticulum, secretory granules) in IDCs, and endocytic vacuoles and lysosomes typically are scarce.

IDCs likely express high levels of Ia. T cell areas contain stellate Ia^+ cells by light-microscopic immunolabeling, and in the case of rodents T cells do not express class II MHC (Dijkstra, 1982; Witmer and Steinman, 1984). The Ia-rich IDC does not express some traditional B cell and macrophage markers, e.g., 2.4G2 anti-Fcγ receptor II (anti-FcγRII), F4/80, Ml/70 or Mac-1, and B220 or $CD45R_A$ (Witmer and Steinman, 1984). Kraal and co-workers have developed two monoclonal antibodies, NL145 (Kraal et al., 1986) and MIDC-8 (Breel et al., 1987), which, while not perfectly restricted to dendritic cells, seem to stain most dendritic cells in T cell areas and lymphoid isolates (Crowley et al., 1989; Breel et al., 1987). Other studies have pointed out that IDCs have certain cytochemical features of dendritic cells—for example, there is little acid phosphatase activity (Eikelenboom, 1978)—and express an antigen termed $S100_\beta$, which is found in LCs but not in other leukocytes (Takahashi et al., 1984).

Two recent studies provide direct evidence that isolated dendritic cells can home to the T area and assume the localization of IDCs. Austyn et al., (1988) labeled highly purified splenic dendritic cells with a Hoechst fluorochrome, injected the cells intravenously, and documented homing by looking for Hoechst-labeled cells (blue emission) in tissue sections of spleen that were double labeled with fluorescein isothiocyanate (FITC) anti-T cell Mab (green emission). Also, it was noted that splenic dendritic cells will bind in vitro to the marginal sinus region of sections of the white pulp nodule. The marginal sinus is the region where the dendritic cells first localized following intravenous injection in situ before entering the T cell areas (Austyn et al., 1988). In contrast to B cells, dendritic cells injected intravenously do not leave the circulation via postcapillary venules to enter lymph nodes (Fossum, 1988). Fossum labeled dendritic cells in rat lymph by giving the animals repeated doses of [^{3}H]thymidine prior to isolation. He also observed homing to the T cell area following intravenous injection. The labeled cells entered the periarteriolar sheaths of spleen as well as the T cell area of the celiac nodes after traversing the liver. Following injection into the footpad, the cells migrated to the paracortex of the popliteal node. The homing of the injected dendritic cells was followed by light-microscopic autoradiography, but serial sections were also examined by electron microscopy to prove that the labeled cells had the ultrastructural characteristics of IDCs (Fossum, 1988).

In the study of homing of spleen-derived murine dendritic cells cited above, migration to the T cell area did not occur in nude mice but could be reconstituted with an injection of T cells (Kupiec-Weglinski et al., 1988). However, dendritic cells are evident in the afferent lymph of nude rats, and IDCs are clearly present in the lymph node cortex of these animals (Fossum et al., 1980). It is possible that there are two pools of dendritic cells in the T cell area: a relatively long-lived, T cell-independent pool of IDCs that functions to present antigens arising from within the lymphoid organ (e.g., when an infectious agent is growing there), and a pool with rapid turnover that migrates with antigen from the tissues into the T cell-dependent areas (see Sections II,D, II,E and VI,B) only in the presence of T cells.

The evidence cited above indicates that the dendritic cells isolated from the spleen are closely related to the IDCs. However, the two cell types may not be identical. For one thing, we find that it is easier to isolate dendritic cells from the spleen than from the lymph node, whereas the density of IDCs is much greater in sections of node. Also, IDCs express the NL145 antigen and lack 33D1, while most isolated spleen dendritic cells express 33D1 but have relatively little NL145. Recent experiments identified an $NL145^+$ $33D1^-$ dendritic cell which could be released into spleen suspensions by collagenase digestion. This cell was larger than the typical dendritic cell and expressed more cell surface MHC molecules (Crowley et al., 1989), but was otherwise similar in overall appearance and cell surface markers. The $NL145^+$ cell most likely corresponds to the IDC in situ, whereas the more easily released dendritic cell may be en route to the T cell area having acquired antigen beforehand, e.g., in the marginal zone. As yet, the two types of dendritic cells isolated from the spleen are not known to be functionally different (R. M. Steinman, unpublished observations).

D. Dendritic Cells and B Lymphocytes in Nonlymphoid Organs

It is difficult to identify small B cells in nonlymphoid organs. However, plasma cells underlie nonkeratinizing external surfaces of the body, such as the gut and exocrine glands. Most of these plasma cells are making IgA (Tomasi and Bienenstock, 1968) and presumably have interacted previously with helper cells capable of enhancing the expression of the

IgA isotype. Since plasma cells likely express little or no class II MHC products, mucosal plasma cells may not present antigens to $CD4^+$ helper cells.

In contrast to B cells, Ia-rich dendritic cells may be present in most nonlymphoid tissues in the steady state. The first evidence was in rats, where Klinkert et al. (1982) identified dendritic cells in skin and liver suspensions and Hart and Fabre (1981) identified dendritic leukocytes (cells that were rich in Ia but lacked typical B cell and macrophage traits) in sections of most tissues. Two sites in which there are few Ia^+ dendritic cells are the brain and the cornea. Findings comparable to those in the rat, i.e., the presence of interstitial dendritic cells in most human organs, were made by Daar et al. (1983), who stained sections of several tissues with Mabs to class II and other leukocyte antigens. Ia^+ dendritic cells in nonlymphoid organs have been described now in several studies (Hart and Fabre, 1981; Mayrhofer et al., 1983; Wilders et al., 1983; McKenzie et al., 1984; Forbes et al., 1986; Sertl et al., 1986; Faustman et al., 1984), including two studies of the 12- to 20-week human fetus (Hofman et al., 1984; Janossy et al., 1986). These studies are hampered by the lack of specific antibodies to identify dendritic cells in tissue section. The use of anti-Ia antibodies also could underestimate the number of dendritic cells, since there may be pools of Ia^- dendritic cell precursors that only express Ia in response to cytokines such as IL-1 (Inaba et al., 1988).

Since the expression of cell surface markers does not establish function, an important approach is to isolate nonlymphoid dendritic cells and compare them with other leukocytes. The most detailed analysis has been in murine epidermis, where it is possible to isolate enriched populations of LCs and maintain these in culture (Schuler and Steinman, 1985; Witmer-Pack et al., 1987; Heufler et al., 1987). In doing so, it has become apparent that freshly isolated LCs can undergo marked changes over 1-3 days in culture. These progressive changes are of several types and are reviewed more extensively elsewhere (Romani et al., 1989d). Briefly, (1) the LCs enlarge over 3 days and develop many long processes (e.g., dendrites, veils). (2) The cell surface is remodeled extensively. Cell surface MHC products and IL-2 receptors are up-regulated, while membrane ATPase and FcR are down-regulated. (3) Freshly isolated LCs can present exogenous protein antigens to T cell clones, whereas cultured LCs do not. However, (4) cultured LCs have powerful sensitizing functions for resting T cells, as in the MLR and oxidative mitogenesis responses. During the latter responses, the LCs exhibit a characteristic feature of dendritic cells, which is the capacity to efficiently bind the T cells that are to be stimulated. This binding seems to occur by an antigen-independent mechanism, to be discussed in Section VI,C. The maturation of LCs in culture depends on cytokines, especially GM-CSF (Witmer-Pack et al., 1987; Heufler et al., 1987). Comparable observations have now been made on cultured human LCs, which lose FcR and staining for ATPase and nonspecific esterase and become active MLR stimulators with abundant cell surface MHC products (Romani et al., 1989b)

Dendritic cells are also evident in the lung, in both tissue sections and single-cell isolates. Holt et al. (1987) have isolated dendritic cells from rat tracheal epithelium and pulmonary interstitium. The dendritic cells are rich in class II MHC products, lack surface Ig and FcRs, and are nonadherent. Sertl et al. (1986) have identified comparable cells in the mouse. It has yet to be determined whether dendritic cells in other nonlymphoid tissues can undergo the process of maturation described above for epidermal LCs.

E. CIRCULATION

B cells recirculate from blood through the B cell areas or follicles of lymphoid organs, then to efferent lymph, and back to blood (Howard et al., 1972; Sprent, 1973). During their circulation through lymph node and Peyer's patch, it would appear that the B cell must exit the blood via postcapillary venules and then traverse the T cell area to move to the B cell follicle. The pathway in the spleen is not clear, but possibly consists of entry into the white pulp from the marginal sinus, traversal of the periarteriolar T cell sheaths, and homing to the B cell follicle. One possible site for B cell-T cell interaction *in situ* would be the lymphoid T cell area, involving B cells in transit to the follicle; another would be the B cell area itself, since immunolabeling of tissue sections identifies some T cells, especially when germinal centers are present (Bhan et al., 1981).

Although B cells recirculate from blood to lymphoid organs, the pathways for dendritic cells seem to be entirely afferent and nonrecirculating. A large number of studies, beginning with the work of Kelly, Balfour, and Drexhage (Kelly et al., 1978; Drexhage et al., 1979), have identified dendritic cells in the afferent lymph of many species (Table I). Lymph draining the skin and the gut have been studied. In each case the dendritic cells have prominent processes or veils, are nonadherent and nonphagocytic, lack Fc receptors and other standard markers of macrophages, and express high levels of class II MHC products. Where analyzed, the lymph dendritic cells are strong stimulators of the growth of resting T lymphocytes in the MLR and polyclonal mitogen responses (Knight et al., 1982; Pugh et al., 1983; Mason et al., 1981). In the case of lymph draining the skin some of the dendritic or veiled cells are noted to contain Birbeck granules (Kelly et al., 1978) and to express the CD1 antigen (Mackay et al., 1988; Hopkins et al., 1989), both characteristics of epidermal LCs (Sullivan et al., 1985; Breathnach, 1964).

The flux of dendritic cells in afferent lymph can be considerable, up to 10^5 per hour in three different species (Pugh et al., 1983; Fossum, 1984; Hopkins et al., 1989). Even before dendritic cells were discovered, a detailed study of several lymphatic beds in the sheep, by Smith et al., reported a lymph flow of 1–10 ml/hr, with 10^5–10^6 cells per milliliter and 20% "macrophages" (Smith et al., 1970). Many of the "macrophages" were noted to be nonadherent and highly motile and had many long processes which could bind lymphocytes. All of these properties subsequently proved typical of dendritic cells and not monocytes or macrophages in many organs and species.

B cells are also present in afferent lymph, but many seem to be expressing CD5 (Mackay et al., 1988; Hopkins et al., 1989). The levels of B cells in lymph are roughly similar to those of dendritic cells, but unlike dendritic cells, B cells are also found in efferent lymph. Since B cells may primarily present specific antigens that have been processed via surface Ig (see Section IV,A), the flow of such antigen-specific B cells in afferent lymph is exceedingly small, given a total flux of about 10^5–10^6 B cells per hour, especially relative to the flux in the recirculating B cell pool in blood and lymphoid organs. In contrast, the movement of dendritic cells in lymph, which are antigen nonspecific in their function and which are only required in small numbers to stimulate T cells, is large.

A notable feature of afferent lymph dendritic cells is their heterogeneity with respect to certain traits (Pugh et al., 1983; Fossum, 1984). Some examples are the levels of nonspecific esterase, Thy-1 and CD4 antigens, and IL-2 receptors. One explanation for this finding is that lymph dendritic cells are derived from nonlymphoid tissue precursors. The latter, at least in the case of murine LCs, undergo marked changes in phenotype upon activation *in vitro*, such as the loss of nonspecific esterase staining and the acquisition of IL-2 receptors (see Section II,D). Possibly, dendritic cells are undergoing comparable changes as they enter the lymph from nonlymphoid tissues.

Given the presence of dendritic cells in the afferent lymph, it is possible that they carry processed antigens picked up in the tissues. Considerable evidence for such a phenomenon is available (see Section VI,B), but the most direct information has come from two recent studies. Macatonia et al. (1987) applied FITC as a contact allergen and recovered FITC-labeled dendritic cells as the major cell type carrying allergen in the draining lymph node. FITC-dendritic cells were detected within

8 hours of applying the allergen, and plateau levels were seen between 24 and 48 hours. Bujdoso *et al.* (1989) boosted ovalbumin-primed sheep with antigen in saline and then found that the dendritic cells in the draining afferent lymph were carrying ovalbumin in a form that is recognized by primed T cells.

Since typical dendritic cells have not been found in efferent lymph, most dendritic cells in afferent lymph must die upon reaching the lymphoid organ, either before or after their encounter with antigen-specific lymphocytes. This would account for the considerable turnover of dendritic cells in lymph and spleen sited above. Less clear is the site at which the dendritic cells in afferent lymph are produced. Given the lack of extensive turnover in epidermal LCs (see Section II,B), it is unlikely that lymph dendritic cells are all derived from the epidermis. More likely, there is a reservoir of immature dendritic cells in the dermis or in the blood, with the latter circulating constantly from blood to tissues to afferent lymph.

Small numbers of typical dendritic cells have been identified in human blood (Table I), but not yet in the blood of other species such as mice (Nussenzweig *et al.*, 1982). The blood dendritic cell is unlikely to be recirculating, since dendritic cells have not been found in efferent lymph. One possibility is that human blood dendritic cells represent cells that, in analogy to the veiled cells of afferent lymph, have been mobilized from tissues and are moving to the spleen to present antigens there. Another is that the blood dendritic cell is part of a pool of cells that moves from blood to tissues to afferent lymph and lymphoid organs, but not back to blood.

In summary, the distribution and circulation pathways for B cells and dendritic cells differ. B cells primarily are in the vascular compartment, recirculating continually from blood to lymphoid follicles to lymph and back to blood. During this pathway, the B cell likely traverses the T cell areas. Mature dendritic cells are infrequent in the blood but can move in substantial numbers via the afferent lymph to the T cell-dependent regions of lymphoid organs. One can speculate from this data as to where these two APCs are likely to encounter antigen and stimulate antigen-specific T cells. Dendritic cells are found in nonlymphoid tissues, where antigens first gain access to the body, from which they may be able to home to the T cell areas of lymphoid organs. In contrast, there seem to be few B cells in nonlymphoid tissues, and most are recirculating continually. B cells are positioned to capture antigens either in the circulation or in germinal centers, where immune complexes are found on follicular dendritic cells (see Section II,B). These contrasting life histories *in situ* are consistent with other sets of observations, to be described below (see

Sections IV–VI), whereby nonlymphoid dendritic cells have been observed to pick up antigens and are important APCs in several primary T cell-dependent responses. B cells likely function in lymphoid organs at later stages of the primary response and in secondary or memory T cell-dependent antibody formation.

F. DELAYED-TYPE HYPERSENSITIVITY (DTH) REACTIONS

DTH reactions, in which a specific antigen elicits a T cell-dependent influx of mononuclear cells in sensitized individuals, provide an opportunity to examine a local immune response *in situ*. The observations of Kaplan, Cohn, and colleagues (Kaplan *et al.*, 1987) are of interest in that they have noted few, if any, B cells in the DTH site, but have seen sizable numbers of dendritic cells. The latter express the CD1 (OKT6) marker found on epidermal LCs, and some of the cells have Birbeck granules, as seen by electron microscopy. These workers suggested that the LCs in the DTH site may not be derived from the epidermis, but from circulating or dermal progenitors (see Section II,E).

III. The Cell Surface of Dendritic Cells and B Lymphocytes

The cell surface phenotypes of these two types of APCs differ considerably (Fig. 1). Many surface components provide important markers for distinguishing these cells and monitoring population purity in experimental studies, and several could contribute to APC function. The latter are reviewed here.

Of some interest (Fig. 1) is the change in phenotype that accompanies the activation of small B cells to large lymphoblasts and the maturation of freshly isolated epidermal LCs upon culture with GM-CSF. The activation of B cells has been studied primarily *in vitro*, using polyclonal mitogens such as anti-Ig and LPS. The activation of dendritic cells refers to the maturation of nonlymphoid dendritic cells to lymphoid dendritic cells, as represented by the maturation of LC in culture. During the activation process, both B cells and dendritic cells process antigens and acquire the capacity to stimulate primary T cells. These functional data are considered below, as are a few papers that deal with B cells and dendritic cells which have been activated *in situ* (see Sections IV and VI).

A. MHC PRODUCTS

Class II MHC products are essential for presentation of antigen to CD4[+] T cells, including T cells with helper function for antibody responses. Lymphoid dendritic cells and freshly isolated epidermal LCs have high levels of class II MHC [I-A and I-E in mice; human leukocyte

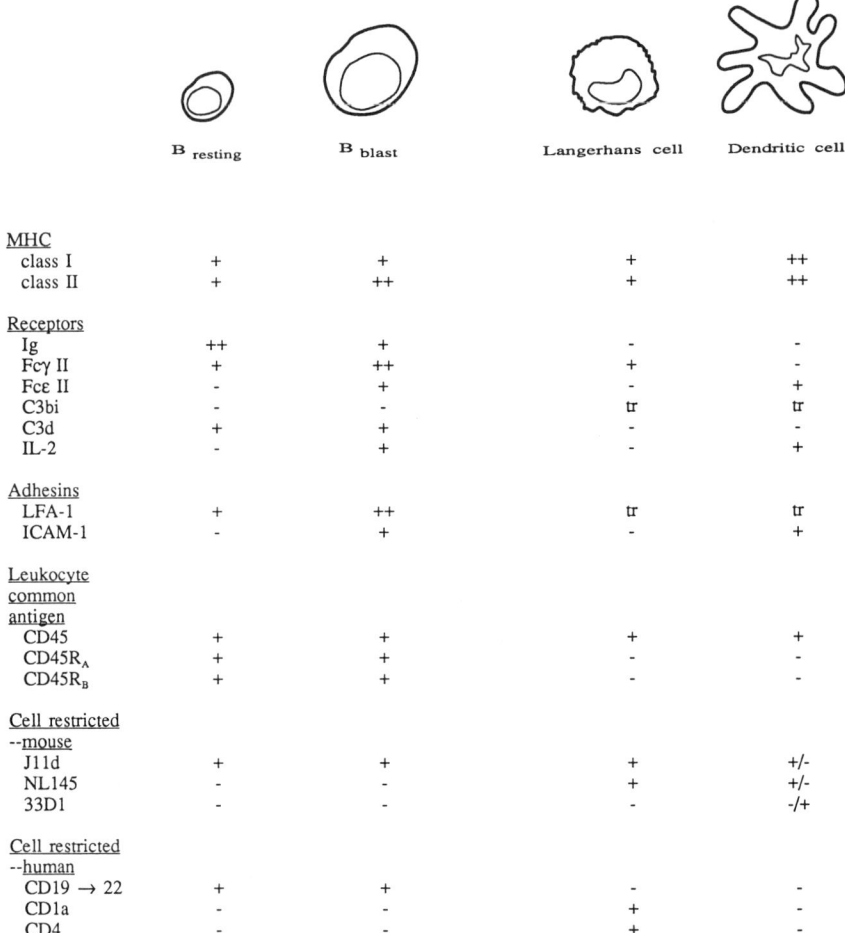

	B resting	B blast	Langerhans cell	Dendritic cell
MHC				
class I	+	+	+	++
class II	+	++	+	++
Receptors				
Ig	++	+	-	-
Fcγ II	+	++	+	-
Fcε II	-	+	-	+
C3bi	-	-	tr	tr
C3d	+	+	-	-
IL-2	-	+	-	+
Adhesins				
LFA-1	+	++	tr	tr
ICAM-1	-	+	-	+
Leukocyte common antigen				
CD45	+	+	+	+
CD45R_A	+	+	-	-
CD45R_B	+	+	-	-
Cell restricted --mouse				
J11d	+	+	+	+/-
NL145	-	-	+	+/-
33D1	-	-	-	-/+
Cell restricted --human				
CD19 → 22	+	+	-	-
CD1a	-	-	+	-
CD4	-	-	+	-

FIG 1. Surface phenotypes of B cells and dendritic cells. The data for B blasts are those observed following stimulation with anti-Ig or LPS in mice and germinal center B cells in humans. The data for dendritic cells are those observed for Langerhans cells that have been maintained in culture, or splenic dendritic cells. Plus or minus signs for dendritic cell expression of 33D1, NL145, and J11d refer to different subpopulations of the dendritic cell family (see text).

antigen (HLA)-DP, -DQ, and -DR in humans]. Quantitative binding studies with an anti-I-A Mab give a minimum of 200,000 antibody binding sites per cell (Nussenzweig *et al.*, 1981; Schuler and Steinman, 1985). Few quantitative data on MHC expression are available for human dendritic cells, but studies of blood (Brooks and Moore, 1988; Knight et al., 1987; Van Voorhis et al., 1983a), inflammatory exudates (Zvaifler et al., 1985), afferent lymph (Spry et al., 1980), and tonsil (Hart and McKenzie, 1988) have emphasized the strong immunolabeling with anti-class II MHC antibodies. The invariant chain, which associates with class II MHC products, also has been detected in epidermal LCs (Claesson-Welsh et al., 1986; Quaranta et al., 1984).

When LCs are cultured, the levels of I-A and I-E increase at least fivefold (Witmer-Pack et al., 1988). The increase in class II MHC is detectable within 3 hours of culture, reaches a plateau within 12–18 hours, and is blocked if cycloheximide is added (Witmer-Pack et al., 1988). Several other surface molecules are not up-regulated, so that the increase in MHC products is selective. Hopkins et al. (1989) have recently reported that, following local administration of antigen in sheep, the dendritic cells in the draining afferent lymph up-regulate the levels of cell surface class II MHC molecules at least fivefold.

Exogenous factors that regulate MHC expression on LCs or other dendritic cells have not been identified, but T cell conditioned media and γ-interferon (IFN-γ) are inactive (Steinman et al., 1980; Schuler and Steinman, 1985). T cell-derived products do not seem to be essential in the case of LCs, since mouse epidermis lacks T cells (Romani et al., 1985), and the suspensions are treated with anti-Thy-1 and complement, which would remove possible contaminants.

Small B cells, like dendritic cells, constitutively express class II MHC products, but the levels on B cells appear to be one fifth of the level on dendritic cells, at most (Nussenzweig et al., 1981). The level of class II MHC on B cells also can be up-regulated markedly, the stimuli being LPS (Monroe and Cambier, 1983a), anti-Ig (Birkeland et al., 1987; Monroe and Cambier, 1983c), IL-4 (Noelle et al., 1984; Roehm et al., 1984), or antigen (Monroe and Cambier, 1983b). The increase is detectable within 6 hours of stimulation, is maximal by 12 hours, and is maintained at high levels for up to 48 hours (E. Puré, unpublished observations).

Expression of class II MHC is essential for antigen presentation to $CD4^+$ cells, but there is no direct correlation of class II MHC levels and overall stimulatory function. For example, B cells that are induced with IL-4 to express more Ia are inactive as MLR stimulators (Krieger et al., 1986). LCs up-regulate their Ia to maximal levels in less than 1 day but only become active MLR stimulators progressively between 1 and 3 days in culture (Witmer-Pack et al., 1987).

Class I MHC products also increase markedly on cultured LCs. Freshly isolated LCs express as much class I MHC as most keratinocytes (Witmer-Pack et al., 1988; Lenz et al., 1989), but with culture, class I, like class II, MHC increases about fivefold (Witmer-Pack et al., 1988). B cells constitutively express class I MHC. It is intriguing that IL-4 up-regulates B cell class II MHC five- to tenfold, with only a twofold increase in class I MHC (Noelle et al., 1984).

Therefore, both dendritic cells and B lymphocytes are lineages that express class I and class II MHC products constitutively. However, the stimuli and factors which up-regulate MHC gene expression seem to differ for each cell type.

B. THE CD45 LEUKOCYTE COMMON ANTIGEN AND ITS RESTRICTED ISOFORMS, CD45R

The gene for the leukocyte common antigen, also referred to as T200 or CD45, encodes (1) a large cytoplasmic region of 705 amino acids, containing two tandem domains of approximately 300 amino acid residues, that has homology to a protein tyrosine phosphatase isolated from human placenta (Charbonneau et al., 1988), (2) a single transmembrane domain, and (3) a large extracellular domain of variable size, depending on the use of three different amino-terminal exons, termed 4, 5, and 6 or A, B, and C. Those antigenic epitopes which are found on all isoform products of this gene and all leukocytes are termed CD45. Other epitopes, which are termed CD45R since they have a more restricted cell distribution, are useful in distinguishing the two types of APCs (see below). The function of CD45 and CD45R isoforms is not yet known, but one possibility is that the different isoforms influence the kinds of cell-cell interactions in which a specific cell type engages.

The leukocyte common CD45 epitope is found on both B cells and dendritic cells, and expression does not vary with different states of activation *in vitro* (Crowley et al., 1989). One of the CD45R epitopes, initially termed B220 (Coffman and Weissman, 1981; Dalchau and Fabre, 1981), is found on B cells at all stages of development but is not found on dendritic cells (Crowley et al., 1989; Romani et al., 1988). The B220 epitope is found on the largest (220-240 kDa) CD45 isoforms and is synthesized when all 3 external exons are spliced into the CD45 transcript (Johnson et al., 1989). B220 expression is unchanged when B cells are stimulated *in vitro* (Metlay et al., 1989).

More recently, another CD45R epitope has been identified in several species. Its expression is B exon dependent (Johnson et al., 1989; Birkeland et al., 1989). Some of the first $CD45R_B$ Mabs are termed OX22 in rats (Spickett et al., 1983) and MB23G2/MB15Cll in mice (Birkeland et al., 1988). The expression of MB23G2 is reduced in one kind of B blast, the proliferating cells of the germinal center (Birkeland et al., 1988), but is not altered on many other kinds of blasts, such as those induced with LPS or with anti-Ig. MB23G2 has not been detected on dendritic cells.

C. Integrins/Adhesins

Leukocytes express a family of three integrins which share a common 95 kDa β chain, CD18. The CD18 β chain is called β_2 to distinguish it from other β chains which define other families of integrins, which include the fibronectin receptor and platelet gpIIb/IIIa. Three different α chains have been described for CD18: a 190-kDa CD11a or LFA-1, a 180-kDa CD11b (C3bi or CR3 receptor; MAC-1), and a 150-kDa CD11c of uncertain function (Sanchez-Madrid et al., 1983a,b). CD11c has yet to be detected on B cells or dendritic cells, but it is found on macrophages and granulocytes (McMichael, 1987). CD11b is missing from most B cells but can be found at low levels on dendritic cells. CD11a is at low levels on B cells and dendritic cells but can be up-regulated on anti-Ig-induced B blasts (J. P. Metlay and E. Puré, unpublished observations).

One of the ligands for CD11a or LFA-1 is a widely distributed 90-kDa glycoprotein called ICAM-1 (Rothlein et al., 1986; Dustin et al., 1986; Marlin and Springer, 1987), which has homology to the neural cell adhesion molecule NCAM (Simmons et al., 1988). B blasts and mature dendritic cells (Romani et al., 1989b) are among the many cell types on which ICAM-1 can be found in humans where anti-ICAM-1 Mabs are available. ICAM-1 is absent or at low levels on resting T cells (Dougherty et al., 1989).

A key step in the function of APCs is the capacity to form stable conjugates with the responding T cell (see Section IV,C). The conjugation of antigen-specific B cells and helper T cell clones is reduced with antibodies to LFA-1 (Sanders et al., 1986, 1987). APC-T cell clustering can be examined in primary immune responses, where it has been shown that clusters are the site for T cell proliferation in the MLR (Inaba and Steinman, 1984; Flechner et al., 1988) and antibody formation in primary T cell-dependent responses (Inaba et al., 1984; Inaba and Steinman, 1985, 1987a). Interestingly, the capacity of B blasts, but not dendritic cells, to bind T cells in the primary MLR is blocked by anti-CD11a (Inaba and Steinman, 1987b; Metlay et al., 1989).

Another pair of molecules that has been implicated in heterotypic cell-cell adhesion is CD2 and LFA-3 (Sanchez-Madrid et al., 1982; Springer et al., 1987). These molecules have not been evaluated during the clustering of APCs and primary T cells.

D. RECEPTORS

A salient difference in receptors is that B cells express an antigen-specific surface Ig receptor and dendritic cells do not. Dendritic cells do not react with antibodies to whole Ig, light chains, or μ and δ heavy chains (Steinman and Cohn, 1974; Nussenzweig et al., 1981). Also, dendritic cells do not react with anti-CD3 or TCR$\alpha\beta$ reagents. Schuler and colleagues (1989) have now shown formally that Ig and TCR genes in dendritic cells are in the germ-line configuration. Thus, B cells are the only APCs that can interact in a monoclonal fashion with antigen. As a result, the same B cell that specifically binds an antigen also presents fragments of that antigen to elicit T cell help.

While dendritic cells lack surface Ig, the manner in which tissue dendritic cells handle antigens still may render these APCs pauciclonal in the sense that they may carry relatively few antigens. Epidermal LCs can take up antigens for about 1 day in culture, but then the LCs are no longer capable of handling additional antigens (Romani et al., 1989c). This being the case, it has been proposed that *in situ* tissue dendritic cells may only be presenting a relatively small number of foreign epitopes acquired at the site of antigen deposition.

FcγRs are found on all small B cells and are up-regulated five- to 20-fold following activation with LPS or anti-Ig (Puré et al., 1984; Viguier et al., 1987). The principal, if not only, FcγR on B cells is termed FcγRII. It is recognized by the Mabs 2.4G2 in mice (Unkeless, 1979) and IV.3 in humans (Rosenfeld et al., 1985). B cell FcγRII is encoded by the β-type transcript of the recently cloned mouse FcR gene (Ravetch et al., 1986). FcγRII binds immune complexes but not soluble IgG. To date, two other FcγRs have not been found on B cells: FcγRI of macrophages, which binds soluble IgG with high affinity, and CD16 FcγRIII, which is found on all natural killer cells and granulocytes and many tissue macrophages.

Dendritic cells in lymph and lymphoid organs lack FcγRs by several criteria: binding of immune complexes or antibody-coated particles (Steinman and Cohn, 1974; Steinman et al., 1979; Kelly et al., 1978; Pugh et al., 1983), reactivity with 2.4G2 or other anti-FcR antibodies (Nussenzweig et al., 1981; Crowley et al., 1989), and capacity to mediate polyclonal responses to anti-CD3 Mab which require FcR on the accessory cell (Young and Steinman, 1988). However, epidermal LCs clearly express FcγRII (Romani et al., 1985, 1989a,b; Rowden, 1981; Stingl et al., 1977; Haines et al., 1983). These FcRs decrease $>90\%$ in expression when the LCs are placed in culture (Schuler and Steinman. 1985; Romani et al., 1989a). Interestingly, although only small numbers remain, about 2000 binding sites for the 2.4G2 Mab per cell, these are sufficient to mediate the mitogenesis of large numbers of T cells in the presence of anti-CD3 (Romani et al., 1989a).

It has been proposed that nonlymphoid dendritic cells express FcRs to acquire antigens in the form of immune complexes, and that both FcR and immune complex uptake is down-regulated when the dendritic cell seeks out antigen-specific T cells (Romani et al., 1989a). However, there is little direct evidence that FcRs on either LCs or B cells function in antigen presentation at this time.

A newly recognized feature of the B blast is the expression of a low affinity FcεR, or CD23, which is up-regulated by IL-4 (DeFrance et al., 1987). This CD23 epitope, which is now known to be homologous to murine Lyb-2, (Nakayama et al., 1989), can also be expressed by epidermal LCs, and in response to IL-4 as well (Bieber et al., 1989). This receptor might account for the finding of IgE on LCs during atopic dermatitis (Bruynzeel-Koomen et al., 1986; Barker et al., 1988).

The receptor for the C3d fragment of C3, also the Epstein–Barr virus (EBV) receptor in humans or CD21 or CR2, is found on B cells but not on other leukocytes (Ling et al., 1987). Except for the $CD5^+$ subset, B cells do not seem to have other complement receptors (CR1 or C3b receptor; CR3 or C3bi receptor). Dendritic cells only express the receptor for C3bi (CR3), but the levels of CR3 in human blood and mouse lymphoid dendritic cells are so low that one often does not detect them in standard immunolabeling approaches. The levels of CR3 on epidermal LCs are higher, as assessed by a sensitive FACscan (Crowley et al., 1989), but still readily missed with two-stage immunofluorescence approaches. The role of C3-coated antigens in antigen presentation has not, to our knowledge, been explored.

Both dendritic cells and B cells can express IL-2 receptors, but only when activated. The p55 or low-affinity IL-2 binding chain is especially abundant on cultured epidermal LCs (Steiner et al., 1986; Crowley et al., 1989). To date, we have been unable to detect an effect of exogenous IL-2 on the growth or function of IL-2 receptor-positive cultured LCs (R. M. Steinman, unpublished observations). G. G. MacPherson (personal communication) has identified IL-2 receptor on rat afferent lymph dendritic cells. Mouse B cells also express p55 when stimulated with LPS (Nakanishi et al., 1984; Monroe and Cambier, 1983a), as do human B cells, such as tonsillar B cells and cells that have been stimulated with the mitogen heat-killed *Staphylococcus aureus* (Saiki et al., 1988). The proliferative response of B cells to IL-2 is weak to modest. Ig secretion can be enhanced by IL-2, but this requires the presence of other lymphokines, such as IL-4 and IL-5 (Purkerson et al., 1988).

Receptors for cytokines other than IL-2 have primarily been studied on B cells. Receptors for IL-4, IL-5, and IL-6 are all up-regulated on the activated B blast (Mita et al., 1988; Yamasaki et al., 1988; Ohara and Paul, 1988; Rolink et al., 1989). Akahoshi et al. (1988) reported that human B cells bind IL-1, but the preparations that were studied would contain dendritic cells which are known to respond functionally to IL-1 (Koide and Steinman, 1988). A determinant called CDw40 is found on both B cells and dendritic cells, particularly following activation (Hart and McKenzie, 1988; Romani et al., 1989b). It has been suggested that CDw40 is a receptor for a B cell growth factor (Ling et al., 1987).

In summary, many of the cell surface molecules of dendritic cells and B lymphocytes are substantially different. The two types of APCs differ with respect to LFA-1, CD45, and receptors such as surface Ig, FcR and C3R. Interesting similarities exist with respect to ICAM-1, IL-2 receptor, CDw40, and CD23, each of which is up-regulated during the activation of both dendritic cells and B cells.

IV. Antigen Presentation

In practice, the measurement of antigen-presenting function requires the induction of a T cell response by the concerted action of antigen and APCs. We prefer to use the term "antigen presentation" in a more restricted and literal sense, i.e., to refer to those events which generate a ligand for the clonotypic T cell receptor. This is currently understood to be the processing of proteins and particulates to form peptides that are associated with MHC molecules on the surface of the APCs. As yet, there is no way to directly monitor the formation and amount of these ligands, i.e., MHC-peptide complexes. In addition to ligand formation, the APC performs other "sensitization" functions, which include binding of the antigen-specific T cell and induction of several T cell genes that are needed to carry out the immune response. As we point out throughout this section, some assays for APC function primarily measure presentation, while others require sensitization functions as well.

In this section, we compare dendritic cells and B cells for their capacity to induce the proliferation of $CD4^+$ helper cells for several different classes of antigens—proteins, MHC, and Mls. We also consider responses that involve graft rejection and the generation of $CD8^+$ cytolytic cells. In Section V we review the more complex system of APC function in the antibody response. In the discussion we attempt to dissect dendritic and B cell function into several components: formation of a ligand for the T cell, including endocytosis and antigen processing; movement in situ such that the APC and the T cell can interact; binding of the APC to the T cell; and initiation of lymphokine production and T cell growth.

A. PRESENTATION OF PROTEIN ANTIGENS

Because of the low frequency of T cells reactive to any given soluble antigen, primary responses to proteins are not readily detectable. Therefore, previously activated and expanded populations of responder cells are utilized. Antigen-primed populations have been prepared at three levels. The first utilizes T cells from lymph nodes draining a depot of antigen plus adjuvant, usually the base of the tail or footpad in mice, and generally at 8-10 days after priming (Corradin and Chiller, 1979). Human blood donors that have been exposed to antigens such as tetanus toxoid (TT) or to *Mycobacteria* also are commonly used. Second, T cells from primed mice and humans can be expanded *in vitro*, and then antigen-specific clones can be isolated (Fathman and Frelinger, 1983; Ottenhoff et al., 1986). A third approach is to fuse antigen-primed T cells to thymoma lines, thus producing stable T cell hybridomas of defined antigen specificities (Haskins et al., 1983).

Because all three experimental approaches utilize T cells that are either recently activated *in vivo* or chronically stimulated *in vitro*, it is possible that steps critical for priming T cells are not being measured during most assays of protein presentation. T cell hybridomas, for example, typically respond to antigen presented by MHC molecules incorporated into otherwise bare lipid bilayers (Watt, 1988), whereas this has not been possible with other T cell populations. Stimulation of many T/T hybrids does reflect the capacity of the APC to generate an effective ligand, but the amount of ligand that is required by T/T hybrids may be much smaller than the amount needed to induce responses in primary cells.

The one system in which APC function for unprimed and sensitized primary T cells has been compared in detail is the MLR (see Section IV,B). It has been shown that primed lymphoblasts, but not unprimed T cells, respond vigorously to allogeneic small B cells as APCs. Even aldehyde-fixed APCs are functional when primed lymphoblasts are the responder T cells (Inaba et al., 1984, 1985). Resting T cells require dendritic cells for stimulation, and the dendritic cells are sensitive to minute exposures to aldehyde fixation. Freshly sensitized T blasts also respond rapidly to growth factors such as IL-2, whereas resting lymphocytes do not. In summary, expanded populations of primed T cells are valuable for detecting responses to specific protein antigens, but such T cells may bypass important requirements for immunogenicity and priming.

Despite the differences in the systems of primed T cells that have been utilized in assays of protein presentation, certain key concepts repeatedly have been evident (Rothbard, 1986; Berzofsky, 1988; Schwartz, 1985; Unanue, 1984; Livingstone and Fathman, 1987). (1) T cells do not respond to soluble antigen but instead recognize antigen when it is presented on the surface of other cells. (2) Most T cells are exquisitely antigen specific and can distinguish between forms of an antigen that differ by as little as one amino acid. (3) T cells are MHC restricted in that they respond to the specific antigen only when presented by cells which express one of the multiple MHC alleles in the populations. (4) This dual recognition of antigen plus MHC is achieved by a single TCR heterodimer. (5) T cells can recognize either native or denatured forms of an antigen. This is because most native antigens must be denatured and/or proteolytically processed by APCs either in an intracellular compartment or extracellularly prior to successful presentation in association with MHC molecules. (6) For the majority of T cell clones and hybrids minimal antigenic peptides often as short as eight to 11 amino acids have been defined (Corradin and Chiller, 1979; Allen *et al.*, 1984; Shimonkevitz *et al.*, 1984; Townsend *et al.*, 1986; Berkower *et al.*, 1984; Rothbard *et al.*, 1988; Maryanski *et al.*, 1988; Guillet *et al.*, 1986), and for bulk T cell populations a single peptide can dominate the repertoire of the responding cells (Kojima *et al.*, 1988).

These concepts have been illuminated and extended by the crystallization of an MHC molecule, the structure of which provides a binding pocket—25 Å in length and about 10 Å in width and depth—for small peptides (Bjorkman *et al.*, 1987a,b). Other MHC molecules can be modeled similarly (Brown *et al.*, 1988). Previously identified polymorphic residues of the MHC molecule can line the binding pocket, and most likely influence peptide binding, or can face outward from the edges of the groove, and most likely contact the TCR (Bjorkman *et al.*, 1987b; Davis and Bjorkman, 1988). Therefore, MHC restriction could operate at the level of the type of peptide that is bound and at the level of MHC-TCR contacts.

1. Early Studies of B Cells

Some of the earliest studies on the presentation of protein suggested that normal B cells could serve as APCs. Kammer and Unanue (1980) tested keyhole limpet hemocyanin (KLH)-primed T cells and found that while spleen-adherent cells or peritoneal cells were, on a per-cell basis, up to 100-fold more potent, spleen-nonadherent cells or sorted Ig^+ B cells could also present antigen. However, as the authors pointed out, the considerable weakness in the potency of B cells made it difficult to rule out a minor contamination of the preparations with non-B stimulators.

To obtain more homogeneous populations of APCs, monoclonal tumor lines were tested. McKean *et al.* (1981) screened several lines for expression of class II MHC molecules as well as the capacity to present soluble protein to chronically stimulated T cell lines. In general, a good correlation existed between expression of Ia and APC function. Some of the lines expressed surface Ig. Glimcher *et al.* (1982) likewise reported that some B cell lymphomas, such as A20, but not other Ia$^+$ B cell tumors, could present proteins.

While studies with monoclonal B cell tumors effectively eliminate the problems of low-level contamination with non-B APCs, tumors are not normal B cells. For example, growing lines may require considerable endocytic activity to obtain essential nutrients by adsorptive endocytosis, and in doing so, may exhibit an antigen-processing capacity that is not representative of resting or even growing primary B cells. Current studies in our laboratory on the presentation of myoglobin or MHC antigens have shown that B cell lines such as A20 are far superior (some 20-fold or more in dose-response studies) to primary activated B cells as APCs, suggesting that B cell tumors are not representative of B cell APCs. EBV-transformed B cell lines can also act as APCs in the human system, and they allow one to generate lines that bind a specific antigen (Lanzavecchia, 1985). There are no studies comparing these lines to activated primary human B cells.

2. *The Role of Surface Ig in B Cell Presentation*

To the degree that presentation in the above studies required processing of the antigen, the efficacy of B cells likely depended on nonspecific endocytosis of the antigen. Yet B cells, unlike other APCs, have specific cell surface receptors for foreign antigens. Chesnut and Grey (1981) addressed the role of surface Ig by testing APC function for T cells from mice that had been immunized to rabbit IgG. Normal rabbit Ig (NRGG) would be expected to be handled like any other soluble protein antigen, but rabbit anti-mouse Ig (RAMIG) would have the capacity to bind to all B cells via membrane Ig. Indeed, enriched B cells failed to present the NRGG but strongly stimulated the T cells when RAMIG was added. Spleen-adherent cells, in contrast, presented both forms of the rabbit Ig equally well. B cell presentation of RAMIG was MHC restricted and was equally effective with $F(ab')_2$ fragments as the antigen, ruling out a special role for FcR-mediated binding by the B cell APCs. Because the spleen-adherent cells presented NRGG, while the B cell preparations did not, a role for contaminating non-B accessory cells was unlikely.

Tony and Parker extended this approach by preparing T cell lines and hybrids that were specific for rabbit Ig. Significant presentation by B cells required microgram- or milligram-per-milliliter levels of NRGG, whereas nanogram-per-milliliter concentrations of RAMIG were active (Tony and Parker, 1985). The presentation of low concentrations of RAMIG also resulted in reciprocal activation of the B cell APCs, as measured by a plaque assay for Ig secretion. In a follow-up study Tony *et al.* (1985) showed that B cells presented monovalent anti-Ig in an essentially equivalent fashion to bivalent anti-Ig. Rabbit Igs that were directed to other B cell structures, i.e., MHC class I molecules, also were presented, although with a fourfold lower efficacy than RAMIG.

More recently, Casten and Pierce (1988; Casten *et al.*, 1988) have extended the above findings by artificially directing a soluble protein, cytochrome *c*, to the B cell surface by coupling the protein to antibodies specific for Ig, I-A, or H-2K. Again, proteins directed to the B cell surface were presented at concentrations one hundredth to one thousandth of those required for unconjugated proteins. It was stated that antigens artificially bound to surface Ig were more efficiently presented than were those bound to surface MHC.

These observations suggest that presentation may gain both a generalized advantage, by concentrating proteins at the APC surface, and a specialized advantage, by binding antigens via surface Ig. While there is long-standing evidence that at least anti-Ig reagents are endocytosed (Unanue *et al.*, 1972; Taylor *et al.*, 1971), it is less clear whether antibodies to other surface molecules can also be endocytosed. There is evidence from studies of macrophages that the endocytic vesicle membrane includes many of the components of the plasma membrane from which the endocytic vesicle derives (Mellman *et al.*, 1980; Muller *et al.*, 1983), so that most antibodies to the cell surface may be internalized to some extent, as long as some other ligand initiates the formation of endocytic vesicles. This might occur if the B cells were exposed to LPS, or if the cells were growing and had to acquire nutrients by adsorptive endocytosis.

Many of the principles concerning the advantage of directing T cell antigens to the B cell surface have been demonstrated utilizing enriched populations of antigen-specific B cells. Rock *et al.* (1984) enriched for TNP-binding B cells from TNP-primed mice. They assayed presentation of TNP coupled to the synthetic terpolymer glutamic acid–lysine–phenylalanine (GAT) to a GAT-reactive hybridoma. The enriched B cells presented unconjugated GAT poorly, but the same B cell populations were strongly stimulatory with TNP–GAT, and at 1000-fold lower concentrations of polymer.

In the human system Lanzavecchia (1985) used EBV to immortalize B cell clones, some of which were specific for TT and could bind the antigen with a K_d of 10^{-8} liters/mol. He then measured the capacity of the lines to present this antigen to TT-specific T cell clones. The

TT-specific B cell line could present the antigen at concentrations one ten-thousandth of those required by B cell lines that were not TT specific. Experiments with antigen-pulsed APCs, blocking with anti-TT antibodies, and inhibition with glutaraldehyde fixation and chloroquine were all consistent with a model of presentation which included surface Ig binding of TT, internalization into an acidic compartment, association of processed antigen with MHC molecules, and recycling to the APC surface.

In all of these experiments binding antigens to surface Ig could signal the B cell to up-regulate APC function, in addition to concentrating the antigen on the B cell surface. Anti-Ig treatment of resting B cells leads to increased synthesis of class II MHC antigens and up-regulation of adhesion molecules such as LFA-1 (see Section III,C), and possibly development of so-called "costimulatory" functions (see MHC and Mls in Section IV,B and C). Indeed, Casten *et al.* (1985) have observed up to a tenfold increase in the capacity of B cells to present cytochrome *c* to a T cell hybridoma when soluble, unlinked anti-Ig is given simultaneously with antigen. However, in the studies by Tony *et al.* (1985), submitogenic doses of RAMIG, monovalent fragments of RAMIG, and antigens directed to MHC molecules all showed enhanced presentation. Such ligands may not activate the B cell to the same extent as intact anti-Ig at high doses. Consequently, the major effect in these systems seems to involve increased antigen binding and uptake by the B cells.

Vitetta and co-workers (Sanders *et al.*, 1987) examined specific TNP-binding B cells (Myers *et al.*, 1986) for the capacity to form conjugates with helper T cell clones. The TNP-binding cells were either from unprimed mice or mice primed with TNP–ovalbumin, and the hybridomas were KLH specific. Virgin B cells required a tenfold higher concentration of TNP–KLH to achieve half-maximal binding (approximately 70,000 conjugates per 10^6 input of B cells after 30 minutes at 37°C). Also, the virgin B cell bound more slowly than did the memory B cell (4–6 versus 2 hours to achieve maximal binding). These studies indicate that when the affinity of the B cell's antigen receptor is increased, as in memory, the increased efficacy of the B cell as an APC is evident in a rapid conjugation assay.

3. B Cell Activation and APC Function

While Chesnut and Grey (1981) initially reported that freshly isolated spleen B cells (Sephadex G10-nonadherent spleen cells depleted of Thy-1$^+$ T cells) could present RAMIG but not nonspecific antigens such as NRGG or ovalbumin, others reported that B cell lymphomas such as A20 could present nonspecific soluble proteins. A follow-up study

(Chesnut et al., 1982a) directly compared fresh B cells, LPS-activated B blasts, and B cell lymphomas as APCs for KLH-primed T cells and TT hybrids. Unstimulated B cells were weak or inactive, but the other forms of B cells were effective APCs. Interestingly, the weak activity of fresh B cells was only seen when T cell hybridomas were evaluated, there being no APC function with primary KLH-sensitized T cells.

Some controversy exists whether true resting B cells can present nonspecific soluble proteins. Ashwell et al. (1984) fractionated fresh B cells on discontinuous gradients and found that their high-density B cells could present soluble antigen to normal primed T cells as well as to T cell hybridomas. A critical point was that, in contrast to the APC function of low-density adherent cells, fresh B cell APC function was ablated by high-dose ionizing radiation (>1500 rad).

Krieger et al. (1985) similarly considered the APC function of resting B cells but arrived at very different conclusions. They subfractionated fresh B cells on discontinuous density gradients and demonstrated very low APC function in the highest density fractions, even if only low-dose irradiation was employed. The APC function of this same high-density population was significantly increased after 48 hours of LPS activation, and the activity was radioresistant. Other investigators (Frohman and Cowing, 1985) have confirmed the weak APC function of small B cells, its sensitivity to high-dose irradiation, and its enhancement by prior activation of the B cells with LPS.

Another approach that might be useful in evaluating the relative contribution of B cells in bulk lymphoid suspensions is to selectively deplete them with a monoclonal antibody to B220, which only reacts with B cells (Coffman and Weissman, 1981). When we do such an experiment with myoglobin-reactive T cell clones (Romani et al., 1989c), we find that B cell depletion enriches the APC function of spleen (exposed to 900 rad of ^{137}Cs) about four- or fivefold (R. M. Steinman et al., unpublished observations). This indicates that, for some combinations of soluble proteins and T cell clones, the B cells that are present in freshly isolated spleen have little, if any, APC function.

At this time, then, the findings from different laboratories on the capacity of small and large B cells to present soluble proteins differ a good deal. In part, these differences reflect the use of surface Ig targeted versus nonspecific antigens. In addition, the different findings may reflect difficulties in defining the APC population in terms of small versus large B cells, as well as the types of responding T cell. Different types of responders may have different requirements in terms of the amount of ligand or other sensitizing functions that are needed to induce a response.

4. Antigen Presentation by Dendritic Cells

The fact that many antigens require intracellular processing prior to presentation to T cells has, for many, called into question the role of nonphagocytic dendritic cells. Dendritic cells are unusually potent in several *in vitro* and *in situ* models of accessory function but yet have no obvious capacity for internalizing many antigens. Sunshine *et al.* (1980) reported presentation of the polymer GAT, as well as purified protein derivative (PPD), by enriched spleen dendritic cells to primed lymph node T cells. They noted that the mechanisms of antigen uptake and processing were unknown. They considered the possibility that other APCs might contaminate the responding T cell population, so that in a follow-up study (Sunshine *et al.*, 1983) T/T hybrids were used as responders. Again, presentation of protein antigens by dendritic cells was detected. Kawai *et al.* (1987) found that dendritic cells could present proteins to freshly sensitized and memory T cells, and more effectively than other APCs. The requirement for spleen dendritic cells in T cell-dependent antibody responses to hapten–carrier conjugates also has suggested presentation by dendritic cells (Inaba *et al.*, 1984; Inaba and Steinman, 1987a).

None of the above studies provides direct evidence that most dendritic cells are internalizing and processing antigens. For example, the dendritic cell populations may have contained a small fraction of actively processing cells, or the antigen preparations under study may have contained denatured or partially degraded material that does not require intracellular processing. There also may have been very low but sufficient levels of endocytosis to provide the necessary MHC–peptide complexes.

Recent studies of the presentation of myoglobin to two class II MHC-restricted CD4$^+$ T cell clones may clarify the presenting function of dendritic cells. Cultured spleen dendritic cells were essentially inactive in presenting native myoglobin, although some presentation of peptide was evident (Romani *et al.*, 1989c). By analogy, cultured epidermal LCs, which have surface and functional properties similar to those of spleen dendritic cells (Schuler and Steinman, 1985; Inaba *et al.*, 1986), could not present myoglobin but could present peptides. The T cell-stimulatory mechanisms of these dendritic cell populations were intact, as evident by their strong accessory function in stimulating the MLR and responses to polyclonal mitogens. However, the capacity to generate an effective peptide ligand from protein was poor. These results indicated that the antigen-presenting (myoglobin presentation to T cell clones) and sensitizing functions (stimulation of resting T cells) of dendritic cells were distinct (Romani *et al.*, 1989c).

Intriguingly, freshly isolated LCs presented native myoglobin to the T cell clones (Romani et al., 1989c). Six thousand to twenty thousand LCs were equal or more active than 500,000 spleen cells. These freshly isolated LCs were weak accessory cells in several primary responses, i.e., the MLR, T cell-dependent antibody response, and polyclonal mitogenesis (Schuler and Steinman, 1985; Inaba et al., 1986), but became active after 1–3 days of culture with the cytokine GM-CSF, which is made by many cells, including keratinocytes (Witmer-Pack et al., 1987; Heufler et al., 1987). Together, the results suggest that dendritic cells in tissues are quantitatively the most active at handling exogenous soluble proteins. Under the influence of cytokines, the nonlymphoid dendritic cells lose the capacity to process exogenous proteins but simultaneously gain the sensitizing functions necessary to bind and stimulate T cells, especially resting T cells. The failure of spleen dendritic cells to present myoglobin to T cell clones represents the final stages in this developmental pathway, when the cells have stopped processing but express all of the other functions needed to sensitize T cells.

More recent experiments (manuscript in preparation) indicate that some dendritic cells in fresh spleen suspensions do present myoglobin. Much like cultured epidermal LCs, the spleen dendritic cells lose this capacity after overnight culture, while maintaining potent accessory function in the assays sited above. Overnight culture is part of the routine protocol for isolating dendritic cells (Steinman et al., 1979; Nussenzweig and Steinman, 1980).

5. Studies in Situ

There is relatively little information comparing dendritic cells and B lymphocytes for the capacity to present protein antigens to T cells *in situ*. One report (Francotte and Urbain, 1985) provides evidence that spleen dendritic cells, but not unfractionated spleen cells or macrophages, actively present an Ig idiotype to induce an antiidiotypic response, but the T cell-dependence and MHC restriction of this phenomenon were not evaluated. There are other studies in which dendritic cells are much more efficient than B cells in presenting cell-associated antigens, and these will be discussed below (see Section IV,D).

A powerful approach would be to selectively deplete an animal of either dendritic cells or B cells prior to immunization. This has been attempted by treating mice from birth with anti-μ antisera. The mice lack mature peripheral B cells as well as serum Ig. Anti-μ-suppressed mice show profound defects in T cell immunity. Several reports establish that these animals do not generate antigen-reactive T cells in lymph nodes, when the nodes are primed with an injection of antigen plus adjuvant (Ron *et al.*, 1981; Kurt-Jones *et al.*, 1988; Janeway *et al.*, 1987). Also, unprimed lymph node cells from anti-μ-suppressed mice show a reduced capacity to present soluble protein antigens to T cell lines (Janeway *et al.*, 1987). On the other hand, some accessory function does persist. The lymph node cells mount normal responses to T cell mitogens, which require accessory cells, and antigen presentation by spleen or peritoneal cells appears normal.

Two groups have reconstituted the deficiency of anti-μ-suppressed mice by the administration of enriched populations of splenic B cells (Ron and Sprent, 1989; Kurt-Jones *et al.*, 1988). Kurt-Jones *et al.* took an elegant approach to try to demonstrate that the infused B cells were independently acting as the APCs. Hapten (FITC)-specific B cells were enriched from primed, parental strain mice by panning on plates coated with FITC-modified gelatin. Parental strain (H-2^d or H-2^a) B cells were then injected into F1 anti-μ-suppressed recipients, which were also immunized with hapten–carrier conjugates. These investigators could then ask whether sensitized F1 T cells were restricted to the MHC of the injected B cells. In one situation the carrier-primed cells were primarily restricted to the B cell MHC when tested for T cell proliferation *in vitro*. This situation involved the use of B cells that were taken from "memory" animals primed 4 months previously; no restriction was observed if the B cells were taken 2 weeks after priming the B cell donor.

Given the fact that the reconstitution of anti-μ-suppressed mice was not consistently restricted to the MHC of the injected B cells, and that very small numbers of mice were evaluated, the basis for the T cell priming deficit in anti-μ-suppressed mice is unclear. In other tests of APC function *in situ* to be described below, primary B cells have not been active in inducing antibody responses, cytotoxic T lymphocyte (CTL) development, or graft rejection *in situ* (see Sections IV,B and D). The effects of anti-μ treatment on dendritic cells have not been documented. For example, priming to protein antigens may require uptake by cells such as epidermal LCs, which have FcRs and might be perturbed by the immune complexes that are present in mice treated with anti-μ. However, anti-μ treatment is a demanding experimental protocol, so that the small numbers of mice that are available for study make it difficult to evaluate dendritic cell function.

B. Allogeneic MHC Products

The strong response to allogeneic MHC products which is observed in higher vertebrates provides an opportunity to study antigen presentation to primary T cells, and therefore the early stages of immunogenicity *in vitro* (the primary MLR) and *in situ* (graft rejection). The antigens presented by allogeneic MHC molecules are probably MHC-peptide complexes. These are recognized as foreign because allogeneic MHC products bind a distinct, restricted set of peptides that is substantially different from the set of peptides bound to self-MHC. Consistent with this hypothesis is the extensive occurrence of T cell clones that see both self-MHC plus peptide and allogeneic MHC (Ashwell et al., 1986), and with a single clonotypic receptor (Malissen et al., 1988). The great abundance of allogeneic MHC-peptide complexes that could be formed would account for the large number of T cell clones that are activated in the MLR (Wilson and Nowell, 1971).

1. Early Experiments on the Primary MLR

At first it was thought that B cells were the major stimulator cells in the MLR. It was known that the MLR was blocked by antibodies to class II MHC products (Fathman et al., 1974) and that B cells were the principal cell type expressing class II MHC antigens. B cell lines, such as EBV-transformed lines in humans and certain B cell lymphomas in mice (Glimcher et al., 1982), were also potent MLR stimulators.

Once dendritic cells were recognized as a distinct class II MHC-bearing cell type, a large number of laboratories reported that these cells are potent MLR stimulators (Steinman and Witmer, 1978; Rollinghoff et al., 1982; Green and Jotte, 1985; Mason et al., 1981; Pugh et al., 1983; Kuntz-Crow and Kunkel, 1982; Naito et al., 1984; Knight et al., 1982; Klinkert et al., 1982; Van Voorhis et al., 1983b). With highly enriched dendritic cell preparations a dose of one dendritic cell per 30–100 allogeneic T cells produced a maximal response. In contrast, dendritic cell-depleted B cell populations from mouse and rat lymphoid organs, rat lymph, and human blood were all weak or inactive as stimulators in the majority of reports (Steinman and Witmer, 1978; Steinman et al., 1983b; Inaba and Steinman, 1984; Pugh et al., 1983; Klinkert et al., 1982; Flechner et al., 1988; Young and Steinman, 1988). The lack of MLR stimulation was evident even when the B cells were not exposed to ionizing irradiation or mitomycin C treatment (Inaba and Steinman, 1984).

Many of the early studies of MLR stimulation by B cells had used populations prepared simply by T cell depletion, e.g., Thy-1$^-$ mouse spleen, or E rosette-negative human blood mononuclear cells. Dendritic cells would be enriched in such preparations. The principal approaches for removing dendritic cells are to pass cell suspensions over Sephadex G10, which retards mouse spleen dendritic cells (Inaba et al., 1983b; Inaba and Steinman, 1984), or to sediment the cells on dense Percoll, which floats cultured but not fresh human blood dendritic cells (Young and Steinman, 1988). These dendritic cell-depleted B cell populations are nonstimulatory in the primary MLR.

2. The Secondary MLR

The secondary MLR has different stimulatory requirements (Inaba and Steinman, 1984). When primed T lymphoblasts are isolated from the primary MLR and rechallenged with B cells, a strong secondary response ensues. If the B cells are mitomycin C-treated or irradiated (900 rad of ^{137}Cs), the T blasts proliferate and release IL-2. If the T blasts are irradiated, the B cells proliferate and at least some begin to secrete antibody. Since restimulation of CD4$^+$ blasts is class II MHC restricted, the observations indicate that small B cells express some alloantigen, but they are only able to induce a secondary versus a primary MLR.

3. MLR Stimulation by B Lymphoblasts

Whereas activated T cells can interact in an MHC-restricted fashion with small B cells, recent data indicate that B blasts activated with either anti-Ig Sepharose or LPS can stimulate a primary MLR (Metlay et al., 1989). By comparing the response to graded doses of stimulator cells, the stimulating activity of B blasts is 3–10% of that of dendritic cells in inducing DNA synthesis or lymphokine release. The lower potency could mean that the B blasts are acting on a small subpopulation of activated T cells or that B blasts are simply 3–10% as active in stimulating the same T cells as dendritic cells.

Several lymphokines have been detected early in the primary MLR that is induced by either dendritic cells or anti-Ig-induced B blasts: IL-2, IL-4, and a B cell growth factor distinct from IL-4 (Puré et al., 1988).

Dendritic cells are capable of stimulating class I MHC-disparate CD8 cells in the apparent absence of CD4$^+$ helper cells. However, B blasts have yet to be evaluated as stimulators of the CD8 MLR.

4. Langerhans Cells

Freshly isolated LCs have as much cell surface class II MHC as spleen dendritic cells, but these LCs are only 3–10% as active as primary MLR stimulators (Schuler and Steinman, 1985; Witmer-Pack et al., 1987). In contrast, fresh LCs are powerful stimulators of sensitized T blasts (Inaba et al., 1986). Once the LCs have been cultured for 2 days in GM-CSF, they become even more active than spleen dendritic cells (Witmer-Pack et al., 1987). A feature that changes in culture is that the LCs become capable of binding the T cells by an antigen-independent mechanism. This binding (see Section VI,C) may be a rate-limiting step in the initiation of the MLR.

5. Rejection of MHC-Incompatible Grafts in Situ

These findings with the MLR have counterparts *in situ*. Lechler and Batchelor (1982) studied a rat transplantation model in which recipients were tolerized to allogeneic kidneys. In the particular strain combination used, it was possible to transplant the accepted kidney into a fresh MHC-incompatible recipient. The graft was accepted, presumably because "passenger leukocytes" had been depleted. One could then rechallenge, with different populations of allogeneic leukocytes bearing the MHC of the accepted kidney. Dendritic cells in small numbers (Knight et al., 1982) induced rejection, whereas much larger numbers of B cells were inactive.

In the mouse Faustman et al. (1984) depleted dendritic cells from mouse pancreatic islets with 33D1 anti-dendritic cell Mab and complement. They were able to transplant the islets across an MHC barrier. Rejection occurred when the recipients were given an infusion of allogeneic dendritic cells. Similar findings were made in a mouse thyroid allograft model, i.e., treatment with 33D1 and complement permitted transplantation across an MHC barrier (Iwai et al., 1989). Knight et al. (1983) injected enriched populations of F1 leukocytes into parental recipients and noted that dendritic cells were some 50 times more potent than unfractionated spleen in stimulating popliteal lymph node enlargement.

More work is needed on the mechanism of allograft immunity *in situ*. The enhanced stimulatory activity of dendritic cells may be due to the fact that dendritic cells home better to the T cell area and thereby gain access to alloreactive T cells. More likely, since B cells do recirculate through the T cell area (see Sections II,C and D), the B cell is less efficient in binding or stimulating alloreactive T cells to initiate the rejection response *in situ*.

In summary, dendritic cells are strong stimulators of responses to allogeneic MHC class I and class II determinants *in vitro* and *in situ*, whereas small B cells are weak or even inactive. There are instances in which B cells actively present MHC determinants at least *in vitro*. One is when the T cell is an activated T lymphoblast; the other is when the B cell is activated following contact with anti-Ig Sepharose or LPS. There may be several levels at which dendritic and B cells differ as stimulator cells: the amounts and varieties of allogeneic MHC–peptide complexes, the capacity to find and bind T cells, and the mechanism used to bind or activate resting T cells. These will be discussed in Section VI.

C. Mls Stimulation

Studies of the MLR were the first to address the distinct APC requirements for activating antigen-specific, resting T cells. This has helped to define dendritic cells as a subset of APCs which were capable of presenting antigen to resting T cells. While the MHC remains the best-characterized antigen system for studying primary T cell activation, in the mouse there is an additional set of loci which leads to T cell proliferative responses as strong, if not stronger, *in vitro*. These are known as the minor lymphocyte-stimulating (Mls) antigens.

1. Mls Antigens

Current evidence indicates that the Mls system involves two separate loci which are either expressed or not expressed in individual inbred strains of mice. Thus, Mls^a mice express only one stimulatory locus for T cells, Mls^c mice express the other, Mls^d mice express both, and Mls^b mice express neither (Abe and Hodes, 1988). Unlike the MHC, stimulation in the Mls is largely unidirectional, i.e., Mls$^+$ strains such as a, c, and d stimulate responses in Mls$^-$ strains such as b (Janeway et al., 1988).

Despite this recent clarification in the genetics of Mls responses, the molecular nature of Mls antigens remains largely obscure. Furthermore, unlike responses to most conventional antigens, Mls responses are not tightly MHC restricted (Molnar-Kimber and Sprent, 1980). However, recognition of specific Mls antigens has recently been associated with particular V_β TCR genes. This implies presentation of Mls antigens to typical TCRs. When T cell hybridomas or clones express either V_β 8.1 (Kappler et al., 1988) or V_β 6 (MacDonald et al., 1988), the T cells preferentially respond to Mls^a stimulators. These T cells, in some cases, are highly MHC restricted and have classical reactivities to antigen plus MHC, but the presence of Mls obviates the need for specific antigen. Similarly, V_β 3-expressing T cells are enriched for Mls^c reactivity (Pullen et al., 1988; Abe et al., 1988). Interestingly, the strains of mice which express specific Mls antigens show a selective deletion of T cells which express the corresponding Mls-reactive TCR elements (Pullen et al., 1988; Kappler et al., 1988). This observation has provided a powerful model for self-tolerance mechanisms and has therefore intensified interest in the question of which cells can present Mls antigens. The utilization of conventional TCRs for Mls recognition, as well as inhibition of the responses by anti-class II MHC Mabs, suggests that Mls antigens are ultimately presented like conventional protein antigens, i.e., as processed peptides associated with MHC molecules. If this proves to be the case, then an analysis of the role of different APCs in stimulating Mls responses may provide an additional system for studying responses of resting T cells to antigen.

2. APC Requirements for Mls Responses

Because of the lack of serological reagents to identify Mls cell surface antigens, measurements of Mls expression by different APCs have relied on proliferative responses by both primary T cells and T cell clones. Such studies have reinforced the concept that, unlike MHC antigens, Mls expression has a restricted tissue distribution. Primary Mls-stimulatory function is enriched in B cell populations, compared to bulk spleen cells (Ahmed *et al.*, 1977; Webb *et al.*, 1985). In the study by Ahmed *et al.* depletion of the peripheral B cell pool by *in vivo* treatment with anti-μ dramatically reduced the capacity of spleen cells to stimulate Mls responses without altering stimulation of allogeneic MHC responses. Together, these results have argued that B cells may be the major, if not only, stimulators of Mls responses *in vitro*.

In contrast, the capacity of dendritic cells to stimulate Mls responses remains controversial. Both Sunshine *et al.* (1985) and Hamilos *et al.* (1989) have reported Mls stimulation by enriched populations of dendritic cells in high doses. However, because of the very strong capacity of B cells to stimulate Mls responses, particularly in primary systems, there remains the possibility of B cell contamination in the dendritic cell preparations. Activated B cells have a low buoyant density (Steinman *et al.*, 1978) and can contaminate spleen dendritic cell preparations, which are routinely selected for their low density on bovine serum albumin (Steinman *et al.*, 1979; Nussenzweig and Steinman, 1980).

Two recent studies have demonstrated that the expression of stimulatory Mls antigens may exclusively be limited to B cells, particularly activated B cells (Webb *et al.*, 1989; Metlay *et al.*, 1989). Macrophages from a variety of tissues, T cells, and, most significantly, highly enriched spleen dendritic cells all failed to stimulate T cell responses to Mls. In contrast, low-density B cells, B cell lines, and B blasts were potent stimulators of the appropriate Mls-reactive T cells. In agreement with the findings of Ahmed *et al.* (1977), splenocytes from anti-μ-suppressed mice failed to stimulate Mls responses (Webb *et al.*, 1989). In keeping with prior observations using B cells as MLR stimulators (see Section IV,B), *in vitro* activated B blasts were at least 30 times more potent than were resting B cells at stimulating primary Mls responses (Metlay *et al.*, 1989). Indeed, some of the primary Mls-stimulatory ability of fresh isolates of B cells might be attributed to contaminating *in vivo* activated B cells.

Some investigators have interpreted these results as suggesting that Mls antigens encode for unique accessory molecules which may enhance T cell responses to self-MHC molecules on B cells (Webb *et al.*, 1989; Janeway *et al.*, 1983; Katz and Janeway, 1985). However, recent studies have failed to demonstrate any enhanced APC function of Mls$^+$- as compared to Mls$^-$-derived APCs (Needleman *et al.*, 1988).

Although B blasts are reproducibly less potent than are dendritic cells at stimulating primary T cells to respond to allogeneic class II MHC, they are dramatically more potent than are dendritic cells at stimulating the same bulk population of resting T cells to respond to Mls antigens. Therefore, one of the key determinants of relative stimulatory ability in a bulk MLR may reside in the capacity of the dendritic cell or the B blast to obtain the appropriate stimulatory peptides. The findings with Mls indicate that B blasts are able to bind primary T cells and elaborate necessary costimulatory functions for activating these cells *in vitro* (Metlay *et al.*, 1989).

3. Studies in Situ

Unlike allogeneic MHC antigens, Mls antigens fail to stimulate graft rejection *in vivo*. When either heart or skin is grafted across Mls barriers, there is no increase in rejection rates as compared to those in matched controls (Sachs *et al.*, 1973; Huber *et al.*, 1973). In retrospect, the possibility that Mls antigens are exclusively expressed on B cells readily explains the failure to find accelerated rejection rates for grafts which are essentially devoid of B cells. On the other hand, the measurements of mortality in lethal graft-versus-host reactions also failed to demonstrate a clear-cut role for Mls antigens, even though B cells should be accessible in the lymphoid organs of the graft recipients. In the study by Nisbet and Edwards (1973), F_1 backcross mice were typed at the Mls by *in vitro* stimulation assays and lethal graft-versus-host disease was followed in parabiosed pairs. Both Mls-compatible and -incompatible pairs showed similar survival rates. Similarly, Korngold and Sprent (1978) found only minimal evidence for graft-versus-host disease with non-T cell-depleted marrow transplants into irradiated, Mls-incompatible recipients. The lack of any *in vivo* correlate to the powerful *in vitro* stimulatory capacity of Mls-incompatible B cells suggests that there are additional limitations on B cell APC function *in vivo*.

D. Viral and Minor Histocompatibility Antigens

In this section we consider a group of papers which indicate that dendritic cells induce CTL responses to simple chemical haptens, minor histocompatibility antigens, and several types of virus. When studied, B cells have been found to be weak or inactive.

1. TNP-modified Syngeneic Cells

One of the first systems in which the accessory function of spleen dendritic cells was studied was the development of CTLs to TNP-modified, high-responder ($H-2K^k$) cells (Nussenzweig *et al.*, 1980). The design of the experiments was to use highly enriched T cells both as responders and as the source of TNP-modified stimulators. When spleen dendritic cells were added in small numbers, hapten-specific CTLs developed. Ia$^+$ macrophages were not active in this assay, and unfractionated spleen cells (60–70% B cells) were weak.

It is possible that the dendritic cells were processing the TNP-modified T cells in these experiments, but in subsequent studies (M. C. Nussenzweig and R. M. Steinman, unpublished observations), antigen-pulsed dendritic cells were inactive as APCs. This suggests that the presence of dendritic cells, and the associated induction of lymphokines in the syngeneic MLR (Inaba et al., 1983a) somehow amplifed CTL development to antigens presented on other TNP-modified cells, which in these experiments were T cells.

2. H-Y Antigens

Boog et al. (1985) reported the abolition of an immune response defect in bm12 mice by injecting antigen on dendritic cells. The bm12 mutation in the class II I-A^b gene reduces presentation of the H-Y male transplantation antigen to CD4$^+$ helper T cells. Female bm12 mice could be primed with male bm12 dendritic cells such that they could reject grafts of male skin *in situ* and form CTLs to male targets upon restimulation *in vitro*. The killer cells were CD8$^+$ but required help from CD4$^+$ cells. As few as 10^4 dendritic cells could prime the animal, while 10^7 LPS-induced B blasts or unfractionated spleen cells were inactive.

In a subsequent series of studies, Boog et al. (1988b) obtained evidence that dendritic cells also could overcome the defect that bm14 mice exhibit in presenting H-Y antigens on class I MHC (D^b) to CD8$^+$ CTLs. Dendritic cells (2×10^5) or normal spleen cells (10^7) could prime mice *in situ* to H-Y, but only dendritic cells could boost the primed cells *in vitro*. However, the defect in another D^b mutant, bm13, could not be abolished with dendritic cells. Another intriguing feature of presentation by dendritic cells was that CD8$^+$ T cells could be restimulated in the absence of CD4$^+$ helpers (Boog et al., 1988a,b), as in the experiments cited above in the primary allogeneic MLR (Inaba et al., 1987).

3. Viral Antigens

Kast et al. (1988) were able to induce CTL responses in wild-type H-2^b mice to Sendai and Moloney leukemia viruses, using small numbers of dendritic cells as APCs *in vitro*. In the case of the bm14 class I MHC mutant, which does not generate a CTL response to Moloney leukemia virus, dendritic cells could overcome the defect. When dendritic cells were compared to LPS-induced B blasts, the former were approximately 30- to 50-fold more active. Dendritic cells could not overcome the defect in bm13 class I MHC molecules to present Sendai virus.

It was concluded that some antigen presentation of Moloney leukemia virus was occurring in bm14 and that the amount of these Moloney leukemia virus–bm14 complexes was either greater or more effective using dendritic cells as APCs. In contrast, too few Sendai virus–bm13 complexes were formed to generate a CTL response, even in the presence of dendritic cells.

Macatonia et al. (1989) have studied the CTL response to influenza antigens. They were able to induce primary responses by using a Terasaki microculture system in which the accessory dendritic cells and responding T cells were maintained in a hanging drop close to an air interface. CTLs would develop when either intact virus or a dominant nucleoprotein peptide was used as antigen.

The diversity of antiviral responses that seem to be enhanced by dendritic cells raises some interesting questions for future work. Will the APC function be even more effective if tissue versus spleen dendritic cells are studied? Is the antigen being presented following processing in an endocytic or cytoplasmic compartment? Can virus in association with dendritic cells induce protective $CD8^+$ T cell-mediated immunity *in situ*?

V. APC Requirements during T Cell-Dependent Antibody Responses

A. The Need for B Cell–T Cell Collaboration

The first evidence for an obligate cooperation of B and T cells was provided by Claman and co-workers (1966). They showed that an antibody response to sheep red blood cells (SRBCs) by lethally irradiated mice could be reconstituted by the adoptive transfer of thymus- and bone marrow-derived cells but not by either cell type alone. Davies et al. (1967) tested the capacity of cells of thymus and bone marrow origin, taken from radiation chimeras, to produce antibody during secondary anti-SRBC responses *in vivo*. Bone marrow-derived cells formed a limited amount of antibody, but thymus-derived cells were inactive. The greatest response was found when *both* cell populations were stimulated. Miller and Mitchell (1968; Mitchell and Miller, 1968) then proved that B cells were the precursors to the antibody-producing cells, while T cells did not produce antibodies but provided help to the B cells.

Two observations indicated that B cell–T cell cooperation required direct cell contact. The first was the hapten–carrier effect, in which determinants, to be recognized by B cells, had to be linked to carrier determinants seen by T cells. Mitchison (1971) showed that different cell populations responded to the carrier and hapten, and that these two determinants had to be physically associated. He concluded that the two interacting cells must engage in a close physical association. Raff (1970) used anti-Thy-1 and complement treatment to prove that the carrier-specific cells were T cells and that Thy-1$^-$ B cells recognized the hapten. Together, this information was interpreted to mean the antigen, here the linked hapten and carrier determinants, provided a bridge between the B and T cells.

It was then shown that B cell–T cell cooperation required MHC histocompatibility between the two cells. Katz et al. (1973) reconstituted the antibody response to hapten–carrier conjugates in irradiated F_1 recipients with separate inocula of carrier-primed, irradiated T cells and hapten-primed, nonirradiated B cells. To produce antibody, the B and T cells had to be MHC compatible, i.e., from the same parental strain, or T cells from one of the parental strains and F_1 B cells. The basis for cooperation between syngeneic, but not allogeneic, cells was postulated to be the engagement of cellular interaction molecules on the surfaces of the B and T cells. In a series of genetic mapping experiments the restriction elements mapped to the class II or immune response regions of the MHC (Katz et al., 1975). In a second set of experiments on the MHC restriction of B cell–T cell cooperation, Sprent and von Boehmer (1976) obviated the potential for alloreactivity by filtering T cells from strain A through (A × B)F_1 recipients. They found that the filtered T cells could only cooperate with B cells that were matched in the K and I regions of the MHC. Following additional experiments (von Boehmer et al., 1975), it was proposed that T_H cells expressed receptors for self-MHC determinants expressed on B cells. The concept of self-recognition was firmly established by a series of subsequent experiments by Sprent (1978) and Swierkosz et al. (1978). (A × B)F_1 helper T cells were positively selected by priming on parental strain APCs in vivo or on accessory cells in vitro. In either case the T cells would cooperate best with B cells that were MHC identical to the APCs used to prime the T cells.

Marrack and Kappler (1978) then studied the antibody response to the synthetic polypeptide TGAL, known to be under control of immune response or class II MHC genes. They found that both B cells and APCs had to be from high-responder mice in order to elicit help from F_1 T cells.

In the context of our current knowledge of T cell recognition of antigen, one can interpret the above observations to mean that antigen-specific B cells process and present carrier peptides to T cells in association with B cell class II MHC molecules. This also accounts for the facts that immune response genes or Ia antigens are expressed on B cells and that B cell–T cell help is MHC restricted.

B. THE ROLE OF DENDRITIC CELLS IN HELPER T CELL PRIMING

The development of *in vitro* culture conditions for generating antibody responses in suspensions of mouse spleen cells led to the recognition of a third, adherent cell requirement for optimal T cell-dependent antibody responses. It was found that the APC–T_H cell interaction was MHC restricted (Singer *et al.*, 1979). In separate experiments aimed at identifying the active adherent cell, dendritic cells were discovered and found to be essential for both primary and secondary responses (Inaba *et al.*, 1983b, 1984). Dendritic cells were required for the initial priming of T cells, which could then help antigen-specific B cells to differentiate into antibody-secreting cells. The latter could occur in the apparent absence of dendritic cells in an antigen-specific, MHC-restricted fashion (Inaba *et al.*, 1984; Inaba and Steinman, 1985).

The initial T cell priming event occurred in prominent dendritic cell–T cell clusters (Inaba *et al.*, 1984; Inaba and Steinman, 1987a). These clusters formed independently of B cells, but when the latter were added, the B cells entered the clusters in an antigen-dependent, MHC-restricted fashion. The clusters were the source of the subsequent antibody-producing cells, as assessed by a plaque assay. When T cells were removed from the clusters at day 1 or 2 of the primary antibody response, the remaining B cells would give rise to antibody-producing cells if supplemented with antigen-nonspecific lymphokines. These factors would help antibody responses to both RBCs and hapten–carrier conjugates, but they could be produced when dendritic cells and T cells were cultured together in the absence of antigen. During such cultures a syngeneic MLR is generated (Nussenzweig and Steinman, 1980) and the clusters of dendritic and T cells release helper factors (Granelli-Piperno *et al.*, 1984).

C. HELPER T CELL SUBSETS

The quality of an antibody response is regulated, at least in part, by the types of lymphokines that are produced by the helper cell. Distinct subsets of $CD4^+$ T cells mediate graft-versus-host disease and antibody responses in rats (Spickett *et al.*, 1983; Streuli *et al.*, 1987) and account for helper–inducer versus suppressor–inducer activity in humans. Long-term murine $CD4^+$ helper T cell clones can also be subsetted based on the lymphokines they produce; T_H1 clones make IL-2 and IFN-γ, while T_H2 clones make IL-4 and IL-5 (Cherwinski *et al.*, 1987). These functional subsets of helper cells can be distinguished on the basis of their CD45R phenotype: OX22 in rats, 2H4 in humans, and 23G2 in mice, the latter being more abundant on T_H2 clones (Birkeland *et al.*, 1988).

These functional subsets arise as the result of antigen-induced differentiation of $CD4^+$ cells *in vitro* (Morimoto *et al.*, 1985; Rudd *et al.*, 1987; Clement *et al.*, 1988) and *in situ*. The latter data from Powrie and Mason (1989) show that $OX22^-$ helper T cells in the rat differentiate from $OX22^+$, $CD4^+$ T cells, indicating that the two functional subsets arise from a common pool of $CD45R^+$, $CD4^+$ T cells. Hayakawa and Hardy (1988) also found that cells with the T_H2 phenotype are part of the memory response. They have categorized murine $CD4^+$ cells using two monoclonal anti-T cell autoantibodies, SM3G11 and SM6C10. The $3G11^-$, $6C10^+$ and $3G11^+$, $6C10^-$ populations exhibit distinct functions. The former secretes IL-4 but not IL-2 when activated by concanavalin A (Con A) and includes memory T cells responsible for secondary antibody formation. In contrast, the other population ($3G11^+$, $6C10^-$) secretes IL-2 but not IL-4 in response to Con A and does not contribute to the secondary antibody response.

A key finding in the study by Hayakawa and Hardy (1988) was that these two populations of $CD4^+$ T cells also exhibited differential accessory cell dependence. $6C10^+$ cells responded when either B cells or non-B cells were used as accessory cells for Con A-induced activation, whereas $3G11^+$ T cells required a non-B accessory cell that has yet to be defined. Many of the $CD4^+$ cells expressed both 3G11 and 6C10 determinants and were *not* distinguishable with regard to lymphokine secretion, accessory cell requirement, or memory T cell activity. The $3G11^-$, $6C10^-$ fraction was unresponsive in any of these assays.

In the MLR, however, both dendritic cells and B blasts induced the release of lymphokines from freshly isolated T cells and *in vitro* primed T lymphoblasts (Metlay *et al.*, 1989). IL-2 secretion was more rapid in the secondary MLR, but comparable levels were observed at the T cell doses used. IL-4 release was more rapid and reached tenfold higher levels in the secondary MLR. A B cell growth factor that is active on anti-Ig-preactivated B blasts reached comparable levels in the primary and secondary MLRs. In contrast to the anti-Ig blasts, resting B cells did not induce lympokine production in the primary MLR.

In summary, both B cells and dendritic cells can stimulate the production of different lymphokines. More work is needed to determine how helper subsets arise, and whether the type of APC influences the generation or stimulation of each subset.

D. B Cells versus Non-B Cells for Antibody Responses *in Situ*

The nature of the APCs required *in vivo* has been addressed using the anti-μ-suppressed or B cell-depleted mice discussed above (see Section IV,A). We have already reviewed the finding that when these mice are primed with antigen plus adjuvant, there are few T cells generated in the draining lymph node that can proliferate in response to antigenic rechallenge *in vitro*. Additional experiments using this model have been done to determine whether helper T cells for antibody responses can be primed in these mice.

Spleen cells from antigen-primed (KLH or fowl γ-globulin), anti-μ-suppressed animals have helper cell function, indicating that a non-B cell can sensitize helper T cells (Ron and Sprent, 1989). Primed helper T cells could also be detected in anti-μ-suppressed nodes when a more sensitive helper T cell assay involving adoptive transfer and antigen challenge *in vivo* was utilized. Ron and Sprent (1989) have suggested that in both the spleen and the lymph node a non-B cell is sufficient for T cell sensitization, but that in the latter, B cells may contribute significantly to the clonal expansion and function of sensitized T cells.

Lassila *et al.* (1988) have obtained evidence that B cells are not the initial APCs for antibody formation *in vivo* in chickens. They depleted B cells from neonatal chickens with cyclophosphamide and reconstituted with bursal cells from MHC-matched or -mismatched donors. In chimeras in which the host and donor strains differed at all known chicken MHC loci, T cell-dependent antibody responses could not be induced. These data could be explained either by the failure to prime T cells in the absence of donor-type accessory cells, or the inability of primed T cells to collaborate with the donor B cells. To distinguish between these two possibilities, donor-type accessory cells (histocompatible with the B cells) were transferred into the chimeras. Now antigenic challenge induced IgM and IgG responses and the formation of germinal centers. Since an allogeneic effect was essentially ruled out in these experiments (by the absence of an antibody response in the original chimeras), it seems likely that donor-type accessory cells were required to prime T cells that could interact with donor B cells in an MHC-restricted fashion. This would support an essential role for a non-B APC as the initial APC for priming the T cell, and it must share the class II MHC of the B cell that is to interact with the helper T cell. The identity of the critical cell(s) in the chicken system is unknown.

In summary, the evidence from *in vitro* experiments indicates that the initial sensitization of T helper cells requires non-B accessory cells, identified as dendritic cells, which first prime helper T cells for subsequent interactions with B cells. The initial APC must be class II MHC histocompatible with the responding B cell. Additional experiments are required to determine whether activated B cells also prime helper T cells for antibody responses to nominal antigens. *In vivo*, there are experiments which indicate that small B cells do not prime helper T cells during a primary response, but there are no definitive experiments to distinguish the role of dendritic cells, macrophages, and activated B cells. The small B cell could also operate *in vivo* to expand responses that are initiated by other APCs.

E. Memory and Germinal Center B Cells as APCs

T cell-dependent antibody responses are accompanied by the formation of germinal centers within the B cell follicles. The germinal centers contain rapidly dividing (Fleidner *et al.*, 1964), antigen-specific (Sordat *et al.*, 1970) B lymphoblasts. Other cellular elements found in the germinal center are macrophages, follicular dendritic cells, and a few T lymphocytes. Tew and co-workers (Kosco *et al.*, 1988) obtained evidence that germinal center B blasts carry antigen, presumably acquired initially from the depots of immune complexes on the follicular dendritic cells shortly after secondary immunization (Nossal *et al.*, 1968; Chen *et al.*, 1978b). The germinal center cells were enriched by flotation on dense Percoll gradients, followed by sorting and/or panning for reactivity to peanut agglutinin, a marker for germinal center B cells. The sorted blasts contained the majority of the recovered antigen, as assessed by using radiolabeled ovalbumin for immunization The sorted blasts also were used to present antigen to ovalbumin-specific T cell hybridomas. At days 1-8 postimmunization the B blasts could induce IL-2 release without the need for additional antigen. At later times, i.e., 3 weeks, germinal center cells would present antigen but only with exogenous ovalbumin (Kosco *et al.*, 1988). These results are consistent with the possibility that germinal center B cells can serve as antigen-presenting cells for T cells.

Long-term antigen-specific memory B cells obtained at least 3 months after immunization have been studied by Hayakawa *et al.* (1987). They used the fluorescent protein phycoerythrin both as the immunizing antigen and as a probe to isolate purified, antigen-binding memory B cells, using multiparameter cell sorting. The memory B cells were $B220^+$ (IgM^-, IgD^-). As few as 500 of the phycoerythrin-binding memory B cells produced strong IgG antiphycoerythrin responses when cultured with $CD4^+$ helper T cells from primed mice. The memory B cells therefore served as the APCs in these cultures. Similar results were obtained with TNP-KLH as the antigen, i.e., with TNP-specific memory B cells and KLH-primed T cells. For both systems low doses of antigen were required. Since the B and T cells used in these experiments were obtained from mice primed at least 3 months earlier, these results demonstrate that a secondary antibody response can be initiated by the presentation of antigen by specific memory B cells to specific T cells.

VI. Discussion—Four Components of APC Function

In Sections IV and V we summarized some of the similarities and differences in the capacity of dendritic cells and B cells to stimulate T cell responses to different groups of antigens. Here, we consider the mechanism of action of these two types of APCs in tissue culture and *in situ* models. We dissect APC function into four steps, of which antigen processing and presentation, i.e., the formation of an MHC–peptide complex to act as the ligand for the TCR, is one. The additional steps we consider are the capacities of APCs to acquire antigens *in situ*, to find and bind antigen-specific T cells *in vitro* and *in situ*, and to induce growth and lymphokine production by T cells that have been bound.

A. Antigen Processing and Presentation

1. Endocytosis and Formation of MHC–Peptide Complexes

Given the identification of a peptide-binding groove on the external surface of the MHC molecule and the capacity of small peptides to substitute for most native antigens in stimulating T cells (see Section IV,A), it is evident that the clonotypic receptor (TCR) for antigen is interacting with an MHC–peptide complex on the APCs. Models depicting this interaction are available (Davis and Bjorkman, 1988).

Peptides and MHC–peptide complexes can be generated by proteases acting extracellularly, since peptides or proteolytic digests of an antigen can be presented by aldehyde-fixed APCs to T/T hybrids (Shimonkevitz et al., 1983, 1984). Extracellular digestion might occur in an acute inflammatory site, where a large number of dying white blood cells that are rich in proteases are found. However, it seems likely that many critical peptides are generated within the cell, either from within endocytic vesicles or from the cytoplasm. This presentation of peptides from within APCs allows the T lymphocyte to recognize targets that are parasitized with an infectious agent, such as a bacterium within an endocytic vacuole, or a virus within the cytoplasm.

The endocytic pathway is one way in which antigens can be processed to form MHC–peptide complexes, particularly for class II MHC products. Processing has been difficult to demonstrate directly, but it has been inferred from several observations made for many antigens. Aldehyde-fixed cells do not present most antigens, but fixed cells can present peptide fragments, particularly to T/T hybridomas (Unanue, 1984; Livingstone and Fathman, 1987; Berzofsky, 1988; Rothbard, 1986). This observation proves that live cells are needed to present intact proteins but does not pinpoint the required function in the live cell. Lysosomotropic agents such as chloroquine block presentation (Unanue,

1984; Ziegler and Unanue, 1982; Chesnut *et al.*, 1982b), although not for all large molecules (Allen and Unanue, 1984; Lee *et al.*, 1988; Buus and Werdelin, 1986b). Since lysosomal hydrolases have an acid pH optimum, the increase in intravacuolar pH that is induced with chloroquine (Wibo and Poole, 1974) should block proteolysis and processing. When chloroquine does not block, as occurs with antigens such as fibrinogen (Lee *et al.*, 1988) and angiotensin (Buus and Werdelin, 1986b), it is assumed that the protein is denatured or unfolded to an extent that permits binding to the MHC molecule and accessibility to the TCR. It is not yet established whether chloroquine only acts at the level of processing, particularly since other lysosomotropic drugs, such as ammonium chloride, may not block presentation (Jensen, 1988). Chloroquine, at least in B cell lines, also alters the association of invariant chains with class II MHC molecules (Nowell and Quaranta, 1985), a step which has recently been implicated in presentation (Stockinger *et al.*, 1989).

Endocytosis could play many roles during antigen presentation. The vacuolar system can provide proteases to cleave proteins into peptides which associate with class II MHC (Buus and Werdelin, 1986a). If a large polypeptide fragment is the first to bind, the proteases may trim it so that T cells can gain access to the MHC-peptide complex. The low pH of the endocytic pathway may influence peptide-class II MHC binding, but this has yet to be demonstrated. Another possibility, before now given little attention, is that the endocytic pathway can intersect with the secretory pathway, possibly in "late endosomes" (Geuze *et al.*, 1988). This would allow access of endocytosed antigens and peptides to newly synthesized, perhaps "unoccupied," MHC molecules. It is noteworthy that the times when both dendritic cells and B cells are best able to acquire antigens for presentation are those when new class II MHC molecules are being synthesized (see Section III,A). Jensen (1988) and Harding and Unanue (1989) recently reported that cycloheximide blocks presentation but not endocytosis of proteins by peritoneal exudate cells. The cycloheximide-sensitive step may be the synthesis of class II MHC products.

There is still no means for identifying specific MHC-peptide complexes (presented antigen) on living APCs, nor for measuring their half-lives once formed. Conceivably, it will be possible to identify these complexes once TCRs for the antigen-MHC complex are solubilized and available as ligands. Once MHC-peptide complexes form intracellularly, it is assumed that they gain access to the cell surface by the recycling of internalized membrane that characteristically occurs from endocytic vacuoles (Steinman *et al.*, 1983a).

In summary, while a general view for antigen processing and presentation is available, there are few specific and direct approaches for monitoring these events. The ensuing analysis of presentation by B cells and dendritic cells therefore must be considered preliminary, and it is for this reason that it is included in a discussion section.

2. Endocytosis and Presentation by B Cells

Neither dendritic cells nor B cells are particularly active in taking up the bulk tracers that are used to detect endocytosis in macrophages or in many cell lines. A soluble protein tracer such as horseradish peroxidase is internalized in large amounts by macrophages (Steinman and Cohn, 1972), to a lesser extent by cultured fibroblasts (Steinman et al., 1974a), and only at trace levels in some dendritic cells (Steinman and Cohn, 1974; Steinman et al., 1974b) and B lymphoblasts (J. P. Metlay and R. M. Steinman, unpublished observations). At a first glance, then, the study of antigen presentation in these APCs might seem misplaced, but the opposite view could be argued. The bulk of an internalized load in an actively endocytic cell such as the macrophage may be digested down to the level of amino acids (Steinman and Cohn, 1972), since these cells are specialized for scavenging and microbicidal activity. In contrast, dendritic cells and B cells, because they show so little bulk endocytic activity, seem to utilize endocytosis primarily as a presentation mechanism and accordingly may prove useful for identifying physiological pathways for the formation of antigen-MHC complexes.

B cells likely use receptor-mediated uptake to endocytose antigens that have been bound to surface Ig molecules. Antibodies directed to surface Ig can be pinocytosed (Taylor et al., 1971; Unanue et al., 1972), but as yet there is little information on the fate of antigens bound to surface Ig. As pointed out by several workers, surface Ig-mediated antigen uptake would enable the specific B cell that binds an antigen to internalize and present fragments (carrier determinants) which in turn attract MHC-restricted helper T cells (Lanzavecchia, 1985; Tony et al., 1985; Rock et al., 1984; Chesnut and Grey, 1981).

Interestingly, Fab fragments of anti-class I MHC antibodies also are efficiently presented (Tony et al., 1985). These ligands may not stimulate uptake, as is thought to be the case with intact anti-Ig reagents, but may enter "piggyback" fashion on B cells that are forming endocytic vesicles for other reasons. The B cells may have been stimulated by antigen *in situ* prior to isolation or by contaminating LPS *in vitro*. B cells may also undergo a low level of constitutive pinocytosis to obtain nutrients such as low-density lipoproteins, transferrin, and vitamins that bind to specific cell surface receptors (Steinman et al., 1983a). This delivery function would be expected to to be enhanced when the B cell is stimulated to grow.

Likewise, formation of an endocytic vesicle during Ig receptor-mediated antigen uptake would also lead to at least some internalization of antigen-nonspecific substrates in the fluid phase. However, there is still little information on many physiological aspects: Do B cells that are stimulated by antigen process immunostimulatory amounts of exogenous, nonspecific proteins, as B cell lines and LPS blasts seem capable of doing (see Section IV,A), and can these B cells present such antigens to primary populations of T cells rather than to T cell lines?

Of some interest is whether the surface Ig molecules themselves are degraded and presented by B cells. When antibody molecules are bound to particles and fed to macrophages, the Ig is rapidly catabolized (Mellman et al., 1983). Given the diverse world of peptide sequences that are inherent in the V domains of surface Ig molecules, Lassila et al. have reasoned that presentation of these molecules would, by cross-reacting with the world of exogenous antigens, essentially tolerize the immune system. There would be few antigen-reactive T cells which would escape tolerization to all of the variable sequences that B cells express (Lassila et al., 1988). This idea and others (see Section VII,B) would argue against a role for constitutive antigen-presenting activity in B cells. For the time being, however, it is clear that one B cell line, A20, can present its idiotope (Weiss and Bogen, 1989).

Another feature of primary B cells, including B cells in the germinal center (Reichert et al., 1982) is that the levels of surface IgD decrease following activation to B blasts. The significance of this decrease is unknown, but it may regulate the capacity to handle antigens via surface Ig.

3. Endocytosis and Presentation by Dendritic Cells

Freshly isolated LCs have been shown to internalize small amounts of peroxidase *in situ* (Wolff and Schreiner, 1970) as well as some adsorbed tracers (Hanau et al., 1987a; Takigawa et al., 1985; Ishii et al., 1984). Birbeck granules have been implicated in the endocytic pathway (Hanau et al., 1987b; Takigawa et al., 1985; Scheynius et al., 1982; Ishii et al., 1984; Ray et al., 1989). However, the absolute levels of endocytosis are low relative to cells that are considered to be "nonprofessional" (keratinocytes) and "professional" (macrophages) in their relative endocytic activity. Interestingly, freshly isolated LCs present protein antigens well (Romani et al., 1989c). Activated or cultured epidermal LCs do not show detectable endocytosis (Schuler and Steinman, 1985) and do not present native myoglobin (Romani et al., 1989c).

These findings suggest that antigen presentation by dendritic cells can be regulated at the level of endocytic activity. Further studies are required in which fresh and cultured LCs are used to present antigens to primary populations rather than to long-term T cell clones and to present antigens other than soluble proteins, e.g., particulates.

Another possibility is that APCs process antigens and release peptides which are then presented on dendritic cell MHC molecules. As yet, this phenomenon has not been demonstrated. Although cultured epidermal LCs present peptides, these peptides cannot be generated by Ia⁻ epidermal cells (Romani et al., 1989c). In ongoing experiments, we have not detected immunostimulatory levels of peptide regurgitation by macrophages either (R. M. Steinman et al., unpublished observations). The cultured epidermal LCs may prove to be a particularly useful biological system to look for transfer of peptides, since these APCs have potent sensitizing functions for T cells but only handle peptides rather than native proteins.

The notion that the endocytic activity of epidermal LCs is regulated for the purposes of antigen presentation extends to other populations of dendritic cells. Veiled cells in afferent lymph do not internalize a variety of substrates when challenged (Pugh et al., 1983; Fossum, 1984). However, these lymph dendritic cells frequently contain what appear to be endocytic inclusions, suggesting that there may have been some endocytic activity while in the tissues prior to entry into the lymph. Spleen dendritic cells do not internalize a number of substrates when challenged in culture, but small amounts of endocytosed material are evident if mice are given colloidal carbon or soluble peroxidase intravenously just prior to isolation of the dendritic cells (Steinman and Cohn, 1974; Steinman et al., 1974b). We have found recently that spleen dendritic cells do present myoglobin when tested immediately after isolation, but they lose this capacity during overnight culture (Steinman et al., 1989). Interdigitating cells do not internalize injected colloids or immune complexes *in situ* (Fossum et al., 1980) but may be able to phagocytose lymphocytes. Electron-microscopic evidence for phagocytosis has been obtained in a situation in which there is considerable death of lymphocytes, the clearance of an inoculum of allogeneic lymphocytes (Fossum and Rolstad, 1986).

Therefore, it is likely that endocytosis by dendritic cells can occur, but this may be relegated to certain stages of the cell's life history and/or to particular ligands such as damaged lymphocytes. More work is required to document the range of antigens that can be presented by dendritic cells, particularly dendritic cells in tissues where antigens gain entry into the body.

4. Biochemistry of MHC Products on Dendritic and B Cells

Potential biochemical differences in the MHC products that are expressed on dendritic cells and B cells require exploration. Boog et al. (1988c) noted that both class I and class II MHC products, when immunoprecipitated from radioiodinated cells and resolved on two-dimensional gels, were less negatively charged on dendritic cells relative to LPS-induced B blasts. Treatment with neuraminidase further reduced the negative charge on MHC products of both B cells and dendritic cells. The basis for the reduced sialylation of dendritic cell MHC molecules is not known, nor is it evident whether it involves all surface glycoproteins or just MHC products. One wonders whether reduced sialylation is due to the activity of sialidases encoded in the neuraminidase locus (Klein, 1986) of the MHC.

Cowing and colleagues (Cowing and Chapdelaine, 1983; Frohman and Cowing, 1985) have found that treatment of B cells with neuraminidase enhances their APC function. Boog et al. (1989) have made similar observations in a system in which spleen cells were used to stimulate CTL responses in enriched populations of $CD8^+$ T cells. Neuraminidase treatment does not enhance presentation by dendritic cells, however (Boog et al., 1989; Hirayama et al., 1988). Boog et al. propose that dendritic cell MHC products are less heavily sialylated and that sialic acid residues on B blasts and other cells may hinder access of the TCR to MHC–peptide complexes (Boog et al., 1989). This suggestion stems from the increased immunolabeling of B cell MHC molecules when anti-MHC antibodies are applied to neuraminidase-treated cells.

Another unknown is the amount of ligand that is needed to stimulate a T cell in the presence of different APCs. So-called costimulatory signals could enhance the efficacy of a small amount of ligand. Recent data suggest that very little ligand on a dendritic cell is stimulatory and that any one dendritic cell simultaneously can stimulate many T cell clones (Romani et al., 1989a). The model involves anti-CD3 stimulation by cultured epidermal LCs. These cells have small numbers of FcγRII, which are essential for APC function in anti-CD3 responses (Smith et al., 1986). It was estimated that only 250 ligands on the LCs (FcR occupied with anti-CD3) were needed to drive a T cell into cycle. In contrast, B lymphoblasts have much higher levels of FcR (ten- to 20-fold) but are one tenth as active in inducing DNA synthesis in the presence of anti-CD3 (Romani et al., 1989a). What then is known about the costimulatory features of dendritic cells and B cells? The information falls into three areas.

B. Interaction of APCs and T Cells in Situ

1. Antigen Capture outside the T Cell Areas of Lymphoid Organs

Where are antigens captured in situ and where do the APCs and T cells interact? Sensitized T cells are most easily identified in lymphoid tissues that drain an antigen depot (Scothorne and McGregor, 1955; Mitchison, 1955), particularly the T cell area (Ford et al., 1975). However, it is difficult to demonstrate antigen in the T cell area. A good example is the study by Fossum (1980), who injected ferritin and colloidal gold into the footpad and observed the tracers in macrophages and on follicular dendritic cells in the presence of antibody, but not in the T area. Likewise, following intravenous administration into mice (Chen et al., 1978a,b), colloidal carbon, colloidal thorium, and horseradish peroxidase are found on follicular dendritic cells and macrophages, but not readily in the T cell area. Clearance of antigens by macrophages, which reside in sites at which antigens first enter the lymphoid organ (subcapsular and marginal sinus regions), may well block significant or prolonged access to the T cell area itself.

Given these findings, and the information that T cells are sensitized in lymphoid organs that drain the site of antigen deposition, it would seem necessary to postulate that foreign antigens can be bound and processed at distal sites and arrive in the T cell area ready to be presented.

2. Capture of Antigens by B Cells in Situ

Since sizable numbers of antigen-specific B cells are not readily found in nonlymphoid tissues or in afferent lymph (Sections II,D, E, and F), one has to consider two other sites where B cells might pick up antigens. One is the circulation, and indeed B cells might be specialized to pick up antigens in the bloodstream. The amount of circulating antigen is likely to be small relative to the high doses (0.1–1.0 mg/ml) that are used when APCs stimulate T cells *in vitro*. However, the efficiency imparted by adsorptive uptake via surface Ig could allow the B cells to acquire antigen from the bloodstream. The B cells would then have to meet helper T cells while circulating through the T or B cell areas.

B cells may also acquire antigen in the germinal center, where there is a depot of extracellular antigen on follicular dendritic cells (see Section II,C) and where $CD4^+$ T cells are also noted (Bhan et al., 1981). B cells in the germinal center may be in transition to the higher-affinity "memory" type. Of some interest are the data that B cells themselves might be necessary to transport immune complexes to the follicular dendritic cells (Heinen et al., 1986). As discussed above (Section V,E), Kosco et al. (1988) have reported that isolates of germinal center B blasts from ovalbumin-immune animals are carrying enough ligand to stimulate an ovalbumin-specific T/T hybridoma.

3. Sites for Antigen Uptake by Dendritic Cells

There are now several examples in which dendritic cells have been shown to be carrying antigens that have been administered *in situ*. The contact sensitivity model has been explored to try to establish that the allergen might be delivered by epidermal LCs which move into the dermis and then into the afferent lymph, eventually to reach the draining lymph node. Early experiments established that afferent lymphatics had to be intact for some 24 hours or more to prime an animal to a contact allergen (Landsteiner and Chase, 1939; Frey and Wenk, 1957). Shelley and Juhlin (1976, 1977) noted that many contact allergens selectively bind to LCs in the epidermis and proposed that these cells were a reticuloepithelial trap. Silberberg-Sinakin *et al.* (1976) identified LCs in electron-microscopic sections of dermal lymphatics underlying the site at which contact allergens had been applied. Macatonia, Knight, and co-workers then proved that the draining lymph node had APCs, probably dendritic cells exclusively, that expressed enough of the contact sensitizer to be visualized in the fluorescence-activated cell sorter (Macatonia *et al.*, 1987) and to stimulate an antigen-specific T cell response (Macatonia *et al.*, 1986).

Protein antigens have also been studied and found to be associated with dendritic cells. Kyewski *et al.* (1986) noted that both spleen and thymic dendritic cells from mice that were given 4 mg of myoglobin intravenously could stimulate a myoglobin-specific $CD4^+$ clone. Holt *et al.* (1987) aerosolized ovalbumin into the rat airway and enriched for dendritic cells that could present to ovalbumin-primed T cells. The enrichment procedure required that macrophages be depleted. Bujdoso *et al.* (1989) showed that dendritic cells in afferent lymph from sheep that were boosted with ovalbumin could also carry enough ligand to stimulate ovalbumin-specific T cell lines. We have recently employed the myoglobin-specific clones of Livingstone and Fathman (Morel *et al.*, 1987) to show that spleen dendritic cells are the major cell type in the spleen that carries myoglobin in an immunostimulatory form following intravenous injection of antigen (Inaba *et al.*, 1989).

These initial considerations on antigen uptake by dendritic cells *in situ*, followed by movement to lymphoid organs, are amenable to some direct experiments. It will be of interest to trace the movements of different types of APCs particularly those laden with antigen, and to relate the localization of injected APCs, to the site at which T cells are actually responding. Also, one needs to evaluate what kinds of antigens can be associated with dendritic cells for immunization *in situ*.

Once lymphoblasts are generated in lymphoid organs, they leave via the efferent lymph. Lymphoblasts do not recirculate, and they seem to preferentially leave the circulation in inflammatory sites (Ottaway and Parrott, 1979; Koster *et al.*, 1971). This would focus the blasts on areas carrying the original antigen and presumably APCs such as macrophages and B cells.

C. APC-T CELL BINDING

1. APC–T Cell Clusters Generate Primary Responses in Vitro

A salient feature of dendritic cell function in primary antibody and MLR responses *in vitro* is that both responses occur in stable aggregates of dendritic cells and lymphocytes (Inaba *et al.*, 1984; Inaba and Steinman, 1984, 1985, 1987a; Flechner *et al.*, 1988). The most obvious parameter that is deficient in the APC function of macrophages, monocytes. and B cells in these primary responses is their inability to form these aggregates. Lipscomb and co-workers have found that HLA-DR$^+$ alveolar macrophages are poor stimulators of the human MLR (Lipscomb *et al.*, 1986) and also attribute this to an inability to cluster T cells (Lyons *et al.*, 1986). Thus, the capacity of dendritic cells to bind T cells may be the rate-limiting step for the onset of many T cell-dependent immune responses.

In the MLR dendritic cells aggregate most of the antigen-reactive T cells within 1 day *in vitro* (Inaba *et al.*, 1984; Flechner *et al.*, 1988). This entry of antigen-reactive T cells into dendritic cell clusters is the only example we know of that illustrates the efficiency of the *in vitro* immune response and does so in a way that is comparable to that which occurs *in situ*. It has been shown that antigen-reactive cells are efficiently depleted from the circulation within a day of exposure to antigen *in situ* (Ford *et al.*, 1975; Rowley *et al.*, 1972), presumably because helper-type T cells are trapped in those lymphoid organs that have APCs bearing the specific ligand.

When B blasts, rather than resting B cells, are used to present MHC or Mls antigens (see Section IV,B and C), the B blasts aggregate the T cells, which then enlarge and synthesize DNA. The efficiency with which B blasts enter clusters is less than that exhibited by dendritic cells, since most B blasts are in the noncluster fraction, whereas most dendritic cells in the culture are in the aggregates (Metlay *et al.*, 1989). What are some of the components that lead to the formation of APC–T cell clusters?

2. Cell Motility

One distinctive feature of dendritic cells, which may influence their capacity to find infrequent clones of antigen-specific T cells, is their capacity to form and retract cell processes, particularly broad veils which are 10 μm or more in extension. This has been evident from the very first observations of living dendritic cells (Steinman and Cohn, 1973; Drexhage *et al.*, 1979). At this time we have not observed the formation of comparable cell processes in B cells, B blasts, macrophages, or monocytes (Freudenthal and R. M. Steinman, unpublished observations). The capacity to form cell processes may allow the dendritic cell to probe for T cells, which then are temporarily immobilized by an antigen-independent mechanism, to be discussed below.

3. Dendritic Cell–T Cell Binding Mechanisms

A critical unknown is whether recognition of antigen on the dendritic cell is the first signal to bring APCs and T cells together. We have reasoned (Inaba and Steinman, 1986, 1987b; Metlay et al., 1989) that antigen recognition may not be the very first step in binding. It may be hard for complementarity to occur when the MHC–peptide complex and TCR are affixed to cell surfaces. There is no freely diffusable ligand, as in many other receptor systems that have been studied. The chance for complementarity would be enhanced if the APCs could actively move about, forming transient conjugates with the T cell, after which recognition might occur. One also must consider the limitations that are imposed if the amount of any one specific MHC–peptide complex on the APCs is low and the frequency of antigen-specific T cells is also low.

That dendritic cell–T cell interactions have an antigen-independent component is manifest in two types of experiment. One involves rapid 10- to 20-minute binding assays between dendritic cells and T blasts that have a defined antigen and MHC specificity (Inaba and Steinman, 1986). When the binding assays are done on ice, the interaction is both efficient and antigen dependent, but when the assays are done at 37°C, extensive binding is observed in the absence of antigen. No signaling, i.e., a T cell response, is evident, however, without antigen (Inaba and Steinman, 1986; Inaba et al., 1985). The dendritic cell–T cell binding at 37°C in the presence or absence of antigen is so rapid that it is hard to determine whether antigen influences the initial binding rate.

Recently, it has been noted that cultured, but not freshly isolated, LCs, can bind small resting T lymphocytes (Inaba et al., 1989a). If one sediments LCs and T cells and incubates them at 37°C for 3 hours, most of the LCs in the tube form conjugates with the T cells. There are about ten to 20 T cells per LC. The clustered T cells can be shown to be competent by adding anti-CD3 Mab and observing lymphoblast formation, DNA synthesis, and mitosis. Over a 3-hour period the extent of clustering in the presence or absence of ligand, here anti-CD3 presented by FcγRII on the LCs, seems equally intense. It is the subsequent induction of T cell growth, not binding, that requires ligation of the TCR. In contrast, macrophages do not bind T cells unless FcγRII and anti-CD3 are available.

Inaba et al. (1986, 1989a) found that LCs only acquired antigen-independent T cell binding capacity after several days in culture.

Therefore, this binding capacity develops after the time that the LCs are capable of processing antigen, which is the first day of culture (Romani *et al.*, 1989c).

We suspect that dendritic cells express an adhesion molecule that allows them to temporarily bind to T cells. This adhesion molecule does not seem to be LFA-1, since antibodies to LFA-1 do not block the initial binding (Inaba and Steinman, 1987b; Metlay *et al.*, 1989). Anti-LFA-1 does affect DNA synthesis and cluster stability after the dendritic cell–T cell aggregate has formed.

The dendritic cell adhesion mechanism may be down-regulated after cluster formation, perhaps after LFA-1 has been engaged. If clusters are allowed to form in the presence of anti-LFA-1, and are then disassembled by pipetting, they do not reform (Inaba and Steinman, 1987b). This implies that the original binding mechanism has been down-regulated, which in turn would limit the dendritic cell from trying to find other T cells after specific antigen-reactive T cells have been identified.

Therefore, the formation and function of dendritic cell–T cell aggregates in the primary MLR may involve at least three molecular interactions acting in sequence (steps 1–3 in Fig. 2): (1) an initial antigen-independent system that is not LFA-1 but has yet to be identified, (2) antigens presented to the T cell clonotypic receptor, and (3) LFA-1/ICAM. The onset of this clustering sequence in turn may be preceded *in situ* by distinct steps involving antigen acquisition/presentation, migration to the T cell area, and motility/cell process formation within the T area.

4. B Cell–T Cell Binding Mechanisms

In contrast to dendritic cell-mediated clustering, the formation of large clusters between B blasts and T cells is fully blocked when anti-LFA-1 is added to the primary MLR (Metlay *et al.*, 1989). Anti-LFA-1 also blocks the binding of hapten (TNP)-specific B cells to carrier-specific T cells in the presence of TNP-KLH (Sanders *et al.*, 1987). The anti-LFA-1 could be acting at the level of the B or T cell, since both express LFA-1. It has been reported that resting human T cells lack ICAM-1 (Dougherty *et al.*, 1989), which would argue that LFA-1 on the T cell is required first. It is also possible that ICAM-1 is found at low levels on T cells or is rapidly up-regulated, in which case LFA-1 on the B cell is important in binding.

As in the case of dendritic cell–T cell binding, LFA-1 may only become functional and stabilize the B cell–T cell interaction after antigen recognition has taken place in the primary MLR (Fig. 2). Wright, Detmers *et al.* have shown that the binding function of the leukocyte integrins, CD11a and CD11b, can be regulated by environmental stimuli. CR3 on

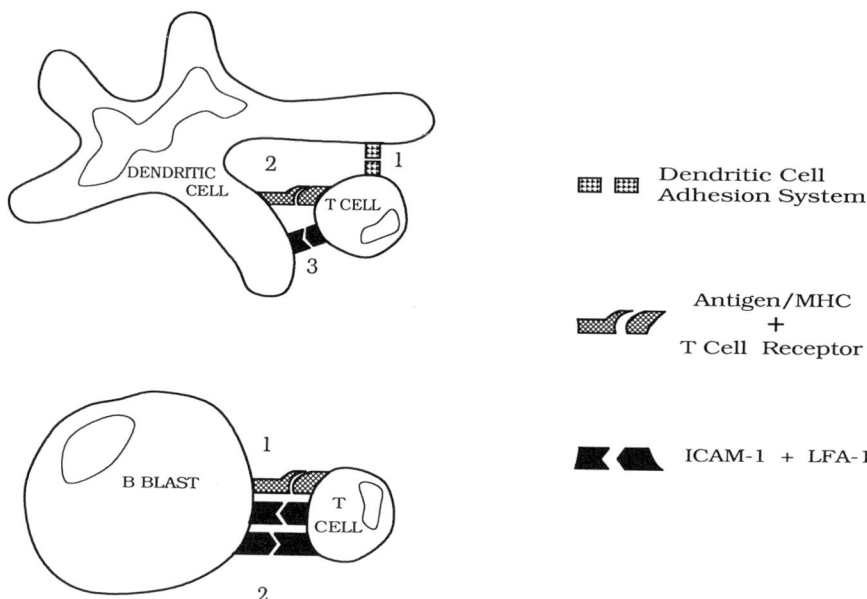

FIG. 2. Diagram of the interactions required for dendritic cells and B cells to form stable aggregates with T cells. As explained in the text, it is thought that the dendritic cell contacts the T cell first by an antigen-independent mechanism. Step 2 involves recognition of presented antigen, and step 3 represents the adhesion via LFA-1 on the T cell. Antigen recognition may be the first step in the B cell–T cell interaction, and this is followed by an interaction between LFA-1 and ICAM-1 which can be expressed on either cell type.

macrophages can be up-regulated by phorbol myristic acetate (PMA) (Wright and Silverstein, 1982) or fibronectin (Wright et al., 1984), and down-regulated by IFN-γ (Wright et al., 1986). Regulation of CR3 on neutrophils involves changes in the state of receptor aggregation more than alterations in receptor numbers (Detmers et al., 1987).

If LFA-1 is nonfunctional on the resting T cell, then T cell recognition of antigen on the B cell may lead to LFA-1 activation and LFA-1-dependent binding between B and T cells. As discussed above, an antigen-dependent binding system would be inefficient if only small amounts of specific MHC–peptide complexes were present on the B blast surface and if one were dealing with infrequent clones of antigen-specific B cells and T cells. These limitations may not pertain to *in vitro* models in which B blast–resting T cell clustering have been identified (Metlay et al., 1989). By using anti-Ig as the activation stimulus, large numbers of presenting B cells are available. Since MLR and Mls loci have been studied, sizable amounts of presented antigen may be present on B blasts, and large numbers of reactive T cell clones recognize allo-MHC and Mls.

The other pathway that generates B cell–T cell conjugates is to activate the T cell with a dendritic cell, and then the T blast can bind and stimulate other APCs, both macrophages and B cells (Inaba and Steinman, 1984, 1985; Koide and Steinman, 1988; Bhardwaj et al., 1989). MHC-restricted T blasts were generated in the primary MLR or in primary responses to carrier proteins such as KLH and ovalbumin. A dose of only 1000–3000 T blasts were then required to trigger an optimal antibody response in cultures of $2-3 \times 10^6$ B cells (Inaba and Steinman, 1984, 1985). Thus, the efficiency of the T blast in functional readouts seems very high. The mechanism of B cell–T blast clustering has not been studied.

Not only can T blasts bind and activate B cells, but the B cells are active APCs for further growth of the T blasts. In this way a response that is initiated by dendritic cells can be further expanded by B cells, as long as the appropriate MHC–peptide complexes are present.

D. Induction of T Cell Growth and Gene Expression

1. Clonal Expansion and Lymphocyte-Activating Factors

In studies of the MLR it has been found that B blasts and dendritic cells, after they have made contact with the T lymphocyte, are roughly similar in their capacity to induce DNA synthesis (Metlay et al., 1989). The MLR studies measured DNA synthesis over a short term. Further studies are needed to test the role of APCs in triggering long-term clonal growth. A recent study indicates that dendritic cells are much more active than are monocytes or small resting B cells in supplying a needed accessory function for T cell cloning (Langhoff and Steinman, 1989). The clones were raised in the presence of a lectin phytohemagglutinin, and exogenous growth factors, so that the dendritic cell may be serving some function in addition to clustering the T cell or inducing lymphokine production. It was suggested that dendritic cells supply a signal that is required for long-term growth. EBV-transformed B cell lines were just as active as dendritic cells in supporting T cell cloning, so that it will be of interest to evaluate primary populations of B lymphoblasts as APCs for clonal expansion.

For some time it has been thought that IL-1 must be produced by the APCs to activate the T cell to produce growth factors or to become responsive to growth factors. More recently, there has been evidence for a more restricted effect of IL-1 on T cells, i.e., that IL-1 only acts on the T_H2 subset of helper cells and only to enhance responsiveness to the growth factor IL-4 (Kurt-Jones et al., 1987; Lightman et al., 1989). As yet, these studies have not been extended to primary cells.

The role of IL-1 in dendritic cell function provides another view on the role of this cytokine. IL-1 is not produced by dendritic cells, from either mice or humans (Bhardwaj et al., 1988, 1989; Koide and Steinman, 1987; Hart and McKenzie, 1988), and a neutralizing anti-IL-1 antibody does not block dendritic cell function (Inaba et al., 1988; Bhardwaj et al., 1989). However, exogenous IL-1 can enhance the function of dendritic cells but at the level of the dendritic cell and not the T cell directly (Koide et al., 1987; Inaba et al., 1988; Heufler et al., 1987). If dendritic cells are cultured in IL-1 for 8 hours or more and washed, their stimulatory function increases some threefold, and this cannot be ascribed to a carryover of IL-1 into the culture with T cells.

The question of there being additional factors that could act independently to activate the T cell has been addressed in recent two-chamber experiments. Clusters of interacting LCs and anti-CD3-stimulated T cells were placed on one side of a 0.4 µm filter, with anti-CD3-coated T cells on the other side. While IL-2 was produced by the clusters and diffused across the filter, the anti-CD3-coated T cells did not blast transform or synthesize DNA (Inaba et al., 1989a). This shows that even when a TCR is occupied by a ligand, one cannot demonstrate soluble dendritic cell-dependent factors that costimulate.

IL-1 production by primary B cell populations has not been detected (Bhardwaj et al., 1988; Koide and Steinman, 1987). There is recent evidence for the production of another cytokine, IL-6, by tonsillar B cells (Schriever et al., 1989). IL-6 has been implicated as a T cell-activating factor for the IL-2-dependent T cell proliferation of mouse T cells in the presence of Con A (Garman et al., 1987).

2. Two Signals for the Induction of Lymphokine Gene Expression

A striking feature to emerge from the study of polyclonal stimuli, i.e., mitogens rather than specific antigens, is that most mitogens require an accessory, or second, signal. Lectins, periodate, and anti-T cell antibodies (including those to the clonotypic receptor and anti-CD3) all require an accessory cell, or the tumor promoter PMA. The critical response that requires two signals is the induction of lymphokine gene expression, including IL-2, IL-4, and IFN-γ (Weiss et al., 1986; Granelli-Piperno et al., 1986; Granelli-Piperno and Keane, 1988). Recent observations reveal that in the primary MLR, both dendritic cells and B blasts are active in inducing the release of active lymphokines into the medium (Puré et al., 1988).

Two broad explanations are often put forth to explain the need for accessory cells or PMA, in addition to MHC–peptide complex, for inducing lymphokine gene expression. One is that those TCRs that have bound ligand must also be cross-linked to signal the cytoplasm. This may occur by clustering of ligands on the APC surface or by some signal that proceeds via an intermediate that is phosphorylated by protein kinase C, the presumed immediate target for PMA. If one places T cells on plates that are coated with anti-CD3, or if one applies anti-CD3 and a cross-linking anti-Ig, extensive DNA synthesis does ensue (Geppert and Lipsky, 1987). Can there be enough antigen on an APC to mimic these experimental models? One could argue that the levels of any one MHC–peptide complex is low, since antigen processing likely generates a large number of different peptides, and many of the MHC molecules on an APC may already be occupied by different peptides produced from within the APC or in its surroundings. On the other hand, one could envisage a relatively high density of MHC–peptide complexes. B cells and dendritic cells may primarily present peptides that they acquire simultaneously with the synthesis of large numbers of new MHC molecules, and the number of different proteins that these APCs internalize may be relatively few (see Sections III,A, IV,A and IV,D).

Another basis for the two-signal requirement is that the accessory cell, or PMA, induces a distinct signal that synergizes with that delivered by antigen and the TCR–CD3ζ complex—in contrast to the first mechanism, whereby the second signal acts to aggregate the TCR complex. There is still little direct evidence on these possibilities with physiological APCs.

Thus, the mechanism of T cell activation, after APC–T cell contacts have been established, is not understood. As yet, there is no evidence that dendritic cells or B blasts differ fundamentally by the criteria that have been analyzed to date, such as production of IL-1 and triggering of T cell growth and lymphokine production. Where dendritic cells and B cells show major differences are in the other aspects of APC function described above, e.g., how and where antigens are acquired, how the expression of class I and class II MHC products are regulated, movements *in situ*, and mechanisms for binding T cells.

VII. Conclusion—Consequences of Having Two Different Types of APCs

A. IMMUNOGENICITY

Both dendritic cells and B lymphocytes play important but distinct roles in immunogenicity. Antigen presentation by dendritic cells provides an efficient pathway for inducing large numbers of active and specific T lymphoblasts, from both $CD4^+$ and $CD8^+$ subsets, while presentation by B cells is essential for helper T cell-dependent antibody formation.

We have reviewed the many specializations that would allow dendritic cells to pick up antigens and initiate immune responses *in situ*. (1) Dendritic cells are widely distributed and are found in many nonlymphoid organs, where antigens typically gain access to the body (see Section II,E). (2) These nonlymphoid dendritic cells in particular can capture antigen (see Sections IV,A and B), and at the same time up-regulate expression of cell surface class I and class II MHC products to levels that are the highest seen on any cell type (see Section III,A). Together, these features should generate relatively high amounts of MHC-peptide complexes at the place where antigens are deposited. However, substantial levels of exogenous antigens may be necessary to charge the dendritic cell, >1 μM, if current *in vitro* data are a guide. An unexplored possibility is that the FcRs on nonlymphoid dendritic cells, perhaps via natural antibodies, can be used to enhance antigen uptake. (3) Dendritic cells are prominent in the afferent lymph and can home to the T cell area via the blood or afferent lymph (see Section II). There is evidence that dendritic cells can carry antigen to the lymphoid organ (see Section VI,B). In the T cell area, these APCs would be in the path of the recirculating T cell pool and thereby in the best position to select antigen-specific clones. There is no evidence that dendritic cells leave the draining lymphoid organ. This would account for the fact that sensitized T cells primarily arise in the lymphoid tissue that drains the site of antigen deposition, but not other lymphoid organs. (4) Dendritic cells can down-regulate antigen uptake and processing (see Section IV,A), perhaps en route to the T cell area, so that antigens acquired in the tissues would not be displaced by endocytosis and processing of self-antigens in the protein-rich fluid of the lymphatic system. (5) Dendritic cells are motile and efficiently capture antigen-specific T cells (see Section VI,C). It is proposed that dendritic cells quickly survey T cells, via a reversible antigen and an LFA-1 independent mechanism, and then retain the T cell if there is complementarity between the presented antigen and the clonotypic receptor.

The initial studies of lymphoid dendritic cells, as in mouse spleen and rat lymph and lymph node, suggested that dendritic cells were constitutively prepared to present antigens. More recent observations on epidermal LCs indicate that many critical aspects of dendritic cell function are regulated at the sites where antigens are deposited. Nonlymphoid dendritic cells, like epidermal LCs, may be immunologically inactive. With the deposition of antigen, many of the specializations in dendritic cell function listed above may come under regulatory controls. GM-CSF and IL-1 are two cytokines that have been implicated in amplifying dendritic cell function *in vitro*. These molecules are inducible products of many different cells such as fibroblasts, endothelium, keratinocytes, and macrophages. We propose that these cytokines need to be induced at the site of antigen deposition in order to activate local dendritic cells and initiate the immune response.

Dendritic cells are not known to have effector functions which would lead to the removal of antigen. Dendritic cells do not make Ig, and they are nonphagocytic. No cytokines are yet known to be produced by these cells. Therefore, when dendritic cells present antigen, the effect seems to be unidirectional on the T cell, generating large numbers of antigen-specific lymphoblasts.

Antigen presentation by B cells is bidirectional in its consequences. Many of the important functions of the B cell can be influenced by the T cell and lymphokine products such as IL-4, IL-5, and IL-6. There is evidence that the B cell must interact with the T cell before that B cell can respond to helper lymphokines (see Section V,B). Presentation in turn triggers the T cell to produce the required lymphokines. The latter would influence clonal growth of the B cell, high-level Ig secretion, switching of Ig isotypes, and perhaps somatic mutation to produce higher-affinity antibodies.

Like the dendritic cell, the APC function of B cells is regulated. The main control involves binding and processing of the specific antigen to which antibody ultimately will be secreted. Binding of antigen may also trigger the B cell to synthesize new class II MHC molecules and cell surface adhesion molecules, such as LFA-1 and ICAM-1.

B cells, by having access to the germinal center, also have access to the most long-lived pool of native antigen that has been described, i.e., immune complexes that persist extracellularly on follicular dendritic cells. B cells also have the receptors that would allow binding of antigens and immune complexes in the circulation, with subsequent carriage to the lymphoid organ. We have reasoned that the occurrence of B cells in the extravascular spaces of nonlymphoid organs may be too infrequent to allow this type of APC to play a major role in capturing antigens in many tissues where antigens are deposited.

The efficacy of B cell presentation can be improved at the level of either the B or T cell. By clonal expansion, and by increasing the affinity of antibodies through somatic mutation, APC function is increased. Both changes are part of the memory, or secondary, response. At the level of the T cell, it is evident that T blasts are much more efficient in at interacting with B cells than with resting T lymphocytes. Another regulation could occur at the level of functional helper T cell subsets and the attendant production of different lymphokines.

What is far from clear is whether B cells participate as APCs in nonspecific antigen presentation, i.e., in triggering immune responses to proteins which the B cell does not bind via surface Ig. Many of the existing data on this question derive from LPS-induced B blasts or transformed B cell lines, rather than from more physiological populations. We have discussed the possibility that primary B cells are not capable of handling nonspecific antigens in the manner shown by dendritic cells, and that this may occur through the weak capacities of B cells to internalize antigens in bulk.

Nor is it clear whether B cells play a role in presenting antigens to those T cells that become CTLs or that mediate macrophage activation and DTH. Again, it may not be possible for the B cell to present particulate and cell-associated antigens in these types of T cell responses.

B. Autoimmunity/Hypersensitivity

An intriguing feature of antigen presentation, as it is now understood, is that exogenous peptides can bind to MHC molecules on the surface of APCs. If small B cells were constitutively active as APCs and had access to peptides, there would be the formation of nonspecific Ig and perhaps autoantibody. That is, helper T cells would react with B cells that were presenting peptides totally unrelated to the antigens whose B cells would specifically bind via surface Ig receptors. A danger for nonspecificity would also occur if macrophages could induce primary immune responses in the same fashion as dendritic cells. For example, macrophages can make cytokines and reactive oxygen intermediates when activated by T cells. Again, it would seem important to restrict the macrophage–T cell interaction to those antigens which the macrophage itself harbors.

Dendritic cells do not have the effector functions of B cells and macrophages, so that when they present antigen, the consequence is the production of T blasts and not the release of Ig or reactive oxygen intermediates, for example. These T blasts very efficiently react with antigens presented by B cells and macrophages, unlike resting T cells. Tissue specificity during an immune response would arise from the property of the T blast to home to inflammatory sites. T blasts generated in lymphoid organs by antigens on dendritic cells would not have ready access to most APCs, but instead would leave the lymphoid organ via the efferent lymph and encounter macrophages and/or B cells in the inflammatory site where the original antigen is found.

What keeps dendritic cells from presenting autoantigens? This is not known. One mechanism is that the dendritic cell may not be actively acquiring antigens when it is resident in a tissue, or even when it courses though the lymph and T cell area. Another is that the self-antigen, in order to be presented, would have to be abundant at the site where the dendritic cell is capturing exogenous antigens. These two controls would not seem fail-safe, so that the presentation of autoantigens on dendritic cells likely can be controlled in other ways.

C. Regulation of the Immune Response at the Level of APC Function

The emphasis in research on immune responsiveness traditionally has been at the levels of the repertoire of antigen receptors expressed by lymphocytes and, in the case of T cells, on the capacity of antigens to associate with MHC products on the APCs. The material presented in this review emphasizes another important level of control, that of APC physiology and the properties of primary cells particularly *in situ*. For an immune response to occur, one needs not only antigen and a T cell repertoire but an appropriate APC. The processing of antigens, the synthesis of MHC products, the capacity of APCs to bind to specific lymphocytes, and the movement of APCs to gain access to T cells can all be induced or modified. There is every reason to believe that immunogenicity and tolerance in large measure reflect the capacity of the antigen in question, or its mode of administration, to influence APC function at each of these levels.

Acknowledgments

The authors very much appreciate the help of N. Bhardwaj, M. Witmer-Pack, J. Ming, M. Birkeland, and R. Camp in reviewing the manuscript. Supported by NIH grants AI13013, 24450, 25185, 24475 and by Medical Science Training Program 5-T32-GM-07739 to J.M. E.P. is a Pew Scholar in the Biomedical Sciences.

References

Abe, R., and Hodes, R. J. (1988). *Immunol. Today* 9, 230.
Abe, R., Vacchio, M. S., Fox, B., and Hodes, R. J. (1988). *Nature (London)* 335, 827.
Ahmed, A., Scher, I., Smith, A. H., and Sell, K. W. (1977). *J. Immunogenet.* 4, 201.
Akahoshi, T., Oppenheim, J. J., and Matsushima, K. (1988). *J. Exp. Med.* 167, 924.
Allen, P. M., and Unanue, E. R. (1984). *J. Immunol.* 132, 1077.
Allen, P. M., Strydom, D. J., and Unanue, E. R. (1984). *Proc. Natl. Acad. Sci. U.S.A.* 81, 2489.
Ashwell, J. D., DeFranco, A. L., Paul, W. E., and Schwartz, R. H. (1984). *J. Exp. Med.* 159, 881.
Ashwell, J. D., Chen, C., and Schwartz, R. H. (1986). *J. Immunol.* 136, 389.

Austyn, J. M. (1987). *Immunology* **62**, 161.
Austyn, J. M., and Steinman, R. M. (1988). *Transplant. Rev.* **2**, 139.
Austyn, J. M., Kupiec-Weglinski, J. W., Hankins, D. F., and Morris, P. J. (1988). *J. Exp. Med.* **167**, 646.
Barker, J. N., Alegre, V. A., and MacDonald, D. M. (1988). *J. Invest. Dermatol.* **90**, 117.
Berkower, I., Matis, L. A., Buckenmeyer, G. K., Gurd, F. R. N., Longo, D. L., and Berzofsky, J. A. (1984). *J. Immunol.* **132**, 1370.
Berzofsky, J. A. (1988). *J. Clin. Invest.* **82**, 1811.
Bhan, A. K., Nadler, L. M., Stashenko, P., McCluskey, R. T., and Schlossman, S. F. (1981). *J. Exp. Med.* **154**, 737.
Bhardwaj, N., Lau, L., Rivelis, M., and Steinman, R. M. (1988). *Cell. Immunol.* **114**, 405.
Bhardwaj, N., Lau, L. L., Friedman, S. M., Crow, M. K., and Steinman, R. M. (1989). *J. Exp. Med.* **169**, 1121.
Bieber, T., Rieger, A., Neuchrist, C., Prinz, J. C., Rieber, E. P., Boltz-Nitulescu, G., Scheiner, O., Kraft, D., Ring, J., and Stingl, G. (1989). *J. Exp. Med.* **170**, 309.
Birkeland, M. L., Simpson, L., Isakson, P. C., and Puré, E. (1987). *J. Exp. Med.* **166**, 506.
Birkeland, M. L., Metlay, J., Saunders, V., Fernandez-Botran, R., Vitetta, E. S., Steinman, R. M., and Puré, E. (1988). *J. Mol. Cell. Immunol.* **4**, 71.
Birkeland, M. L., Johnson, P., Trowbridge, I. S., and Puré, E. (1989). *Proc. Natl. Acad. Sci. U.S.A.* (in press).
Bjorkman, P. J., Saper, M. A., Samraoui, B., Bennett, W. S., Strominger, J. L., and Wiley, D. C. (1987a). *Nature (London)* **329**, 506.
Bjorkman, P. J., Saper, M. A., Samraoui, B., Bennett, W. S., Strominger, J. L., and Wiley, D. C. (1987b). *Nature (London)* **329**, 512.
Boog, C. J. P., Kast, W. M., Timmers, H. Th. M., Boes, J., De Waal, L. P., and Melief, C. J. M. (1985). *Nature (London)* **318**, 59.
Boog, C. J. P., Boes, J., and Melief, C. J. M. (1988a). *Eur. J. Immunol.* **18**, 219.
Boog, C. J. P., Boes, J., and Melief, C. J. M. (1988b). *J. Immunol.* **140**, 3331.
Boog, C. J. P., Neefjes, J. J., Boes, J., Ploegh, H. L., and Melief, C. J. M. (1989). *Eur. J. Immunol.* **19**, 537.
Bowers, W. E., and Berkowitz, M. R. (1986). *J. Exp. Med.* **163**, 872.
Breathnach, A. S. (1964). *J. Anat.* **98**, 265.
Breel, M., Mebius, R. E., and Kraal, G. (1987). *Eur. J. Immunol.* **17**, 1555.
Brooks, C. F., and Moore, M. (1988). *Immunology* **63**, 303.
Brown, J. H., Jardetzky, T., Saper, M. A., Samraoui, B., Bjorkman, P. J., and Wiley, D. C. (1988). *Nature (London)* **332**, 845.
Bruynzeel-Koomen, C., van Wichen, D. F., Toonstra, J., Berrens, L., and Bruynzeel, P. L. B. (1986). *Arch. Dermatol. Res.* **278**, 199.
Bujdoso, R., Hopkins, J., Dutia, B. M., Young, P., and McConnell, I. (1989). *J. Exp. Med.* (Submitted for publication).
Buus, S., and Werdelin, O. (1986a). *J. Immunol.* **136**, 452.
Buus, S., and Werdelin, O. (1986b). *J. Immunol.* **136**, 459.
Caernielewski, J., Vaigot, P., and Prunieras, M. (1985). *J. Invest. Dermatol.* **84**, 424.
Casten, L. A., and Pierce, S. K. (1988). *J. Immunol.* **140**, 404.
Casten, L. A., Lakey, E. K., Jelachich, M. L., Margoliash, E., and Pierce, S. K. (1985). *Proc. Natl. Acad. Sci. U.S.A.* **17**, 5890.
Casten, L. A., Kaumaya, P., and Pierce, S. K. (1988). *J. Exp. Med.* **168**, 171.
Charbonneau, H., Tonks, N. K., Walsh, K. A., and Fischer, E. H. (1988). *Proc. Natl. Acad. Sci. U.S.A.* **85**, 7182.
Chen, L. L., Adams, J. C., and Steinman, R. M. (1978a). *J. Cell Biol.* **77**, 148.

Chen, L. L., Frank, A. M., Adams, J. C., and Steinman, R. M. (1978b). *J. Cell Biol.* **79**, 184.
Cherwinski, H. M., Schumacher, J. H., Brown, K. D., and Mossman, T. R. (1987). *J. Exp. Med.* **166**, 1229.
Chesnut, R. W., and Grey, H. M. (1981). *J. Immunol.* **126**, 1075.
Chesnut, R. W., and Grey, H. M. (1986). *Adv. Immunol.* **39**, 51.
Chesnut, R. W., Colon, S. M., and Grey, H. M. (1982a). *J. Immunol.* **128**, 1764.
Chesnut, R. W., Colon, S. M., and Grey, H. M. (1982b). *J. Immunol.* **129**, 2382.
Claesson-Welsh, L., Scheynius, A., Tjernlund, U., and Peterson, P. A. (1986). *J. Immunol.* **136**, 484.
Claman, H. N., Chaperon, E. A., and Triplett, R. F. (1966). *Proc. Soc. Exp. Biol. Med.* **122**, 1167.
Clement, L. T., Yamashita, N., and Martin, A. M. (1988). *J. Immunol.* **141**, 1464.
Coffman, R. L., and Weissman, I. L. (1981). *Nature (London)* **289**, 681.
Corradin, G., and Chiller, J. M. (1979). *J. Exp. Med.* **149**, 436.
Cowing, C., and Chapdelaine, J. N. (1983). *Proc. Natl. Acad. Sci. U.S.A.* **80**, 6000.
Crowley, M., Inaba, K., Witmer-Pack, M., and Steinman, R. M. (1989). *Cell. Immunol.* **118**, 108.
Daar, A., Fuggle, S., Hart, D. N. J., Dalchau, R., Abdulaziz, Z., Fabre, J. W., Ting, A., and Morris, P. J. (1983). *Transplantation* **15**, 311.
Dalchau, R., and Fabre, J. W. (1981). *J. Exp. Med.* **153**, 753.
Davies, A. J. S., Leuchers, E., Wallis, V., Marchant, R., and Elliot, E. V. (1967). *Transplantation* **5**, 222.
Davis, M. M., and Bjorkman, P. J. (1988). *Nature (London)* **334**, 395.
DeFrance, T., Aubry, J. P., Rousset, F., Vanbervliet, B., Bonnefoy, J. Y., Arai, N., Takebe, Y., Yokota, T., Lee, F., Arai, K., DeVries, J., and Banchereau, J. (1987). *J. Exp. Med.* **165**, 1459.
Detmers, P. A., Wright, S. D., Olsen, E., Kimball, B., and Cohn, Z. A. (1987). *J. Cell Biol.* **105**, 1137.
Dijkstra, C. D. (1982). *Res: J. Reticuloendothel. Soc.* **32**, 167.
Dougherty, G. J., Murdoch, S., and Hogg, N. (1989). *Eur. J. Immunol.* **18**, 35.
Drexhage, H. A., Mullink, H., de Groot, J., Clarke, J., and Balfour, B. M. (1979). *Cell Tissue Res.* **202**, 407.
Duijvestijn, A. M., Schutte, R., Kohler, Y. G., Korn, C., and Hoefsmit, E. C. M. (1983). *Cell Tissue Res.* **231**, 313.
Dustin, M. L., Rothlein, R., Bhan, A. K., Dinarello, C. A., and Springer, T. A. (1986). *J. Immunol.* **137**, 245.
Eikelenboom, P. (1978). *Cell Tissue Res.* **195**, 445.
Fathman, C. G., and Frelinger, J. G. (1983). *Annu. Rev. Immunol.* **1**, 633.
Fathman, C. G., Handwerger, B. S., and Sachs, D. A. (1974). *J. Exp. Med.* **140**, 853.
Faustman, D. L., Steinman, R. M., Gebel, H. M., Hauptfeld, V., Davie, J. M., and Lacy, P. E. (1984). *Proc. Natl. Acad. Sci. U.S.A.* **81**, 3864.
Flechner, E., Freudenthal, P., Kaplan, G., and Steinman, R. M. (1988). *Cell. Immunol.* **111**, 183.
Fleidner, T. M., Kesse, M., Cronkite, E. P., and Robertson, J. S. (1964). *Ann. N. Y. Acad. Sci.* **113**, 578.
Forbes, R. D. C., Parfrey, N. A., Gomersall, M., Darden, A. G., and Guttmann, R. D. (1986). *J. Exp. Med.* **164**, 1239.
Ford, W. L., Simmonds, S. J., and Atkins, R. C. (1975). *J. Exp. Med.* **141**, 681.
Fossum, S. (1980). *Scand. J. Immunol.* **12**, 433.

Fossum, S. (1984). *Scand. J. Immunol.* **19**, 49.
Fossum, S. (1988). *Scand. J. Immunol.* **27**, 97.
Fossum, S. (1989). *In* "Current Topics in Pathology" (O. H. Ivessen, ed.), p. 101. Springer-Verlag, Berlin.
Fossum, S., and Rolstad, B. (1986). *Eur. J. Immunol.* **16**, 440.
Fossum, S., Smith, M. E., Bell, E. B., and Ford, W. L. (1980). *Scand. J. Immunol.* **12**, 421.
Francotte, M., and Urbain, J. (1985). *Proc. Natl. Acad. Sci. U.S.A.* **82**, 8149.
Freitas, A. A., and Coutinho, A. (1981). *J. Exp. Med.* **154**, 994.
Frelinger, J. G., Hood, L., Hill, S., and Frelinger, J. A. (1979). *Nature (London)* **282**, 321.
Frey, J. R., and Wenk, P. (1957). *Int. Arch. Allergy Appl. Immunol.* **11**, 81.
Frohman, M., and Cowing, C. (1985). *J. Immunol.* **134**, 2269.
Garman, R. D., Jacobs, K. A., Clark, S. C., and Raulet, D. H. (1987). *Proc. Natl. Acad. Sci. U.S.A.* **84**, 7629.
Gaudernack, G., and Bjercke, S. (1985). *Scand. J. Immunol.* **21**, 493.
Geppert, T. D., and Lipsky, P. E. (1987). *J. Immunol.* **138**, 1660.
Geuze, H. J., Stoorvogel, W., Strous, G. J., Slot, J. W., Bleekemolen, J. E., and Mellman, I. (1988). *J. Cell Biol.* **107**, 2491.
Glimcher, L. H., Kim, K.-J., Green, I., and Paul, W. E. (1982). *J. Exp. Med.* **155**, 445.
Granelli-Piperno, A., and Keane, M. (1988). *Transplant. Proc.* **20**, 136.
Granelli-Piperno, A., Inaba, K., and Steinman, R. M. (1984). *J. Exp. Med.* **160**, 1792.
Granelli-Piperno, A., Andrus, L., and Steinman, R. M. (1986). *J. Exp. Med.* **163**, 922.
Green, J., and Jotte, R. (1985). *J. Exp. Med.* **162**, 1546.
Gschnait, F., and Brenner, W. (1979). *J. Invest. Dermatol.* **73**, 566.
Guillet, J.-G., Lai, M.-Z., Briner, T. J., Smith, J. A., and Gefter, M. L. (1986). *Nature (London)* **324**, 260.
Haines, K. A., Flotte, T. J., Springer, T. A., Gigli, I., and Thorbecke, G. J. (1983). *Proc. Natl. Acad. Sci. U.S.A.* **80**, 3448.
Hamilos, D. L., Mascali, J. J., Chesnut, R. W., Young, R. M., Ishioka, G., and Grey, H. M. (1989). *J. Immunol.* **142**, 1069.
Hanau, D., Fabre, M., Schmitt, D. A., Garaud, J.-C., Pauly, G., Tongio, M.-M., Mayer, S., and Cazenave, J.-P. (1987a). *Proc. Natl. Acad. Sci. U.S.A.* **84**, 2901.
Hanau, D., Fabre, M., Schmitt, D. A., Stampf, J. L., Garaud, J. D., Bieber, T., Grosshans, E., Benezra, C., and Cazenave, J. P. (1987b). *J. Invest. Dermatol.* **89**, 172.
Harding, C. V., and Unanue, E. R. (1989). *J. Immunol.* **142**, 12.
Hart, D. N. J., and McKenzie, J. L. (1988). *J. Exp. Med.* **168**, 157.
Hart, D. N. J., and Fabre, J. W. (1981). *J. Exp. Med.* **154**, 347.
Haskins, K., Kubo, R., White, J., Pigeon, M., Kappler, J., and Marrack, P. (1983). *J. Exp. Med.* **157**, 1149.
Hayakawa, K., and Hardy, R. R. (1988). *J. Exp. Med.* **168**, 1825.
Hayakawa, K., Ishii, R., Yamasaki, K., Kishimoto, T., and Hardy, R. (1987). *Proc. Natl. Acad. Sci. U.S.A.* **84**, 1379.
Heinen, E., Braun, N., Couile, P. G., van Snick, J., Moeremans, M., Cormann, N., Kinet-Denoel, C., and Simar, L. J. (1986). *Eur. J. Immunol.* **16**, 167.
Herzenberg, L. A., Stall, A. M., Lalor, P. A., Sidman, C., Moore, W. A., and Parks, D. R. (1986). *Immunol. Rev.* **93**, 81.
Heufler, C., Koch, F., and Schuler, G. (1987). *J. Exp. Med.* **167**, 700.
Heusermann, U., Stutte, H. J., and Muller-Hermelink, H. K. (1974). *Cell Tissue Res.* **153**, 415.

Hirayama, Y., Inaba, K., Inaba, M., Kato, T., Kitaura, M., Hosokawa, T., Ikehara, S., and Muramatsu, S. (1988). *J. Exp. Med.* **168**, 1443.
Hofman, F. M., Danilovs, J. A., and Taylor, C. R. (1984). *Transplantation* **37**, 590.
Holt, P. G., Schon-Hegrad, M. A., and Oliver, J. (1987). *J. Exp. Med.* **167**, 262.
Hopkins, J., Dutia, B. M., Bujdoso, R., and McConnell, I. (1989). *J. Exp. Med.* (submitted for publication).
Howard, J. C. (1972). *J. Exp. Med.* **135**, 185.
Howard, J. C., Hunt, S. V., and Gowans, J. L. (1972). *J. Exp. Med.* **135**, 200.
Huber, B., Demant, P., and Festenstein, H. (1973). *Transplant. Proc.* **4**, 1377.
Humphrey, J. H., Grennan, D., and Sundaram, V. (1984). *Eur. J. Immunol.* **14**, 859.
Inaba, K., and Steinman, R. M. (1984). *J. Exp. Med.* **160**, 1717.
Inaba, K., and Steinman, R. M. (1985). *Science* **229**, 475.
Inaba, K., and Steinman, R. M. (1986). *J. Exp. Med.* **163**, 247.
Inaba, K., and Steinman, R. M. (1987a). *Cell. Immunol.* **105**, 432.
Inaba, K., and Steinman, R. M. (1987b). *J. Exp. Med.* **165**, 1403.
Inaba, K., Granelli-Piperno, A., and Steinman, R. M. (1983a). *J. Exp. Med.* **158**, 2040.
Inaba, K., Steinman, R. M., Van Voorhis, W. C., and Muramatsu, S. (1983b). *Proc. Natl. Acad. Sci. U.S.A.* **80**, 6041.
Inaba, K., Witmer, M. D., and Steinman, R. M. (1984). *J. Exp. Med.* **160**, 858.
Inaba, K., Koide, S., and Steinman, R. M. (1985). *Proc. Natl. Acad. Sci. U.S.A.* **82**, 7686.
Inaba, K., Schuler, G., Witmer, M. D., Valinsky, J., Atassi, B., and Steinman, R. M. (1986). *J. Exp. Med.* **164**, 605.
Inaba, K., Young, J. W., and Steinman, R. M. (1987). *J. Exp. Med.* **166**, 182.
Inaba, K., Witmer-Pack, M. D., Inaba, M., Muramatsu, S., and Steinman, R. M. (1988). *J. Exp. Med.* **167**, 149.
Inaba, K., Romani, N., and Steinman, R. M. (1989a). *J. Exp. Med.* (in press).
Inaba, K. *et al.* (1989b). In preparation.
Ishii, M., Terao, Y., Kitajima, J., and Hamada, T. (1984). *J. Invest. Dermatol.* **82**, 28.
Iwai, H., Kuma, S. I., Inaba, M. M., Good, R. A., Yamashita, T., Kumazawa, T., and Ikehara, S. (1989). *Transplantation* **47**, 45.
Jacobson, E. B., Caporale, L. H., and Thorbecke, G. J. (1974). *Cell. Immunol.* **13**, 416.
Janeway, C. A., Jr., Conrad, P. J., Tite, J., Jones, B., and Murphy, D. B. (1983). *Nature (London)* **306**, 80.
Janeway, C. A., Jr., Ron, J., and Katz, M. E. (1987). *J. Immunol.* **138**, 1051.
Janeway, C. A., Jr., Fischer-Lindahl, K., and Hammerling, U. (1988). *Immunol. Today* **9**, 125.
Janossy, G., Bofill, M., Poulter, L. W., Rawlings, E., Burford, G. D., Navarrete, C., Ziegler, A., and Kelemen, E. (1986). *J. Immunol.* **136**, 4354.
Jensen, P. E. (1988). *J. Immunol.* **141**, 2545.
Johnson, P., Greenbaum, L., Bottomly, K., and Trowbridge, I. S. (1989). *J. Exp. Med.* **169**, 1179.
Kaiserling, E., Stein, H., and Mueller-Hermelink, H. K. (1974). *Cell Tissue Res.* **155**, 47.
Kammer, G. M., and Unanue, E. R. (1980). *Clin. Immunol. Immunopathol.* **15**, 434.
Kaplan, G., Nusrat, A., Witmer, M. D., Nath, I., and Cohn, Z. A. (1987). *J. Exp. Med.* **165**, 763.
Kappler, J. W., Staerz, U., White, J., and Marrack, P. C. (1988). *Nature (London)* **332**, 35.
Kast, W. M., Boog, C. J. P., Roep, B. O., Voordouw, A. C., and Melief, C. J. M. (1988). *J. Immunol.* **140**, 3186.
Katz, D. H., Hamaoka, T., and Benacerraf, B. (1973). *J. Exp. Med.* **137**, 1405.

Katz, D. H., Graves, M., Dorf, M. E., Dimuzio, H., and Benacerraf, B. (1975). *J. Exp. Med.* **141**, 263.
Katz, M. E., and Janeway, C. A., Jr. (1985). *J. Immunol.* **134**, 2064.
Katz, S. I., Tamaki, K., and Sachs, D. H. (1979). *Nature (London)* **282**, 324.
Kawai, J., Inaba, K., Komatusbara, S., Hirayama, Y., Naito, K., and Muramatsu, S. (1987). *Cell. Immunol.* **109**, 1.
Kelly, R. H., Balfour, B. M., Armstrong, J. A., and Griffiths, S. (1978). *Anat. Rec.* **190**, 5.
Kinashi, T., Inaba, K., Tsubata, T., Tashiro, K., Palacios, R., and Honjo, T. (1988). *Proc. Natl. Acad. Sci. U.S.A.* **85**, 4473.
Klein, J. (1986). "Natural History of the Major Histocompatibility Complex." Wiley, New York.
Klinkert, W. E. F., Labadie, J. H., O'Brien, J. P., Beyer, C. F., and Bowers, W. E. (1978). *Proc. Natl. Acad. Sci. U.S.A.* **77**, 5414.
Klinkert, W. E. F., Labadie, J. H., and Bowers, W. E. (1982). *J. Exp. Med.* **156**, 1.
Knight, S. C., Balfour, B. M., O'Brien, J., Buttifant, L., Sumerska, T., and Clark, J. (1982). *Eur. J. Immunol.* **12**, 1057.
Knight, S. C., Mertin, J., Stackpoole, A., and Clark, J. (1983). *Proc. Natl. Acad. Sci. U.S.A.* **80**, 6032.
Knight, S. C., Farrant, J., Bryant, A., Edwards, A. J., Burman, S., Lever, A., Clark, J., and Webster, A. D. B. (1986). *Immunology* **57**, 595.
Knight, S. C., Fryer, P., Griffiths, S., and Harding, B. (1987). *Immunology* **61**, 21.
Koide, S. L., and Steinman, R. M. (1988). *J. Exp. Med.* **168**, 409.
Koide, S. L., and Steinman, R. M. (1987). *Proc. Natl. Acad. Sci. U.S.A.* **84**, 3802.
Koide, S. L., Inaba, K., and Steinman, R. M. (1987). *J. Exp. Med.* **165**, 515.
Kojima, M., Cease, K. B., Buckenmeyer, K., and Berzofsky, J. A. (1988). *J. Exp. Med.* **167**, 1100.
Korngold, R., and Sprent, J. (1978). *J. Exp. Med.* **148**, 1687.
Kosco, M. H., Szakal, A. K., and Tew, J. G. (1988). *J. Immunol.* **140**, 354.
Koster, F. T., McGregor, D. D., and Mackaness, G. B. (1971). *J. Exp. Med.* **133**, 400.
Kraal, G., Breel, M., Janse, M., and Bruin, G. (1986). *J. Exp. Med.* **163**, 981.
Krieger, J. I., Grammer, S. F., Grey, H. M., and Chesnut, R. W. (1985). *J. Immunol.* **135**, 2937.
Krieger, J. I., Chesnut, R. W., and Grey, H. M. (1986). *J. Immunol.* **137**, 3117.
Kuntz-Crow, M., and Kunkel, H. G. (1982). *Clin. Exp. Immunol.* **49**, 338.
Kupiec-Weglinski, J. W., Austyn, J. M., and Morris, P. J. (1988). *J. Exp. Med.* **167**, 632.
Kurt-Jones, E. A., Hamberg, S., O'Hara, J., Paul, W. E., and Abbas, A. K. (1987). *J. Exp. Med.* **166**, 1774.
Kurt-Jones, E. A., Liano, D., HayGlass, K. A., Benacerraf, B., Sy, M.-S., and Abbas, A. K. (1988). *J. Immunol.* **140**, 3773.
Kyewski, B. A., Fathman, C. G., and Rouse, R. V. (1986). *J. Exp. Med.* **163**, 231.
Landsteiner, K., and Chase, M. W. (1939). *J. Exp. Med.* **69**, 767.
Langhoff, E., and Steinman, R. M. (1989). *J. Exp. Med.* **169**, 315.
Lanzavecchia, A. (1985). *Nature (London)* **314**, 537.
Lassila, O., Vainio, O., and Matzinger, P. (1988). *Nature (London)* **334**, 253.
Lechler, R. I., and Batchelor, J. R. (1982). *J. Exp. Med.* **155**, 31.
Lee, P., Matsueda, G. R., and Allen, P. M. (1988). *J. Immunol.* **140**, 1063.
Lenz, A., Heufler, C., Hammensee, H. G., Glassl, H., Koch, F., Romani, N., and Schuler, G. (1989). *Proc. Natl. Acad. Sci. U.S.A.* (submitted for publication).
Lightman, A. H., Chin, J., Schmidt, J. A., and Abbas, A. K. (1989). *Proc. Natl. Acad. Sci. U.S.A.* **85**, 9699.

Ling, N. R., Maclennan, I. C. M., and Mason, D. Y. (1987). In "Leukocyte Typing III: White Cell Differentiation Antigens" (A. J. McMichael et al., eds.). Oxford Univ. Press, London and New York.
Lipscomb, M. F., Lyons, C. R., Nunez, G., Ball, E. J., Stastny, P., Vial, W., Lem, V., Weissler, J., Miller, L. M., and Toews, G. B. (1986). J. Immunol. 136, 497.
Livingstone, A. M., and Fathman, C. G. (1987). Annu. Rev. Immunol. 5, 477.
Lyons, C. R., Ball, E. J., Toews, G. B., Weissler, J. C., Stastny, P., and Lipscomb, M. F. (1986). J. Immunol. 137, 1173.
Macatonia, S. E., Edwards, A. J., and Knight, S. C. (1986). Immunology 59, 509.
Macatonia, S. E., Knight, S. C., Edwards, A. J., Griffiths, S., and Fryer, P. (1987). J. Exp. Med. 166, 1654.
Macatonia, S. E., Taylor, P. M., Knight, S. D., and Askonas, B. A. (1989). J. Exp. Med. 169, 1255.
MacDonald, H. R., Schneider, R., Lees, R. K., Howe, R. C., Acha-Orbea, H., Festenstein, H., Zinkernagel, R. M., and Hengartner, H. (1988). Nature (London) 332, 40.
Mackay, C. R., Kimpton, W. G., Brandon, M. R., and Cahill, R. N. P. (1988). J. Exp. Med. 167, 1755.
MacKenzie, I. C. (1975). Am. J. Anat. 144, 127.
MacLennan, I. C. M., and Gray, D. (1986). Immunol. Rev. 91, 61.
MacLennan, I. C. M., Gray, D., Kumararatne, D. S., and Bazin, H. (1982). Immunol. Today 3, 305.
Malissen, M., Trucy, J., Letourneur, F., Rebai, N., Dunn, D. E., Fitch, F. W., Hood, L., and Malissen, B. (1988). Cell (Cambridge, Mass.) 55, 49.
Marlin, S. D., and Springer, T. A. (1987). Cell (Cambridge, Mass.) 51, 813.
Marrack, P., and Kappler, J. W. (1978). J. Exp. Med. 147, 1596.
Maryanski, J. L., Pala, P., Cerottini, J.-C., and Corradin, G. J. (1988). J. Exp. Med. 167, 1391.
Mason, D. W., Pugh, C. W., and Webb, M. (1981). Immunology 44, 75.
Mayrhofer, G., Pugh, C. W., and Barclay, A. N. (1983). Eur. J. Immunol. 13, 112.
Mayrhofer, P., Holt, P. G., and Papdimitriou, J. M. (1986). Immunology 58, 379.
McKean, D. J., Infante, A. J., Nilson, A., Kimoto, M., Fathman, C. G., Walker, E., and Warner, N. (1981). J. Exp. Med. 154, 1419.
McKenzie, J. L., Beard, M. E. J., and Hart, D. N. J. (1984). Transplant. Proc. 38, 371.
McMichael, A. et al. (1987). In "Leukocyte Typing III: White Cell Differentiation Antigens" (A. J. McMichael et al., eds.). Oxford Univ. Press, London and New York.
Mellman, I. S., Steinman, R. M., Unkeless, J. C., and Cohn, Z. A. (1980). J. Cell Biol. 86, 712.
Mellman, I. S., Plutner, H., Steinman, R. M., Unkeless, J. C., and Cohn, Z. A. (1983). J. Cell Biol. 96, 887.
Metlay, J. P., Puré, E., and Steinman, R. M. (1989). J. Exp. Med. 169, 239.
Miller, J. F. A. P., and Mitchell, G. F. (1968). J. Exp. Med. 128, 801.
Mita, S., Harada, N., Naomi, S., Hitoshi, Y., Sakamoto, K., Akagi, M., Tominaga, A., and Takatsu, K. (1988). J. Exp. Med. 168, 863.
Mitchell, G. F., and Miller, J. F. A. P. (1968). J. Exp. Med. 128, 821.
Mitchison, N. A. (1955). J. Exp. Med. 102, 157.
Mitchison, N. A. (1971). Eur. J. Immunol. 1, 18.
Miyama-Inaba, M., Kuma, S.-I., Inaba, K., Ogata, H., Iwai, H., Yasumizu, R., Muramatsu, S., Steinman, R. M., and Ikehara, S. (1988). J. Exp. Med. 168, 811.
Molnar-Kimber, K., and Sprent, J. (1980). J. Exp. Med. 151, 407.
Monroe, J. G., and Cambier, J. C. (1983a). J. Immunol. 130, 626.
Monroe, J. G., and Cambier, J. C. (1983b). J. Immunol. 131, 2641.
Monroe, J. G., and Cambier, J. C. (1983c). J. Exp. Med. 158, 1589.

Morel, P. A., Livingstone, A. M., and Fathman, C. G. (1987). *J. Exp. Med.* **166**, 583.
Morimoto, C., Letvin, N. L., Boyd, A. W., Hagan, M., Brown, H. M., Kornacki, M. M., and Schlossman, S. F. (1985). *J. Immunol.* **134**, 3762.
Muller, W. A., Steinman, R. M., and Cohn, Z. A. (1983). *J. Cell Biol.* **96**, 29.
Myers, C. D., Sanders, V. M., and Vitetta, E. S. (1986). *J. Immunol. Methods* **92**, 45.
Naito, K., Komatsubara, S., Kawai, J., Mori, K., and Muramatsu, S. (1984). *Cell. Immunol.* **88**, 361.
Nakanishi, K., Malek, T. R., Smith, K. A., Hamaoka, T., Shevach, E. M., and Paul, W. E. (1984). *J. Exp. Med.* **160**, 1605.
Nakayama, E., von Heogen, I., and Parnes, J. R. (1989). *Proc. Natl. Acad. Sci. U.S.A.* **86**, 1352.
Needleman, B. W., Lynch, D. H., and Hodes, R. J. (1988). *J. Immunol.* **141**, 3760.
Nisbet, N. W., and Edwards, J. (1973). *Transplant. Proc.* **4**, 1411.
Noelle, R., Krammer, P. H., Ohara, J., Uhr, J. W., and Vitetta, E. S. (1984). *Proc. Natl. Acad. Sci. U.S.A.* **81**, 6149.
Nossal, G. J. V., Abbot, A., Mitchell, J., and Lummus, Z. (1968). *J. Exp. Med.* **127**, 277.
Nowell, J., and Quaranta, V. (1985). *J. Exp. Med.* **162**, 1371.
Nussenzweig, M. C., and Steinman, R. M. (1980). *J. Exp. Med.* **151**, 1196.
Nussenzweig, M. C., Steinman, R. M., Gutchinov, B., and Cohn, Z. A. (1980). *J. Exp. Med.* **152**, 1070.
Nussenzweig, M. C., Steinman, R. M., Unkeless, J. C., Witmer, M. D., Gutchinov, B., and Cohn, Z. A. (1981). *J. Exp. Med.* **154**, 168.
Nussenzweig, M. C., Steinman, R. M., Witmer, M. D., and Gutchinov, B. (1982). *Proc. Natl. Acad. Sci. U.S.A.* **79**, 161.
Nussenzweig, M. C., Shaw, A. C., Sinn, E., Danner, D. B., Holmes, K. L., Morse, H. C., III, and Leder, P. (1987). *Science* **236**, 816.
Ohara, J., and Paul, W. E. (1988). *Proc. Natl. Acad. Sci. U.S.A.* **85**, 8221.
Oliver, P. D., and LeDourain, N. M. (1984). *J. Immunol.* **132**, 1748.
Osmond, D. G., and Nossal, G. J. V. (1974). *Cell. Immunol.* **13**, 132.
Ottaway, C. A., and Parrott, D. M. V. (1979). *J. Exp. Med.* **150**, 218.
Ottenhoff, T. H. M., Neuteboom, S., Elferink, D. G., and De Vries, R. R. P. (1986). *J. Exp. Med.* **164**, 1923.
Pelletier, M., Tautu, C., Landry, D., Montplaisir, S., Chartrand, C., and Perreault, C. (1986). *Immunology* **58**, 263.
Powrie, F., and Mason, D. (1989). *J. Exp. Med.* **169**, 653.
Pugh, C. W., MacPherson, G. G., and Steer, H. W. (1983). *J. Exp. Med.* **157**, 1758.
Pullen, A. M., Marack, P., and Kappler, J. W. (1988). *Nature (London)* **335**, 796.
Puré, E., Durie, C. J., Summerill, C. K., and Unkeless, J. C. (1984). *J. Exp. Med.* **160**, 1836.
Puré, E., Inaba, K., and Metlay, J. (1988). *J. Exp. Med.* **168**, 795.
Purkerson, J. M., Newberg, M., Wise, G., Lynch, K. R., and Isakson, P. C. (1988). *J. Exp. Med.* **168**, 1175.
Quaranta, V., Majdic, O., Stingl, G., Liszka, K., Honigsmann, H., and Knapp, W. (1984). *J. Immunol.* **132**, 1900.
Raff, M. C. (1970). *Nature (London)* **226**, 1257.
Ravetch, J. V., Luster, A. D., Weinshank, R., Kochan, J., Pavlovec, A., Portnoy, D. A., Hulmes, J., Pan, Y.-C. E., and Unkeless, J. C. (1986). *Science* **234**, 718.
Ray, A., Schmitt, D., Dezutter-Dambuyant, C., Fargier, M.-C., and Thivolet, J. (1989). *J. Invest. Dermatol.* **92**, 217.
Reichert, R. A., Gallatin, W. M., Weissman, I. L., and Butcher, E. C. (1982). *J. Exp. Med.* **157**, 813.

Rhodes, J. M., and Agger, R. (1987). *Immunol. Lett.* **16**, 107.
Rock, K. L., Benacerraf, B., and Abbas, A. K. (1984). *J. Exp. Med.* **4**, 1102.
Roehm, N. W., Leibson, J., Zlotnick, A., Kappler, J., Marrack, P., and Cambier, J. C. (1984). *J. Exp. Med.* **160**, 679.
Rolink, A. G., Melchers, F., and Palacios, R. (1989). *J. Exp. Med.* **169**, 1693.
Rollinghoff, M., Pfizenmaier, K., and Wagner, H. (1982). *Eur. J. Immunol.* **12**, 337.
Romani, N., Stingl, G., Tschachler, E., Witmer, M. D., Steinman, R. M., Shevach, E. M., and Schuler, G. (1985). *J. Exp. Med.* **161**, 1368.
Romani, N., Inaba, K., Witmer-Pack, M., Crowley, M., Puré, E., and Steinman, R. M. (1989a). *J. Exp. Med.* **169**, 1153.
Romani, N., Lenz, A., Glassl, H., Stossl, H., Stanzl, Y., Majdic, O., and Schuler, G. (1989b). *J. Invest. Dermatol.* (submitted for publication).
Romani, N., Koide, S., Crowley, M., Witmer-Pack, M., Livingstone, A. M., Fathman, C. G., Inaba, K., and Steinman, R. M. (1989c). *J. Exp. Med.* **169**, 1169.
Romani, N., Witmer-Pack, M., Crowley, M., Koide, S., Schuler, G., Inaba, K., and Steinman, R. M. (1989d). *CRC Crit. Rev. Immunol.* (in press).
Ron, Y., and Sprent, J. (1985). *J. Exp. Med.* **161**, 1581.
Ron, Y., and Sprent, J. (1989). *J. Immunol.* **138**, 2848.
Ron, Y., DeBaetselier, P., Gordon, J., Feldman, M., and Segal, S. (1981). *Eur. J. Immunol.* **11**, 964.
Rosenfeld, S. I., Looney, R. J., Leddy, J. P., Phillips, D. C., Abraham, G. N., and Anderson, C. L. (1985). *J. Clin. Invest.* **76**, 2317.
Rothbard, J. B. (1986). *Ann. Immunol. (Paris)* **137**, 518.
Rothbard, J. B., Lechler, R. I., Howland, K., Bal, V., Eckels, D. D., Sekaly, R., Long, E. O., Taylor, W. R., and Lamb, J. R. (1988). *Cell (Cambridge, Mass.)* **52**, 515.
Rothlein, R., Dustin, M. L., Marlin, S. D., and Springer, T. A. (1986). *J. Immunol.* **137**, 1270.
Rowden, G. (1981). *CRC Crit. Rev. Immunol.* **3**, 95.
Rowley, D. A., Gowans, J. L., Atkins, R. C., Ford, W. L., and Smith, M. E. (1972). *J. Exp. Med.* **136**, 499.
Rudd, C. E., Morimoto, C., Wong, L. L., and Schlossman, S. (1987). *J. Exp. Med.* **166**, 1758.
Sachs, J. A., Huber, B., Pena-Martinez, J., and Festenstein, H. (1973). *Transplant. Proc.* **4**, 1385.
Saiki, O., Tanaka, T., Doi, S., and Kishimoto, S. (1988). *J. Immunol.* **140**, 853.
Sanchez-Madrid, F., Kresnky, A. M., Ware, C. F., Robbins, E., Strominger, J. L., Burakoff, S. J., and Springer, T. A. (1982). *Proc. Natl. Acad. Sci. U.S.A.* **79**, 7489.
Sanchez-Madrid, F., Simon, P., Thompson, S., and Springer, T. A. (1983a). *J. Exp. Med.* **158**, 586.
Sanchez-Madrid, F., Nagy, J. A., Robbins, E., Simon, P., and Springer, T. A. (1983b). *J. Exp. Med.* **158**, 1785.
Sanders, V. M., Synder, J. M., Uhr, J. W., and Vitetta, E. S. (1986). *J. Immunol.* **137**, 2395.
Sanders, V. M., Uhr, J. W., and Vitetta, E. S. (1987). *Cell. Immunol.* **104**, 419.
Santiago-Schwartz, F., Bakke, A. C., Woodward, J. G., O'Brien, R. L., and Horwitz, D. A. (1985). *J. Immunol.* **134**, 779.
Scheynius, A., Klareskog, L., Forsum, U., Masson, P., Karlsson, L., Peterson, P. A., and Sundstrom, C. (1982). *J. Invest. Dermatol.* **78**, 452.
Schnizlein, C. T., Kosco, M. H., Szakal, A. K., and Tew, J. G. (1985). *J. Immunol.* **134**, 1360.
Schriever, F., Freedman, A. S., Freeman, G., Messner, E., Daley, J., and Nadler, L. M. (1989). *J. Exp. Med.* **169**, 2043.

Schuler, G., and Steinman, R. M. (1985). *J. Exp. Med.* **161**, 526.
Schuler, G. *et al.* (1989). In preparation.
Schwartz, R. H. (1985). *Annu. Rev. Immunol.* **3**, 237.
Scollay, R. G., Butcher, E. C., and Weissman, I. L. (1980). *Eur. J. Immunol.* **10**, 210.
Scothorne, R. J., and McGregor, I. A. (1955). *J. Anat.* **89**, 283.
Sertl, K., Takemura, T., Tschachler, E., Ferrans, V. J., Kaliner, M. A., and Shevach, E. M. (1986). *J. Exp. Med.* **163**, 436.
Shelley, W. B., and Juhlin, L. (1976). *Nature (London)* **261**, 46.
Shelley, W. B., and Juhlin, L. (1977). *Arch. Dermatol.* **113**, 187.
Shimonkevitz, R., Kappler, J., Marrack, P., and Grey, H. (1983). *J. Exp. Med.* **158**, 303.
Shimonkevitz, R., Colon, S., Kappler, J. W., Marrack, P., and Grey, H. M. (1984). *J. Immunol.* **133**, 2067.
Silberberg-Sinakin, I., Thorbecke, G. J., Baer, R. L., Rosenthal, S. A., and Berezowsky, V. (1976). *Cell. Immunol.* **25**, 137.
Simmons, D., Makgoba, M. W., and Seed, B. (1988). *Nature (London)* **331**, 624.
Singer, A., Hathcock, K. S., and Hodes, R. (1979). *J. Exp. Med.* **149**, 1208.
Smith, J. B., McIntosh, G. H., and Morris, B. (1970). *J. Anat.* **107**, 87.
Smith, K. G. C., Austyn, J. M., Hariri, G., Beverley, P. C. L., and Morris, P. J. (1986). *Eur. J. Immunol.* **16**, 478.
Sordat, B., Sordat, M., Hess, W., Stoner, R. D., and Cottier, H. (1970). *J. Exp. Med.* **131**, 77.
Spalding, D., Koopman, W. J., Eldridge, J. H., McGhee, J. R., and Steinman, R. M. (1983). *J. Exp. Med.* **157**, 1646.
Spickett, G. P., Brandon, M. R., Mason, D. W., Williams, A. F., and Woollett, G. R. (1983). *J. Exp. Med.* **158**, 795.
Sprent, J. (1973). *Cell. Immunol.* **7**, 10.
Sprent, J. (1978). *J. Exp. Med.* **147**, 1142.
Sprent, J., and von Boehmer, H. (1976). *J. Exp. Med.* **144**, 617.
Springer, T. A., Dustin, M. L., Kishimoto, T. K., and Marlin, S. D. (1987). *Annu. Rev. Immunol.* **5**, 223.
Spry, C. J. F., Pflug, A. J., Janossy, G., and Humphrey, J. H. (1980). *Clin. Exp. Immunol.* **39**, 750.
Steiner, G., Tschachler, E., Tani, M., Malek, T. R., Shevach, E. M., Holter, W., Knapp, W., Wolff, K., and Stingl, G. (1986). *J. Immunol.* **137**, 155.
Steinman, R. M., and Cohn, Z. A. (1972). *J. Cell Biol.* **55**, 186.
Steinman, R. M., and Cohn, Z. A. (1973). *J. Exp. Med.* **137**, 1142.
Steinman, R. M., and Cohn, Z. A. (1974). *J. Exp. Med.* **139**, 380.
Steinman, R. M., and Inaba, K. (1989). *BioEssays* **10**, 145.
Steinman, R. M., and Witmer, M. D. (1978). *Proc. Natl. Acad. Sci. U.S.A.* **75**, 5132.
Steinman, R. M., Silver, J. M., and Cohn, Z. A. (1974a). *J. Cell Biol.* **63**, 949.
Steinman, R. M., Lustig, D. S., and Cohn, Z. A. (1974b). *J. Exp. Med.* **139**, 1431.
Steinman, R. M., Machtinger, B. G., Fried, J., and Cohn, Z. A. (1978). *J. Exp. Med.* **147**, 279.
Steinman, R. M., Kaplan, G., Witmer, M. D., and Cohn, Z. A. (1979). *J. Exp. Med.* **149**, 1.
Steinman, R. M., Nogueira, N., Witmer, M. D., Tydings, J. D., and Mellman, I. S. (1980). *J. Exp. Med.* **152**, 1248.
Steinman, R. M., Mellman, I. S., Muller, W. A., and Cohn, Z. A. (1983a). *J. Cell Biol.* **96**, 1.
Steinman, R. M., Gutchinov, B., Witmer, M. D., and Nussenzweig, M. C. (1983b). *J. Exp. Med.* **157**, 613.

Steinman, R. M., Inaba, K., Schuler, G., Witmer, M. D., Koide, S., Flechner, E., Bhardwaj, M., and Young, J. W. (1987). In "Progress in Immunology VI" (B. Cinader and R. G. Miller, eds), p. 1013. Academic Press, San Diego, California.

Steinman, R. M., et al. (1989). In preparation.

Stingl, G., Wolff-Schreiner, E. C., Pichler, W. J., Gschnait, F., and Knapp, W. (1977). Nature (London) 268, 245.

Stockinger, B., Pessara, U., Lin, R. H., Habicht, J., Grez, M., and Koch, N. (1989). Cell (Cambridge, Mass.) 56, 683.

Streuli, M., Matsuyama, T., Morimoto, C., Schlossman, S. F., and Saito, H. (1987). J. Exp. Med. 166, 1567.

Sullivan, S., Bergstresser, P. R., Tigelaar, R. E., and Streilein, J. W. (1985). J. Invest. Dermatol. 84, 491.

Sunshine, G. H., Katz, D. R., and Feldmann, M. (1980). J. Exp. Med. 152, 1817.

Sunshine, G. H., Gold, D. P., Wortis, H. H., Marrack, P., and Kappler, J. W. (1983). J. Exp. Med. 158, 1745.

Sunshine, G. H., Mitchell, T. J., Czitrom, A. A., Edwards, S., Glasebrook, A. L., Kelso, A., and MacDonald, H. R. (1985). Cell. Immunol. 91, 60.

Swierkosz, J. E., Rock, K., Marrack, P., and Kappler, J. W. (1978). J. Exp. Med. 147, 554.

Szakal, A. K., and Hanna, M. G., Jr. (1968). Exp. Mol. Pathol. 8, 75.

Takahashi, K., Isobe, T., Ohtsuki, Y., Sonobe, H., Takeda, I., and Akagi, T. (1984). Am. J. Pathol. 116, 497.

Takigawa, M., Iwatsuki, K., Yamada, M., Okamoto, H., and Imamura, S. (1985). J. Invest. Dermatol. 85, 12.

Taylor, R. B., Duttus, P. H., Raff, M. C., and de Petris, S. (1971). Nature (London), New Biol. 233, 225.

Tew, J. G., Thorbecke, J., and Steinman, R. M. (1982). Res: J. Reticuloendothel. Soc. 31, 371.

Tomasi, T. B., Jr., and Bienenstock, J. (1968). Adv. Immunol. 9, 1.

Tony, H. P., and Parker, D. C. (1985). J. Exp. Med. 161, 223.

Tony, H. P., Phillips, N. E., and Parker, D. C. (1985). J. Exp. Med. 162, 1695.

Townsend, A. R. M., Rothbard, J., Gotch, F. M., Bahadur, G., Wraith, D., and McMichael, A. J. (1986). Cell (Cambridge, Mass.) 44, 959.

Unanue, E. R. (1984). Annu. Rev. Immunol. 2, 395.

Unanue, E. R., Perkins, W. D., and Karnovsky, M. J. (1972). J. Exp. Med. 136, 885.

Unkeless, J. C. (1979). J. Exp. Med. 150, 580.

Vakkila, J., Lehtonen, E., Koskimies, S., and Hurme, M. (1987). Immunol. Lett. 15, 229.

Van Voorhis, W. C., Hair, L. S., Steinman, R. M., and Kaplan, G. (1982). J. Exp. Med. 155, 1172.

Van Voorhis, W. C., Steinman, R. M., Hair, L. S., Luban, J., Witmer, M. D., Koide, S., and Cohn, Z. A. (1983a). J. Exp. Med. 158, 126.

Van Voorhis, W. C., Valinsky, J., Hoffman, E., Luban, J., Hair, L. S., and Steinman, R. M. (1983b). J. Exp. Med. 158, 174.

Veerman, A. J. P. (1974). Cell Tissue Res. 148, 247.

Veerman, A. J. P., and Van Ewijk, W. (1974). Cell Tissue Res. 156, 427.

Veldman, J. E., and Kaiserling, E. (1980). In "The Reticuloendothelial System: Morphology" (I. Carr and W. T. Daems, eds), p. 381. Plenum, New York.

Viguier, M., Lotteau, V., Charron, D., and Debre, P. (1987). Eur. J. Immunol. 17, 1540.

von Boehmer, H., Hudson, L., and Sprent, J. (1975). J. Exp. Med. 142, 989.

Watt, T. H. (1988). J. Immunol. 141, 3708.

Webb, S. R., Li, J. H., Wilson, D. B., and Sprent, J. (1985). Eur. J. Immunol. 15, 92.

Webb, S. R., Okamoto, A., Ron, Y., and Sprent, J. (1989). J. Exp. Med. 169, 1.

Weiss, A., Imboden, J., Hardy, K., Manger, B., Terhorst, C., and Stobo, J. (1986). *Annu. Rev. Immunol.* **4**, 593.
Weiss, S., and Bogen, B. (1989). *Proc. Natl. Acad. Sci. U.S.A.* **86**, 282.
Wibo, M., and Poole, B. (1974). *J. Cell Biol.* **63**, 430.
Wilders, M. M., Sminia, T., and Janse, E. M. (1983). *Immunology* **50**, 303.
Wilson, D. B., and Nowell, P. C. (1971). *J. Exp. Med.* **133**, 442.
Witmer, M. D., and Steinman, R. M. (1984). *Am. J. Anat.* **170**, 465.
Witmer-Pack, M. D., Olivier, W., Valinsky, J., Schuler, G., and Steinman, R. M. (1987). *J. Exp. Med.* **166**, 1484.
Witmer-Pack, M. D., Valinsky, J., Olivier, W., and Steinman, R. M. (1988). *J. Invest. Dermatol.* **90**, 387.
Wolff, K., and Schreiner, E. (1970). *J. Invest. Dermatol.* **54**, 37.
Wright, S. D., and Silverstein, S. C. (1982). *J. Exp. Med.* **156**, 1149.
Wright, S. D., Licht, M. R., Craigmyle, L. S., and Silverstein, S. C. (1984). *J. Cell Biol.* **99**, 336.
Wright, S. D., Detmers, P. A., Jong, M. T. C., and Meyer, B. C. (1986). *J. Exp. Med.* **163**, 1245.
Yamasaki, K., Taga, T., Hirata, Y., Yawata, H., Kawanishi, Y., Seed, B., Taniguchi, T., Hirano, T., and Kishimoto, T. (1988). *Science* **241**, 825.
Young, J. W., and Steinman, R. M. (1988). *Cell. Immunol.* **111**, 167.
Ziegler, H. K., and Unanue, E. R. (1982). *Proc. Natl. Acad. Sci. U.S.A.* **79**, 175.
Zvaifler, N. J., Steinman, R. M., Kaplan, G., Lau, L. L., and Rivelis, M. (1985). *J. Clin. Invest.* **76**, 789.

This article was accepted for publication on 20 March 1989.

The CD5 B Cell

THOMAS J. KIPPS

*Department of Molecular and Experimental Medicine,
Scripps Clinic and Research Foundation,
La Jolla, California 92037*

I. Introduction

Few lymphocyte subpopulations have evoked such controversy as the CD5 B cell. After it finally was accepted that normal B lymphocytes may coexpress CD5, it was disputed whether CD5 B cells constituted a distinct B cell subset. It still is debated whether this cell type represents a discrete B cell lineage or more simply a stage in B cell activation and/or maturation. The relationship between the CD5 B cell and autoimmune disease and/or autoantibodies also is controversial. This chapter will review current ideas concerning the CD5 B cell, hoping to resolve some of the controversy. However, some issues still remain unanswered and are the topic of current research.

In this review, the international nomenclature established for cell differentiation antigens will be used. Historically, the CD5 B cell in mice or humans has been referred to as the Ly-1 B cell or Leu-1 B cell, respectively. Although these terms are still in use, all defined surface differentiation antigens, including CD5, will be referred to by their assigned CD (cluster of differentiation) number. Whenever appropriate, the monoclonal antibodies (Mabs) employed to define surface expression of a particular CD antigen will be listed in brackets along with reference to contributing investigators. This will not be a complete listing of all Mabs reactive with a particular CD antigen, but rather the Mab(s) utilized in the study reviewed.

Since its initial description, the cell subset(s) thought exclusively to express the CD5 surface antigen has undergone repeated modification. In the mid-1970s the CD5 surface antigen, then known as Lyt-1, was defined using alloantisera raised in inbred strains of mice. Utilizing these antisera with complement to deplete Lyt-1-bearing lymphocytes prior to *in vitro* assays or cell transfer experiments, the CD5 antigen originally was thought to be a surface marker for the helper–inducer T lymphocyte subpopulation (Cantor and Boyse, 1975a,b). However, with the advent of anti-CD5 Mabs and sensitive flow-cytometric analyses, CD5 was noted to be expressed by all T lymphocytes (Ledbetter *et al.*, 1980).

Almost concomitantly, CD5 was detected on certain B cell tumors in both mice (Lanier et al., 1981a,b, 1983) and humans (Gough et al., 1980; Wang et al., 1980; Martin et al., 1980, 1981; Royston et al., 1980). At first thought perhaps to represent examples of neoplastic cell "lineage infidelity," it soon was discovered in both mice and humans that CD5 may be expressed by normal B lymphocytes (Manohar et al., 1982; Hayakawa et al., 1983; Caligaris-Cappio et al., 1982).

II. CD5 B Cells Defined

CD5 B cells are lymphocytes that coexpress a 67-kDa pan-T lymphocyte surface glycoprotein, designated CD5, and surface antigens restricted to the B lymphocyte lineage (Hayakawa et al., 1983; Herzenberg et al., 1986; Hardy and Hayakawa, 1986; Gadol and Ault, 1986). Surface expression of CD5 is defined by the reactivity of cells with Mabs Ly-1 [53-7.3 (Ledbetter and Herzenberg, 1979)] in mice, or Leu-1 or its equivalent (see Martin et al., 1981) in humans. Both murine and human CD5 B cells express roughly 20% of the level of CD5 expressed by most T lymphocytes (Manohar et al., 1982; Hayakawa et al., 1985; Gadol and Ault, 1986; Hardy and Hayakawa, 1986; Kipps and Vaughan, 1987). However, these cells lack expression of other T cell-associated differentiation antigens, such as CD4, CD8, and CD3, and, in the mouse, Thy-1.

In addition to surface immunoglobulin (sIg), these cells express other surface antigens at levels comparable to B cells considered CD5$^-$ (Hayakawa et al., 1983; Hardy et al., 1984, 1986; Gadol and Ault, 1986; Kipps and Vaughan, 1987). This includes CD19, CD20, and CD21, antigens that are expressed exclusively by lymphocytes of the B cell lineage (Ling et al., 1987). Murine CD5 B cells coexpress other B cell surface antigens, such as ThB [49-H4 (Eckhardt and Herzenberg, 1980)], the B cell isomer of Ly-5 [B220, RA3-6B2 (Coffman, 1983)], and a receptor for Ig Fc (Dexter and Corley, 1987) that is recognized by the Mab 2.4G2 (Unkeless, 1979).

Detection and enumeration of CD5 B cells require sensitive immunofluorescence or immunohistochemical methods. Even with the brightest of fluorochrome-labeled anti-CD5 Mabs and the most sensitive of immunofluorescence techniques, B cells expressing CD5 cannot be delineated into a separate subpopulation distinct from B cells that lack expression of this marker (Fig. 1). Because of this, subtraction methods must be used to enumerate these cells within a mixed cell population. Generally, the percentage of CD5 B cells is defined as the percentage of B cells stained with a fluorochrome-labeled anti-CD5 Mab minus the percentage of B cells stained with a fluorochrome-labeled isotype control Mab above a given fluorescence threshold.

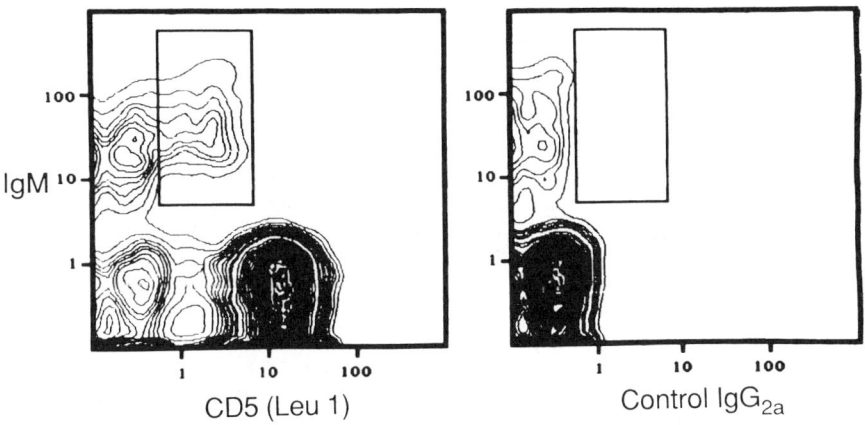

FIG. 1. Immunofluorescence of PBLs from a normal adult stained with biotin-labeled anti-IgM and either FITC-labeled anti-CD5 [Leu-1] (left) or an FITC-labeled control antibody of the same murine Ig isotype [IgG$_{2a}$] (right). The biotin-labeled anti-IgM was developed by second-step staining with Texas red–avidin. The boxed areas represent the region of integration used to calculate the percentage of CD5 B cells. The percentage of cells in the box of the control panel (left) is subtracted from the percentage of cells in the box of cells stained with anti-CD5 (right).

Other characteristics may help to distinguish the CD5 B cell. Flow-cytometric analyses of CD5 B cells from both mice and humans demonstrate these cells to have larger forward- and side-angle light scatter than CD5$^-$ B cells, consistent with the cells having a greater size than most other B lymphocytes. Murine CD5 B cells especially express higher levels of sIgM and lower levels of sIgD than do other B lymphocytes (Hayakawa et al., 1984; Hardy et al., 1983). Human CD5 B cells may comprise the B cell subpopulation noted spontaneously to form rosettes with mouse erythrocytes (MRBCs) (Gobbi et al., 1983; Lydyard et al., 1987). Human tonsillar CD5 B cells also may coexpress 4F2, a surface antigen associated with cellular activation (Haynes et al., 1981). Demonstration that 4F2 and CD5 are coexpressed on B cells, however, was not performed directly, but rather through inference from studies on the B cell growth factor (BCGF) response of various B lymphocyte populations selectively depleted of B cells expressing either 4F2 or CD5 (Richard et al., 1987). Finally, in contrast to most other B cells, human (Kipps and Vaughan, 1987) and mouse (Herzenberg et al., 1987) CD5 B cells may express low levels of CD11b [Leu-15, MAC-1 (Springer et al., 1978, 1979)], the receptor for C3bi that commonly is expressed by cells of the myelomonocytic lineage (Beller et al., 1982; Hogg and Horton, 1987). In addition, human CD5 B cells may express low levels of other myelomonocytic-associated surface antigens, such as CD14 [MY4, Mo2 (Griffin et al., 1981; Elias et al., 1985; Todd et al., 1981)]. Expression of such surface antigens commonly is not detected on most other B lymphocytes (Hogg and Horton, 1987).

CD5 B cells apparently are more resilient to *in vitro* cell culture than are CD5$^-$ B cells. Murine B cells survive for a few days *in vitro* without exogenous cytokines or viral transformation. Most of the B cells that are viable after prolonged culture are noted to coexpress the CD5 surface antigen (Hardy and Hayakawa, 1986; Herzenberg et al., 1986). That the CD5 B cell phenotype simply is not acquired *in vitro* is suggested by cell-sorting experiments in which CD5 B and CD5$^-$ murine splenic B cells are separated prior to culture. In such experiments, separated CD5 B cells survive significantly longer than do CD5$^-$ B cells. The capacity of CD5 B cells to survive for prolonged periods *in vitro* has permitted some investigators to establish CD5 B cell lines for biochemical and molecular studies (Braun, 1983; Braun et al., 1984, 1986).

III. Anatomic Localization of CD5 B Cells

Studies of inbred mice have discerned an anatomic distribution of CD5 B cells that is not random. Although demonstrable as a rare splenic B cell subpopulation in most normal inbred mice, murine CD5 B cells normally are not found in lymph nodes, blood, or bone marrow (Hayakawa et al., 1983). In contrast, CD5 B cells constitute a major lymphoid subpopulation in the murine peritoneal cavity (Hayakawa et al., 1986a). In general, B cells comprise approximately 30-60% of the harvested peritoneal cells of most inbred strains of mice, T cells constitute 10%, and monocytes and macrophages comprise the remainder. Approximately one half of the peritoneal B cells coexpress CD5 and share phenotypic characteristics with splenic CD5 B cells (Hayakawa et al., 1986a).

Recently, one group of investigators reported finding CD5 B cells in the thymus of normal mice (Miyama-Inaba et al., 1988). About 1% of the cells in most thymic cell suspensions are B lymphocytes. In order to study the phenotype of these thymic B cells, thymocytes were depleted of T cells by treatment with anti-Thy-1.2 [F7D5 or 30-H12], anti-CD4 [GK1.5 (Dialynas et al., 1983)], and anti-CD8 [Lyt-2.2 or HO-2.2] and rabbit complement, and then layered onto 65% Percoll for discontinuous density gradient centrifugation. Cells enriched for sIgM-bearing B lymphocytes were found in the low-density fraction at the media–Percoll interface. These cells could be stimulated to proliferate by treatment with both interleukin-4 (IL-4) and anti-IgM or *Escherichia coli* lipopolysaccharide (LPS), but not concanavalin A. Flow-cytometric analyses demonstrated that greater than 70% of these thymic B cells expressed CD5, in addition to CD11b [MAC-1], sIgM [14-8], Ia [M5/114.15.2], CD45R [RA3-3A1/6.1], and low-density B220. As such, these cells have the phenotype of CD5 B cells found in the spleen or the peritoneal cavity of normal mice. To be sure, earlier studies failed to detect CD5 B cells within the thymus (Hayakawa et al., 1983). These studies analyzed whole thymic cell preparations in which CD5 B cells are below the limits of detection. This emphasizes that CD5 B cells at best constitute a rare subpopulation within the thymus.

In humans, distinctions in the anatomic distribution of CD5 B cells are less well resolved. In normal adults, CD5 B cells have been reported to comprise anywhere from less than 1% to 30% of the B cells circulating in the peripheral blood (Plater-Zyberk et al., 1985; Maini et al., 1987; Lydyard et al., 1987; Taniguchi et al., 1987; Hardy and Hayakawa, 1986; Dauphinee et al., 1988; Hardy et al., 1987; Casali et al., 1987; Gadol and Ault, 1986; Kipps and Vaughan, 1987). CD5 B cells constitute less than 10% of the splenic B cells of most adults tested (Freedman et al., 1987a) but may account for up to 30% of the B cells in lymph nodes and inflamed tonsils. Using immunohistochemistry to identify cells positioned within the lymph node, CD5 B cells are identifiable as a small subpopulation of cells scattered around the edge of the germinal center (Caligaris-Cappio et al., 1982; Gobbi et al., 1983). CD5 B cells generally are not detectable in the adult bone marrow (T. J. Kipps, unpublished observations; M. Loken, personal communication). In only a few cases examined CD5 B cells have not been detected among the mononuclear cells present in peritoneal washings of patients undergoing gynecological procedures.

IV. CD5 B Cells in Ontogeny

CD5 B cells appear early in development. CD5 B cells in mice can be detected with the first appearance of IgD-bearing B lymphocytes in neonatal spleen. Unlike other lymphocytes, the absolute number of CD5 B cells rapidly reaches near-adult levels early in lymphocyte ontogeny (Hayakawa et al., 1986a). Thus, the proportion of CD5 B cells relative to other splenic lymphocyte subpopulations decreases with age. In BALB/c mice CD5 B cells constitute approximately 20% of the sIgM$^+$ splenic B cells 5 days after birth (Dexter and Corley, 1987). The percentage of sIgM$^+$ splenic B cells that coexpress CD5 progressively diminishes from this level to roughly 9% at 22 days and approximately 5% at 3 months of age. Similarly, the frequency of peritoneal B cells that coexpress CD5 diminishes from nearly 100% at 7 days after birth to 46% at 3 weeks and 16% at 3 months of age (Hayakawa et al., 1986a; Dexter and Corley, 1987). The reduction in the proportion of splenic and peritoneal B cells that coexpress CD5, however, is not due to a reduction in the absolute number of CD5 B cells, but rather is secondary to an increase in the absolute number of B cells that do not coexpress CD5. In fact, the absolute numbers of CD5 B cells found in the spleen more than double between 1 and 3 weeks of age (Dexter and Corley, 1987). Similarly, there is approximately a ninefold increase in the absolute numbers of CD5 B cells found in the peritoneum between 3 weeks and 3 months of age.

In humans, CD5 B cells constitute a major B cell subpopulation in fetal spleen and newborn cord blood. Examination of the cell surface phenotype of splenic lymphocytes from fetuses at 19-22 weeks of gestation revealed that 40-60% of the total B lymphocyte population coexpresses CD5 along with other B cells surface antigens, i.e., HLA-DR, CD19 [B4 or Leu-12 (Nadler et al., 1983; Meeker et al., 1984)], CD20 [B1 (Stashenko et al., 1980)], and sIgM and sIgD (Bofill et al., 1985; Antin et al., 1986). At birth most of the B lymphocytes in cord blood coexpress CD5 (Hardy and Hayakawa, 1986; Hardy et al., 1987). However, by young adulthood CD5 B cells constitute less than 10-30% of the B cells in normal spleen, lymph nodes, and peripheral blood (Gobbi et al., 1983; Kipps and Vaughan, 1987).

V. CD5 B Cells in Aging

Aging may affect the levels of CD5 B cells. Recent studies of mice indicate that aging is associated with an increase in the absolute numbers and/or relative proportions of CD5 B cells in the peritoneum, lymphoid organs, and peripheral blood. In normal BALB/c mice, the number of peritoneal CD5 B cells increases slowly but steadily, from approximately 3×10^6 in 6- to 8-week-old mice to greater than 3×10^7 in mice greater than 1 year of age (Stall et al., 1988). This increase appears secondary to oligoclonal expansions of CD5 B cells, in that clusters of cells expressing homogenous levels of sIgM sharing the same Ig light chain can be detected using multiparameter flow-cytometric analyses (Stall et al., 1988; Tarlinton et al., 1988). Subsequent to 5-7 months of age, similar expansions often can be detected in the spleen and, later, lymph nodes, peripheral blood, and bone marrow of normal mice of all strains tested (BALB/c, C57BL/6, or CBA). All mice over 18 months of age had phenotypically homogenous expansions of CD5 B cells in lymphoid organs and peripheral blood. Similar apparent clonal expansions of CD5 B cells may be detected in autoimmune strains of NZB or (NZB × NZW)F_1

(B/W) mice, but at an accelerated rate (Raveche et al., 1981; Stall et al., 1988; Seldin et al., 1987; Wofsy and Chiang, 1987). The latter mice, however, generally succumb to autoimmune disease prior to developing large expansions of such cells, unless they are treated with weekly injections of anti-CD4 [GK1.5] to ameliorate their autoimmune disease (Wofsy and Chiang, 1987).

Long-term studies in humans, examining the effect that aging has on the relative proportions of circulating CD5 B cells, are ongoing. To be sure, malignancies of the CD5 B cell (discussed below), such as chronic lymphocytic leukemia (CLL) and small-cell lymphocytic non-Hodgkin's lymphoma (NHL), are most common in older age groups. These diseases have peak incidences in the sixth or seventh decades of life. Perhaps an age-related increase in the proportion of CD5 B cells may predispose to malignant transformation of CD5 B cells.

VI. CD5 B Cell Malignancies

Several murine B cell lymphomas that have developed in aging mice have been noted to coexpress CD5. The BCL_1 leukemia that occurred spontaneously in an aging BALB/c mouse (Slavin and Strober, 1978) subsequently was found to express CD5, in addition to other B cell surface antigens (Hardy et al., 1984). That CD5 B cell lymphomas may arise from chronic antigenic stimulation associated with aging was suggested by studies of the CH series of lymphomas in $BI0.H-2^aH-4^b$ p/Wts mice. These lymphomas arise in aging recipients of adoptively transferred syngeneic spleen cells after hyperimmunization with sheep erythrocytes (SRBCs) (Lanier et al., 1978, 1982). In addition to sIgM, these lymphomas also coexpress CD5 (Lanier et al., 1982; Pennell et al., 1985). Finally, many B cell lymphomas arising in aging NFS/N v-congenic mice also express CD5 (Davidson et al., 1984). Many of these lymphomas have been adapted for *in vitro* culture. In particular, the CH series of lymphomas has proven to be a highly interesting model with which to study CD5 B cell Ig gene expression (discussed in Section XIV).

In humans, the most common malignancy of the CD5 B cell is CLL. Early attempts to devise a hypothetical model of B cell development by drawing analogy to B cell malignancies positioned the CLL cell as representative of an early stage in B cell differentiation (Anderson et al., 1984). This schema, however, is not compatible with the observation that approximately 95% of the patients with B cell CLL have leukemic cells that coexpress CD5 in addition to other B cell surface antigens (Martin et al., 1980; Royston et al., 1980; Wang et al., 1980; Boumsell et al., 1980). This trait is shared neither by early B lymphocytes found within the bone marrow (as discussed in Section III) nor by other "immature" B cell malignancies (Melink and LeBien, 1983; Caligaris-Cappio and Janossy, 1985). Further, leukemic CD5 B cells generally form rosettes with MRBCs (Forbes et al., 1982), a trait apparently shared by normal CD5 B cells (Gobbi et al., 1983; Lydyard et al., 1987). In contrast to other B cell leukemias, leukemic CD5 B cells also are noted to express myelomonocytic surface antigens (den Ottolander et al., 1985: Kipps and Vaughan, 1987; Morabito et al., 1987), similar to the normal CD5 B cell. In a recent survey of 31 cases of $CD5^+$ CLL, 29 (94%) coexpressed CD5 [Leu-1], 26 (84%) were positive for CD14 [MY4], 22 (71%) were reactive with a Mab specific for the monocyte Fc receptor [MFC-1], 22 (71%) were positive for CD11b [OKM1], and eight (26%) expressed CD15 [Leu-M1] (Morabito et al., 1987). In addition, many of the cases with leukemic cells reactive with anti-CD14 [MY4] also stained with MY7. These many shared phenotypic characteristics make a strong argument that B cell CLL, the most common adult leukemia in Western societies, is a malignancy of the relatively uncommon CD5 B cell.

Solid tissue human B cell lymphomas also may express the CD5 surface antigen. Malignant B cells of small-cell lymphocytic lymphoma (SL) morphologically resemble the leukemic cells seen in the peripheral blood of patients with CLL and, in contrast to lymphomas of follicular center cell origin, frequently coexpress B cell surface antigens and CD5 (Burns et al., 1983; Knowles et al., 1983; Cossman et al., 1984; Al Saati et al., 1984; Delia et al., 1986; van den Oord et al., 1986b; Spier et al., 1986; Medeiros et al., 1987). Patients with CLL often develop lymphadenopathy secondary to a small lymphocytic infiltrate that histologically resembles SL. In a study of 16 patients with SL, the ten patients with B lymphomas that expressed CD5 also were noted to have a peripheral lymphocytosis of malignant CD5 B cells. This led the authors of this study to classify CD5 as a marker for lymphomas associated with CLL (Harris and Bhan, 1985a). A more recent and larger study of 48 patients, however, revealed that 14 of 32 patients (44%) with B cell SL without associated leukemia had lymphoma cells that expressed the CD5 surface marker (Medeiros et al., 1987).

Included within the broad category of SL not generally associated with peripheral lymphocytosis are the subtypes mantle-zone lymphoma (MZL) (Weisenburger et al., 1982; van den Oord et al., 1986b; Weisenburger, 1986; Ellison et al., 1987; Samoszuk et al., 1986; Harris and Bhan, 1985b), and intermediate lymphocytic lymphoma (ILL) or intermediately differentiated lymphocytic lymphoma (Weisenburger, et al., 1981, 1987; Jaffe et al., 1987; Burke et al., 1985). Strict morphological criteria for MZL requires histological presence of clear-cut, reactive germinal centers surrounded by well-defined, broad, expanding mantle zones of monoclonal B lymphocytes (Ellison et al., 1987). In contrast, ILL is characterized by atypical monoclonal expansions of small lymphoid cells, with slightly irregular and indented nuclear contours (Weisenburger et al., 1987). The histology of these lymphomas suggests that they may be derived from malignant transformation of lymphocytes normally residing within the marginal zone surrounding the germinal center (van den Oord et al., 1986a). Although there is not universal agreement concerning the origin of such cells (Harris and Bhan, 1985b; Weisenburger, 1986; Manconi et al., 1987), it generally is agreed that these tumors are B cell lymphomas that often express CD5.

VII. CD5 as a Marker for B Cell Activation

Several investigators have suggested that B cell expression of CD5 is an indicator of B cell activation. This view was supported by studies demonstrating that phorbol myristate acetate (PMA) can induce malignant and normal $CD5^-$ human B lymphocytes to express CD5 (Miller and Gralow, 1984). PMA is a potent inducer of protein kinase C, and has been used in many different systems to trigger cellular activation and/or differentiation (Abb et al., 1979; Nagasawa and Mak, 1980; Diamond et al., 1980; Ralph and Kishimoto, 1981; Nagasawa et al., 1981; Cossman et al., 1982; LeBien et al., 1982; Nadler et al., 1982; Bertoglio, 1983; Weinstein et al., 1983; Yamasaki et al., 1983; Miyake et al., 1983; Mastro, 1983; Aman et al., 1984; Nishizuka, 1984; Guy et al., 1985; Wolf et al., 1985; Castagna, 1987; Harnett and Klaus, 1988). When cultured with PMA at 10 ng/ml for 48 hours, approximately 50% of the peripheral lymphocytes expressing the pan-B lymphocyte antigen CD19 [Leu-12] also were noted to coexpress CD5 [Leu-1]. However, without addition of PMA to the culture, fewer than 1% of the CD19-expressing B cells coexpressed CD5. Examination of cell yields and viabilities indicated that the change in the percentage of cells coexpressing CD5 and B cell surface markers could not be explained simply by the outgrowth or differential survival of a subpopulation of CD5 B cells within the culture. This finding has been corroborated by other investigators (Hardy and Hayakawa, 1986; Youinou et al., 1986, 1987; Freedman et al., 1987a). Highly purified splenic B cell populations with fewer than 1% detectable CD5 B cells could be stimulated to express CD5 by treatment with PMA, indicating that induction of CD5 expression does not require accessory T cells or monocytes (Freedman et al., 1987a). Other surface antigens associated with B cell activation (Tsudo et al., 1984; Clark et al., 1985; Boyd et al., 1985a; Freedman et al., 1987b; Friedman et al., 1986;

Crow et al., 1986), such as CD25 [anti-Tac (Waldmann et al., 1984; Boyd et al., 1985b)] and CD23 [Blast-2 (Thorley-Lawson et al., 1985)], also are induced by coculture with PMA. Together, these findings are interpreted to indicate that CD5 is a B cell activation antigen *and* that CD5 B cells are activated B lymphocytes (Freedman et al., 1987b, 1989).

Whether PMA can induce all B cells to express detectable levels of CD5 is not resolved. Usually, the percentage of cells coexpressing CD5 and B cell surface antigens does not exceed 50% of the B cells stimulated. This may reflect heterogeneity within the prestimulated population in the ability of B cells to augment or acquire CD5 surface antigen expression. For example, PMA may increase the level of CD5 expression on a subpopulation of cells, allowing for the detection of cells that previously expressed undetectable levels of CD5. Alternatively, PMA may augment CD5 antigen expression on all B cells (Hardy and Hayakawa, 1986). In any case, it is noteworthy that populations of human lymphocytes that have the highest initial proportions of CD5 B cells also generally have the highest proportions of CD5 B cells subsequent to culture with PMA (Youinou et al., 1986; Hara et al., 1988).

That PMA can induce CD5 expression on human B cells, however, does not prove that CD5 is a marker for activated B cells. Indeed, PMA treatment results in enhanced surface expression of a variety of surface antigens on both T and B lymphocytes that are not considered markers of cellular activation (Kikutani et al., 1986b; Hardy and Hayakawa, 1986; Noonan et al., 1987). More importantly, B lymphocytes do not express enhanced levels of CD5 when when activated by treatment with anti-Ig (Freedman et al., 1987a), *Staphylococcus aureus* protein A (Hardy and Hayakawa, 1986), pokeweed mitogen (Miller and Gralow, 1984), Epstein–Barr virus (EBV) (Youinou et al., 1986, 1987), *E. coli* LPS (Hayakawa et al., 1984), purified or recombinant ILs (Freedman et al., 1989), or anti-Ig plus media conditioned by phytohemagglutinin (PHA)-stimulated T cells (Kikutani et al., 1986a). Thus, activation of human B cells by selective methods does not stimulate B cells to express higher levels of CD5. Although treatment with LPS may augment the expression of CD5 on some CD5-expressing murine B cell tumors (Ovnic and Corley, 1987), none of the measures commonly used to activate murine B lymphocytes, including treatment with LPS or phorbol esters, induces $CD5^-$ murine B cells to express CD5 (Hayakawa et al., 1984; Hardy and Hayakawa, 1986). Together, these data argue that CD5 B cells are not simply activated B lymphocytes.

Another argument used to support the concept that CD5 B cells are activated B cells is derived from studies examining the response of B cell subpopulations to exogenous agents. CD5 B cells apparently respond to exogenous cytokines and phorbol esters differently than $CD5^-$ B cells. Murine splenocytes, for example, generally are not stimulated by phorbol ester to initiate DNA synthesis without a second signal, such as that provided by a calcium ionophore. Populations of peritoneal B lymphocytes enriched with CD5 B cells, however, incorporate tritiated thymidine after treatment with phorbol esters without the need for a second signal (Rothstein and Kolber, 1988). In humans there exists apparent heterogeneity between B cells in their ability to respond to BCGFs. Small (and presumably resting) B cells respond to low-molecular-weight BCGF (of 18-20 kDa) only in the presence of anti-IgM antibody, whereas large (and presumably preactivated) B cells respond to this BCGF even in the absence of anti-IgM antibody (Muraguchi et al., 1983; Dugas et al., 1985). Tonsillar and peripheral blood B cells also are heterogeneous with respect to their response capacities to the high-molecular-weight BCGF of approximately 50 kDa (Ambrus et al., 1985). CD5 B cells apparently initiate DNA synthesis in response to this factor alone, while small (presumably $CD5^-$) B cells require prestimulation with anti-IgM antibodies in order to respond substantially to this factor (Richard et al., 1987). The tonsillar cells responsive to high-molecular-weight BCGF without anti-IgM also coexpressed 4F2, a surface antigen associated with activated cells (Haynes et al., 1981). Through inference, it was reasoned that CD5 and 4F2 were coexpressed by a subpopulation of "activated" tonsillar B cells able to respond to high-molecular-weight BCGF without supplemental stimulation. However, CD5 B cells inherently may respond differently to exogenous cytokines and phorbol esters because they have a distinctive physiology. Consistent with this notion, stimulation of B lymphocytes with any of the different agents that provide the "first signal" (i.e., anti-IgM or calcium ionophore) does not induce $CD5^-$ B cells to coexpress CD5 (discussed above). Thus, one cannot conclude from such studies that CD5 B cells are a subpopulation of activated normal B cells.

Finally, flow-cytometric analyses of murine CD5 B cells using simultaneous two-color surface immunofluorescence and the fluorescent dye 7-amino-actinomycin D (7AAD) also apparently provided support for the notion that CD5 is a marker for activated B cells (Rabinovitch et al., 1986). Cell staining with the latter supposedly is dependent on the chromatin conformation, activated cells having greater 7AAD fluorescence than nonactivated cells. Analyses of SM/J, NZB, or BALB/c mouse splenocytes demonstrated that cells coexpressing CD5 and sIgM had greater 7AAD fluorescence than sIgM-bearing cells that were $CD5^-$. From their studies, these authors concluded that the CD5 B cell subpopulation was enriched for cells in the S or G_2-M phase of the cell cycle, and that the $CD5^-$ subpopulation was composed of essentially nondividing cells.

However, subsequent and more direct study of BALB/c or NZB lymphocyte populations that were enriched for CD5 B cells demonstrated that less than 2% of CD5 B cells *in vivo* normally are found in the S and G_2 phases of the cell cycle (Förster and Rajewsky, 1987). As such, either a few cells within the CD5 B cell population are dividing rapidly or all CD5 B cells are cycling at a slow rate. Nevertheless, these studies indicate that the vast majority of CD5 B cells are in the resting G_0 or G_1 stage of the cell cycle and thus most likely are not activated B lymphocytes.

VIII. CD5 B Cells Define a Distinct B Cell Lineage

Early work examining the ability of adult bone marrow allografts to reconstitute B cells in lethally irradiated mice indicated that the CD5 B cell may constitute a lineage distinct from CD5⁻ B lymphocytes. By transplanting cells from Ig allotype-congenic donor mice, the B lymphocytes within the host can be identified as being of either host or donor origin. Using these methods in conjunction with multiparameter flow-cytometric analyses, it was demonstrated that the lymphoid populations of mice reconstituted with adult bone marrow had virtually no CD5 B cells of donor origin (Hayakawa *et al.*, 1985; Herzenberg *et al.*, 1986). On the other hand, such reconstituted animals had high proportions of CD5⁻ B cells in the spleen that were of donor origin.

That donor CD5 B cells could grow in an Ig allotype-congenic environment was demonstrated in transplantation experiments using donor populations enriched for CD5 B cells. Transfer of neonatal bone marrow or splenocytes into lethally irradiated mice allowed for the emergence of CD5 B cells of donor origin (Hayakawa *et al.*, 1985). The neonatal cells responsible for transfer of CD5 B cells did not necessarily coexpress sIg or CD5 and likely represented CD5 B cell progenitors. Transfer of lymphocytes from the adult mouse peritoneum, on the other hand, also resulted in the colonization of donor-type CD5 B cells within irradiated recipient mice. In contrast to the CD5 B cell progenitors in neonatal spleen, however, the peritoneal cells responsible for transfer of donor-type CD5 B cells to irradiated recipients coexpressed both sIgM and CD5 at the time of cell transfer (Hayakawa *et al.*, 1986b). Furthermore, $\varkappa$ light chain-expressing CD5 B cells reconstituted $\varkappa$ light chain-expressing CD5 B cells, and $\varkappa$ light chain-negative CD5 B cells reconstituted λ light chain-expressing CD5 B cells. As such, CD5 B lymphocytes in the adult mouse peritoneum apparently constitute a self-renewing cell subpopulation.

Further support for this concept was provided by adoptive transfer studies of peritoneal lymphocytes injected into allotype-congenic neonatal mice (Förster and Rajewsky, 1987). Peritoneal B lymphocytes from CB.20 adult mice of the IgH^b allotype were found to propagate in neonatal BALB/c mice expressing the IgH^a allotype. Survival of the transferred cells was not dependent on the presence of donor T cells in the transferred cell population. However, the source of the donor lymphocyte population was critical in that bone marrow-derived lymphocytes from adult animals could not colonize such neonatal recipients. Dual immunofluorescence studies demonstrated that most, if not all, of the IgH^b allotype-expressing cells in the recipient mice expressed CD5 [53-7.3] but not CD8 [53-6.7]. In fact, CD5 B cells expressing the IgH^b allotype accounted for over half of the peritoneal CD5 B cells of recipient mice several months after cell transfer. These animals also had elevated levels of serum IgM that increased over time. Interestingly, at 20 weeks after cell transfer, nearly 50% of the serum antibody was of the IgH^b allotype, suggesting that CD5 B cells may be a major source of serum IgM antibody. Recipient animals produced antigen-specific IgM antibodies of the IgH^b allotype in response to thymus-independent antigens, such as $\alpha(1 \to 3)$ dextran, but not in response to thymus-dependent antigens. In total, these studies strengthen the hypothesis that the CD5 B cells form a distinct B cell lineage.

IX. CD5 B Cells after Human Bone Marrow Transplantation

Unlike the mouse, adult human bone marrow apparently contains cells that may reconstitute the CD5 B cell population. Following bone marrow transplantation, most circulating B cells have been reported to express CD5. This was first indicated by a serial study of four acute myelogenous leukemia patients who received bone marrow transplants (Ault et al., 1985). When in clinical remission, the patients were treated with cytosine arabinoside and whole-body irradiation. One patient received bone marrow from an identical twin donor. The other three patients received HLA-matched sibling marrow allografts depleted of donor T cells using anti-CD5 Mab [Leu-1] and complement. These three patients also were given methotrexate in prophylaxis against graft-versus-host disease (GVHD). One of these subsequently developed grade II acute GVHD that successfully was treated with infusions of anti-CD5 Mab. This patient, however, failed to produce detectable B lymphocytes in the peripheral blood at any time after transplantion. The other three patients all developed circulating B cells approximately 30 days after transplantation. These B cells all coexpressed both CD5 and pan-B lymphocyte surface antigens, such as CD19 [Leu-12]. Conventional CD5$^-$ B cells appeared in the peripheral blood 2-6 weeks later. CD5 B cells, however, remained the predominant B cell subpopulation for several weeks, accounting for over half of all the circulating B cells. In a subsequent study, the same investigators examined the recovering B cells of a heterogenous group of 46 patients who received bone marrow grafts (Antin et al., 1987). Again, CD5 B cells accounted for more than half of the circulating B lymphocytes in patients following bone marrow transplantation. Recovery of CD5 B cells, however, was reduced significantly in patients with acute or chronic GVHD, but apparently was unaffected by patient age, disease, or *ex vivo* treatment of the marrow with anti-CD5 Mab and complement. Thus, for longer than one year after bone marrow transplantation, CD5 B cells constituted the predominant circulating B lymphocyte subpopulation in patients without GVHD.

Conflicting results, however, were obtained in a study of 21 leukemic patients who underwent allogenic bone marrow transplantation with bone marrow depleted of T cells by treatment with anti-CD8 [RFT8] and anti-CD6 [RFT12] Mabs (Drexler et al., 1987). Although only five of these patients had GVHD, the percentage of circulating lymphocytes that reacted with anti-CD5 [RFT1] and an anti-pan-B Mab [RFB7] never exceeded 2% from any one patient. Collectively, the average proportion of lymphocytes that were CD5 B cells was not greater than that of normal control subjects. From their data, these investigators concluded that bone marrow transplant recipients actually may lack circulating CD5 B cells. These authors suggested that the earlier studies described above may have been artifactual secondary to nonspecific binding of the IgG$_{2a}$ anti-CD5 Mab used [Leu-1]. However, these earlier studies apparently were well controlled. Alternative explanations are possible. For example, differences in the methods used for purging T cells from the donor marrow or in the treatment of GVHD may influence the relative proportions of CD5 B cells after bone marrow transplantation. Resolution of this issue will require further study.

X. CD5 B Cell Physiology

A. Autoantibody Production

The first indication that CD5 B cells may constitute a functionally distinct subset of autoantibody-producing cells was presented by Hayakawa and co-workers in the Herzenberg laboratory. These investigators demonstrated that splenic CD5 B cells were enriched for spontaneous plaque-forming cells (PFCs) producing IgM antibodies to isologous RBCs pretreated with the proteolytic enzyme bromelain (Hayakawa et al., 1984). Previously, such PFCs to bromelain-treated RBCs (brmRBCs) were detected among B cells from either the spleen or the peritoneum of normal nonimmunized mice (Cunningham, 1974;

Lord and Dutton, 1975; Pages and Bussard, 1975; Bussard et al., 1977; Steele and Cunningham, 1978). The B lymphocytes responsible for these PFCs were found to make IgM "autoantibodies" to self-erythrocyte membrane antigens, more specifically trimethylammonium determinants or phosphatidyl choline (PtC), exposed on senescent RBCs or normal RBCs after treatment with bromelain (Pages and Bussard, 1978; Pages et al., 1982; Cox and Hardy, 1985; Kawaguchi, 1987). The numbers of such B lymphocytes are noted to increase with advancing age, reminiscent of the age-related expansions of CD5 B cells discussed in Section V (Errington and Cox, 1986). That these PFCs are in fact CD5 B cells is indicated by cell-sorting experiments in which CD5 B cells were found to be enriched and CD5$^-$ B cells were found to be depleted of PFCs to brmRBCs (Hayakawa et al., 1984).

CD5 B cells also were implicated in the pathogenesis of autoimmune disease. Several mouse strains that develop autoimmune pathology have elevated numbers of splenic and peritoneal CD5 B cells. NZB and related strains characteristically produce high serum levels of pathological autoantibodies reactive with autologous erythrocytes, thymocytes, and single-stranded DNA (ssDNA) (Shirai and Mellors, 1971; DeHeer et al., 1978; Izui et al., 1978; Andrews, et al., 1978; Smith and Steinberg, 1983; Theofilopoulos and Dixon, 1985). The anti-DNA antibodies produced by such animals are cross-reactive with a remarkable array of different compounds, such as multiple polynucleotides, cardiolipin and other phospholipids proteoglycans, and some intracellular proteins (Eilat, 1982; Pisetsky, 1984; Schwartz and Stollar, 1985). That these antibodies are produced by CD5 B cells was implied by the finding that NZB and related mice have dramatically increased numbers of splenic CD5 B cells compared to normal BALB/c mice (Hayakawa et al., 1983, 1984). Such mice also have the highest percentages of CD5 B cells in the peritoneum of several mouse strains tested, with 25–70% of NZB peritoneal cells coexpressing B cell surface antigens and CD5 (Hayakawa et al., 1986a).

That pathogenic autoantibodies may be produced by CD5 B cells in NZB mice was suggested further by cell-sorting experiments in which pure populations of CD5 B cells or CD5$^-$ B cells were isolated for in vitro culture (Hayakawa et al., 1983, 1984). In these experiments only CD5 B cells were found to secrete IgM antibodies reactive with either autologous T lymphocytes or ssDNA in vitro. However, most, if not all, of the splenic B cells that produced antibodies in vitro after in vivo immunization with exogenous antigens were found in the isolated CD5$^-$ B cell population. From such studies, these investigators postulated that CD5 B cells constitute a functionally distinct B cell subpopulation involved in autoimmune pathogenesis.

Other mouse strains genetically programmed to develop autoimmune disease also were found to have elevated numbers of CD5 B cells. Mice homozygous for the viable motheaten (me^v) or motheaten (me) gene(s) located on chromosome 6 have severe autoimmune disease and a markedly shortened life span (Green and Shultz, 1975; Shultz and Green, 1976; Rossi et al., 1985). These animals have hypergammaglobulinemia, primarily resulting from elevated levels of IgM and IgG_3 antibodies (Sidman et al., 1986), and high titers of IgM autoantibodies (Sidman et al., 1984; McCoy et al., 1985). In addition, the sera contain high concentrations of factors capable of stimulating B cell maturation (Sidman et al., 1984) and/or activation (Sidman et al., 1985). Such factors are produced by B cells (Sidman et al., 1984) and by large numbers of activated macrophages (McCoy et al., 1984). Presumably secondary to such factors, these animals have increased numbers of plasma cells in the spleen, lymph nodes, lung and other organs, and reduced numbers of circulating B cells (Sidman et al., 1978a,b; McCoy et al., 1985; Davidson et al., 1979; Rossi et al., 1985). Almost all of the B cells from C57BL/6 (me/me) mice are large by forward-angle light scatter and coexpress normal to high levels of sIgM, low levels of sIgD and CD5, and thus phenotypically are CD5 B cells (Sidman et al., 1986).

In contrast, some strains which lack detectable CD5 B cells are immunodeficient. CBA/N mice are immunodeficient secondary to a gene(s), designated *xid*, located on the X chromosome (Berning et al., 1980; Cohen et al., 1985a,b). These mice are deficient in mature B lymphocytes, nonresponsive to soluble polysaccharides (type 2 antigens) and PtC on any carrier, and hypogammaglobulinemic, particularly with respect to IgM (Amsbaugh et al., 1972; Scher et al., 1973, 1975a,b; Mond et al., 1977; Kincade, 1977; Huber et al., 1977; Ahmed et al., 1977). In addition, CBA/N mice have depressed numbers of cells in the spleen or the peritoneum that spontaneously form plaques with isologous brmRBCs (Rosenberg, 1979). That the CD5 B cell may regulate or provide for some of these immune functions was suggested when CBA/N mice were found to be devoid of detectable CD5 B cells in the spleen (Hardy et al., 1983) and the peritoneum (Hayakawa et al., 1986a; Herzenberg et al., 1986). These mice, however, may develop CD5 B cells if reconstituted with autologous bone marrow after treatment with the immunosuppressant cyclosporine A (de la Hera et al., 1987), indicating that precursors for CD5 B cells may exist in CBA/N mice. Such treatment also may enhance the numbers of spontaneous brmRBC PFCs detected in the spleen and the peritoneum of such animals.

In order to examine the effects of the *xid* and *me* mutant genes together in the same animal, the *me* gene first was bred into NFS and C3H/HeN mice, resulting in new strains of mice that had a motheaten phenotype similar to that of C57BL/6 (*me/me*) mice (Scribner *et al.*, 1987). The *xid* gene then was bred into such (*me/me*) mice. The survival of (*me/me*) homozygous mice was not altered by the introduction of the *xid* gene. However, compared to mice of the same genetic background that lack the *xid* gene(s), (*me/me*) animals carrying the *xid* gene(s) had markedly reduced levels of circulating IgM autoantibodies to ssDNA, self-T lymphocyte surface antigens, and isologous brmRBCs (Scribner *et al.*, 1987). Furthermore, NFS (*me/me*) *xid* mice did not have detectable CD5 B cells in the spleen, in contrast to NFS (*me/me*) mice, in which greater than 80% of the splenic B cells were noted to express CD5. As such, either the *xid* gene(s) or a closely linked gene(s) may suppress CD5 B cell development and the associated production of IgM autoantibodies.

Whether CD5 B cells are responsible for production of pathogenic autoantibodies, however, remains controversial. Using a 3T3 fibroblast-filler cell-supported cloning system (Pike and Nossal, 1985), sorted splenic or peritoneal B cells were stimulated with LPS and then distributed into separate wells of 60-well Terasaki trays at one to 600 cells per well. After several days' culture, supernatants from individual wells were assayed via enzyme-linked immunosorbent assay for nonspecific mouse Ig and specific anti-DNA or anti-fluorescein isothiocyanate (FITC) Ig. Using the Poisson equation, the total number of antibody-forming cells (AFCs) and the numbers of AFCs producing anti-DNA or anti-FITC antibodies were calculated. In agreement with earlier studies on splenocytes from normal mouse strains (Pisetsky and Caster, 1982), splenocytes of three normal mouse strains (i.e., CBA, BALB/c, and C57BL/6) and the autoimmune NZB strain were found to have relatively high proportions of AFCs reactive with denatured DNA. Generally, the numbers of anti-DNA AFCs exceeded the numbers of anti-FITC AFCs by 2:1 or 3:1. Curiously, populations enriched for CD5 B cells (i.e., CBA peritoneal cells or NZB splenocytes) did not have increased frequencies of anti-DNA AFCs compared to populations with few detectable CD5 B cells (i.e., BALB/c splenocytes). Furthermore, in limited cell-sorting experiments, isolated CD5$^-$ B lymphocytes from NZB spleen were found to have greater proportions of anti-DNA AFCs than that of separated NZB CD5 B cells (Conger *et al.*, 1987).

That the population of CD5 B cells may not be enriched for cells producing anti-DNA autoantibodies also is supported by recent studies examining the antibodies produced by hundreds of hybridomas derived from splenocytes or peritoneal B lymphocytes of BALB/c or NZB mice (Kaushik *et al.*, 1988). Although many of the hybridomas generated from peritoneal cells of either strain produced Mabs that reacted with brmRBCs, none produced Mab with anti-DNA or anticytoskeletal protein autoreactivity. Furthermore, although splenic B cells have proportionately fewer CD5 B cells, several hybridomas derived from fusion with splenic B lymphocytes of either strain produced Mabs reactive with DNA and self-cytoskeletal proteins.

Fusion of splenocytes from CD5 B cell-enriched motheaten viable mice, however, yielded proportionately greater numbers of hybridomas producing anti-DNA and other autoantibodies, compared to hybridomas derived from fusion of spleen cells from other mouse strains. LPS-stimulated splenocytes from 1- and 2-month-old C57BL/6 me^v mice were fused with Sp2/0, to generate Mab-producing hybridomas (Painter *et al.*, 1988). Although the numbers of clones generated were small compared to the numbers of splenocytes fused, greater than 50% (17 of 33) of the hybridomas produced autoantibodies reactive with syngenetic thymocytes, erythrocytes, kidney, skin, IgG, or other self-antigens. The majority of these (11 of 16) demonstrated multispecificity for more than one self-antigen. As such, the frequency of hybridomas producing multispecific autoantibodies (11 of 33) far exceeded that of hybridomas produced by these same investigators from LPS-stimulated splenocytes of normal BALB/c mice (two of 356) (Bellon *et al.*, 1987) or normal C57BL/6 mice not possessing the me^v gene(s) (two of 144) (Mills *et al.*, 1985).

C57BL/6 me^v autoantibody-producing hybridomas were found to utilize a variety of different V_H genes and a restricted set of V_κ genes (Painter *et al.*, 1988). The V_H genes utilized by each of 16 independent autoantibody-producing hybridomas were studied by Northern blot analyses and were found to be heterogenous. Three of these V_H genes apparently belonged to the V_H J606 gene family, one to V_H X24, four belonged to V_H J558 subgroup, three were from V_H Sl07, two were from V_H 7183, and three utilized a V_H gene cross-hybridizing with V_H X24 and V_H 7183 gene family probes. In contrast, autoantibody-producing hybridomas generated from LPS-stimulated splenocytes of BALB/c mice utilized primarily V_H genes belonging to V_H 7183, V_H QPC52, and V_H 7183 (Monestier *et al.*, 1986), V_H gene families most proximal to the Ig heavy-chain J gene segments (Yancopoulos *et al.*, 1984; Yancopoulos and Alt, 1986). An apparent restriction was noted, however, in the antibody light-chain V genes expressed by C57BL/6 me^v-derived hybridomas. Of the V_κ genes expressed by sixteen different hybridomas, four were of the $V_\kappa 1$ subgroup, another four were of the $V_\kappa 9$ family, two were of the $V_\kappa 4$ subgroup, and another two were of the $V_\kappa 19$ family. V_κ genes from these four V_κ gene subgroups frequently are used to encode the light chain of mouse autoantibodies produced in other mouse strains (Shlomchik *et al.*, 1986; Kasturi *et al.*, 1988). From their data, the authors reasoned that the heavy chains of the autoantibodies produced in C57BL/6 me^v mice apparently are encoded by a random assortment of V_H genes, similar to that observed encoding antibodies obtained from LPS-stimulated lymphocytes from normal mouse strains (Dildrop et al., 1985). However, the light chains of the such autoantibodies apparently are encoded by a restricted set of V_χ genes that commonly are associated with autoantibodies produced in other mouse strains.

However, caution must be exercised in extrapolating from data obtained from analyses of antibodies produced by hybridomas, as the process of cell fusion may be nonrandom. An acknowledged problem with the previously described study is the apparent bias introduced by cell fusion. Perhaps because C57BL/6 me^v mice produce high amounts of B cell maturation factors and primarily have mostly CD5 B cells, it was not possible to obtain many hybridomas from fusion experiments with splenocytes from these mice. That the small number of hybridomas generated may not be representative of the entire population of C57BL/6 me^v B cells is indicated by the fact that no λ light chain-producing hybridomas were generated, even though almost one third of the total me^v-derived serum IgM antibodies have λ light chains (Sidman et al., 1986). Thus, the B cells amenable to cell fusion may not be representative of the entire B cell population.

Another important question is whether antibodies produced by CD5 B cells from autoimmune strains of mice differ from the antibodies expressed by CD5 B cells from normal mice. Multiparameter flow-cytometric analyses of whole lymphocyte populations using fluorochrome-conjugated antigen suggest that the spectrum of autoantibodies expressed by CD5 B cells from normal mice actually may differ from that of CD5 B cells present in motheaten mice. Using fluorescent liposomes composed of synthetic distearoylphosphatidyl choline to label cells expressing antibody reactive with PtC, it was found that 5-15% of peritoneal lymphocytes from normal adult B10.H-2^aH-4^b p/Wts mice were reactive with PtC (Mercolino et al., 1988). Virtually all of the PtC-reactive cells were large by light scatter and coexpressed bright sIgM, dull sIgD, and CD5 [53-7.3]. As such, these cells phenotypically were CD5 B cells. Included in the population of CD5 B cells reactive with PtC were essentially all of the precursors to cells that, upon LPS stimulation, secrete antibody hemolytic for brmRBCs. However, motheaten mice were found to have very low frequencies of PtC liposome-binding cells within the peritoneum, despite having proportionately large numbers of CD5 B lymphocytes. Whether this discrepancy relates to differences in the fine specificities of antibodies produced by CD5 B cells from motheaten mice compared to those of BALB/c mice is unresolved.

In humans, CD5 B cells apparently are enriched for cells producing IgM autoantibodies. Earlier studies indicated that the human peripheral B cells that rosette with MRBCs were enriched for cells that synthesize IgM anti-IgG autoantibodies [rheumatoid factor (RF)] after stimulation with EBV (Fong et al., 1983). That such B lymphocytes likely were CD5 B cells was indicated by EBV transformation experiments on sorted $CD5^+$ and $CD5^-$ B cell populations isolated from the peripheral blood of normal volunteers that recently were vaccinated with tetanus toxoid (TT) (Casali et al., 1987). Analyses of the resulting lymphoblastoid colonies revealed that many produced antibodies reactive with TT. Colonies producing IgM anti-TT were derived primarily from the transformed CD5 B cell population, while clones synthesizing IgG anti-TT were generated from the $CD5^-$ B cell subset. In addition, many of the lymphoblastoid colonies derived from transformed CD5 B cells produced IgM antibodies with low affinity for ssDNA or for the Fc of IgG (RF) (Casali et al., 1987). Although not elaborated on in the text, many of these autoantibodies were polyreactive with a wide array of compounds. In contrast, none of the lymphoblastoid colonies derived from transformed $CD5^-$ B cells produced such IgM autoantibodies. Although these studies may be difficult to interpret secondary to the bias that transformation with EBV may introduce, studies performed independently on freshly isolated B cells of normal individuals or from patients with rheumatoid arthritis (RA) supported the notion that CD5 B cells are enriched for cells producing IgM autoantibody (Hardy et al., 1987). After stimulation with S. aureus Cowan I (SAC) cells, sorted CD5 B cells produced high levels of RF. In contrast, $CD5^-$ B cells isolated from the same individuals failed to produce RF, even after in vitro stimulation with SAC cells. Together, these observations indicate that the CD5 B cells in both RA patients and normal individuals are enriched for cells capable of synthesizing RF and perhaps other autoantibodies.

CLL B cells also may share with normal CD5 B cells the capacity to express autoreactive IgM antibodies, particularly RF. Thirteen of 65 patients (20%) with CLL were noted to have leukemic cells that formed rosettes with human IgG-coated autologous erythrocytes (Preud'homme and Seligmann, 1972). Moreover, in a limited study of 13 patients, four (30%) were found to express sIgM capable of binding fluorescein-conjugated human IgG (Kipps et al., 1987b). These observations are supported by more recent studies on IgM antibodies secreted by leukemic B cells after stimulation with pokeweed mitogen (Sthoeger et al., 1989). In this analysis, 53% of the 17 antibody-producing leukemic cell populations secreted IgM reactive with IgG, ssDNA, or double-stranded DNA (dsDNA). In total, these studies indicate that the antibodies produced by leukemic CD5 B cells often have reactivity for self-antigens.

B. Helper B Cell Activity

Studies by Okumura and colleagues first indicated that there may exist a functional subset of CD5 B cells with apparent immunoregulatory activities (Okumura et al., 1982). Thy-1⁻ hapten-primed splenic B cells require T cells from carrier-primed mice to produce antihapten antibodies in response to the hapten–carrier conjugate *in vitro*. When such splenic B cells were depleted of CD5-bearing lymphocytes, using anti-CD5 Mab Ly-1 [53-76.6] and complement, the number of added carrier-primed T cells required for an optimal antibody response increased significantly. Addition of Thy⁻ B lymphocytes from nonprimed donor mice to the cultures, however, significantly augmented the antihapten antibody production, particularly when the numbers of added carrier-primed T cells in the culture were limiting. The ability of the nonprimed B lymphocytes to facilitate hapten-specific antibody production was abrogated by removal of the 2–3% of the splenic non-T cell population that expressed CD5. This helper activity required that the nonprimed B cells be syngeneic with the hapten-primed B cells at the Ig V_H gene locus.

Functional studies of murine CD5 B cells were extended using an *in vitro* model system to examine the secondary antibody response of hapten-primed C57BL/6 B splenocytes to a hapten, 4-hydroxy-3-nitrophenyl acetyl (NP), coupled to Ficoll, a T cell-independent carrier (Sherr and Dorf, 1984). Generation of PFCs producing anti-NP antibodies bearing the major IgH^b-linked idiotypic determinants, designated NP^b, was reduced significantly if T cell-depleted splenocytes also were depleted of CD5-bearing lymphocytes. Generation of NP^b idiotype PFCs could be restored by adding nylon wool-adherent and Thy-1⁻ B cells from normal or athymic mice. B cells responsible for this helper activity in the donor B cell population were designated B_H cells. Priming the B_H cell donor mice with antigen was not required. However, the donor mice had to be syngeneic with C57BL/6 mice at both the IgV_H region and the I–A locus of the major histocompatibility complex (MHC) in order to provide effective B_H cells (Sherr and Dorf, 1984, 1985).

The restriction of B_H cells for interacting only with cells that share identity at the V_H gene locus may be related to the specificity of the response measured, i.e., generation of antibodies bearing NP^b idiotype in response to the hapten NP. Antibodies bearing NP^b idiotype in C57BL/6 mice are λ light chain-bearing molecules with variable regions apparently encoded by a single pair of V_L and V_H genes that have not diversified from the germ-line DNA (Reth et al., 1978, 1979; Bothwell et al., 1981, 1982). Studies examining the immune response against NP^b idiotope(s) demonstrated that the expression of NP^b idiotope and its association with NP-binding activity are strain specific (Takemori et al., 1982). Such strain specificity apparently reflects the polymorphism seen in inbred strains of mice within the Ig V region, resulting in genetic differences in the inherited germ line-encoded antibody repertoire.

These B_H cells were presumed to be CD5 B cells. Such cells are resistant to treatment with anti-Thy-1 and complement, nonadherent, and depleted by treatment with anti-CD5 [53-76.6] and complement (Sherr and Dorf, 1984). Furthermore, mice that have elevated numbers of splenic CD5 B cells, such as viable motheaten mice, discussed in Section X,A (Sidman et al., 1986), also have elevated numbers of splenic B_H cells (Sherr et al., 1987b).

The B_H cells active in this system apparently express sIgM/sIgD with λ but not $\varkappa$ light chains. Pretreatment of the cell population containing B_H activity with complement and antibodies specific for IgM [78/25 (Stall and Loken, 1984)], IgD [AFG/222.5 (Stall and Loken, 1984)] or λ light chain [JC5.1], but not $\varkappa$ light chain [187.1 (Yelton et al., 1981)] depleted the population of detectable B_H activity (Sherr and Ju, 1986). Furthermore, nylon-adherent Thy-1.2$^-$ cell populations could be enriched for B_H activity by selecting for cells adhering to anti-λ light chain-coated petri dishes. This finding suggested that the B_H cells express a repertoire of Ig molecules distinct from that of conventional B lymphocytes for which expression of immunoglobulin with $\varkappa$ light chains is predominant.

For unexplained reasons, augmentation of the NP^b idiotypic antibody response was abrogated by pretreatment of the B_H cell population with complement and antibodies specific for CD4 [GK1.5 (Dialynas et al., 1983), 2B6 (Logdberg et al., 1985; Wassmer et al., 1985)] or CD11a [LFA-1, M17/5.1.4 (Sanchez-Madrid et al., 1982; Davignon et al., 1981)] but not CD11b [MAC-1], indicating that lymphocyte function-associated antigens also may play a role in B_H cell-dependent helper activity (Sherr and Ju, 1986). However, as discussed earlier, CD5 B cells do not coexpress detectable amounts of CD4 by sensitive flow-cytometric analyses.

The helper activity provided by such cells apparently consists of at least two components. One of these is antiidiotypic immunoglobulin and another is a late-acting B cell maturation factor (Sherr et al., 1987b). Previously, it was noted that B_H cells may produce antiidiotypic antibodies capable of binding anti-NP antibodies bearing NP^b idiotypic determinants, even though they were derived from donor mice that were not primed with antigen (Sherr and Dorf, 1984). To investigate this further, hybridomas were generated from splenic B_H cells by fusion with 750-6, a C3H-derived B lymphoblastoid cell line (Sherr et al., 1987a). Hybridomas were selected that produced IgAλ antiidiotypic antibodies specific for NP^b idiotypic determinants. Media conditioned by such hybridomas could substitute for B_H cells in the cultures of hapten-primed CD5 B cell-depleted lymphocytes to achieve comparable levels of NP^b idiotype expression in response to NP–Ficoll. Such conditioned media evidently contained two discrete factors that were required for stimulation of NP^b idiotypic antibody production in these cultures. One factor was anti-NP^b idiotypic antibody, and the other was a nonantibody cytokine of undetermined molecular weight. Antiidiotypic antibodies had been noted to enhance the proliferative cell and PFC capacity of idiotype-bearing B cells cultured with suboptimal concentrations of functionally efficient T helper cells by other investigators (Pereira *et al.*, 1986a) (discussed further in Section XVI). Also, neoplastic CD5 B cell lines, such as BCL_1, have been noted to secrete soluble factors that stimulate B cell growth and differentiation (Brooks *et al.*, 1984). Together, these data suggest that the immunoregulatory potential of CD5 B cells may be mediated by an unidentified cytokine(s) and secreted antibody with anti-Ig reactivity.

Studies of humans, testing whether CD5 B cells could augment Ig secretion by conventional B cells in the presence of suboptimal numbers of T cells, failed to demonstrate any enhancing activity (Antin *et al.*, 1986). Whether this indicates a true distinction between human and mouse CD5 B cells is not clear. To be sure, the studies of humans were performed using fetal CD5 B cells that were tested for their ability to augment the primary antigen response to antigens *in vitro*. Studies in mice, on the other hand, examined the ability of CD5 B cells from adult mice to augment IgG antibody secondary antibody responses *in vitro*.

That the human CD5 B cells may have immunoregulatory function, however, is indicated by work by MacKenzie and colleagues, who examined for immunoregulatory cells in multiple myeloma (MM). This malignancy often is associated humoral immune dysfunction (Cone and Uhr, 1964; Fahey *et al.*, 1963; Cwynarski and Cohen, 1971; Pilarski *et al.*, 1984; MacKenzie *et al.*, 1987; Paglieroni *et al.*, 1988). Some patients with MM have peripheral blood cells that can suppress the *in vitro* antibody synthesis of pokeweed mitogen (PWM)-stimulated normal PBLs from unrelated donors (Paglieroni and MacKenzie, 1977, 1980). These cells apparently form rosettes with human IgG-coated human RBCs (EA). PWM-stimulated cultures of PBLs produced two thirds to one half as much antibody when mitomycin C-treated EA^+ cells from MM patients were added to the cultures within 2 hours after mitogen stimulation (MacKenzie *et al.*, 1987). Media conditioned by such EA^+ MM cells also could suppress the PWM-induced antibody secretion by normal PBLs. This suppression was mediated by a factor of 10–20 kDa that was trypsin sensitive and nuclease resistant. In contrast to other factors that act late after mitogen stimulation (Bich-Thuy et al., 1984), suppression by EA+ cells requires early addition of cells or conditioned media to the PWM-stimulated cultures. The EA+ cells producing this factor were nonadherent and negative for nonspecific esterase. Also, these immunoregulatory cells were not stimulated to proliferate or produce antibody in response to PWM or PHA. Using sensitive flow-cytometric analyses, these investigators demonstrated these cells to coexpress low levels of sIgM and CD5 [Leu-1], in addition to CD19 [Leu-12], low-density CD20 [Leu-16], CD21 [B2, HB-5 (Tedder et al., 1984)], CD22 [Leu-14], and HLA-DR and -DQ [Leu-10] (MacKenzie et al., 1987). These cells, however, did not express T cell-associated antigens CD8 [Leu-2], CD4 [Leu-3], CD3 [Leu-4], or CD2 [Leu-5]; NK cell-associated antigens CD16 [Leu-11] or Leu-7; monocyte-associated antigen CD15 [Leu-M1]; or the early B progenitor antigen CD10 [J5, CALLA]. These cells phenotypically resembled CD5 B cells. Interestingly, although isolated from the peripheral blood of patients with monoclonal B cell malignancies, the cells from any one patient were not monoclonal with respect to Ig light-chain expression. Regulatory cells from any one patient were noted to express either $\varkappa$ or λ Ig light chains. This indicates that these immunoregulatory cells probably are not derived from the malignant myeloma cell clone.

Patients with CLL may have leukemic CD5 B cells with immunoregulatory activity. One patient with severe hypogammaglobulinemia had leukemic CD5 B cells that suppressed PWM-induced Ig synthesis of normal PBLs by over 80% (Paglieroni et al., 1988). Like most CLL cells, these leukemic cells coexpressed CD5 [Leu-1], CD19 [Leu-12], CD20 [B1], and HLA-DR, but not CD10 [J5], CD21 [B2], CD22 [Leu-14], CD25 [Tac, p55 chain of the receptor for IL-2 (Waldmann et al., 1984)], or PCA-1. Suppression of Ig synthesis by normal PBLs apparently was mediated by a protease-sensitive but nuclease-resistant factor of approximately 10–20 kDa (Paglieroni et al., 1988). Another patient with B cell CLL was noted to have leukemic cells that apparently secreted BCGF upon stimulation with anti-IgM (Kawamura et al., 1986). This factor did not induce proliferation of nonstimulated or PHA-stimulated T cells. However, this BCGF induced the proliferation of B cell blasts that previously had been stimulated by treatment with anti-IgM antibodies or SAC. BCGF also could induce proliferation of autologous leukemic cells that had been prestimulated with anti-IgM antibody, indicating that such a factor could operate in an autocrine fashion on leukemic CD5 B cells expressing antigen or self-reactive sIg. This may not apply to all leukemic CD5 B cell populations, however. Other investigators, for example, have reported that CLL B cells have impaired responsiveness to T cell-derived BCGF, even after prior stimulation with anti-IgM antibodies (Perri, 1986). Such discrepancies suggest that leukemic CD5 B cell populations from different patients may have different functional activities.

C. MONOCYTOID FEATURES

B cells and monocyte/macrophages may share a curious developmental relationship. Certain myeloid cell lines produce immunoglobulin μ chain constant-region gene transcripts, suggesting that they originated from precursor cells of the B lineage (Kemp et al., 1980). Other studies demonstrate that certain pre-B cell lines may differentiate into monocytes or macrophages. One such line is ABLS 8.1, a pre-B cell tumor with rearranged Ig heavy-chain genes that was derived from a BALB/c mouse infected with Abelson leukemia virus (Sklar et al., 1975; Cory et al., 1980). When treated with the demethylating drug 5-azacytidine, these cells differentiate into functional macrophagelike cell lines (Boyd and Schrader, 1982). Similarly, a human pre-B cell line, RS4;11, derived from a patient with acute lymphoblastic leukemia, can differentiate into a phagocytic monocytoid cell line after treatment with PMA (Stong et al., 1985). Although these examples may represent the lineage infidelity of neoplastic cells (Smith et al., 1983), an alternative hypothesis is that such cases represent a transient phase of limited promiscuity in gene expression occurring in normal bipotential progenitor cells (Greaves et al., 1986). The latter would argue that monocyte/macrophagelike cells may be derived from a pre-B cell precursor that may be poised to undergo Ig heavy-chain gene rearrangement.

More recent studies have indicated that certain pre-B cells capable of developing along the myelocyte lineage in fact may be CD5 B cell precursors. Several pre-B cell lines capable of spontaneously differentiating into macrophagelike lines coexpress CD5 (Holmes et al., 1986; Davidson et al., 1988). A well-studied example is HAFTL-1, a cell line derived from murine fetal liver cells transformed with v-Ha-*ras* (Holmes et al., 1986). HAFTL-1 cells express CD5 [NEI-017] and B cell-associated differentiation antigens Lyb-2 [10.1-D2 (Subbarao and Mosier, 1983)], Ly-5 [B220, RA3-6B2 (Coffman, 1983)], Lyb-8 [CY-34-1.1 (Symington et al., 1982)], and Ly-17, the FcR [2.4G2 (Unkeless, 1979)]. They also produce terminal deoxynucleotidyl transferase and have either nonrearranged Ig heavy-chain genes or DJ_H rearrangements (Holmes et al., 1986; Alessandrini et al., 1987). However, these cells lack expression of ThB [53-9.2 (Ledbetter and Herzenberg, 1979)], CD11b [MAC-1, M1/70 (Springer et al., 1978, 1979)], Ia [10-3.6 (Oi et al.,

1978)], and 6C3 (Pillemer *et al.*, 1984). As such, HAFTL-1 cells resemble early B cell progenitors, or pre-B cells. In contrast to bone marrow-derived pre-B cells (Dasch and Jones, 1986) or pre-B cell lines (Paige *et al.*, 1978), however, HAFTL-1 could be induced by treatment with LPS to express Ia and differentiate along either the monocyte/macrophage or B cell pathway. In differentiating from lymphoidlike precursors into macrophages, HAFTL-1 cells lost surface expression of Lyb-8, Lyb-2, and the B cell-associated isoform of Ly-5, B220. Instead, they expressed CD11b, MAC-2 [M3/38 (Ho and Springer, 1982)], and the 204-kDa monocyte-associated form of Ly-5 (Tung *et al.*, 1981). Consistent with this monocyte/macrophage surface antigen phenotype, these cells also produced high levels of nonspecific esterase and lysozyme and became phagocytic for latex beads (Davidson *et al.*, 1988). Some LPS-stimulated HAFTL-1 cells, however, differentiated further along the B cell pathway to express ThB and higher levels of B220, rearrange their Ig heavy-chain genes, and produce immunoglobulin gene transcripts. Both macrophage and pre-B cell lines continued to coexpress CD5. In each case, induced macrophages and pre-B cells were found to share identical v-*ras* genomic integration sites, indicating a common clonal origin for both macrophage and CD5 pre-B cell lines.

That mature Ig-expressing CD5 B cells may be derived from a common myeloid–B cell progenitor is suggested by studies of a methylcholanthrene-induced lymphoblastic B cell line, P388 (Nadler *et al.*, 1983). This cell line was found to express surface CD5 and to be related clonally to a macrophage cell line, designated P388D1, derived from the same animal. Together, these data suggest that there may exist a close developmental relationship among monocytes, macrophages, and CD5 B cells.

B cells, and CD5 B cells in particular, also share several functional properties with monocytes and macrophages. B cells coexpress class II MHC surface antigens and may serve, like macrophages, as antigen-presenting cells (Chesnut and Grey, 1981; Glimcher *et al.*, 1982; Issekutz *et al.*, 1982; Chesnut *et al.*, 1982a,b; Grey *et al.*, 1982; Walker *et al.*, 1982; Birmingham *et al.*, 1982; Lanzavecchia, 1985). Monocytes and macrophages are the primary source of IL-1, a polypeptide cytokine and T cell mitogen that plays a pivotal role in inducing the cellular immune response to infection, injury, or antigenic challenge (Mizel *et al.*, 1978; Kronheim *et al.*, 1985; Dinarello, 1988). Several reports indicate that normal peripheral B cells, as well as leukemic CD5 B cells, also may synthesize IL-1 of 15–20 kDa that is biochemically and functionally indistinguishable from that synthesized by monocytes and macrophages (Durum *et al.*, 1985; Pistoia *et al.*, 1986; Matsushima *et al.*, 1985; Morabito *et al.*, 1987). As discussed earlier, both normal and leukemic

CD5 B cells, in contrast to other B cells, may express low levels of myelomonocytic surface antigens, such as CD11b, CD14, and CD15. It is not known whether expression of such surface antigens imparts peculiar functional activities onto the CD5 B cell. However, it is interesting to note that only those CD5 B leukemic cell populations found to express myelomonocytic surface antigens produce IL-1 *in vitro*, either spontaneously or after stimulation with LPS or LPS plus indomethacin (Morabito *et al.*, 1987). Whether the IL-1 produced by normal peripheral B cells is the exclusive product of CD5 B cells within the population of peripheral B cells is not known. However, it is tempting to speculate that several of the above-mentioned B cell myeloid characteristics are peculiar to the CD5 B cell.

XI. Physiology of the CD5 Surface Antigen

Whether the CD5 surface molecule is important to the physiology of the CD5 B cell will require resolution of the structure and function of the CD5 surface molecule. Indeed, expression of CD5 on the surface of these cells may be an epiphenomenon not intricately related to the peculiar physiology of the CD5 B cell. In this case, characteristics other than expression of CD5, such as Ig gene expression or helper B cell activity, eventually may prove better suited to delineate the true CD5 B cell. On the other hand, delineating the function of the CD5 surface molecule may lead to a clearer understanding of CD5 B cell physiology.

Most of the studies of the CD5 surface antigen have been performed on T lymphocytes. Since the CD5 molecules expressed by B and T cells appear to be biochemically similar (Fox *et al.*, 1982), it is conceivable that conclusions made from studies on CD5 expressed by T cells may be extrapolated to apply for CD5 expressed by B lymphocytes. However, some caution is warranted. Aside from expressing different levels of CD5, T and B cells also express a different constellation of surface antigens. Association of any of these surface antigens with CD5 may uniquely affect the physiology of the CD5 surface molecule. Nevertheless, studies of the function of this molecule expressed by T lymphocytes are reviewed here, as they may be relevant to that of CD5 expressed by the CD5 B cell.

CD5 may function as a receptor molecule. This is indicated by studies with anti-CD5 monoclonal antibodies. Such antibodies may affect the physiology of T lymphocytes or cultured T cell lines. This was first demonstrated by using a rat IgG_{2a} anti-mouse CD5 Mab [α Ly-1 (Hollander *et al.*, 1981; Hollander, 1982)]. This Mab could augment cell proliferation and cytotoxic T cell generation when added to mixed-lymphocyte cultures without complement. This effect required that the antibody be added during the first 24 hours of the mixed-lymphocyte reaction. Addition of this Mab to the culture stimulated production of growth factor(s) by the responding lymphocytes (Hollander et al., 1981). Subsequently, it was demonstrated that anti-CD5 Mab [53-7.3] induced increases in cytosolic calcium concentration, cell surface IL-2 receptor levels, and IL-2 production of thymocytes or T cell lines that previously had been activated with suboptimal concentrations of PHA (Ledbetter et al., 1987).

Anti-CD5 Mabs also can affect human lymphocytes. Addition of intact IgG_1 [OKT1] or $F(ab')_2$ anti-CD5 Mab to mixtures of human B cells and irradiated autologous CD4 T lymphocytes enhanced the generation of PFCs measured in a reverse hemolytic plaque assay (Thomas et al., 1984). These antibody preparations had no significant effect on mixtures of B cells and autologous irradiated CD8 T lymphocytes. Anti-CD5 also stimulated cultures of CD4 T cells to produce helper factor(s) capable of inducing B cell proliferation. Interestingly, the production of such helper factor(s) required that the CD4 T cells be cocultured with irradiated autologous non-T (E rosette-negative) cells (Thomas et al., 1984). This suggests that either anti-CD5 stimulates CD4 T cells to produce stimulatory factors that, in turn, induce non-T cells to produce other helper factor(s) or that triggering of CD4 T cells by anti-CD5 requires an additional signal provided by a non-T cell (perhaps a CD5 B cell?). In addition, a number of different anti-CD5 Mabs apparently may augment proliferation of PBLs and purified T cell preparations after they have been preactivated with free or Sepharose-bound anti-CD3 Mab [G19-4 (Ledbetter et al., 1985; Ceuppens and Baroja, 1986; Geppert and Lipsky, 1988)].

Extensive evaluation of the physiological effects of anti-CD5 Mab was performed on the Jurkat human T cell line by Ledbetter et al. (1986). These investigators monitored changes in the levels of cyclic nucleotides, cAMP and cGMP, and cytoplasmic calcium upon binding of the anti-CD5 Mab to the cell surface. They demonstrated that anti-CD5 Mabs caused an increase in cytoplasmic free calcium concentration within 3 minutes of the addition of antibody, accompanied by a rapid threefold increase in cGMP levels. The levels of cAMP were unaffected. These data suggest that both cGMP and cytoplasmic free calcium are involved in signal transduction upon binding of the CD5 surface molecule to its appropriate ligand.

Human cytolytic T lymphocyte (CTL) lines that do not express CD5 were compared with $CD5^+$ CTL lines to examine the functional significance of the CD5 surface antigen (Bierer et al., 1988). In limiting concentrations of anti-CD3 Mab, anti-CD5 Mab stimulated increases in cytoplasmic free calcium levels in $CD5^+$ CTLs, but not $CD5^-$ CTLs. As noted in earlier studies, anti-CD5 Mab alone had no effect. More recently, a subclone of the Jurkat human T cell line was selected for loss of the CD5 surface antigen. In the presence of anti-CD3 Mab linked to Sepharose beads, anti-CD5 Mab stimulated IL-2 production of the parent Jurkat cell line but not of the variant $CD5^-$ Jurkat cell line (Nishimura et al., 1988a). Retroviral-mediated gene transfer of CD5 cDNA into $CD5^-$ Jurkat cells or $CD5^-$ CTL lines restored CD5 surface expression. Infected cells that expressed CD5 produced IL-2 in response to anti-CD5 Mab added in the presence of suboptimal amounts of anti-CD3 Mab.

These experiments indicate that the CD5 surface antigen most likely is a cytokine receptor or a receptor-associated molecule. Speculation that CD5 may serve as the receptor for IL-1 was stimulated by findings that IL-1 and anti-CD5 Mab have similar activities *in vitro* (Ceuppens and Baroja, 1986). Indeed, both IL-1 and anti-CD5 Mabs induce cell surface expression of IL-2 receptors and IL-2 production by T cells preactivated with anti-CD3 Mab bound to Sepharose beads (Williams et al., 1985; Ledbetter et al., 1985; Ceuppens and Baroja, 1986).

However, functionally the IL-1 receptor and CD5 are not one and the same. The stimulatory signal provided by anti-CD5 Mab apparently is distinct from that provided by IL-1, in that the two together in culture have additive effects in inducing T cell proliferation (Ledbetter et al., 1985). In contrast to IL-1, anti-CD5 Mab does not enhance the proliferation of T cells preactivated with suboptimal concentrations of PHA (Ledbetter et al., 1986; Ceuppens and Baroja, 1986). Furthermore, although expression of CD5 apparently is restricted to lymphocytes, IL-1 receptors also have been found in the brain (Katsuura et al., 1988), fibroblasts (Akahoshi et al., 1988a; Bonin and Singh, 1988), natural killer-like cells (Lubinski et al., 1988), mammary and colon carcinoma cell lines (Gaffney et al., 1988), cultured synovial cells (Chin et al., 1988), and polymorphonuclear leukocytes (Rhyne et al., 1988). Moreover, gluococorticoids, which hardly affect the level of CD5 surface membrane expression, increase the surface expression of the IL-1 receptor on peripheral lymphocytes, particularly B cells (Akahoshi et al., 1988b).

Isolation of the cDNA encoding human (Jones et al., 1986) or mouse (Huang et al., 1987) CD5 has demonstrated the molecule to have structural features common to other receptor molecules encoded by members of the Ig supergene family. The human CD5 has a large extracellular segment of 347 amino acid residues, a short transmembrane region of 30 residues, and an intracellular domain of 93 amino acid residues. The mouse molecule shares extensive homology with the human molecule in both amino acid constitution and deduced secondary structure (Huang et al., 1987), confirming earlier predictions that the CD5 surface antigens of mice and humans are homologs (Ledbetter et al., 1981).

Although the receptor for the IL-1 receptor molecule also is encoded by a member of the Ig supergene family, it is distinct from CD5. Recent studies have distinguished two types of IL-1, designated IL-1α (Auron et al., 1984) and IL-1β (Lomedico et al., 1984). Although they have similar molecular weights and biological activities, these two types of IL-1 have a markedly different primary structure and most likely a different tertiary structure (Priestle et al., 1988). Nevertheless, both IL-1α and IL-1β molecules apparently bind to a single 70- to 80-kDa receptor glycoprotein (Rhyne et al., 1988) with K_ds of 6.6×10^{-11} M and 4×10^{-12} M, respectively (Chin et al., 1988). The cDNA encoding this receptor glycoprotein in the mouse has been isolated (Sims et al., 1988). From the nucleic acid sequence, one can deduce this receptor to have a protein backbone of 65 kDa, with a 319-amino acid extracellular portion, a 21-amino acid hydrophobic transmembrane segment, and a 217-amino acid cytoplasmic domain. Although the IL-1 receptor has many structural features in common with other molecules encoded by the Ig supergene family, including CD5, it is clearly distinct from CD5.

It is possible, however, that coexpression of CD5 may influence the binding activity of the IL-1 receptor for IL-1. Recent experiments have increased speculation that the IL-1 receptor actually may be comprised of two or more chains that together have higher or more selective IL-1-binding affinities (Bird et al., 1987; Kroggel et al., 1988; Dinarello et al., 1989). Through cross-linking studies, other protein chains of 23, 43, 110, and 220 kDa apparently may be associated with the IL-1 receptor molecule. Because of the similarity in size of the cloned IL-1 receptor and CD5, association of the IL-1 receptor with CD5 may not have been apparent. However, recent data indicate that CD5, in fact, may influence the binding activity of the IL-1 receptor (Nishimura et al., 1988b). Mutant CD5$^-$ Jurkat cells (discussed above) apparently do not respond to or bind IL-1, even after prior stimulation with anti-CD3 Mab. However, infection of these cells with a retroviral vector that restored CD5 surface expression restored the ability of these cells to bind and internalize IL-1. As such, CD5 may facilitate the binding activity of the IL-1 receptor when coexpressed on the cell membrane.

The CD5 surface molecule also may induce activation signals in CD5 B cells when attached to its specific ligand. The CD5 molecule expressed by T cells is biochemically similar to the CD5 molecule expressed in T or B cell CLL (Martin et al., 1981; Fox et al., 1982). Furthermore, induction of CD5 antigen expression on human B cells with phorbol esters is associated with increased levels of mRNA complementary to the T cell-derived CD5 cDNA (Freedman et al., 1987a). Finally, anti-CD5 Mabs [SC-1, Leu-1] are noted to enhance the proliferation of purified B cells isolated from the peripheral blood of rheumatoid arthritis patients with high levels of circulating CD5 B cells, suggesting that anti-CD5 Mab may be weakly mitogenic for CD5 B lymphocytes (Hara et al., 1988). These studies suggest that the CD5 molecule also may be a physiological receptor molecule for the CD5 B cell.

Recent data suggest that CD5 may complex with other surface molecules on the B cell surface. CD5 is reported to cap with anti-CD5 Mabs on the surface of leukemic cells from patients with CLL (Bergui et al., 1988). Anti-CD5 Mab-induced capping results in comodulation of CD21 [HB-5], the receptor for C3d (Weis et al., 1984; Fingeroth et al., 1984; Iida et al., 1983). However, such treatment with anti-CD5 did not comodulate CD19 [B4], CD20 [B1], or sIgM. Moreover, anti-CD21 Mab induced comodulation of CD5. Subsequent to capping with either CD5 or CD21, leukemic cells no longer adhered to plates coated with C3d. These data suggest that CD5 and CD21 may be associated on the leukemic cell membrane, perhaps forming a complex receptor for complement fragments. As CD21 generally is not expressed by T lymphocytes, such a complex may endow the B cell surface-associated CD5 molecule with a unique physiology. Also, coexpression of both CD21 and CD5 by the CD5 B cell may allow this cell type to respond differently to complement fragments, or other soluble factors, than do B lymphocytes that only express CD21.

XII. Genetic Influence on the Relative Numbers of CD5 B Cells

Comparison of inbred mouse strains indicate that the level of CD5 B cells may be under genetic control. As discussed in Section X,A, NZB and (NZB × NZW)F_1 mice have increased numbers and frequencies of CD5 B cells in both the spleen and the peritoneum compared to other mouse strains. The absolute numbers of splenic and peritoneal CD5 B cells also vary among other inbred strains of mice. Most mouse strains, including nude (nu/nu) mice and the autoimmune MRL mice (Murphy and Roths, 1978), have approximately the same low numbers of splenic CD5 B cells, comprising roughly 2% of the total splenic B cells in the adult animal (Hayakawa et al., 1983). Other mouse strains, such as CBA/N (discussed in Section X,A), do not have detectable splenic CD5 B cells (Hardy et al., 1983). Greater strain variation is seen in the proportions of peritoneal cells that coexpress CD5. Some 10–35% of peritoneal cells from BALB/c and related strains are CD5 B cells. CD5 B cells represent only 5–20% of the peritoneal cells from CBA, NFS, CSW, C57BL/10, A.TH, A.TL, or 129/Sv mice. In contrast, less than 1% of the peritoneal cells from SJL and related strains are CD5 B cells. Backcross experiments between SJL and BALB/c mice demonstrated that the gene(s) regulating the differences in the levels of peritoneal CD5 B cells of these two strains segregate independently from the Ig heavy-chain locus (Hayakawa et al., 1986a). This is consistent with the backcross experiments described in Section X,A, in which the introduction of the X chromosome-linked *xid* gene(s) into C57BL/6 (*me/me*) mice resulted in marked reduction in the number of detectable CD5 B cells (Scribner et al., 1987). Together, these observations indicate that strain-specific variations in the CD5 B cell level may be under genetic control.

In humans, the relative proportion of CD5 B cells circulating in the peripheral blood also appears to be influenced genetically (Kipps and Vaughan, 1987). Among normal young adults there exists heterogeneity in the proportion of PBLs that coexpress B cell surface antigens and CD5, such cells representing between 0% and 6% of PBLs. Despite such discrepancies between unrelated persons, the level of circulating CD5 B cells for any one individual is constant over at least several months. Studies of related family members indicated that the relative numbers of circulating CD5 B cells segregated in a non-Mendelian fashion. However, in contrast to ordinary siblings that may have disparate proportions of circulating CD5 B cells, monozygotic twins or triplets share identical CD5 B cell levels. These studies are consistent with the notion that, as in inbred mouse strains, the relative numbers of CD5 B cells are under multifactorial genetic control.

XIII. CD5 B Cells in Human Autoimmune Diseases

Persons with autoimmune diseases were speculated to have elevated numbers of CD5 B cells (Hayakawa et al., 1984). Such speculation originated from observations that the numbers of CD5 B cells are increased in certain strains of mice, such as NZB, that genetically are programmed to develop systemic autoimmune pathology. This resulted in several studies investigating the levels at which CD5 B cells are found in the peripheral blood of patients with autoimmune diseases. Several such studies indicated that the levels of circulating CD5 B cells may be elevated in patients with RA (Plater-Zyberk et al., 1985; Maini et al., 1987; Lydyard et al., 1987; Taniguchi et al., 1987; Hardy and Hayakawa, 1986; Dauphinee et al., 1988; Hardy et al., 1987). However, patients with systemic lupus erythematosus (SLE), an autoimmune disease that most resembles the autoimmune pathology afflicting NZB mice, do not have elevated levels of CD5 B cells. For example, using fluorescence-microscopic techniques, CD5 B cells were found to comprise an average of 20% of the circulating B cells of RA patients compared to less than 5% of the B cells of normal controls or patients with SLE (Plater-Zyberk et al., 1985). The average absolute numbers of circulating B cells, however, were comparable among each of the three groups. Using more sensitive flow-cytometric techniques, these investigators detected coexpression of CD5 on a greater proportion of B cells from persons of all three groups. However, the average proportions of B cells that expressed CD5 still were greatest in the PBLs of RA patients (Maini et al., 1987). Similar results were reported by Okumura's group in their comparative analyses of 13 RA patients and a comparable number of age-matched controls (Taniguchi et al., 1987). Although both groups had comparable absolute numbers of circulating B cells, these comprising 16% ($\pm$ 5% SD) and 14% ($\pm$ 5% SD) of the circulating lymphocytes, respectively, the proportions of B cells found to express CD5 tended to be higher in RA patients (20 $\pm$ 9%) than in normal controls (14 $\pm$ 6%).

Autoimmune diseases other than RA also may be associated with elevated levels of circulating CD5 B cells. CD5 B cells have been found in increased numbers in patients with primary Sjögren's syndrome (1° SS) (Dauphinee et al., 1988; Hardy et al., 1987) and progressive systemic sclerosis (Hardy et al., 1987). In a study of 19 patients with 1° SS, the mean percentage of B cells with detectable surface expression of CD5 was 46% in 1° SS patients, compared to only 26% in normal control subjects.

When examined, the levels of CD5 B cells in the peripheral blood of patients with RA or 1° SS generally are stable over time (Kipps and Vaughan, 1987; Taniguchi et al., 1987; Dauphinee et al., 1988). The few exceptions were patients treated with high-dose corticosteroids or combined immunosuppressive chemotherapy and irradiation (Taniguchi et al., 1987; Dauphinee et al., 1988). Two patients with 1° SS whose levels of CD5 B cells dropped significantly subsequent to such therapy also had clinical remissions in their autoimmune pathology (Dauphinee et al., 1988). Of note, however, there was no apparent relationship to the relative CD5 B cell level and the titer of RF (Kipps and Vaughan, 1987; Plater-Zyberk et al., 1985), except for patients with extremely high titers ($>5 \times 10^{12}$) of RF (Taniguchi et al., 1987).

Whether circulating CD5 B cells play a role in the pathophysiology of RA is uncertain. To be sure, not all RA patients have high levels of circulating CD5 B cells and normal unaffected individuals without high-titer RF may have high levels of circulating CD5 B cells (Kipps and

Vaughan, 1987; Maini et al., 1987; Hardy et al., 1987). Moreover, monozygotic twins discordant for RA have identical levels of CD5 B cells in the peripheral blood (Kipps and Vaughan, 1987). Also, CLL patients, with monoclonal expansions of CD5 B cells, do not develop classical RA pathology more frequently than does the general population. Perhaps these apparent discrepancies are secondary to the fact that the population of circulating lymphocytes in the peripheral blood is not representative of the cells found at sites of primary disease activity (i.e., the peripheral joints). It is possible that closer examination of the cells within these sites will reveal a more definitive relationship between the CD5 B cell and autoimmune disease. Alternatively, CD5 B cells may have little to do with autoimmune pathogenesis.

XIV. Immunoglobulin Gene Expression in Murine CD5 B Cell Lymphomas

Spontaneous murine CD5 B cell lymphomas may express Igs with antigenic specificities shared by antibodies produced by nonmalignant CD5 B lymphocytes. As mentioned in Section VI, the CH lymphomas arise in B10.H-2^aH-4^b p/Wts mice after adoptive spleen cell transfer and hyperimmunization with SRBCs (Lanier et al., 1978, 1982). As they coexpress both sIgM and CD5 (Lanier et al., 1982; Pennell et al., 1985), they possibly are derived from neoplastic transformation of CD5 B cells. Because many were found to express sIg reactive with SRBCs, it first was speculated that hyperimmunization with SRBCs contributed to lymphomagenesis through chronic antigenic stimulation of SRBC-reactive B cell clones (LoCascio et al., 1984; Lynes et al., 1978; Arnold et al., 1983). In closer analyses of 27 such lymphomas, however, only six produced antibody reactive with SRBCs (Pennell et al., 1985). However, an even greater number (nine) of the 27 lymphomas formed rosettes with brmRBCs. Several such lymphomas expressed sIg specific for PtC (Mercolino et al., 1986). Moreover, many of the lymphomas that produced antibody reactive with SRBCs also formed rosettes with brmRBCs. In this regard, the sIg of many of these lymphomas had binding specificity in common with that of normal CD5 B cells found within the spleen or the peritoneum of nonimmunized mice (discussed in Section X,A).

In order to examine the structural basis for the autoantibodies produced by CH lymphomas, heterologous antiidiotypic antibodies were prepared against the detergent-solubilized affinity-purified sIg expressed by each of several tumors (Pennell et al., 1985). Following extensive absorption with isotype-matched Ig myeloma protein, the antisera were tested for binding to each of the various lymphomas. Cross-reactive idiotypes (CRIs) were identified on 21 of 27 independently derived CH lymphomas. These 21 CH lymphomas could be categorized into five partially overlapping sets based upon idiotypic cross-reactivity. A minimum of 16 idiotopes were detected on 23 of the 27 CH lymphomas. Only four of these idiotopes were confined to a single tumor; the rest were all shared. Some of these CRIs apparently were V_H specific, in that they were present on both λ- and ϰ-expressing tumors. As such, the frequencies of CRIs were greater than the frequency at which a given lymphoma reacted with the immunogen used to induce these lymphomas, namely SRBCs. Because of this, these authors proposed that the tumors were selected by virtue of their expressed Ig idiotype(s) rather than their specific reactivity for antigen, namely SRBCs.

Nucleic acid sequence analyses of the antibody V genes expressed by these CH lymphomas, however, revealed that the frequent occurrence of CRIs was secondary to the fact that CH lymphomas express a highly restricted set of antibody V genes with little somatic diversification (Pennell et al., 1988). Ten independently derived CH lymphomas, representing each of the five previously defined groups of major CRIs (Pennell et al., 1985), were found to utilize only five different V_H and seven different V_L genes (Pennell et al., 1988). Lymphomas within each of the five groups expressed identical V_H genes.

The V_H genes expressed by several of the CH lymphomas could not be assigned strictly to any of the ten previously defined murine V_H gene families (Brodeur and Riblet, 1984; Winter et al., 1985; Kofler, 1988). Such assignment generally requires that a given V gene share greater than 80% homology with representative genes of a given subgroup (Brodeur and Riblet, 1984). The V_H gene expressed by each of three CH lymphomas had closest similarity with members of the X24 or 7183 V_H gene families, but at only 72 or 75% homology, respectively (Yancopoulos et al., 1984; Hartman and Rudikoff, 1984). Remarkably, this expressed V_H gene is identical to the V_H genes expressed by three clonally unrelated anti-brmRBC antibody-producing hybridomas generated from autoimmune NZB mice (Reininger et al., 1987). As such, this V_H gene most likely is conserved between NZB and Bl0.H-2^aH-4^b p/Wts mice and expressed without somatic diversification. Because it lacks better than 80% homology with any of the previously described V_H genes, this V_H gene may define a new V_H gene family. Furthermore, the $V_ϰ$ gene expressed by one these three CH lymphomas also is identical to that of the $V_ϰ$ gene expressed by the NZB hybridomas. Another two CH lymphomas expressed identical V_H genes that also apparently were derived from an as yet undefined V_H gene family, sharing only seventy-five percent similarity with members of the 36-60 V_H gene family (Near et al., 1984; Dzierzak et al., 1986). Two sets of two other lymphomas each expressed identical V_H genes belonging to the J558 and S107 V_H gene families, respectively.

Studies on apparent oligoclonal expansions of normal murine CD5 B cells have revealed these cells also may express a limited repertoire of Ig V genes that have not diversified from the germ-line DNA. As discussed in Section V, oligoclonal expansions of CD5 B cells can be detected in older mice or in younger NZB mice (Stall et al., 1988; Tarlinton et al., 1988). This is particularly apparent when CD5 B cells are passaged in allotype-congenic neonatal mice in which donor CD5 B cells expressing an Ig allotype different from that of the host can be monitored (Förster and Rajewsky, 1987). In such recipients, apparent clonal expansions of donor CD5 B cells can be detected in the peritoneum. B cells of such expansions coexpress CD5 and a distinctive density of donor-allotype sIgM. Cell fusion of peritoneal or spleen cells from mice with such noted oligoclonal donor CD5 B cell expansions generated hybridomas producing antibodies of donor allotype that had limited variable-region diversity (Förster et al., 1988). Among 17 hybridomas thus generated, eight were progeny of only three different B cell clones, consistent with these hybridomas' being derived from only a few clonal precursors. Surprisingly, however, clonally independent hybridomas expressed identical V genes. As such, the expanded CD5 B cell clones apparently utilized a limited set of antibody V genes. Moreover, the lack of sequence differences between independent clones indicated that the expressed V genes were not diversified through the process of somatic hypermutation. Interestingly, the V genes utilized by several of these hybridomas were identical to V genes concomitantly reported to be expressed by several of the CH lymphomas described above. Furthermore, some of the expressed $V_\varkappa$ genes shared greater than 99% nucleic acid sequence identity to a $V_\varkappa$ gene repeatedly expressed by hybridomas generated from NZB B lymphocytes producing antibodies specific for brmRBCs (Reininger et al., 1987). As such, the antibody V genes utilized by normal, as well as malignant, CD5 B cells apparently are expressed with little somatic diversification. Furthermore, the mechanism(s) responsible for the restriction in the expressed antibody V gene repertoire seemingly operates in a reproducible fashion in both normal and autoimmune mouse strains.

XV. Immunoglobulin Gene Expression in Human CD5 B Cell Malignancies

Despite the enormous potential for diversity in immunoglobulin V gene expression through human genetic polymorphisms, antibodies produced by B cell malignancies of unrelated persons may share common idiotypic determinants. Initially defined by using absorbed heterologous antisera (Kunkel et al., 1974a,b), and then more recently by using murine Mabs (Carson and Fong, 1983; Mageed et al., 1986; Posnett et al., 1986), these common idiotopes, or CRIs, were identified initially on IgM autoantibodies, such as RF. That such CRIs were not merely the tertiary reflections of a common binding activity, however, was suggested by protein sequence data. These data demonstrated that the light- or heavy-chain variable regions of CRI-bearing Igs may have conserved primary structure (Kunkel et al., 1974b; Andrews and Capra, 1981; Ledford et al., 1983; Capra and Kehoe, 1974; Pons-Estel et al., 1984; Capra et al., 1972).

Human CD5 B cell malignancies frequently express antibodies bearing major CRIs. In a study of over 30 CLL patients, five of 20 (25%) patients with $\varkappa$ light chain-expressing leukemic cells had malignant lymphocytes that expressed a CRI defined by reactivity with a Mab, designated 17.109 (Kipps et al., 1987a,b). This antibody, prepared against an IgM RF, recognizes a $\varkappa$ light chain-associated CRI present on many human IgM RF paraproteins isolated from patients with Waldenstrom's macroglobulinemia (Carson and Fong, 1983; Carson et al., 1987a,b). Furthermore, over 20% (eight of 34) of all sIg-expressing CLLs were found to react with G6 (Kipps et al., 1988a), a Mab specific for an Ig heavy chain-associated CRI present on several RF paraproteins (Mageed et al., 1986). Interestingly, nearly one half of the CLL cases with leukemic cells reactive with 17.109 also reacted with G6, reflecting a biased coexpression of these CRIs.

Flow-cytometric analyses indicated that CRI expression by leukemic cells is not qualitatively heterogeneous (Kipps et al., 1988b). Dual immunofluorescence studies using fluorescein-labeled antibodies specific for the antibody constant region and phycoerythrin-conjugated anti-CRI antibodies demonstrated that the relative staining intensities of anti-CRI Mabs correlated directly with the relative number of expressed sIg molecules. CRI^- but sIg^+ leukemic cells were not detected in any leukemic cell population expressing a particular CRI. Moreover, differences in the relative staining intensities of an anti-CRI Mab on different leukemic cell populations were found secondary to differences in relative amounts of expressed sIg. These data indicated that different levels of CRI expression by cells within or between leukemic populations are not secondary to qualitative structural differences in the epitopes comprising the CRI, but rather are secondary to the level of sIg expressed by the leukemic cells. As such, these data suggest that antibody gene expression in CLL is stable.

In order to examine the molecular basis for the 17.109 CRI expression in CLL, the $\varkappa$ variable-region genes from unrelated CLL patients with 17.109-reactive lymphocytes were isolated (Kipps et al., 1988b).

Analyses of multiple independent cDNA clones did not reveal any sequence heterogeneity among the V_x genes expressed within a leukemic cell population from any one patient. In addition, 17.109-reactive leukemic cells from unrelated patients were found to express nearly identical V_x genes, these belonging to the V_x IIIb subsubgroup. The V_x genes expressed by 17.109-reactive leukemic cells were found to share greater than 99% nucleic acid sequence identity to a germ-line V_x III gene isolated from placental DNA, designated *Humkv325* (Radoux et al., 1986). Thus, the 17.109 CRI in CLL apparently is secondary to the expression of a highly conserved x variable gene with little or no somatic mutation.

Similarly, analyses of the molecular basis for the G6 CRI in CLL revealed the G6 idiotope(s) to be a serological marker for expression of a conserved V_H gene of the V_H1 subgroup (Kipps et al., 1989b). Protein sequence data of Waldenstrom's RF paraproteins demonstrated that G6-reactive IgM RFs share considerable sequence homology in the first, second and fourth frameworks of the heavy-chain variable region (Newkirk et al., 1987). From these data, it had been deduced that the heavy-chain variable regions of G6-reactive RFs were encoded by a V_H gene(s) of the V_H1 subgroup, a relatively short D segment, and the J_H4 gene segment. Nucleic acid sequence analyses confirmed that G6-reactive leukemic cells express V_H genes belonging to the V_H1 subgroup. Importantly, the V_H genes expressed by G6-reactive leukemic cells from unrelated CLL patients were found to share greater than 99% nucleic acid sequence homology (Kipps et al., 1989b). Despite expressing near-identical V_H genes, however, G6-reactive leukemic cells may express markedly different D segments and utilize J_H6 or J_H4 gene segments. Comparisons of the deduced amino acid sequences of G6-reactive CLL and that of G6$^-$ antibody heavy chains encoded by V_H1 genes suggests that the G6 CRI in CLL is relatively resilient to substitutions within CDR3 but is affected by permutations within CDR1 and CDR2. Together, these data argue that the G6 CRI in CLL also is a serological marker for a conserved V_H1 gene expressed with little or no somatic mutation.

Solid-tissue B cell lymphomas that frequently express CD5, such as SL (discussed in Section VI), also express these CRIs at frequencies comparable to that noted in CLL (Kipps et al., 1989a). Five of 12 examined x light chain-positive SL lymphomas from patients without associated CLL were noted to react to the 17.109 Mab. Moreover, over 10% of all SL cases examined expressed sIg with the G6 CRI. Recently, molecular analyses revealed that the V_x genes rearranged, and presumably expressed, by 17.109-reactive SL are homologous to *Humkv325* and to V_x genes expressed by 17.109-reactive CLL (Pratt et al., 1989).

These studies indicate that, as in CLL, malignant B cells in SL may express Ig V genes that have not diversified from the germ-line DNA.

However, other human B cell malignancies do not express these CRIs at comparable frequencies. Although CRIs have been detected on B cell NHLs of follicular center-cell origin (Stevenson et al., 1986), expression of the CRIs defined by 17.109 or G6 is rare in such lymphomas that ordinarily do not express CD5. Of over 30 $\varkappa$ light chain-expressing follicular NHLs, only one reacted with 17.109, and none reacted with the G6 Mab (Kipps et al., 1988a). These studies indicate that $CD5^+$ and $CD5^-$ human B cell lymphomas may be distinguished with respect to the expression of autoantibody-associated CRIs. As such, these two categories of B cell malignancies may differ in their utilization and/or diversification of expressed Ig V genes.

Support for the notion that there exists a distinction between $CD5^+$ and $CD5^-$ B cell malignancies in their respective rates of somatic hypermutation comes from analyses of the relative expression frequencies of variable-region framework determinants. Somatic mutation in the expressed antibody V gene may permute and distort antigenic determinants that form the CRIs. However, variable-region framework determinants may be relatively resilient to the process of somatic hypermutation. For our studies, we stained cells with a Mab specific for $V_\varkappa$ IIIb $\varkappa$ light-chain framework determinants (Greenstein et al., 1984). Of the CD5 B cell neoplasms, we noted that the anti-$V_\varkappa$ IIIb antibody reacts exclusively with cells bearing the 17.109 CRI, suggesting that the $Humkv325$ gene is the predominant $V_\varkappa$ IIIb gene expressed in these malignancies. In contrast, only one of the three $CD5^-$ NHLs found to react with the $V_\varkappa$ IIIb Mab expressed the 17.109 CRI. The proportion of $\varkappa$ light chain-expressing, $CD5^-$ NHLs that reacted with the anti-$V_\varkappa$ IIIb Mab, however, did not differ significantly from the frequencies with which the anti-$V_\varkappa$ IIIb framework Mab reacted with $\varkappa$ light chain-expressing CLL or CD5 B cell NHL. These results are consistent with the notion that the relatively low-expression frequencies of CRI by $CD5^-$ NHL of follicular center-cell origin may be related in part to differences in the degree to which the expressed antibody V genes have diversified from inherited germ-line repertoire.

In contrast to CLL, malignant B cell NHLs of follicular center-cell origin may permute their expressed Ig V genes through somatic hypermutation. Follicular B cell NHLs frequently may escape from passive immunotherapy with monoclonal antiidiotypic antibodies through the spontaneous generation of idiotype variants. Somatic mutation affecting expression of idiotype apparently may operate independently of the selection imposed by monoclonal antiidiotypic antibodies, as idiotypic heterogeneity is noted in such lymphomas even prior to passive immunotherapy (Raffeld et al., 1985; Carroll et al., 1986). Idiotype variant tumor populations generally express sIg at amounts comparable to that of the original tumor population (Levy et al., 1987; Meeker et al., 1985; Sklar et al., 1984). Molecular analyses of the expressed immunoglobulin genes of parent and variant populations reveal that the V–D and D–J junctions of the antibody heavy chain-variable region and the V–J junction of the antibody light chain are conserved, indicating that the tumor populations of any one patient are clonally related. Furthermore, lymphoma subpopulations also are noted to share chromosomal translocations that have identical molecular breakpoints, confirming the clonal origin of both parent and idiotype-negative variant populations (Cleary et al., 1988). However, nucleic acid sequence analyses of the Ig V genes expressed by individual cells of a given lymphoma reveal extensive V gene heterogeneity. In fact, no two hybridomas generated from such lymphomas express identical heavy- or light-chain V genes (Levy et al., 1987; Cleary et al., 1986). Nucleic acid base differences are concentrated in the V gene, but also are noted in the 5' untranslated region. Overall, the pattern of substitutions seen suggests that the process(es) of somatic hypermutation noted in V genes expressed during secondary immune responses is operating in these lymphomas (Griffiths et al., 1984; Clarke et al., 1985; Rajewsky et al., 1987). In this regard the stability of Ig V gene expreesion in $CD5^-$ NHLs of follicular center-cell origin apparently differs from that of B cell neoplasms that commonly express the CD5 surface antigen, namely CLL and SL NHLs.

Aside from expressing V genes that have not diversified from the germline DNA, however, the high-frequency expression of the 17.109 or G6 CRIs in CD5 B cell malignancies also indicates that V gene utilization by these neoplasms is nonrandom. Estimates of the number of disparate $V_\varkappa$ genes in humans range from 35 to 70 (Bentley, 1984; Klobeck et al., 1984; Jaenichen et al., 1984; Pech and Zachau, 1984). To date, over 35 $V_\varkappa$ genes have been distinguished (Bentley, 1984; Klobeck et al., 1984; Jaenichen et al., 1984; Pech and Zachau, 1984; Chen et al., 1987a,b). Of these, eight belong to the $V_\varkappa$ III subgroup (Chen et al., 1987a,b). However, only one of these, *Humkv325*, has nucleic acid sequence homology with the $V_\varkappa$ gene expressed by the 17.109 CRI-bearing leukemic cells. Moreover, only *Humkv325* can encode the $\varkappa$ light chain paraproteins that are recognized by 17.109 without sequence permutation. Similarly, V_H1 gene(s) encoding the G6 CRI apparently also is present in single copy in the human haploid genome. Expression of this particular V_H1 gene(s) in greater than 10% of the malignant CD5 B cell populations examined would not be expected if the utilization of V_H genes in CD5 B cell malignancies were random.

The apparent restriction in the repertoire of V genes expressed in CD5 B cell malignancies may reflect in part a genetically programmed restriction in the expression of antibody V genes by the CD5 B cell. Certain V genes may have a greater propensity for Ig gene rearrangement, resulting in a disproportionate expression of such V genes in the leukemic cell repertoire. However, since Ig gene rearrangement may not be successful in generating a functional Ig gene, the rearrangement frequency of commonly utilized V genes may exceed the frequency at which these V genes actually are expressed. Some preliminary data support this notion. The *Humkv325* $V_\varkappa$ gene encoding the 17.109 CRI is rearranged abortively in many CLLs that express λ light chains (Kipps *et al.*, 1988c). The mechanism(s) accounting for this is not known. One hypothesis is that the relative order of V genes positioned along the chromosome may affect their relative expression frequencies, as has been demonstrated in the mouse (Alt *et al.*, 1984, 1987; Yancopoulos and Alt, 1985). However, mapping studies of the human Ig $\varkappa$ light-chain locus demonstrates that many functional $V_\varkappa$ genes are located between the $J_\varkappa$ locus and *Humkv325* (Pohlenz *et al.*, 1987). Thus, frequent abortive rearrangements of *Humkv325* in CLL cannot be explained simply by chromosomal order. In this regard, the rearrangement of *Humkv325* in CLL may be similar to that of a recently identified $V_H 5$ gene, designated $V_H 251$ (Humphries *et al.*, 1988). Although not the most proximal V_H gene to the D and J regions, this gene was found to be rearranged with the D-J segment in the leukemic cells from greater than 20% of the 30 patients studied (Humphries *et al.*, 1988).

A mechanism(s) providing for preferential V gene rearrangement alone, however, may not account for the frequent expression of autoantibody CRIs in CD5 B cell neoplasms. Recent studies have demonstrated that the 17.109 or G6 CRIs are expressed by a small subpopulation of normal B cells in the human tonsil and spleen, but rarely by PBLs. Cells expressing these CRIs constitute a small lymphocyte subpopulation confined to the mantle zone and interfollicular region surrounding the germinal center (Fig. 2) (Kipps *et al.*, 1989c). Dual-immunofluorescence analyses indicate that a large proportion of such CRI-bearing cells coexpress CD5. Coexpression of both 17.109 and G6 CRIs, however, is detected only on a small subset of such cells. In fact, the frequency at which these CRIs are coexpressed within a given lymphocyte population is comparable to the product of frequencies at which each CRI is expressed alone. However, as mentioned above, over 40% of the CLLs and SLs that are 17.109 CRI$^+$ also coexpress the G6 CRI. This indicates that there exists a bias toward coexpression of *Humkv325*, with the $V_H 1$ gene(s) encoding the G6 CRI in CD5 B cell malignancies.

This raises the possibility that the variable-region protein structures recognized by Mabs 17.109 or G6 actually may affect leukemogenesis indirectly. Both CRIs commonly are present on IgM autoantibodies, particularly RF (Carson et al., 1987a,b; Mageed et al., 1986). Furthermore, when both CRIs are coexpressed on the same IgM molecule, the antibody invariably has been found to have RF activity (Silverman et al., 1988). Moreover, leukemic cells coexpressing both CRIs also have sIgM with IgG-binding activity. Perhaps B lymphocytes with such self-reactive sIg may be stimulated to divide constitutively, thereby increasing the likelihood for chance transformation. Alternatively, such autoreactive sIg may serve to focus a transforming agent onto the cell, for example, by binding a leukemogenic virus or antigen–antibody complexes containing such a transforming agent (Mann et al., 1987). Whatever the mechanism, however, it appears that both preferential rearrangement and selected coexpression of particular antibody V genes may occur in CD5 B cell malignancies.

The conservation in the primary sequence of V genes encoding the G6 or 17.109 CRIs suggests that the proteins they encode subserve an important physiology. This physiology may be related to the autoreactivity frequently noted for antibodies encoded by these conserved V genes. Such autoreactive antibodies may function to trap antigen–antibody complexes, increasing the capacity of such cells to present antigen to appropriate effector cells. Alternatively, early expression of autoreactive antibodies in development by the CD5 B cell may stimulate clonal expansion in the sterile fetal environment. The continued expression of such autoreactive antibodies may endow the CD5 B cell with constitutive stimulation. As such, the self-reactive Ig may stimulate the cell in an autocrinelike manner, allowing these cells to persist as a self-renewing cell subpopulation. Another possibilty, though not exclusive of the rest, is that expression of such conserved V genes may allow the CD5 B cell to establish a primordial network of idiotypic and antiidiotypic interactions that may regulate the humoral, and perhaps cellular, immune systems.

Consistent with this notion, the $V_H 1$ gene utilized by G6-reactive CLL is homologous to $51p1$, a $V_H 1$ gene expressed during early human B cell ontogeny. This is noteworthy in that the set of V_H genes expressed during early fetal development is highly restricted (Schroeder et al., 1987). Of the V_H genes isolated from the fetal liver library, one V_H gene accounted for the expression of over 20% (three of 14) of the heavy-chain sequences, while three others each accounted for 14% (two of 14) of the expressed variable-region genes. Through statistical analyses of these data, the total size of the fetal V_H repertoire has been inferred to consist of only nine to 39 disparate-antibody V_H genes. Early restriction in human fetal

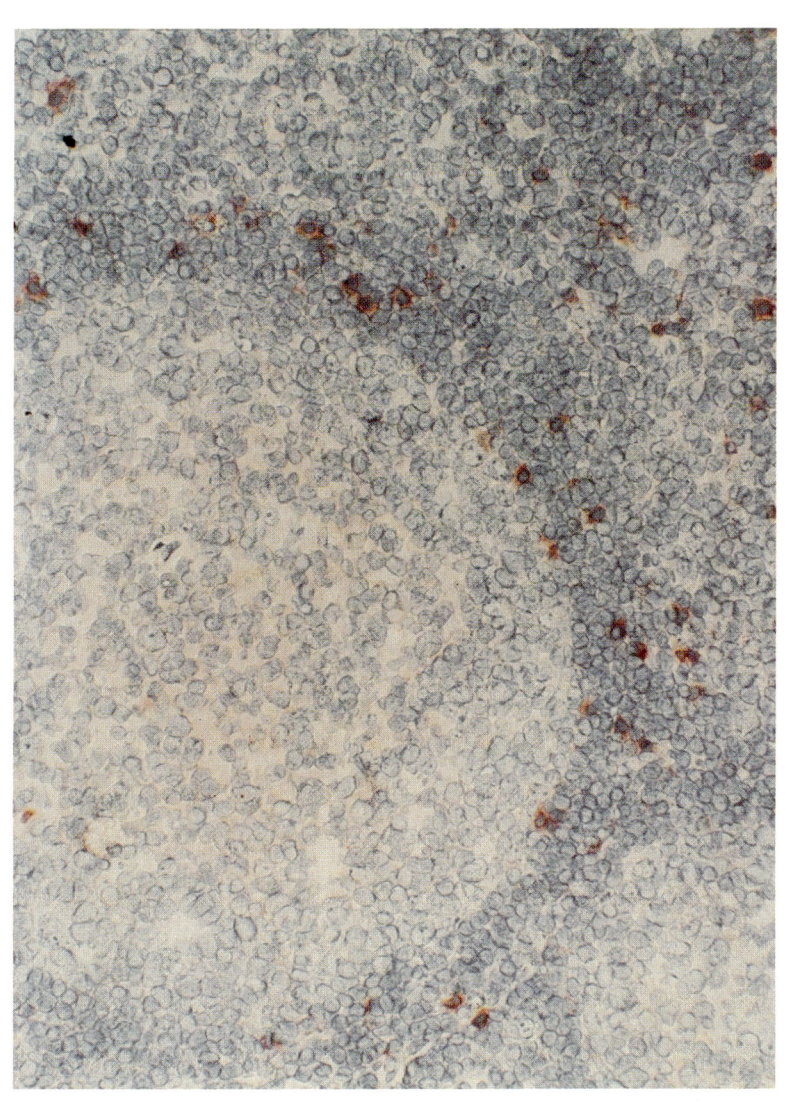

FIG. 2. Immunohistochemical staining of tonsillar cells reactive with 17.109 was performed as described elsewhere (Kipps et al., 1988a). Dark red cells are lymphocytes reactive with the 17.109 Mab.

V gene expression is noted prior to development of mature sIg-expressing B cells and, hence, may be programmed genetically (Schroeder et al., 1987). The homology between the V_H gene expressed by G6-reactive CLL and a V_H gene frequently utilized in the highly restricted fetal repertoire suggests that the set of V genes expressed in CLL may be comparable to that utilized during early B cell development.

XVI. CD5 B Cells and the Primordial Immune Network

Many of the antibodies produced in early B cell ontogeny apparently have autoreactivity (Kearney and Vakil, 1986; Holmberg et al., 1986a). The antibodies produced by hybridomas generated from nonstimulated splenocytes of newborn mice frequently produce antibodies that react with self-antigens, such as actin, myosin, tubulin, or isologous brmRBCs (Dighierio et al., 1983, 1985; Freitas et al., 1986; Araujo et al., 1987). In two studies, the noted frequencies of hybridomas producing autoreactive antibodies were quite high (20–30%), considering the limited panel of self-antigens that were used for screening (Holmberg et al., 1986a; Freitas et al., 1986). The occurrence of such "natural" autoantibodies apparently is not dependent on exogenous antigen stimulation, as they may be detected in the sera of mice raised in either antigen- or germ-free environments (Hooijkaas et al., 1984). Indeed, the proportion of anti-self-"activated" B cells may be increased in such germ-free animals compared to normally raised mice, presumably because such cells are not diluted out by B cells producing antibodies to exogenous antigens (Pereira et al., 1986b; Forni et al., 1988). Similar autoantibodies have been detected in normal human sera (Guilbert et al., 1982; Dighiero et al., 1982).

The antibodies produced during early B cell ontogeny may form an immune network of idiotypic and antiidiotypic reactivities. Hybridomas generated from splenocytes of newborn nonprimed BALB/c mice differ from hybridomas made from LPS-stimulated spleen cells of adult mice, in that a high frequency of the former produces antiidiotypic antibodies specific for immunoglobulins encoded by nondiversified antibody V genes (Holmberg et al., 1986b; Vakil and Kearney, 1986; Kearney and Vakil, 1986; Araujo et al., 1987). These antiidiotypic antibodies characteristically are IgM antibodies with low affinity for one or more idiotopes present on germ-line-encoded antibodies. There exists an apparent high degree of interconnectivity in that antiidiotypic antibodies react with idiotopes encoded by seemingly disparate-antibody variable-region genes. Moreover, present in this neonatal repertoire are anti-antiidiotypic antibodies capable of reacting with one or several of the neonatal

B cell-derived monoclonal antiidiotypes. Assuming that both antiidiotypic and anti-antiidiotypic antibodies are products of nondiversified antibody V genes, the humoral immune system apparently may be genetically programmed to generate a primordial network of idiotypic and antiidiotypic specificities during early B cell ontogeny (Jerne, 1984, 1985).

That this hypothetical immune network may have physiological significance for the normal development of the adult T and B cell repertoire was indicated by studies testing the effect of these neonatal B cell-derived monoclonal antibodies *in vivo* (Vakil and Kearney, 1986; Vakil *et al.*, 1986; Martinez *et al.*, 1986a; Araujo *et al.*, 1987). Timed administration of any of the monoclonal antiidiotypic antibodies to neonatal mice could influence profoundly the subsequent adult B cell repertoire by either enhancing or suppressing the utilization of idiotope-bearing antibodies in adult humoral immune responses (Vakil and Kearney, 1986; Vakil *et al.*, 1986).

Whether such antiidiotypic antibodies could enhance or suppress the subsequent expression of idiotope-bearing antibodies depended on the time at which they were administered during the prenatal or neonatal period. Indeed, the early-appearing, multispecific, antiidiotypic antibodies had profound effects on the development of the normal adult B cell repertoire (Vakil *et al.*, 1986). Examination of the immune response to bacterial dextrans, for example, revealed a discordance between the developmental period that dextran-specific precursors first were detected and the much later age at which dextran-specific antibody responses could be elicited in C57BL/6 mice. Also, administration of antiidiotype at or around the time respective idiotope(s)-bearing cells first are detected during development profoundly suppressed the ability of such cells to produce anti-dextran antibody. This was interpreted to suggest that the late development of the dextran-specific antibody response is regulatory rather than due to late rearrangement and activation of appropriate V genes in ontogeny (Lundkvist *et al.*, 1987).

Such a primordial immune network also may influence the T cell specificities for antigen (Martinez *et al.*, 1988). BALB/c helper T cells generated against 2,4,6-trinitrophenyl (TNP)-derivatized syngeneic splenocytes proliferate and induce antibody secretion of syngeneic B lymphocytes in response to TNP-modified self (Martinez *et al.*, 1986b). This specific T helper cell response could be blocked by monoclonal antibodies directed against either TNP or MHC class II antigens. Interestingly, this response also could be diminished by a monoclonal antiidiotypic antibody, designated F6(51), that is specific for an idiotope expressed by the TNP-binding myeloma protein MOPC 460 (Martinez *et al.*, 1986b). In contrast, TNP self-responsive T helper cells derived from IgH-congenic mouse strains, like CB.20, were not affected by the F6(51) antiidiotype. These data suggested that T helper cells may express T cell receptors that bear idiotypic determinants recognized by F6(51). This notion was supported by experiments indicating that the F6(51) antiidiotypic antibodies can induce IL-2 production in BALB/c T helper cells responsive to TNP-modified self, presumably by binding the T cell's receptor for antigen (Martinez *et al.*, 1984, 1986c).

Accumulating data in this system indicate that immunoglobulins may affect the postthymic maturation of the T cell antigen receptor repertoire. TNP self-responsive T helper cells from mice treated in the prenatal or neonatal period with the F6(51) antiidiotypic antibody are resistant to inhibition with the F6(51) antibody and presumably lack the F6(51) idiotope(s) (Martinez *et al.*, 1986a). These animals apparently express a different repertoire of T cell receptor specificities with respect to TNP-modified self-determinants (Martinez *et al.*, 1987). Also lacking the F6(51) idiotope(s) are TNP self-reactive T helper cells derived from adult BALB/c mice that previously had been treated with anti-IgM antibodies during the first 4 weeks of life (Martinez *et al.*, 1986b). Similarly, TNP self-responsive T helper cells derived from mice reconstituted with autologous bone marrow apparently also lack expression of the F6(51) idiotope(s). However, reconstitution of such mice with syngeneic Thy-1$^-$ but CD5$^+$ peritoneal cells restored the ability of such animals to generate TNP self-responsive T helper cells bearing the F6(51) idiotope(s) (Marcos *et al.*, 1988). These data are consistent with the notion that the Igs expressed by the CD5 B cell may influence directly the postthymic maturation of T cell receptor specificities.

XVII. Conclusion

Cells that coexpress B cell surface antigens and CD5 apparently constitute a self-renewing lymphocyte subpopulation endowed with distinctive physiology. These cells may regulate Ig expression by other B lymphocytes and may assist in the processing, presentation, and/or recognition of antigen. Apparently, these activities in part are mediated by the Igs produced by the CD5 B cell. Such Igs frequently are noted to have reactivity to a variety of self proteins, including Igs, proteolytically processed erythrocyte membranes, and denatured DNA. Such autoreactive antibodies, however, do not contribute necessarily to autoimmune pathology and may be physiological. Although CD5 B cells are distinguished by their expression of CD5, the relationship between the expression of this surface molecule and CD5 B cell physiology is ambiguous and requires resolution. Indeed, expression of CD5 may be fortuitous. If so, CD5 B cells may be defined better through the Igs that they produce. These antibodies apparently are encoded by a restricted set of highly conserved Ig V genes. Expression of antibodies encoded by these antibody V genes without somatic hypermutation may account in part for the peculiar physiology of the CD5 B cell. Recent studies suggest that such antibodies possibly may contribute to a hypothetical network of idiotypic and antiidiotypic antibody interactions that can pattern the expression of both T and B cell receptor specificities. As such, the CD5 B cell may play a pivotal role in the ontogeny and homeostasis of the humoral immune system.

Acknowledgments

The author appreciates the many helpful discussions with Dennis A. Carson of the Scripps Clinic and Research Foundation. This work was supported in part by National Institutes of Health Grants AG04100, AR38475 (First Award), and RR00833. T.J.K. is a Scholar of the Leukemia Society of America, supported in part by the Scott Helping Hand Fund. This is Publication 5821-BCR from the Research Institute of Scripps Clinic.

References

Abb, J., Bayliss, G. J., and Deinhardt, F. (1979). Lymphocyte activation by the tumor-promoting agent 12-O-tetradecanoylphorbol-13-acetate (TPA). *J. Immunol.* **122**, 1639.

Ahmed, A., Scher, I., Sharrow, S. O., Smith, A. H., Paul, W. E., Sachs, D. H., and Sell, K. W. (1977). B-lymphocyte heterogeneity: Development and characterization of an alloantiserum which distinguishes B-lymphocyte differentiation alloantigens. *J. Exp. Med.* **145**, 101.

Akahoshi, T., Oppenheim, J. J., and Matsushima, K. (1988a). Interleukin 1 stimulates its own receptor expression on human fibroblasts through the endogenous production of prostaglandin(s). *J. Clin. Invest.* **82**, 1219.

Akahoshi, T., Oppenheim, J. J., and Matsushima, K. (1988b). Induction of high-affinity interleukin 1 receptor on human peripheral blood lymphocytes by glucocorticoid hormones. *J. Exp. Med.* **167**, 924.

Alessandrini, A., Pierce, J. H., Baltimore, D., and Desiderio, S. V. (1987). Continuing rearrangement of immunoglobulin and T-cell genes in a Ha-*ras*-transformed lymphoid progenitor cell line. *Proc. Natl. Acad. Sci. U.S.A.* **84**, 1799.

Al Saati, T., Laurent, G., Caveriviere, P., Rigal, F., and Delsol, G. (1984). Reactivity of Leu 1 and T101 monoclonal antibodies with B cell lymphomas (correlations with other immunological markers). *Clin. Exp. Immunol.* **58**, 631.

Alt, F. W., Yancopoulos, G. D., Blackwell, T. K., Wood, C., Thomas, E., Boss, M., Coffman, R., Rosenberg, N., Tonegawa, S., and Baltimore, D. (1984). Ordered rearrangement of immunoglobulin heavy chain variable region segments. *EMBO J.* **3**, 1209.

Alt, F. W., Blackwell, T. K., and Yancopoulos, G. D. (1987). Development of the primary antibody repertoire. *Science* **238**, 1079.

Aman, P., Gordon, J., and Klein, G. (1984). TPA (12-O-tetradecanoyl-phorbol-13-acetate) activation and differentiation of human peripheral B lymphocytes. *Immunology* **51**, 27.

Ambrus, J. L., Jr., Jurgensen, C. H., Brown, E. J., and Fauci, A. S. (1985). Purification to homogeneity of a high molecular weight human B cell growth factor; demonstration of specific binding to activated B cells; and development of a monoclonal antibody to the factor. *J. Exp. Med.* **162**, 1319.

Amsbaugh, D. F., Hansen, C. T., Prescott, B., Stashak, P. W., Barthold, D. R., and Baker, P. J. (1972). Genetic control of the antibody response to type 3 pneumococcal polysaccharide in mice. I. Evidence that an X-linked gene plays a decisive role in determining responsiveness. *J. Exp. Med.* **136**, 931.

Anderson, K. C., Bates, M. P., Slaughenhoupt, B. L., Pinkus, G. S., Schlossman, S. F., and Nadler, L. M. (1984). Expression of human B cell-associated antigens on leukemias and lymphomas: A model of human B cell differentiation. *Blood* **63**, 1424.

Andrews, B. S., Eisenberg, R. A., Theofilopoulos, A. N., Izui, S., Wilson, C. B., McConahey, P. J., Murphy, E. D., Roths, J. B., and Dixon, F. J. (1978). Spontaneous murine lupus-like syndromes. Clinical and immunopathological manifestations in several strains. *J. Exp. Med.* **148**, 1198.

Andrews, D. W., and Capra, J. D. (1981). Complete amino acid sequence of variable domains from two monoclonal human anti-gamma globulins of the Wa crossidiotypic group: Suggestion that the J segments are involved in the structural correlate of the idiotype. *Proc. Natl. Acad. Sci. U.S.A.* **78**, 3799.

Antin, J. H., Emerson, S. G., Martin, P., Gadol, N., and Ault, K. A. (1986). Leu-1+ (CD5+) B cells. A major lymphoid subpopulation in fetal spleen: Phenotypic and functional studies. *J. Immunol.* **136**, 505.

Antin, J. H., Ault, K. A., Rappeport, J. M., and Smith, B. R. (1987). B lymphocyte reconstitution after human bone marrow transplantation. Leu-1 antigen defines a distinct population of B lymphocytes. *J. Clin. Invest.* **80**, 325.

Araujo, P. M., Holmberg, D., Martinez-A, C., and Coutinho, A. (1987). Idiotypic multireactivity of "natural" antibodies. "Natural" anti-idiotypes also inhibit helper cells with cross-reactive clonotypes. *Scand. J. Immunol.* **25**, 497.

Arnold, L. W., LoCascio, N. J., Lutz, P. M., Pennell, C. A., Klapper, D., and Haughton, G. (1983). Antigen-induced lymphomagenesis: Identification of a murine B cell lymphoma with known antigen specificity. *J. Immunol.* **131**, 2064.

Ault, K. A., Antin, J. H., Ginsburg, D., Orkin, S. H., Rappeport, J. M., Keohan, M. L., Martin, P., and Smith, B. R. (1985). Phenotype of recovering lymphoid cell populations after marrow transplantation. *J. Exp. Med.* **161**, 1483.

Auron, P. E., Webb, A. C., Rosenwasser, L. J., Mucci, S. F., Rich, A., Wolff, S. M., and Dinarello, C. A. (1984). Nucleotide sequence of human monocyte interleukin 1 cDNA. *Proc. Natl. Acad. Sci. U.S.A.* **81**, 7907.

Beller, D. I., Springer, T. A., and Schreiber, R. D. (1982). Anti-Mac-1 selectively inhibits the mouse and human type three complement receptor. *J. Exp. Med.* **156**, 1000.

Bellon, B., Manheimer-Lory, A., Monestier, M., Moran, T., Dimitriu-Bona, A., Alt, F., and Bona, C. (1987). High frequency of autoantibodies bearing cross-reactive idiotopes among hybridomas using VH7183 genes prepared from normal and autoimmune murine strains. *J. Clin. Invest.* **79**, 1044.

Bentley, D. L. (1984). Most kappa immunoglobulin mRNA in human lymphocytes is homologous to a small family of germ-line V genes. *Nature (London)* **307**, 77.

Bergui, L., Tesio, L., Schena, M., Riva, M., Malavasi, F., and Schulz, T. (1988). CD5 and CD21 molecules are a functional unit in the cell/substrate adhesion of B-chronic lymphocytic leukemia cells. *Eur. J. Immunol.* **18**, 89.

Berning, A. K., Eicher, E. M., Paul, W. E., and Scher, I. (1980). Mapping of the X-linked immune deficiency mutation (*xid*) of CBA/N mice. *J. Immunol.* **124**, 1875.

Bertoglio, J. H. (1983). Monocyte-independent stimulation of human B lymphocytes by phorbol myristate acetate. *J. Immunol.* **131**, 2279.

Bich-Thuy, L. T., Banchereau, J., and Revillard, J. P. (1984). Suppression of polyclonal human B cell activation by IgG binding factors: Interference with the maturation of Ig-containing cells into Ig-secreting cells. *Cell. Immunol.* **87**, 231.

Bierer, B. E., Nishimura, Y., Burakoff, S. J., and Smith, B. R. (1988). Phenotypic and functional characterization of human cytolytic T cells lacking expression of CD5. *J. Clin. Invest.* **81**, 1390.

Bird, T. A., Gearing, A. J., and Saklatvala, J. (1987). Murine interleukin-1 receptor: Differences in binding properties between fibroblastic and thymoma cells and evidence for a two-chain receptor model. *FEBS Lett.* **225**, 21.

Birmingham, J. R., Chesnut, R. W., Kappler, J. W., Marrack, P., Kubo, R., and Grey, H. M. (1982). Antigen presentation to T cell hybridomas by a macrophage cell line: An inducible function. *J. Immunol.* **128**, 1491.

Bofill, M., Janossy, G., Janossa, M., Burford, G. D., Seymour, G. J., Wernet, P., and Kelemen, E. (1985). Human B cell development. II. Subpopulations in the human. *J. Immunol.* **134**, 1531.

Bonin, P. D., and Singh, J. P. (1988). Modulation of interleukin-1 receptor expression and interleukin-1 response in fibroblasts by platelet-derived growth factor. *J. Biol. Chem.* **263**, 11052.

Bothwell, A. L., Paskind, M., Reth, M., Imanishi-Kari, T., Rajewsky, K., and Baltimore, D. (1981). Heavy chain variable region contribution to the NP^b family of antibodies: Somatic mutation evident in a $\gamma 2a$ variable region. *Cell (Cambridge, Mass.)* **24**, 625.

Bothwell, A. L., Paskind, M., Reth, M., Imanishi-Kari, T., Rajewsky, K., and Baltimore, D. (1982). Somatic variants of murine immunoglobulin lambda light chains. *Nature (London)* **298**, 380.

Boumsell, L., Coppin, H., Pham, D., Raynal, B., Lemerle, J., Dausset, J., and Bernard, A. (1980). An antigen shared by a human T cell subset and B cell chronic lymphocytic leukemic cells. Distribution on normal and malignant lymphoid cells. *J. Exp. Med.* **152**, 229.

Boyd, A. W., and Schrader, J. W. (1982). Derivation of macrophage-like lines from the pre-B lymphoma 8.1 using 5-azacytidine. *Nature (London)* **297**, 691.

Boyd, A. W., Anderson, K. C., Freedman, A. S., Fisher, D. C., Slaughenhoupt, B., Schlossman, S. F., and Nadler, L. M. (1985a). Studies of in vitro activation and differentiation of human B lymphocytes. I. Phenotypic and functional characterization of the B cell population responding to anti-Ig antibody. *J. Immunol.* **134**, 1516.

Boyd, A. W., Fisher, D. C., Fox, D. A., Schlossman, S. F., and Nadler, L. M. (1985b). Structural and functional characterization of IL 2 receptors on activated human B cells. *J. Immunol.* **134**, 2387.

Braun, J. (1983). Spontaneous *in vitro* occurrence and long-term culture of murine B lymphoblast cell lines. *J. Immunol.* **130**, 2113.

Braun, J., Kiely, J. M., and Unanue, E. R. (1984). Propagation of B lymphocytes *in vitro*. *Curr. Top. Microbiol. Immunol.* **113**, 237.

Braun, J., Citri, Y., Baltimore, D., Forouzanpour, F., King, L., Teheranizadeh, K., Bray, M., and Kliewer, S. (1986). B-Lyl cells: Immortal Ly-1+ B lymphocyte cell lines spontaneously arising in murine splenic cultures. *Immunol. Rev.* **93**, 5.

Brodeur, P. H., and Riblet, R. (1984). The immunoglobulin heavy chain variable region

(Igh-V) locus in the mouse. I. One hundred Igh-V genes comprise seven families of homologous genes. *Eur. J. Immunol.* **14**, 922.

Brooks, K. H., Uhr, J. W., and Vitetta, E. S. (1984). A B cell growth factor-like activity is secreted by cloned, neoplastic B cells. *J. Immunol.* **133**, 3133.

Burke, J. S., Warnke, R. A., Connors, J. M., and Beckstead, J. H. (1985). Diffuse malignant lymphoma with cerebriform nuclei: A B-cell lymphoma studied with monoclonal antibodies. *Am. J. Clin. Pathol.* **83**, 753.

Burns, B. F., Warnke, R. A., Doggett, R. S., and Rouse, R. V. (1983). Expression of a T-cell antigen (Leu-1) by B-cell lymphomas. *Am. J. Pathol.* **113**, 165.

Bussard, A. E., Vinit, M. A., and Pages, J. M. (1977). Immunochemical characterization of the auto antibodies by mouse peritoneal cells in culture. *Immunochemistry* **14**, 1.

Caligaris-Cappio, F., and Janossy, G. (1985). Surface markers in chronic lymphoid leukemias of B cell type. *Semin. Hematol.* **22**, 1.

Caligaris-Cappio, F., Gobbi, M., Bofill, M., and Janossy, G. (1982). Infrequent normal B lymphocytes express features of B-chronic lymphocytic leukemia. *J. Exp. Med.* **155**, 623.

Cantor, H., and Boyse, E. A. (1975a). Functional subclasses of T-lymphocytes bearing different Ly antigens. I. The generation of functionally distinct T-cell subclasses is a differentiative process independent of antigen. *J. Exp. Med.* **141**, 1376.

Cantor, H., and Boyse, E. A. (1975b). Functional subclasses of T lymphocytes bearing different Ly antigens. II. Cooperation between subclasses of Ly+ cells in the generation of killer activity. *J. Exp. Med.* **141**, 1390.

Capra, J. D., and Kehoe, J. M. (1974). Structure of antibodies with shared idiotypy: The complete sequence of the heavy chain variable regions of two immunoglobulin M anti-gamma globulins. *Proc. Natl. Acad. Sci. U.S.A.* **71**, 4032.

Capra, J. D., Kehoe, J. M., Williams, R. C., Jr., Feizi, T., and Kunkel, H. G. (1972). Light chain sequences of human IgM cold agglutinins. *Proc. Natl. Acad. Sci. U.S.A.* **69**, 40.

Carroll, W. L., Lowder, J. N., Streifer, R., Warnke, R., Levy, S., and Levy, R. (1986). Idiotype variant cell populations in patients with B cell lymphoma. *J. Exp. Med.* **164**, 1566.

Carson, D. A., and Fong, S. (1983). A common idiotope on human rheumatoid factors identified by a hybridoma antibody. *Mol. Immunol.* **20**, 1081.

Carson, D. A., Chen, P. P., Kipps, T. J., Radoux, V., Jirik, F., Goldfien, R. D., Fox, R. I., Silverman, G. J., and Fong, S. (1987a). Molecular basis for the cross-reactive idiotypes on human anti-IgG autoantibodies (rheumatoid factors). *Ciba Found. Symp.* **129**, 123.

Carson, D. A., Chen, P. P., Kipps, T. J., Radoux, V., Jirik, F. R., Goldfien, R. D., Fox, R. I., Silverman, G. J., and Fong, S. (1987b). Idiotypic and genetic studies of human rheumatoid factors. *Arthritis Rheum.* **30**, 1321.

Casali, P., Burastero, S. E., Nakamura, M., Inghirami, G., and Notkins, A. L. (1987). Human lymphocytes making rheumatoid factor and antibody to belong to Leu-1+ B-cell subset. *Science* **236**, 77.

Castagna, M. (1987). Phorbol esters as signal transducers and tumor promoters. *Biol. Cell.* **59**, 3.

Ceuppens, J. L., and Baroja, M. L. (1986). Monoclonal antibodies to the CD5 antigen can provide the necessary second signal for activation of isolated resting T cells by solid-phase-bound OKT3. *J. Immunol.* **137**, 1816.

Chen, P. P., Albrandt, K., Kipps, T. J., Radoux, V., Liu, F. T., and Carson, D. A. (1987a). Isolation and characterization of human VkIII germ-line genes. Implications for the molecular basis of human VkIII light chain diversity. *J. Immunol.* **139**, 1727.

Chen, P. P., Robbins, D. L., Jirik, F. R., Kipps, T. J., and Carson, D. A. (1987b). Isolation and characterization of a light chain variable region gene for human rheumatoid factors. *J. Exp. Med.* **166**, 1900.

Chesnut, R. W., and Grey, H. M. (1981). Studies on the capacity of B cells to serve as antigen-presenting cells. *J. Immunol.* **126**, 1075.

Chesnut, R. W., Colon, S. M., and Grey, H. M. (1982a). Antigen presentation by normal B cells, B cell tumors and macrophages: Functional and biochemical comparison. *J. Immunol.* **128**, 1764.

Chesnut, R. W., Colon, S. M., and Grey, H. M. (1982b). Requirements for the processing of antigens by antigen-presenting B cells. I. Functional comparison of B cell tumors and macrophages. *J. Immunol.* **129**, 2382.

Chin, J., Rupp, E., Cameron, P. M., MacNaul, K. L., Lotke, P. A., Tocci, M. J., Schmidt, J. A., and Bayne, E. K. (1988). Identification of a high-affinity receptor for interleukin 1 alpha and interleukin 1 beta on cultured human rheumatoid synovial cells. *J. Clin. Invest.* **82**, 420.

Clark, E. A., Shu, G., and Ledbetter, J. A. (1985). Role of the Bp35 cell surface polypeptide in human B-cell activation. *Proc. Natl. Acad. Sci. U.S.A.* **82**, 1766.

Clarke, S. H., Huppi, K., Ruezinsky, D., Staudt, L., Gerhard, W., and Weigert, M. (1985). Inter- and intraclonal diversity in the antibody response to influenza hemagglutinin. *J. Exp. Med.* **161**, 687.

Cleary, M. L., Meeker, T. C., Levy, S., Lee, E., Trela, M., Sklar, J., and Levy, R. (1986). Clustering of extensive somatic mutations in the variable region of an immunoglobulin heavy chain gene from a human B cell lymphoma. *Cell (Cambridge, Mass.)* **44**, 97.

Cleary, M. L., Galili, N., Trela, M., Levy, R., and Sklar, J. (1988). Single cell origin of bigenotypic and biphenotypic B cell proliferations in human follicular lymphomas. *J. Exp. Med.* **167**, 582.

Coffman, R. L. (1983). Surface antigen expression and immunoglobulin gene rearrangement during mouse pre-B cell development. *Immunol. Rev.* **69**, 5.

Cohen, D. I., Hedrick, S. M., Nielsen, E. A., D'Eustachio, P., Ruddle, F., Steinberg, A. D., Paul, W. E., and Davis, M. M. (1985a). Isolation of a cDNA clone corresponding to an X-linked gene family (XLR) closely linked to the murine immunodeficiency disorder *xid*. *Nature (London)* **314**, 369.

Cohen, D. I., Steinberg, A. D., Paul, W. E., and Davis, M. M. (1985b). Expression of an X-linked gene family (XLR) in late-stage B cells and its alteration by the *xid* mutation. *Nature (London)* **314**, 372.

Cone, L., and Uhr, J. W. (1964). Immunological deficiency disorders associated with chronic lymphocytic leukemia and multiple myeloma. *J. Clin. Invest.* **43**, 2241.

Conger, J. D., Pike, B. L., and Nossal, G. J. (1987). Clonal analysis of the anti-DNA repertoire of murine B lymphocytes. *Proc. Natl. Acad. Sci. U.S.A.* **84**, 2931.

Cory, S., Adams, J. M., and Kemp, D. J. (1980). Somatic rearrangements forming active immunoglobulin mu genes in B and T lymphoid cell lines. *Proc. Natl. Acad. Sci. U.S.A.* **77**, 4943.

Cossman, J., Neckers, L. M., Arnold, A., and Korsmeyer, S. J. (1982). Induction of differentiation in a case of common acute lymphoblastic leukemia. *N. Engl. J. Med.* **307**, 1251.

Cossman, J., Neckers, L. M., Hsu, S., Longo, D., and Jaffe, E. S. (1984). Low-grade lymphomas. Expression of developmentally regulated B-cell antigens. *Am. J. Pathol.* **115**, 117.

Cox, K. O., and Hardy, S. J. (1985). Autoantibodies against mouse bromelain-modified RBC are specifically inhibited by a common membrane phospholipid, phosphatidylcholine. *Immunology* **55**, 263.

Crow, M. K., Jover, J. A., and Friedman, S. M. (1986). Direct T helper-B cell interactions induce an early B cell activation antigen. *J. Exp. Med.* **164**, 1760.

Cunningham, A. J. (1974). Large numbers of cells in normal mice produce antibody components of isologous erythrocytes. *Nature (London)* **252**, 749.

Cwynarski, M. T., and Cohen, S. (1971). Polyclonal immunoglobulin deficiency in myelomastosis and macroglobulinemia. *Clin. Exp. Immunol.* **8**, 237.

Dasch, J. R., and Jones, P. P. (1986). Independent regulation of IgM, IgD, and Ia antigen expression in cultured immature B lymphocytes. *J. Exp. Med.* **163**, 938.

Dauphinee, M., Tovar, Z., and Talal, N. (1988). B cells expressing CD5 are increased in Sjogren's syndrome. *Arthritis Rheum.* **31**, 642.

Davidson, W. F., Morse, H. C., 3rd, Sharrow, S. O., and Chused, T. M. (1979). Phenotypic and functional effects of the motheaten gene on murine B and T lymphocytes. *J. Immunol.* **122**, 884.

Davidson, W. F., Fredrickson, T. N., Rudikoff, E. K., Coffman, R. L., Hartley, J. W., and Morse, H. C., 3rd (1984). A unique series of lymphomas related to the Ly-1+ lineage of B lymphocyte differentiation. *J. Immunol.* **133**, 744.

Davidson, W. F., Pierce, J. H., Rudikoff, S., and Morse, H. C., 3rd (1988). Relationships between B cell and myeloid differentiation. Studies with a B lymphocyte progenitor line, HAFTL-1. *J. Exp. Med.* **168**, 389.

Davignon, D., Martz, E., Reynolds, T., Kurzinger, K., and Springer, T. A. (1981). Monoclonal antibody to a novel lymphocyte function-associated antigen (LFA-1): Mechanism of blockade of T lymphocyte-mediated killing and effects on other T and B lymphocyte functions. *J. Immunol.* **127**, 590.

DeHeer, D. H., Linder, E. J., and Edgington, T. S. (1978). Delineation of spontaneous erythrocyte autoantibody responses of NZB and other strains of mice. *J. Immunol.* **120**, 825.

de la Hera, A., Marcos, M. A., Toribio, M. L., Marquez, C., Gaspar, M. L., and Martinez, C. (1987). Development of Ly-1+ B cells in immunodeficient CBA/N mice. *J. Exp. Med.* **166**, 804.

Delia, D., Bonati, A., Giardini, R., Villa, S., De Braud, F., Cattoretti, G., and Rilke, F. (1986). Expression of the T1 (CD5, p67) surface antigen in B-CLL and B-NHL and its correlation with other B-cell differentiation markers. *Hematol. Oncol.* **4**, 237.

den Ottolander, G. J., Schuit, H. R., Waayer, J. L., Huibregtsen, L., Hijmans, W., and Jansen, J. (1985). Chronic B-cell leukemias: Relation between morphological and immunological features. *Clin. Immunol. Immunopathol.* **35**, 92.

Dexter, C. M., and Corley, R. B. (1987). Expression of the Fc gamma receptor on Ly-1+ B lymphocytes. *Eur. J. Immunol.* **17**, 867.

Dialynas, D. P., Wilde, D. B., Marrack, P., Pierres, A., Wall, K. A., Havran, W., Otten, G., Loken, M. R., Pierres, M., Kappler, J., and Fitch, F. W. (1983). Characterization of the murine antigenic determinant, designated L3T4a, recognized by monoclonal antibody GK1.5: Expression of L3T4a by functional T cell clones appears to correlate primarily with class II MHC antigen-reactivity. *Immunol. Rev.* **74**, 29.

Diamond, L., O'Brien, T. G., and Baird, W. M. (1980). Tumor promoters and the mechanism of tumor promotion. *Adv. Cancer Res.* **32**, 1.

Dighiero, G., Guilbert, B., and Avrameas, S. (1982). Naturally occurring antibodies against nine common antigens in humans sera. II. High incidence of monoclonal Ig exhibiting antibody activity against actin and tubulin and sharing antibody specificities with natural antibodies. *J. Immunol.* **128**, 2788.

Dighiero, G., Lymberi, P., Mazie, J. C., Rouyre, S., Butler-Browne, G. S., Whalen, R. G., and Avrameas, S. (1983). Murine hybridomas secreting natural monoclonal antibodies reacting with self antigens. *J. Immunol.* **131**, 2267.

Dighiero, G., Lymberi, P., Holmberg, D., Lundquist, I., Coutinho, A., and Avrameas, S. (1985). High frequency of natural autoantibodies in normal newborn mice. *J. Immunol.* **134**, 765.

Dildrop, R., Krawinkel, U., Winter, E., and Rajewsky, K. (1985). V_H-gene expression in murine lipopolysaccharide blasts distributes over the nine known V_H-gene groups and may be random. *Eur. J. Immunol.* **15**, 1154.

Dinarello, C. A. (1988). Biology of interleukin 1. *FASEB J.* **2**, 108.

Dinarello, C. A., Clark, B. D., Puren, A. J., Savage, N., and Rosoff, P. M. (1989). The interleukin 1 receptor. *Immunol. Today* **10**, 49.

Drexler, H. G., Brenner, M. K., Wimperis, J. Z., Gignac, S. M., Janossy, G., Prentice, H. G., and Hoffbrand, A. V. (1987). CD5-positive B cells after T cell depleted bone marrow transplantation. *Clin. Exp. Immunol.* **68**, 662.

Dugas, B., Vazquez, A., Gérard, J. P., Richard, Y., Auffredou, M. T., Delfraissy, J. F., Fradelizi, D., and Galanaud, P. (1985). Functional properties of two human B cell growth factor species separated by lectin affinity column. *J. Immunol.* **135**, 333.

Durum, S. K., Schmidt, J. A., and Oppenheim, J. J. (1985). Interleukin 1: An immunological perspective. *Annu. Rev. Immunol.* **3**, 263.

Dzierzak, E. A., Janeway, C. A., Jr., Richard, N., and Bothwell, A. (1986). Molecular characterization of antibodies bearing Id-460. I. The structure of two highly homologous V_H genes used to produce idiotype positive immunoglobulins. *J. Immunol.* **136**, 1864.

Eckhardt, L. A., and Herzenberg, L. A. (1980). Monoclonal antibodies to ThB detect close linkage of Ly-6 and a gene regulating ThB expression. *Immunogenetics* **11**, 275.

Eilat, D. (1982). Monoclonal autoantibodies: An approach to studying autoimmune disease. *Mol. Immunol.* **19**, 943.

Elias, J. A., Schreiber, A. D., Gustilo, K., Chien, P., Rossman, M. D., Lammie, P. J., and Daniele, R. P. (1985). Differential interleukin 1 elaboration by unfractionated and density fractionated human alveolar macrophages and blood monocytes: Relationship to cell maturity. *J. Immunol.* **135**, 3198.

Ellison, D. J., Turner, R. R., van Antwerp, R., Martin, W. E., and Nathwani, B. N. (1987). High-grade mantle zone lymphoma. *Cancer (Philadelphia)* **60**, 2717.

Errington, S. L., and Cox, K. O. (1986). Limiting dilution analysis of age- and gender-related differences in autoantibody production against bromelain-modified RBC. *Int. Arch. Allergy Appl. Immunol.* **79**, 276.

Fahey, J. L., Scoggins, R., Utz, J. P., and Szwed, C. P. (1963). Infection, antibody response and gamma globulin components in multiple myeloma and macroglobulinemia. *Am. J. Med.* **35**, 698.

Fingeroth, J. D., Weis, J. J., Tedder, T. F., Strominger, J. L., Biro, P. A., and Fearon,

D. T. (1984). Epstein–Barr virus receptor of human B lymphocytes is the C3d receptor CR2. *Proc. Natl. Acad. Sci. U.S.A.* **81**, 4510.

Fong, S., Vaughan, J. H., and Carson, D. A. (1983). Two different rheumatoid factor-producing cell populations distinguished by the mouse erythrocyte receptor and responsiveness to polyclonal B cell activators. *J. Immunol.* **130**, 162.

Forbes, I. J., Zalewski, P. D., Valente, L., and Gee, D. (1982). Two maturation-associated mouse erythrocyte receptors of human B cells. I. Identification of four human B-cell subsets. *Clin. Exp. Immunol.* **47**, 396.

Forni, L., Heusser, C., and Coutinho, A. (1988). Natural lymphocyte activation in postnatal development of germ-free and conventional mice. *Ann. Immunol. (Paris)* **139**, 245.

Förster, I., and Rajewsky, K. (1987). Expansion and functional activity of Ly-1+ B cells upon transfer of peritoneal cells into allotype-congenic, newborn mice. *Eur. J. Immunol.* **17**, 521.

Förster, I., Gu, H., and Rajewsky, K. (1988). Germline antibody V regions as determinants of clonal persistence and malignant growth in the B cell compartment. *EMBO J.* **7**, 3693.

Fox, R. I., Harlow, D., Royston, I., and Elder, J. (1982). Structural characterization of the human T cell surface antigen (p67) isolated from normal and neoplastic lymphocytes. *J. Immunol.* **129**, 401.

Freedman, A. S., Boyd, A. W., Bieber, F. R., Daley, J., Rosen, K., Horowitz, J. C., Levy, D. N., and Nadler, L. M. (1987a). Normal cellular counterparts of B cell chronic lymphocytic leukemia. *Blood* **70**, 418.

Freedman, A. S., Boyd, A. W., Berrebi, A., Horowitz, J. C., Levy, D. N., Rosen, K. J., Daley, J., Slaughenhoupt, B., Levine, H., and Nadler, L. M. (1987b). Expression of B cell activation antigens on normal and malignant B cells. *Leukemia* **1**, 9.

Freedman, A. S., Freeman, G., Whitman, J., Segil, J., Daley, J., and Nadler, L. M. (1989). Studies of *in vitro* activated CD5+ B cells. *Blood* **73**, 202.

Freitas, A. A., Guilbert, B., Holmberg, D., Wennerstrom, G., Coutinho, A., and Avrameas, S. (1986). Analysis of autoantibody reactivities in hybridoma collections derived from normal adult BALB/c mice. *Ann. Immunol. (Paris)* **137**, 33.

Friedman, S. M., Jover, J. A., Chartash, E. K., and Crow, M. K. (1986). Antigen-specific, MHC nonrestricted T helper cell-induced B cell activation. *J. Exp. Med.* **164**, 1773.

Gadol, N., and Ault, K. A. (1986). Phenotypic and functional characterization of human Leu1 (CD5) cells. *Immunol. Rev.* **93**, 23.

Gaffney, E. V., Koch, G., Tsai, S. C., Loucks, T., and Lingenfelter, S. E. (1988). Correlation between human cell growth response to interleukin 1 and receptor binding. *Cancer Res.* **48**, 5455.

Geppert, T. D., and Lipsky, P. E. (1988). Activation of T lymphocytes by immobilized monoclonal antibodies to CD3. Regulatory influences of monoclonal antibodies to additional T cell surface determinants. *J. Clin. Invest.* **81**, 1497.

Glimcher, L. H., Kim, K. J., Green, I., and Paul, W. E. (1982). Ia antigen-bearing B cell tumor lines can present protein antigen and alloantigen in a major histocompatibility complex-restricted fashion to antigen-reactive T cells. *J. Exp. Med.* **155**, 445.

Gobbi, M., Caligaris-Cappio, F., and Janossy, G. (1983). Normal equivalent cells of B cell malignancies: Analysis with monoclonal antibodies. *Br. J. Haematol.* **54**, 393.

Gough, N. M., Kemp, D. J., Tyler, B. M., Adams, J. M., and Cory, S. (1980). Intervening sequences divide the gene for the constant region mouse immunoglobulin

mu chains into segments, each encoding a domain. *Proc. Natl. Acad. Sci. U.S.A.* **77**, 554.
Greaves, M. F., Chan, L. C., Furley, A. J., Watt, S. M., and Molgaard, H. V. (1986). Lineage promiscuity in hemopoietic differentiation and leukemia. *Blood* **67**, 1.
Green, M. C., and Schultz, L. D. (1975). Motheaten, an immunodeficient mutant of the mouse. I. Genetics and pathology. *J. Hered.* **66**, 250.
Greenstein, J. L., Solomon, A., and Abraham, G. N. (1984). Monoclonal antibodies reactive with idiotypic and variable-region specific determinants on human immunoglobulins. *Immunology* **51**, 17.
Grey, H. M., Colon, S. M., and Chesnut, R. W. (1982). Requirements for the processing of antigen by antigen-presenting B cells. II. Biochemical comparison of the fate of antigen in B cell tumors and macrophages. *J. Immunol.* **129**, 2389.
Griffin, J. D., Ritz, J., Nadler, L. M., and Schlossman, S. F. (1981). Expression of myeloid differentiation antigens on normal and malignant myeloid cells. *J. Clin. Invest.* **68**, 932.
Griffiths, G. M., Berek, C., Kaartinen, M., and Milstein, C. (1984). Somatic mutation and the maturation of immune response to 2-phenyl oxazolone. *Nature (London)* **312**, 271.
Guilbert, B., Dighiero, G., and Avrameas, S. (1982). Naturally occurring antibodies against nine common antigens in human sera. I. Detection, isolation and characterization. *J. Immunol.* **128**, 2779.
Guy, G. R., Bunce, C. M., Gordon, J., Michell, R. H., and Brown, G. (1985). A combination of calcium ionophore and 12-O-tetradecanoyl-phorbol-13-acetate (TPA) stimulates the growth of purified resting B cells. *Scand. J. Immunol.* **22**, 591.
Hara, M., Kitani, A., Hirose, T., Norioka, K., Harigai, M., Suzuki, K., Tabata, H., Kawakami, M., Kawagoe, M., and Nakamura, H. (1988). Stimulatory effect of CD5 antibody on B cells from patients with rheumatoid arthritis. *Clin. Immunol. Immunopathol.* **49**, 223.
Hardy, R. R., and Hayakawa, K. (1986). Development and physiology of Ly-1 B and its human homolog, Leu-1 B. *Immunol. Rev.* **93**, 53.
Hardy, R. R., Hayakawa, K., Parks, D. R., and Herzenberg, L. A. (1983). Demonstration of B-cell maturation in X-linked immunodeficient mice by simultaneous three-colour immunofluorescence. *Nature (London)* **306**, 270.
Hardy, R. R., Hayakawa, K., Herzenberg, L. A., Morse, H. C., 3rd, and Davidson, W. F. (1984). Ly-1 as a differentiation antigen on normal and neoplastic B cells. *Curr. Top. Microbiol. Immunol.* **113**, 231.
Hardy, R. R., Dangl, J. L., Hayakawa, K., Jager, G., and Herzenberg, L. A. (1986). Frequent lambda light chain gene rearrangement and expression in a Ly-1 B lymphoma with a productive kappa chain allele. *Proc. Natl. Acad. Sci. U.S.A.* **83**, 1438.
Hardy, R. R., Hayakawa, K., Shimizu, M., Yamasaki, K., and Kishimoto, T. (1987). Rheumatoid factor secretion from human Leu-1+ B cells. *Science* **236**, 81.
Harnett, M. M., and Klaus, G. G. (1988). Protein kinase C activators inhibit the antigen receptor-coupled polyphosphoinositide phosphodiesterase in murine B lymphocytes. *FEBS Lett.* **239**, 281.
Harris, N. L., and Bhan, A. K. (1985a). Mantle-zone lymphoma. A pattern produced by lymphomas of more than one cell type. *Am. J. Surg. Pathol.* **9**, 872.
Harris, N. L., and Bhan, A. K. (1985b). B-cell neoplasms of the lymphocytic, lymphoplasmacytoid, and plasma cell types: Immunohistologic analysis and clinical correlation. *Hum. Pathol.* **16**, 829.

Hartman, A. B., and Rudikoff, S. (1984). V$_H$ genes encoding the immune response to beta-(1,6)-galactan: Somatic mutation in IgM molecules. *EMBO J.* **3**, 3023.

Hayakawa, K., Hardy, R. R., Parks, D. R., and Herzenberg, L. A. (1983). The "Ly-1 B" Cell subpopulation in normal immunodefective, and autoimmune mice. *J. Exp. Med.* **157**, 202.

Hayakawa, K., Hardy, R. R., Honda, M., Herzenberg, L. A., and Steinberg, A. D. (1984). Ly-1 B cells: Functionally distinct lymphocytes that secrete IgM autoantibodies. *Proc. Natl. Acad. Sci. U.S.A.* **81**, 2494.

Hayakawa, K., Hardy, R. R., and Herzenberg, L. A. (1985). Progenitors for Ly-1 B cells are distinct from progenitors for other B cells. *J. Exp. Med.* **161**, 1554.

Hayakawa, K., Hardy, R. R., and Herzenberg, L. A. (1986a). Peritoneal Ly-1 B cells: Genetic control, autoantibody production, increased lambda light chain expression. *Eur. J. Immunol.* **16**, 450.

Hayakawa, K., Hardy, R. R., Stall, A. M., and Herzenberg, L. A. (1986b). Immunoglobulin-bearing B cells reconstitute and maintain the murine Ly-1 B cell lineage. *Eur. J. Immunol.* **16**, 1313.

Haynes, B. F., Hemler, M., Cotner, T., Mann, D. L., Eisenbarth, G. S., Strominger, J. L., and Fauci, A. S. (1981). Characterization of a monoclonal antibody (5E9) that defines a human cell surface antigen of cell activation. *J. Immunol.* **127**, 347.

Herzenberg, L. A., Stall, A. M., Lalor, P. A., Sidman, C., Moore, W. A., and Parks, D. R. (1986). The Ly-1 B cell lineage. *Immunol. Rev.* **93**, 81.

Herzenberg, L. A., Stall, A. M., Braun, J., Weaver, D., Baltimore, D., and Grosschedl, R. (1987). Depletion of the predominant B-cell population in mu heavychain transgenic mice. *Nature (London)* **329**, 71.

Ho, M. K., and Springer, T. A. (1982). MAC-2, a novel 32,000 M$_r$ mouse macrophage subpopulation-specific antigen defined by monoclonal antibodies. *J. Immunol.* **128**, 1221.

Hogg, N., and Horton, M. A. (1987). Myeloid antigens: New and previously defined clusters. In "Leukocyte Typing III" (A. J. McMichael, P. C. L. Beverley, S. Cobbold, et al., eds.), p. 576. Oxford Univ. Press, London and New York.

Hollander, N. (1982). Effects of anti-Lyt antibodies on T-cell functions. *Immunol. Rev.* **68**, 43.

Hollander, N., Pillemer, E., and Weissman, I. L. (1981). Effects of Lyt antibodies on T-cell functions: Augmentation by anti-Lyt-1 as opposed to inhibition by anti-Lyt-2. *Proc. Natl. Acad. Sci. U.S.A.* **78**, 1148.

Holmberg, D., Freitas, A. A., Portnoi, D., Jacquemart, F., Avrameas, S., and Coutinho, A. (1986a). Antibody repertoires of normal BALB/c mice: B lymphocyte populations defined by state of activation. *Immunol. Rev.* **93**, 147.

Holmberg, D., Wennerström, G., Andrade, L., and Coutinho, A. (1986b). The high idiotypic connectivity of "natural" newborn antibodies is not found in adult mitogenreactive B cell repertoires. *Eur. J. Immunol.* **16**, 82.

Holmes, K. L., Pierce, J. H., Davidson, W. F., and Morse, H. C., 3rd (1986). Murine hematopoietic cells with pre-B or pre-B/myeloid characteristics are generated by in vitro transformation with retroviruses containing *fes*, *ras*, *abl*, and *src* oncogenes. *J. Exp. Med.* **164**, 443.

Hooijkaas, H., Benner, R., Pleasants, J. R., and Wostmann, B. S. (1984). Isotypes and specificities of immunoglobulins produced by germ-free mice fed chemically defined ultrafiltered "antigen-free" diets. *Eur. J. Immunol.* **14**, 1124.

Huang, H. J., Jones, N. H., Strominger, J. L., and Herzenberg, L. A. (1987). Molecular cloning of Ly-1, a membrane glycoprotein of mouse T lymphocytes and a subset of B cells: Molecular homology to its human counterpart Leu-1/T1 (CD5). *Proc. Natl. Acad. Sci. U.S.A.* **84**, 204.

Huber, B., Gershon, R. K., and Cantor, H. (1977). Identification of a B-cell surface structure involved in antigen-dependent triggering: Absence of this structure on B cells from CBA/N mutant mice. *J. Exp. Med.* **145**, 10.

Humphries, C. G., Shen, A., Kuziel, W. A., Capra, J. D., Blattner, F. R., and Tucker, P. W. (1988). A new human immunoglobulin V_H family preferentially rearranged in immature B-cell tumours. *Nature (London)* **331**, 446.

Iida, K., Nadler, L., and Nussenzweig, V. (1983). Identification of the membrane receptor for the complement fragment C3d by means of a monoclonal antibody. *J. Exp. Med.* **158**, 1021.

Issekutz, T., Chu, E., and Geha, R. S. (1982). Antigen presentation by human B cells: T cell proliferation induced by Epstein Barr virus B lymphoblastoid cells. *J. Immunol.* **129**, 1446.

Izui, S., McConahey, P. J., and Dixon, F. J. (1978). Increased spontaneous polyclonal activation of B lymphocytes in mice with spontaneous autoimmune disease. *J. Immunol.* **121**, 2213.

Jaenichen, H. R., Pech, M., Lindenmaier, W., Wildgruber, N., and Zachau, H. G. (1984). Composite human V_K genes and a model of their evolution. *Nucleic Acids Res.* **12**, 5249.

Jaffe, E. S., Bookman, M. A., and Longo, D. L. (1987). Lymphocytic lymphoma of intermediate differentiation — Mantle zone lymphoma: A distinct subtype of B-cell lymphoma. *Hum. Pathol.* **18**, 877.

Jerne, N. K. (1984). Idiotypic networks and other preconceived ideas. *Immunol. Rev.* **79**, 5.

Jerne, N. K. (1985). The generative grammar of the immune system. *Science* **229**, 1057.

Jones, N. H., Clabby, M. L., Dialynas, D. P., Huang, H. J., Herzenberg, L. A., and Strominger, J. L. (1986). Isolation of complementary DNA clones encoding the human lymphocyte glycoprotein T1/Leu-1. *Nature (London)* **323**, 346.

Kasturi, K., Monestier, M., Mayer, R., and Bona, C. (1988). Biased usage of certain Vk gene families by autoantibodies and their polymorphism in autoimmune mice. *Mol. Immunol.* **25**, 213.

Katsuura, G., Gottschall, P. E., and Arimura, A. (1988). Identification of a high-affinity receptor for interleukin-1 beta in rat brain. *Biochem. Biophys. Res. Commun.* **156**, 61.

Kaushik, A., Lim, A., Poncet, P., Ge, X. R., and Dighiero, G. (1988). Comparative analysis of natural antibody specifications among hybridomas originating from spleen and peritoneal cavity of adult NZB and BALB/c mice. *Scand. J. Immunol.* **27**, 461.

Kawaguchi, S. (1987). Phospholipid epitopes for mouse antibodies against bromelain-treated mouse erythrocytes. *Immunology* **62**, 11.

Kawamura, N., Muraguchi, A., Hori, A., Horii, Y., Mutsuura, S., Hardy, R. R., Kikutani, H., and Kishimoto, T. (1986). A case of human B cell leukemia that implicates an autocrine mechanism in the abnormal growth of Leu 1 B cells. *J. Clin. Invest.* **78**, 1331.

Kearney, J. F., and Vakil, M. (1986). Idiotype-directed interactions during ontogeny play a major role in the establishment of the adult B cell repertoire. *Immunol. Rev.* **94**, 39.

Kemp, D. J., Harris, A. W., Cory, S., and Adams, J. M. (1980). Expression of the immunoglobulin C mu gene in mouse T and B lymphoid and myeloid cell lines. *Proc. Natl. Acad. Sci. U.S.A.* **77**, 2876.

Kikutani, H., Kimura, R., Nakamura, H., Sato, R., Muraguchi, A., Kawamura, N., Hardy, R. R., and Kishimoto, T. (1986a). Expression and function of an early activation marker restricted to human B cells. *J. Immunol.* **136**, 4019.

Kikutani, H., Nakamura, H., Sato, R., Kimura, R., Yamasaki, K., Hardy, R. R., and Kishimoto, T. (1986b). Delineation and characterization of human B cell subpopulations at various stages of activation by using a B cell-specific monoclonal antibody. *J. Immunol.* **136**, 4027.

Kincade, P. W. (1977). Defective colony formation by B lymphocytes from CBA/N and C3H/HeJ mice. *J. Exp. Med.* **145**, 249.

Kipps, T. J., and Vaughan, J. H. (1987). Genetic influence on the levels of circulating CD5 B lymphocytes. *J. Immunol.* **139**, 1060.

Kipps, T. J., Fong, S., Tomhave, E., Chen, P. P., Goldfien, R. D., and Carson, D. A. (1987a). High-frequency expression of a conserved kappa light-chain variable-region gene in chronic lymphocytic leukemia. *Proc. Natl. Acad. Sci. U.S.A.* **84**, 2916.

Kipps, T. J., Fong, S., Tomhave, E., Chen, P. P., Goldfien, R. D., and Carson, D. A. (1987b). Immunoglobulin V gene utilization in CLL. In "Chronic Lymphocytic Leukemia: Recent Progress and Future Direction" (R. P. Gale and K. R. Rai, eds.), p. 115. Liss, New York.

Kipps, T. J., Robbins, B. A., Kuster, P., and Carson, D. A. (1988a). Autoantibody-associated cross-reactive idiotypes expressed at high frequency in chronic lymphocytic leukemia relative to B-cell lymphomas of follicular center cell origin. *Blood* **72**, 422.

Kipps, T. J., Tomhave, E., Chen, P. P., and Carson, D. A. (1988b). Autoantibody-associated kappa light chain variable region gene expressed in chronic lymphocytic leukemia with little or no somatic mutation. Implications for etiology and immunotherapy. *J. Exp. Med.* **167**, 840.

Kipps, T. J., Rassenti, L. A., Pratt, L. F., Chen, P. P., and Carson, D. A. (1988c). Frequent immunoglobulin gene rearrangement of a conserved kappa light chain variable region in chronic lymphocytic leukemia. *Blood* **72s**, 208a (abstr.).

Kipps, T. J., Robbins, B. A., Tefferi, A., Meisenholder, G. W., Carson, D. A., and Banks, P. (1989a). Autoantibody-associated cross reactive idiotypes frequently expressed in CD5 B cell non-Hodgkin's lymphomas. *J. Clin. Invest.* (in press).

Kipps, T. J., Tomhave, E., Pratt, L. F., Chen, P. P., and Carson, D. A. (1989b). Developmentally restricted V_H gene expressed at high frequency in chronic lymphocytic leukemia. *Proc. Natl. Acad. Sci. U.S.A.* (in press).

Kipps, T. J., Robbins, B. A., Meisenholder, G. W., and Carson, D. A. (1989c). Anatomic localization of cells expressing major autoantibody-associated cross-reactive idiotypes. Submitted for publication.

Klobeck, H. G., Solomon, A., and Zachau, H. G. (1984). Contribution of human V kappa II germ-line genes to light-chain diversity. *Nature (London)* **309**, 73.

Knowles, D. M., 2nd, Halper, J. P., Azzo, W., and Wang, C. Y. (1983). Reactivity of monoclonal antibodies Leu 1 and OKT1 with malignant human lymphoid cells. Correlation with conventional cell markers. *Cancer (Philadelphia)* **52**, 1369.

Kofler, R. (1988). A new murine Ig V_H gene family. *J. Immunol.* **140**, 4031.

Kroggel, R., Martin, M., Pingoud, V., Dayer, J. M., and Resch, K. (1988). Two-chain structure of the interleukin 1 receptor. *FEBS Lett.* **229**, 59.

Kronheim, S. R., March, C. J., Erb, S. K., Conlon, P. J., Mochizuki, D. Y., and Hopp, T. P. (1985). Human interleukin 1. Purification to homogeneity. *J. Exp. Med.* **161**, 490.

Kunkel, H. G., Agnello, V., Winchester, R. J., Capra, J. D., and Kehoe, J. M. (1974a). Cross-idiotypic specificity among monoclonal IgM proteins with anti-globulin activity. *Proc. Natl. Acad. Sci. U.S.A.* **71**, 4032.

Kunkel, H. G., Winchester, R. J., Joslin, F. G., and Capra, J. D. (1974b). Similarities in the light chains of anti-gamma-globulins showing cross-idiotypic specificities. *J. Exp. Med.* **139**, 128.

Lanier, L. L., Lynes, M. A., Haughton, G., and Wettstein, P. (1978). Novel type of murine B-cell lymphoma. *Nature (London)* **271**, 554.

Lanier, L. L., Warner, N. L., Ledbetter, J. A., and Herzenberg, L. A. (1981a). Expression of Lyt-1 antigen on certain murine B cell lymphomas. *J. Exp. Med.* **153**, 998.

Lanier, L. L., Warner, N. L., Ledbetter, J. A., and Herzenberg, L. A. (1981b). Quantitative immunofluorescent analysis of surface phenotypes of murine B cell lymphomas and plasmacytomas with monoclonal antibodies. *J. Immunol.* **127**, 1691.

Lanier, L. L., Arnold, L. W., Raybourne, R. B., Russell, S., Lynes, M. A., Warner, N. L., and Haughton, G. (1982). Transplantable B-cell lymphomas in B10.H-2^a H-4^b p/Wts mice. *Immunogenetics* **16**, 367.

Lanier, L. L., Richie, E. R., Howell, A. L., and Allison, J. P. (1983). Expression of Ly-1 and Ly-2 on a spontaneous AKR B-cell lymphoma. *Immunogenetics* **17**, 655.

Lanzavecchia, A. (1985). Antigen-specific interaction between T and B cells. *Nature (London)* **314**, 537.

LeBien, T. W., Bollum, F. J., Yasmineh, W. G., and Kersey, J. H. (1982). Phorbol ester-induced differentiation of a non-T, non-B leukemic cell line: Model for human lymphoid progenitor cell development. *J. Immunol.* **128**, 1316.

Ledbetter, J. A., and Herzenberg, L. A. (1979). Xenogeneic monoclonal antibodies to mouse lymphoid differentiation antigens. *Immunol. Rev.* **47**, 63.

Ledbetter, J. A., Rouse, R. V., Micklem, H. S., and Herzenberg, L. A. (1980). T cell subsets defined by expression of Lyt-1,2,3 and Thy-1 antigens. Two-parameter immunofluorescence and cytotoxicity analysis with monoclonal antibodies modifies current views. *J. Exp. Med.* **152**, 280.

Ledbetter, J. A., Evans, R. L., Lipinski, M., Cunningham-Rundles, C., Good, R. A., and Herzenberg, L. A. (1981). Evolutionary conservation of surface molecules that distinguish T lymphocyte helper/inducer and cytotoxic/suppressor subpopulations in mouse and man. *J. Exp. Med.* **153**, 310.

Ledbetter, J. A., Martin, P. J., Spooner, C. E., Wofsy, D., Tsu, T. T., Beatty, P. G., and Gladstone, P. (1985). Antibodies to Tp67 and Tp44 augment and sustain proliferative responses of activated T cells. *J. Immunol.* **135**, 2331.

Ledbetter, J. A., Parsons, M., Martin, P. J., Hansen, J. A., Rabinovitch, P. S., and June, C. H. (1986). Antibody binding to CD5 (Tp67) and Tp44 T cell surface molecules: Effects on cyclic nucleotides, cytoplasmic free calcium, and cAMP-mediated suppression. *J. Immunol.* **137**, 3299.

Ledbetter, J. A., June, C. H., Grosmaire, L. S., and Rabinovitch, P. S. (1987). Crosslinking of surface antigens causes mobilization of intracellular ionized calcium in T lymphocytes. *Proc. Natl. Acad. Sci. U.S.A.* **84**, 1384.

Ledford, D. K., Goni, F., Pizzolato, M., Franklin, E. C., Solomon, A., and Frangione, B. (1983). Preferential association of kappa IIIb light chains with monoclonal human IgM kappa autoantibodies. *J. Immunol.* **131**, 1322.

Levy, R., Levy, S., Cleary, M. L., Carroll, W., Kon, S., Bird, J., and Sklar, J. (1987). Somatic mutation in human B-cell tumors. *Immunol. Rev.* **96**, 43.

Ling, N. R., MacLennan, I. C. M., and Mason, D. Y. (1987). B-cell and plasma cell antigens: New and previously defined clusters. In "Leukocyte Typing III"

(A. J. McMichael, P. C. L. Beverley, S. Cobbold, *et al.*, eds), p. 302. Oxford Univ. Press, London and New York.

LoCascio, N. J., Haughton, G., Arnold, L. W., and Corley, R. B. (1984). Role of cell surface immunoglobulin in B-lymphocyte activation. *Proc. Natl. Acad. Sci. U.S.A.* 81, 2466.

Logdberg, L., Wassmer, P., and Shevach, E. M. (1985). Role of the L3T4 antigen in T-cell activation. I. Description of a monoclonal IgM antibody to a distinct epitope (L3T4b) of the L3T4 antigen and its effect on interleukin 1-induced thymocyte proliferation. *Cell. Immunol.* 94, 299.

Lomedico, P. T., Gubler, U., Hellmann, C. P., Dukovich, M., Giri, J. G., Pan, Y. C., Collier, K., Semionow, R., Chua, A. O., and Mizel, S. B. (1984). Cloning and expression of murine interleukin-1 cDNA in *Escherichia coli. Nature (London)* 312, 458.

Lord, E. M., and Dutton, R. W. (1975). The properties of plaque-forming cells from autoimmune and strains of mice with specificity for autologous erythrocyte antigens. *J. Immunol.* 115, 1199.

Lubinski, J., Fong, T. C., Babbitt, J. T., Ransone, L., Yodoi, J. J., and Bloom, E. T. (1988). Increased binding of IL-2 and increased IL-2 receptor mRNA synthesis are expressed by an NK-like cell line in response to IL-1. *J. Immunol.* 140, 1903.

Lundkvist, I., Ivars, F., Holmberg, D., and Coutinho, A. (1987). The immune response to bacterial dextrans. V. A "dominant" idiotype in IgCHb mice. *J. Immunol.* 138, 4395.

Lydyard, P. M., Youinou, P. Y., and Cooke, A. (1987). CD5-positive B cells in rheumatoid arthritis and chronic lymphocytic leukemia. *Immunol. Today* 8, 37.

Lynes, M. A., Lanier, L. L., Babcock, G. F., Wettstein, P. J., and Haughton, G. (1978). Antigen-induced murine B cell lymphomas. I. Induction and characterization of CH1 and CH2. *J. Immunol.* 122, 2352.

MacKenzie, M. R., Paglieroni, T. G., and Warner, N. L. (1987). Multiple myeloma: An immunologic profile. IV. The EA rosette-forming cell is a Leu-1 positive immunoregulatory B cell. *J. Immunol.* 139, 24.

Mageed, R. A., Dearlove, M., Goodall, D. M., and Jefferis, R. (1986). Immunogenic and antigenic epitopes of immunoglobulins: XVII—Monoclonal antibodies reactive with common and restricted idiotopes to the heavy chain of human rheumatoid factors. *Rheumatol. Int.* 6, 179.

Maini, R. N., Plater-Zyberk, C., and Andrew, E. (1987). Autoimmunity in rheumatoid arthritis. An approach via a study B lymphocytes. *Rheum. Dis. Clin. North Am.* 13, 319.

Manconi, R., Poletti, A., Volpe, R., Carbone, A., and De Paoli, P. (1987). Mantle-zone lymphoma: Additional arguments for its origin [letter]. *Am. J. Surg. Pathol.* 11, 333.

Mann, D. L., DeSantis, P., Mark, G., Pfeifer, A., Newman, M., Gibbs, N., Popovic, M., Sarngadharan, M. G., Gallo, R. C., Clark, J., and Blattner, W. (1987). HTLV-I-associated B-cell CLL: Indirect role for retrovirus in leukemogenesis. *Science* 236, 1103.

Manohar, V., Brown, E., Leiserson, W. M., and Chused, T. M. (1982). Expression of Lyt-1 by a subset of B lymphocytes. *J. Immunol.* 129, 532.

Marcos, M. A., de la Hera, A., Pereira, P., Marquez, C., Toribio, M., Coutinho, A., and Martinez, C. (1988). B cell participation in the recursive selection of T cell repertoires. *Eur. J. Immunol.* 18, 1015.

Martin, P. J., Hansen, J. A., Nowinski, R. C., and Brown, M. A. (1980). A new human T-cell differentiation antigen: Unexpected expression on chronic lymphocytic leukemia cells. *Immunogenetics* 11, 429.

Martin, P. J., Hansen, J. A., Siadak, A. W., and Nowinski, R. C. (1981). Monoclonal antibodies recognizing normal human T lymphocytes and malignant human B lymphocytes: A comparative study. *J. Immunol.* **127**, 1920.

Martinez, C., Pereira, P., Bernabe, R., Bandeira, A., Larsson, E. L., Cazenave, P. A., and Coutinho, A. (1984). Internal complementarities in the immune system: Regulation of the expression of helper T-cell idiotypes. *Proc. Natl. Acad. Sci. U.S.A.* **81**, 4520.

Martinez, C., Pereira, P., Cazenave, P. A., and Coutinho, A. (1986a). The mutual selective influences of T- and B-cell repertoires: The idiotypic net (at) work. *Ann. Immunol. (Paris)* **137**, 82.

Martinez, C., Pereira, P., de la Hera, A., Bandeira, A., Marquez, C., and Coutinho, A. (1986b). The basis for major histocompatibility complex (MHC) and immunoglobulin gene control of helper T cell idiotopes. *Eur. J. Immunol.* **16**, 417.

Martinez, C., Toribio, M. L., de la Hera, A., Cazenave, P. A., and Coutinho, A. (1986c). Maternal transmission of idiotypic network interactions selecting available T cell repertoires. *Eur. J. Immunol.* **16**, 1445.

Martinez, C., Marcos, M. A., Pereira, P., Marquez, C., Toribio, M., de la Hera, A., Cazenave, P. A., and Coutinho, A. (1987). Turning (Ir gene) low responders into high responders by manipulation of the developing immune system. *Proc. Natl. Acad. Sci. U.S.A.* **84**, 3812.

Martinez, C., Pereira, P., Toribio, M. L., Marcos, M. A., Bandeira, A., de la Hera, A., Marquez, C., Cazenave, P. A., and Coutinho, A. (1988). The participation of B cells and antibodies in the selection and maintenance of T cell repertoires. *Immunol. Rev.* **101**, 191.

Mastro, A. M. (1983). Phorbol ester tumor promoters and lymphocyte proliferation. *Cell Biol. Int. Rep.* **7**, 881.

Matsushima, K., Procopio, A., Abe, H., Scala, G., Ortaldo, J. R., and Oppenheim, J. J. (1985). Production of interleukin 1 activity by normal human peripheral blood B lymphocytes. *J. Immunol.* **135**, 1132.

McCoy, K. L., Nielson, K., and Clagett, J. (1984). Spontaneous production of colony-stimulating activity by splenic Mac-1 antigen-positive cells from autoimmune motheaten mice. *J. Immunol.* **132**, 272.

McCoy, K. L., Clagett, J., and Rosse, C. (1985). Effects of the motheaten gene on murine B-cell production. *Exp. Hematol.* **13**, 554.

Medeiros, L. J., Strickler, J. G., Picker, L. J., Gelb, A. B., Weiss, L. M., and Warnke, R. A. (1987). "Well-differentiated" lymphocytic neoplasms. Immunologic findings correlated with clinical presentation and morphologic features. *Am. J. Pathol.* **129**, 523.

Meeker, T. C., Miller, R. A., Link, M. P., Bindl, J., Warnke, R., and Levy, R. (1984). A unique human B lymphocyte antigen defined by a monoclonal antibody. *Hybridoma* **3**, 305.

Meeker, T. C., Lowder, J., Cleary, M. L., Stewart, S., Warnke, R., Sklar, J., and Levy, R. (1985). Emergence of idiotype variants during treatment of B-cell lymphoma with anti-idiotype antibodies. *N. Engl. J. Med.* **312**, 1658.

Melink, G. B., and LeBien, T. W. (1983). Construction of an antigenic map for human B-cell precursors. *J. Clin. Immunol.* **3**, 260.

Mercolino, T. J., Arnold, L. W., and Haughton, G. (1986). Phosphatidyl choline is recognized by a series of Ly-1+ murine B cell lymphomas specific for erythrocyte membranes. *J. Exp. Med.* **163**, 155.

Mercolino, T. J., Arnold, L. W., Hawkins, L. A., and Haughton, G. (1988). Normal mouse peritoneum contains a large population of Ly-1+ (CD5) B cells that recognize phosphatidyl choline. Relationship to cells that secrete hemolytic antibody specific for autologous erythrocytes. *J. Exp. Med.* **168**, 687.

Miller, R. A., and Gralow, J. (1984). The induction of Leu-1 antigen expression in human malignant and normal B cells by phorbol myristic acetate (PMA). *J. Immunol.* **133**, 3408.

Mills, L. E., O'Donnell, J. F., Guyre, P. M., LeMarbre, P. J., Miller, J. D., and Bernier, G. M. (1985). Spurious E rosette formation in B cell chronic lymphocytic leukemia due to monoclonal anti-sheep RBC antibody. *Blood* **65**, 270.

Miyake, R., Tanaka, Y., Tsuda, T., Yamanishi, J., Kikkawa, U., and Nishizuka, Y. (1983). Membrane phospholipid turnover in signal transduction; protein kinase C and mechanism of action of tumor promoters. *Proc. Int. Symp. Princess Takamatsu Cancer Res. Fund., 14th*, 167.

Miyama-Inaba, M., Kuma, S., Inaba, K., Ogata, H., Iwai, H., Yasumizu, R., Muramatsu, S., Steinman, R. M., and Ikehara, S. (1988). Unusual phenotype of B cells in the thymus of normal mice. *J. Exp. Med.* **168**, 811.

Mizel, S. B., Rosenstreich, D. L., and Oppenheim, J. J. (1978). Phorbol myristic acetate stimulates LAF production by the macrophage cell line, P388D. *Cell. Immunol.* **40**, 230.

Mond, J. J., Lieberman, R., Inman, J. K., Mosier, D. E., and Paul, W. E. (1977). Inability of mice with a defect in B-lymphocyte maturation to respond to phosphorycholine on immunogenic carriers. *J. Exp. Med.* **146**, 1138.

Monestier, M., Manheimer-Lory, A., Bellon, B., Painter, C., Dang, H., Talal, N., Zanetti, M., Schwartz, R., Pisetsky, D., Kuppers, R., Rose, N., Brochier, J., Klareskog, L., Holmdahl, R., Erlanger, B., Alt, F., and Bona, C. (1986). Shared idiotypes and restricted immunoglobulin variable region heavy chain genes characterize murine autoantibodies of various specificities. *J. Clin. Invest.* **78**, 753.

Morabito, F., Prasthofer, E. F., Dunlap, N. E., Grossi, C. E., and Tilden, A. B. (1987). Expression of myelomonocytic antigens on chronic lymphocytic leukemia B cells correlates with their ability to produce interleukin 1. *Blood* **70**, 1750.

Muraguchi, A., Butler, J. L., Kehrl, J. H., and Fauci, A. S. (1983). Differential sensitivity of human B cell subsets to activation signals delivered by anti-mu antibody and proliferative signals delivered by a monoclonal B cell growth factor. *J. Exp. Med.* **157**, 530.

Murphy, E. D., and Roths, J. B. (1978). Autoimmunity and lymphoproliferation: Induction by mutant gene *lpr*, and acceleration by a male-associated factor in strain BXSB mice. In "Genetic Control of Autoimmune Disease" (N. R. Rose, P. E. Bigazzi, and N. L. Warner, eds.), p. 207. Elsevier/North-Holland, New York.

Nadler, L. M., Ritz, J., Bates, M. P., Park, E. K., Anderson, K. C., Sallan, S. E., and Schlossman, S. F. (1982). Induction of human B cell antigens in non-T cell acute lymphoblastic leukemia. *J. Clin. Invest.* **70**, 433.

Nadler, L. M., Anderson, K. C., Marti, G., Bates, M., Park, E., Daley, J. F., and Schlossman, S. F. (1983). B4, a human B lymphocyte-associated antigen expressed on normal, mitogen-activated, and malignant B lymphocytes. *J. Immunol.* **131**, 244.

Nagasawa, K., and Mak, T. W. (1980). Phorbol esters induce differentiation in human malignant T lymphoblasts. *Proc. Natl. Acad. Sci. U.S.A.* **77**, 2964.

Nagasawa, K., Howatson, A., and Mak, T. W. (1981). Induction of human malignant T-lymphoblastic cell lines MOLT-3 and Jurkat by 12-O-tetradecanoylphorbol-13-acetate: Biochemical, physical, and morphological characterization. *J. Cell. Physiol.* **109**, 181.

Near, R. I., Juszczak, E. C., Huang, S. Y., Sicari, S. A., Margolies, M. N., and Gefter,

M. L. (1984). Expression and rearrangement of homologous immunoglobulin V_H genes in two mouse strains. *Proc. Natl. Acad. Sci. U.S.A.* **81**, 2167.

Newkirk, M. M., Mageed, R. A., Jefferis, R., Chen, P. P., and Capra, J. D. (1987). Complete amino acid sequences of variable regions of two human IgM rheumatoid factors, BOR and KAS of the Wa idiotypic family, reveal restricted use of heavy and light chain variable and joining region gene segments. *J. Exp. Med.* **166**, 550.

Nishimura, Y., Bierer, B. E., Jones, W. K., Jones, N. H., Strominger, J. L., and Burakoff, S. J. (1988a). Expression and function of a CD5 cDNA in human and murine T cells. *Eur. J. Immunol.* **18**, 747.

Nishimura, Y., Bierer, B. E., and Burakoff, S. J. (1988b). Expression of CD5 regulates responsiveness to IL-1. *J. Immunol.* **141**, 3438.

Nishizuka, Y. (1984). The role of protein kinase C in cell surface signal transduction and tumour promotion. *Nature (London)* **308**, 693.

Noonan, D. J., Isakov, N., Theofilopoulos, A. N., Dixon, F. J., and Altman, A. (1987). Protein kinase C-activating phorbol esters augment expression of T cell receptor genes. *Eur. J. Immunol.* **17**, 803.

Oi, V. T., Jones, P. P., Goding, J. W., and Herzenberg, L. A. (1978). Properties of monoclonal antibodies to mouse Ig allotypes, H-2, and Ia antigens. *Curr. Top. Microbiol. Immunol.* **81**, 115.

Okumura, K., Hayakawa, K., and Tada, T. (1982). Cell-to-cell interaction controlled by immunoglobulin genes of Thy-1-, Lyt-1+, Ig+ (B') cell in allotype-restricted antibody production. *J. Exp. Med.* **156**, 443.

Ovnic, M., and Corley, R. B. (1987). Quantitation of cell surface molecules on a differentiating, Ly-1+ B cell lymphoma. *J. Immunol.* **138**, 3075.

Pages, J. M., and Bussard, A. E. (1975). Precommitment of normal mouse peritoneal cells by erythrocyte antigens in relation to auto-antibody production. *Nature (London)* **257**, 316.

Pages, J. M., and Bussard, A. E. (1978). Establishment and characterization of permanent murine hybridoma secreting monoclonal autoantibodies. *Cell. Immunol.* **41**, 188.

Pages, J. M., Poncet, P., Serban, D., Witz, I. P., and Bussard, A. E. (1982). Relationship between choline derivatives and mouse erythrocyte membrane antigens revealed by mouse monoclonal antibodies. I. Anticholine activity of anti-mouse erythrocyte monoclonal antibodies. *Immunol. Lett.* **5**, 167.

Paglieroni, T., and MacKenzie, M. R. (1977). Studies on the pathogenesis of an immune defect in multiple myeloma. *J. Clin. Invest.* **59**, 1120.

Paglieroni, T., and MacKenzie, M. R. (1980). Multiple myeloma: An immunologic profile. Cytotoxic and suppressive effects of the EA rosette-forming cell. *J. Immunol.* **124**, 2563.

Paglieroni, T., Caggiano, V., and MacKenzie, M. (1988). CD5 positive immunoregulatory B cell subsets. *Am. J. Hematol.* **28**, 276.

Paige, C. J., Kincade, P. W., and Ralph, P. (1978). Murine B cell leukemia line with inducible surface immunoglobulin expression. *J. Immunol.* **121**, 641.

Painter, C. J., Monestier, M., Chew, A., Bona-Dimitriu, A., Kasturi, K., Bailey, C., Scott, V. E., Sidman, C. L., and Bona, C. A. (1988). Specificities and V genes encoding monoclonal autoantibodies of viable motheaten mice. *J. Exp. Med.* **167**, 1137.

Pech, M., and Zachau, H. G. (1984). Immunoglobulin genes of different subgroups are interdigitated within the V_K locus. *Nucleic Acids Res.* **12**, 9229.

Pennell, C. A., Arnold, L. W., Lutz, P. M., LoCascio, N. J., Willoughby, P. B., and

Haughton, G. (1985). Cross-reactive idiotypes and common antigen binding specificities expressed by a series of murine B-cell lymphomas: Etiological implications. *Proc. Natl. Acad. Sci. U.S.A.* **82**, 3799.

Pennell, C. A., Arnold, L. W., Haughton, G., and Clarke, S. H. (1988). Restricted Ig variable region gene expression among Ly-1+ B cell lymphomas. *J. Immunol.* **141**, 2788.

Pereira, P., Forsgren, S., Portnoi, D., Bandeira, A., Martinez, C., and Coutinho, A. (1986a). The role of immunoglobulin receptors in "cognate" T-B cell collaboration. *Eur. J. Immunol.* **16**, 355.

Pereira, P., Forni, L., Larsson, E. L., Cooper, M., Heusser, C., and Coutinho, A. (1986b). Autonomous activation of B and T cells in antigen-free mice. *Eur. J. Immunol.* **16**, 685.

Perri, R. T. (1986). Impaired expression of cell surface receptors for B cell growth factor by chronic lymphocytic leukemia B cells. *Blood* **67**, 943.

Pike, B. L., and Nossal, G. J. (1985). A high-efficiency cloning system for single hapten-specific B lymphocytes that is suitable for assay of putative growth and differentiation factors. *Proc. Natl. Acad. Sci. U.S.A.* **82**, 3395.

Pilarski, L. M., Mant, M. J., Ruether, B. A., and Belch, A. (1984). Severe deficiency of B lymphocytes in peripheral blood from multiple myeloma patients. *J. Clin. Invest.* **74**, 1301.

Pillemer, E., Whitlock, C., and Weissman, I. L. (1984). Transformation-associated proteins in murine B-cell lymphomas that are distinct from Abelson virus gene products. *Proc. Natl. Acad. Sci. U.S.A.* **81**, 4434.

Pisetsky, D. S. (1984). Hybridoma SLE autoantibodies: Insights for the pathogenesis of autoimmune disease. *Clin. Immunol. Rev.* **3**, 169.

Pisetsky, D. S., and Caster, S. A. (1982). The B-cell repertoire for autoantibodies: Frequency of precusor cells for anti-DNA antibodies. *Cell. Immunol.* **72**, 294.

Pistoia, V., Cozzolino, F., Rubartelli, A., Torcia, M., Roncella, S., and Ferrarini, M. (1986). *In vitro* production of interleukin 1 by normal and malignant human B lymphocytes. *J. Immunol.* **136**, 1688.

Plater-Zyberk, C., Maini, R. N., Lam, K., Kennedy, T. D., and Janossy, G. (1985). A rheumatoid arthritis B cell subset expresses a phenotype similar to that in chronic lymphocytic leukemia. *Arthritis Rheum.* **28**, 971.

Pohlenz, H. D., Straubinger, B., Thiebe, R., Pech, M., Zimmer, F. J., and Zachau, H. G. (1987). The human V kappa locus. Characterization of extended immunoglobulin gene regions by cosmid cloning. *J. Mol. Biol.* **193**, 241.

Pons-Estel, B., Goni, F., Solomon, A., and Frangione, B. (1984). Sequence similarities among kappa IIIb chains of monoclonal human IgM kappa autoantibodies. *J. Exp. Med.* **160**, 893.

Posnett, D. N., Wisniewolski, R., Pernis, B., and Kunkel, H. G. (1986). Dissection of the human antigammaglobulin idiotype system with monoclonal antibodies. *Scand. J. Immunol.* **23**, 169.

Pratt, L. F., Rassenti, L., Larrick, J., Robbins, B., Banks, P., and Kipps, T. J. (1989). Immunoglobulin gene expression in small lymphocytic lymphoma with little or no somatic hypermutation. *J. Immunol.* (in press).

Preud'homme, J. L., and Seligmann, M. (1972). Anti-human immunoglobulin G activity of membrane-bound immunoglobulin M in lymphoproliferative disorders. *Proc. Natl. Acad. Sci. U.S.A.* **69**, 2132.

Priestle, J. P., Schar, H. P., and Grutter, M. G. (1988). Crystal structure of the cytokine interleukin-1 beta. *EMBO J.* **7**, 339.

Rabinovitch, P. S., Torres, R. M., and Engel, D. (1986). Simultaneous cell cycle analysis and two-color surface immunofluorescence using 7-amino-actinomycin D and single laser excitation: Applications to study of cell activation and the cell cycle of murine Ly-1 B cells. *J. Immunol.* **136**, 2769.

Radoux, V., Chen, P. P., Sorge, J. A., and Carson, D. A. (1986). A conserved human germline V kappa gene directly encodes rheumatoid factor light chains. *J. Exp. Med.* **164**, 2119.

Raffeld, M., Neckers, L., Longo, D. L., and Cossman, J. (1985). Spontaneous alteration of idiotype in a monoclonal B-cell lymphoma. Escape from detection by anti-idiotype. *N. Engl. J. Med.* **312**, 1653.

Rajewsky, K., Forster, I., and Cumano, A. (1987). Evolutionary and somatic selection of the antibody repertoire in the mouse. *Science* **238**, 1088.

Ralph, P., and Kishimoto, T. (1981). Tumor promoter phorbol myristic acetate stimulates secretion correlated with growth cessation in human B cell lines. *J. Clin. Invest.* **68**, 1093.

Raveche, E. S., Alabaster, O., Tjio, J. H., Taurog, J., and Steinberg, A. D. (1981). Analysis of NZB hyperdiploid spleen cells. *J. Immunol.* **126**, 154.

Reininger, L., Ollier, P., Poncet, P., Kaushik, A., and Jaton, J. C. (1987). Novel V genes encode virtually identical variable regions of six murine monoclonal anti-bromelain-treated red blood cell autoantibodies. *J. Immunol.* **138**, 316.

Reth, M., Hämmerling, G. J., and Rajewsky, K. (1978). Analysis of the repertoire of anti-NP antibodies in C57BL/6 mice by cell fusion. I. Characterization of antibody families in the primary and hyperimmune response. *Eur. J. Immunol.* **8**, 393.

Reth, M., Imanishi-Kari, T., and Rajewsky, K. (1979). Analysis of the repertoire of anti-(4-hydroxy-3-nitrophenyl)acetyl (NP) antibodies in C57BL/6 mice by cell fusion. II. Characterization of idiotopes by monoclonal anti-idiotope antibodies. *Eur. J. Immunol.* **9**, 1004.

Rhyne, J. A., Mizel, S. B., Taylor, R. G., Chédid, M., and McCall, C. E. (1988). Characterization of the human interleukin 1 receptor on human polymorphonuclear leukocytes. *Clin. Immunol. Immunopathol.* **48**, 354.

Richard, Y., Leprince, C., Dugas, B., Treton, D., and Galanaud, P. (1987). Reactivity of Leu-1+ tonsillar B cells to a high molecular weight B cell growth factor. *J. Immunol.* **139**, 1563.

Rosenberg, Y. J. (1979). Influence of the sex-linked defect in CBA/N mice on responses to isologous erythrocytes. Ability to overcome the defect with age. *J. Exp. Med.* **150**, 1561.

Rossi, G. A., Hunninghake, G. W., Kawanami, O., Ferrans, V. J., Hansen, C. T., and Crystal, R. G. (1985). Motheaten mice—An animal model with an inherited form of interstitial lung disease. *Am. Rev. Respir. Dis.* **131**, 150.

Rothstein, T. L., and Kolber, D. L. (1988). Peritoneal B cells respond to phorbol esters in the absence of co-mitogen. *J. Immunol.* **140**, 2880.

Royston, I., Majda, J. A., Baird, S. M., Meserve, B. L., and Griffiths, J. C. (1980). Human T cell antigens defined by monoclonal antibodies: The 65,000-dalton antigen of T cells (T65) is also found on chronic lymphocytic leukemia cells bearing surface immunoglobulin. *J. Immunol.* **125**, 725.

Samoszuk, M. K., Epstein, A. L., Said, J., Lukes, R. J., and Nathwani, B. N. (1986). Sensitivity and specificity of immunostaining in the diagnosis of mantle zone lymphoma. *Am. J. Clin. Pathol.* **85**, 557.

Sanchez-Madrid, F., Davignon, D., Martz, E., and Springer, T. A. (1982). Antigens involved in mouse cytolytic T-lymphocyte (CTL)-mediated killing: Functional screening and topographic relationship. *Cell. Immunol.* **73**, 1.

Scher, I., Frantz, M. M., and Steinberg, A. D. (1973). The genetics of the immune response to a synthetic double-stranded RNA in a mutant CBA mouse strain. *J. Immunol.* **110**, 1396.

Scher, I., Ahmed, A., Strong, D. M., Steinberg, A. D., and Paul, W. E. (1975a). X-linked B-lymphocyte immune defect in CBA/N mice. I. Studies of the function and composition of spleen cells. *J. Exp. Med.* **141**, 788.

Scher, I., Steinberg, A. D., Berning, A. K., and Paul, W. E. (1975b). X-linked B-lymphocyte immune defect in CBA/N mice. II. Studies of the mechanisms underlying the immune defect. *J. Exp. Med.* **142**, 637.

Schroeder, H. W., Jr., Hillson, J. L., and Perlmutter, R. M. (1987). Early restriction of the human antibody repertoire. *Science* **238**, 791.

Schwartz, R. S., and Stollar, B. D. (1985). Origins of anti-DNA autoantibodies. *J. Clin. Invest.* **75**, 321.

Scribner, C. L., Hansen, C. T., Klinman, D. M., and Steinberg, A. D. (1987). The interaction of the *xid* and *me* genes. *J. Immunol.* **138**, 3611.

Seldin, M. F., Conroy, J., Steinberg, A. D., D'Hoosteleare, L. A., and Raveche, E. S. (1987). Clonal expansion of abnormal B cells in old NZB mice. *J. Exp. Med.* **166**, 1585.

Sherr, D. H., and Dorf, M. E. (1984). An idiotype-specific helper population that bears immunoglobulin, Ia, and Lyt-1 determinants. *J. Exp. Med.* **159**, 1189.

Sherr, D. H., and Dorf, M. E. (1985). H-2-restricted helper activity mediated by immunoglobulin-bearing lymphocytes. *J. Immunol.* **134**, 2084.

Sherr, D. H., and Ju, S. T. (1986). Idiotype-specific helper cells (B_H) express immunoglobulin markers and employ T cell function-associated molecules. *J. Immunol.* **137**, 3406.

Sherr, D. H., Braun, J., and Dorf, M. E. (1987a). Idiotype-specific Ly-1 B cell-mediated helper activity: Hybridomas that produce anti-idiotype antibody and nonimmunoglobulin lymphokine(s) 1. *J. Immunol.* **138**, 2057.

Sherr, D. H., Dorf, M. E., Gibson, M., and Sidman, C. L. (1987b). Ly-1 B helper cells in autoimmune "viable motheaten" mice. *J. Immunol.* **139**, 1811.

Shirai, T., and Mellors, R. C. (1971). Natural thymocytotoxic autoantibody and reactive antigen in New Zealand black and other mice. *Proc. Natl. Acad. Sci. U.S.A.* **68**, 1412.

Shlomchik, M. J., Nemazee, D. A., Sato, V. L., Van Snick, J., Carson, D. A., and Weigert, M. G. (1986). Variable region sequences of murine IgM anti-IgG monoclonal autoantibodies (rheumatoid factors). A structural explanation for the high frequency of IgM anti-IgG B cells. *J. Exp. Med.* **164**, 407.

Shultz, L. D., and Green, M. C. (1976). Motheaten, an immunodeficiency mutant of the mouse. II. Depressed immune competence and elevated serum immunoglobulins. *J. Immunol.* **116**, 936.

Sidman, C. L., Shultz, L. D., and Unanue, E. R. (1978a). The mouse mutant "motheaten." I. Development of lymphocyte populations. *J. Immunol.* **121**, 2392.

Sidman, C. L., Shultz, L. D., and Unanue, E. R. (1978b). The mouse mutant "motheaten." II. Functional studies of the immune system. *J. Immunol.* **121**, 2399.

Sidman, C. L., Marshall, J. D., Masiello, N. C., Roths, J. B., and Shultz, L. D. (1984). Novel B-cell maturation factor from spontaneously autoimmune viable motheaten mice. *Proc. Natl. Acad. Sci. U.S.A.* **81**, 7199.

Sidman, C. L., Shultz, L. D., and Evans, R. (1985). A serum-derived molecule from autoimmune viable motheaten mice potentiates the action of a B cell maturation factor. *J. Immunol.* **135**, 870.

Sidman, C. L., Shultz, L. D., Hardy, R. R., Hayakawa, K., and Herzenberg, L. A.

(1986). Production of immunoglobulin isotypes by Ly-1+ B cells in viable motheaten and normal mice. *Science* **232**, 1423.
Silverman, G. J., Goldfien, R. D., Chen, P., Mageed, R. A., Jefferis, R., Goni, F., Frangione, B., Fong, S., and Carson, D. A. (1988). Idiotypic and subgroup analysis of human monoclonal rheumatoid factors. Implications for structural and genetic basis of autoantibodies in humans. *J. Clin. Invest.* **82**, 469.
Sims, J. E., March, C. J., Cosman, D., Widmer, M. B., MacDonald, H. R., McMahan, C. J., Grubin, C. E., Wignall, J. M., Jackson, J. L., Call, S. M., Friend, D., Alpert, A. R., Gillis, S., Urdal, D. L., Dower, S. K. (1988). cDNA expression cloning of the IL-1 receptor, a member of the immunoglobulin superfamily. *Science* **241**, 585.
Sklar, J., Cleary, M. L., Thielemans, K., Gralow, J., Warnke, R., and Levy, R. (1984). Biclonal B-cell lymphoma. *N. Engl. J. Med.* **311**, 20.
Sklar, M. D., Shevach, E. M., Green, I., and Potter, M. (1975). Transplantation and preliminary characterisation of lymphocyte surface markers of Abelson virus-induced lymphomas. *Nature (London)* **253**, 550.
Slavin, S., and Strober, S. (1978). Spontaneous murine B-cell leukaemia. *Nature (London)* **272**, 624.
Smith, H. R., and Steinberg, A. D. (1983). Autoimmunity—A perspective. *Annu. Rev. Immunol.* **1**, 175.
Smith, L. J., Curtis, J. E., Messner, H. A., Senn, J. S., Furthmayr, H., and McCulloch, E. A. (1983). Lineage infidelity in acute leukemia. *Blood* **61**, 1138.
Spier, C. M., Grogan, T. M., Fielder, K., Richter, L., and Rangel, C. (1986). Immunophenotypes in "well-differentiated" lymphoproliferative disorders, with emphasis on small lymphocytic lymphoma. *Hum. Pathol.* **17**, 1126.
Springer, T., Galfré, G., Secher, D. S., and Milstein, C. (1978). Monoclonal xenogeneic antibodies to murine cell surface antigens: Identification of novel leukocyte differentiation antigens. *Eur. J. Immunol.* **8**, 539.
Springer, T., Galfré, G., Secher, D. S, and Milstein, C. (1979). Mac-1: A macrophage differentiation antigen identified by monoclonal antibody. *Eur. J. Immunol.* **9**, 301.
Stall, A. M., and Loken, M. R. (1984). Allotypic specificities of murine IgD and IgM recognized by monoclonal antibodies. *J. Immunol.* **132**, 787.
Stall, A. M., Farinas, M. C., Tarlinton, D. M., Lalor, P. A., Herzenberg, L. A., and Strober, S. (1988). Ly-1 B-cell clones similar to human chronic lymphocytic leukemia routinely develop in older normal mice and young autoimmune Zealand black-related animals. *Proc. Natl. Acad. Sci. U.S.A.* **85**, 7312.
Stashenko, P., Nadler, L. M., Hardy, R., and Schlossman, S. F. (1980). Characterization of a human B lymphocyte-specific antigen. *J. Immunol.* **125**, 1678.
Steele, E. J., and Cunningham, A. J. (1978). High proportion of Ig-producing cells making autoantibody in normal mice. *Nature (London)* **274**, 483.
Stevenson, F. K., Wrightham, M., Glennie, M. J., Jones, D. B., Cattan, A. R., Feizi, T., Hamblin, T. J., and Stevenson, G. T. (1986). Antibodies to shared idiotypes as agents for analysis and therapy for human B cell tumors. *Blood* **68**, 430.
Sthoeger, Z. M., Waki, M., Tse, D. B., Vinciguerra, V. P., Allen, S. L., Budman, D. R., Lichtman, S. M., Schulman, P., Weiselberg, L. R., and Chiorazzi, N. (1989). Production of autoantibodies by CD5-expressing B lymphocytes from patients with chronic lymphocytic leukemia. *J. Exp. Med.* **169**, 255.
Stong, R. C., Korsmeyer, S. J., Parkin, J. L., Arthur, D. C., and Kersey, J. H. (1985). Human acute leukemia cell line with the t(4;11) chromosomal rearrangement exhibits B lineage and monocytic characteristics. *Blood* **65**, 21.
Subbarao, B., and Mosier, D. E. (1983). Induction of B lymphocyte proliferation by

monoclonal anti-Lyb 2 antibody. *J. Immunol.* **130**, 2033.

Symington, F. W., Subbarao, B., Mosier, D. E., and Sprent, J. (1982). Lyb-8.2: A new B cell antigen defined and characterized with a monoclonal antibody. *Immunogenetics* **16**, 381.

Takemori, T., Tesch, H., Reth, M., and Rajewsky, K. (1982). The immune response against anti-idiotope antibodies. I. Induction of idiotope-bearing antibodies and analysis of the idiotope repertoire. *Eur. J. Immunol.* **12**, 1040.

Taniguchi, O., Miyajima, H., Hirano, T., Noguchi, M., Ueda, A., Hashimoto, H., Hirose, S., and Okumura, K. (1987). The Leu-1 B-cell subpopulation in patients with rheumatoid arthritis. *J. Clin. Immunol.* **7**, 441.

Tarlinton, D., Stall, A. M., and Herzenberg, L. A. (1988). Repetitive usage of immunoglobulin V_H and D gene segments in CD5+ Ly-1 B clones of (NZB × NZW)F1 mice. *EMBO J.* **7**, 3705.

Tedder, T. F., Clement, L. T., and Cooper, M. D. (1984). Expression of C3d receptors during human B cell differentiation: Immunofluorescence analysis with the HB-5 monoclonal antibody. *J. Immunol.* **133**, 678.

Theofilopoulos, A. N., and Dixon, F. J. (1985). Murine models of systemic lupus erythematosus. *Adv. Immunol.* **37**, 269.

Thomas, Y., Glickman, E., DeMartino, J., Wang, J., Goldstein, G., and Chess, L. (1984). Biologic functions of the OKT1 T cell surface antigen. I. The T1 molecule is involved in helper function. *J. Immunol.* **133**, 724.

Thorley-Lawson, D. A., Nadler, L. M., Bhan, A. K., and Schooley, R. T. (1985). BLAST-2 [EBVCS], an early cell surface marker of human B cell activation, is superinduced by Epstein Barr virus. *J. Immunol.* **134**, 3007.

Todd, R. F., 3rd, Nadler, L. M., and Schlossman, S. F. (1981). Antigens on human monocytes identified by monoclonal antibodies. *J. Immunol.* **126**, 1435.

Tsudo, M., Uchiyama, T., and Uchino, H. (1984). Expression of Tac antigen on activated normal human B cells. *J. Exp. Med.* **160**, 612.

Tung, J. S., Scheid, M. P., Pierotti, M. A., Hämmerling, U., and Boyse, E. A. (1981). Structural features and selective expression of three Ly-5+ cell-surface molecules. *Immunogenetics* **14**, 101.

Unkeless, J. C. (1979). Characterization of a monoclonal antibody directed against mouse macrophage and lymphocyte Fc receptors. *J. Exp. Med.* **150**, 580.

Vakil, M., and Kearney, J. F. (1986). Functional characterization of monoclonal auto-anti-idiotype antibodies isolated from the early B cell repertoire of BALB/c mice. *Eur. J. Immunol.* **16**, 1151.

Vakil, M., Sauter, H., Paige, C., and Kearney, J. F. (1986). In vivo suppression of perinatal multispecific B cells results in a distortion of the adult B cell repertoire. *Eur. J. Immunol.* **16**, 1159.

van den Oord, J. J., de Wolf-Peeters, C., and Desmet, V. J. (1986a). The marginal zone in the human reactive lymph node. *Am. J. Clin. Pathol.* **86**, 475.

van den Oord, J. J., de Wolf-Peeters, C., Pulford, K. A., Mason, D. Y., and Desmet, V. J. (1986b). Mantle zone lymphoma. Immuno- and enzymehistochemical studies on the cell of origin. *Am. J. Surg. Pathol.* **10**, 780.

Waldmann, T. A., Goldman, C. K., Robb, R. J., Depper, J. M., Leonard, W. J., Sharrow, S. O., Bongiovanni, K. F., Korsmeyer, S. J., and Greene, W. C. (1984). Expression of interleukin 2 receptors on activated human B cells. *J. Exp. Med.* **160**, 1450.

Walker, E. B., Lanier, L. L., and Warner, N. L. (1982). Characterization and functional properties of tumor cell lines in accessory cell replacement assays. *J. Immunol.* **128**, 852.

Wang, C. Y., Good, R. A., Ammirati, P., Dymbort, G., and Evans, R. L. (1980). Identification of a p69,71 complex expressed on human T cells sharing determinants with B-type chronic lymphatic leukemic cells. *J. Exp. Med.* **151**, 1539.

Wassmer, P., Chan, C., Logdberg, L., and Shevach, E. M. (1985). Role of the L3T4-antigen in T cell activation. II. Inhibition of T cell activation by monoclonal anti-L3T4 antibodies in the absence of accessory cells. *J. Immunol.* **135**, 2237.

Weinstein, I. B., Arcoleo, J., Backer, J., Jeffrey, A., Hsiao, W. L., Gattoni-Celli, S., Kirschmeier, P., and Okin, E. (1983). Molecular mechanisms of tumor promotion and multistage carcinogenesis. *Proc. Int. Symp. Princess Takamatsu Cancer Res. Fund. 14th*, 59.

Weis, J. J., Tedder, T. F., and Fearon, D. T. (1984). Identification of a 145,000 M_r membrane protein as the C3d receptor (CR2) of human B lymphocytes. *Proc. Natl. Acad. Sci. U.S.A.* **81**, 881.

Weisenburger, D. D. (1986). Mantle-zone lymphoma: Another opinion [letter]. *Am. J. Surg. Pathol.* **10**, 733.

Weisenburger, D. D., Nathwani, B. N., Diamond, L. W., Winberg, D. D., and Rappaport, H. (1981). Malignant lymphoma, intermediate lymphocytic type: A clinicopathologic study of 42 cases. *Cancer (Philadelphia)* **48**, 1415.

Weisenburger, D. D., Kim, H., and Rappaport, H. (1982). Mantle zone lymphoma: A follicular variant of intermediate lymphocytic lymphoma. *Cancer (Philadelphia)* **49**, 1429.

Weisenburger, D. D., Linder, J., Daley, D. T., and Armitage, J. O. (1987). Intermediate lymphocytic lymphoma: An immunohistologic study with comparison to other lymphocytic lymphomas. *Hum. Pathol.* **18**, 781.

Williams, J. M., Deloria, D., Hansen, J. A., Dinarello, C. A., Loertscher, R., Shapiro, H. M., and Strom, T. B. (1985). The events of primary T cell activation can be staged by use of Sepharose-bound anti-T3 (64.1) monoclonal antibody and purified interleukin 1. *J. Immunol.* **135**, 2249.

Winter, E., Radbruch, A., and Krawinkel, U. (1985). Members of novel V_H gene families are found in VDJ regions of polyclonally activated B-lymphocytes. *EMBO J.* **4**, 2861.

Wofsy, D., and Chiang, N. Y. (1987). Proliferation of Ly-1 B cells in autoimmune NZB and (NZB × NZW)F1 mice. *Eur. J. Immunol.* **17**, 809.

Wolf, M., Cuatrecasas, P., and Sahyoun, N. (1985). Interaction of protein kinase C with membranes is regulated by Ca^{2+}, phorbol esters, and ATP. *J. Biol. Chem.* **260**, 15718.

Yamasaki, H., Enomoto, T., Hamel, E., and Kanno, Y. (1983). Membrane interaction and modulation of gene expression by tumor promoters. *Proc. Int. Symp. Princess Takamatsu Cancer Res. Fund., 14th*, 221.

Yancopoulos, G. D., and Alt, F. W. (1985). Developmentally controlled and tissue-specific expression of unrearranged V_H gene segments. *Cell (Cambridge, Mass.)* **40**, 271.

Yancopoulos, G. D., and Alt, F. W. (1986). Regulation of the assembly and expression of variable-region genes. *Annu. Rev. Immunol.* **4**, 339.

Yancopoulos, G. D., Desiderio, S. V., Paskind, M., Kearney, J. F., Baltimore, D., and Alt, F. W. (1984). Preferential utilization of the most J_H-proximal V_H gene segments in pre-B-cell lines. *Nature (London)* **311**, 727.

Yelton, D. E., Desaymard, C., and Scharff, M. D. (1981). Use of monoclonal anti-mouse immunoglobulin to detect mouse antibodies. *Hybridoma* **1**, 5.

Youinou, P., Mackenzie, L., Bourbigot, B., Le Saout, J., Le Goff, P., Jouquan, J., and Lydyard, P. M. (1986). Expression of T-lymphocyte antigens by serum B lymphocytes rheumatoid polyarthritis. *Rev. Rhum. Mal. Osteo-Articulaires* **53**, 643.

Youinou, P., Mackenzie, L., Jouquan, J., Le Goff, P., and Lydyard, P. M. (1987). CD5 positive B cells in patients with rheumatoid arthritis: Phorbol ester mediated enhancement of detection. *Ann. Rheum. Dis.* **46**, 17.

This article was accepted for publication on 13 February 1989.

Biology of Natural Killer Cells

GIORGIO TRINCHIERI

Wistar Institute of Anatomy and Biology,
Philadelphia, Pennsylvania 19104

I. Introduction

In 1960 Govaerts (1) observed that thoracic duct lymphocytes of dogs carrying a kidney transplant were cytotoxic *in vitro* for kidney cells of the donor animal. Since then the study of cytotoxic lymphocytes has been extended to various cellular reactions of adaptive immunity, directed against transplantation antigens on allogeneic cells, viral antigens, tumor-associated antigens, and self-antigens in autoimmune pathology (2, 3). The specific adaptive cytotoxic response against transplantation alloantigens is mediated by thymus-dependent effector T lymphocytes. The alloantigens recognized by the cytotoxic T lymphocytes (CTLs) were shown to be encoded by genes of the major histocompatibility complex (MHC) (4) and were later identified as the products of MHC class I and class II genes (5–7).

Numerous studies of humans and experimental animals have tested the hypothesis that CTLs directed against antigens expressed *de novo* on syngeneic tumor cells were responsible for the immune surveillance against growth of neoplastic cells (8). In these studies, cytotoxicity mediated by lymphocytes of cancer patients was demonstrated on both autologous and allogeneic tumor target cells. However, Zinkernagel and Doherty (9) showed that CTLs recognize viral antigens on target cells only in association with products of syngeneic MHC, and this MHC restriction of CTLs was also then demonstrated for tumor-associated antigens (10).

On the other hand, studies of cytotoxicity by human lymphocytes revealed not only that both allogeneic and syngeneic tumor cells were lysed in a non-MHC-restricted fashion, but also that lymphocytes from normal donors were often cytotoxic. Lymphocytes from any healthy donor, as well as peripheral blood and spleen lymphocytes from several experimental animals, in the absence of known or deliberate sensitization, were found to be spontaneously cytotoxic *in vitro* for some normal fresh cells, most cultured cell lines, immature hematopoietic cells, and tumor cells (11–16). This type of nonadaptive, non-MHC-restricted cell-mediated cytotoxicity was defined as "natural" cytotoxicity, and the effector cells mediating natural cytotoxicity were functionally defined as natural killer (NK) cells. The existence of NK cells has prompted a reinterpretation of both the studies of specific cytotoxicity against spontaneous human tumors (17) and the theory of immune surveillance, at least in its most restrictive interpretation, based on a predominant role of adaptive immunity and tumor antigen-specific CTLs (18, 19).

For many years a major difficulty in the study of NK cells stemmed from the fact that they were functionally defined, i.e., cells that mediate natural, non-MHC-restricted cytotoxicity. It is now known that different types of lymphocytes and other leukocytes can mediate non-MHC-restricted cytotoxicity either spontaneously or upon activation. However, most cells mediating natural cytotoxicity in humans and many other species share similar functional characteristics, and the cells appear to constitute a discrete cell subset. Unlike cytotoxic T cells, NK cells cannot be demonstrated to have clonally distributed specificity, restriction for MHC products at the target cell surface, or immunological memory. NK cells cannot as yet be formally assigned to a single lineage based on the definitive identification of a stem cell, a distinct anatomical location of maturation, or unique genotypic rearrangements. Thus, some investigators have suggested that NK cells be defined operationally, referring to any lymphoid cell from an unimmunized host mediating MHC-unrestricted cytotoxicity (20, 21).

Nevertheless, it is possible to (1) unequivocally distinguish mature NK cells from T, B, and myeloid cells; (2) distinguish NK progenitors from those of T, B, and myeloid cells; and (3) suggest that NK cells are dependent on intact bone marrow and not on thymus for their differentiation (22, 23). NK cells, therefore, represent a discrete leukocyte subset, possibly constituting a third lineage of lymphoid cells (22-25). Although the exact characterization of the NK cell subset and its possible heterogeneity still requires detailed analysis, a consensus on an operational definition of NK cells was reached at the Fifth International Workshop on Natural Killer Cells in 1988 (26). NK cells have been defined as large granular lymphocytes (LGLs) that do not express on their surface the CD3 antigen or any of the known T cell receptor chains (i.e., α, β, γ, or δ) but do express CD16 and NKH-1 (Leu-19) cell surface markers in humans and NK-1.1/NK-2.1 in mice and mediate cytolytic reactions even in the absence of MHC class I or class II expression on the target cells (26).

Certain T lymphocytes that are either $\alpha\beta^+$ or $\gamma\delta^+$ may express, particularly upon activation, a cytolytic activity that resembles that of NK cells; these T lymphocytes are more appropriately described as displaying "NK-like" activity or "non-MHC-requiring" cytolysis (26). The lymphokine-activated killer (LAK) cells, which have recently received much attention for their possible therapeutic use (27), are interleukin-2 (IL-2)-activated lymphocytes that are NK cells or non-MHC-requiring T cells. The relative contribution of the respective cell type depends on the source of lymphocytes and conditions for activation (26).

One of the surface receptors that were identified on NK cells since their original description (11) is a low-affinity receptor for the Fc fragment of immunoglobulin G (IgG) (FcR) or CD16 antigen (28). Through their FcR (CD16), NK cells can interact with and lyse IgG antibody-coated target cells. Although antibody-dependent cell-mediated cytotoxicity (ADCC) can be mediated by a variety of cell types, including monocyte/macrophages and polymorphonucleated leukocytes (PMNs), the lymphocyte subset that mediates ADCC has been operationally defined as killer (K) cells and is identical or largely overlapping with the NK cell subset (29–33).

Although NK cells were named on the basis of the cytotoxic activity that initially served to identify them, this cell type exerts a variety of functions, including production of lymphokines, regulatory functions on the adaptive immune system and on hematopoiesis, and natural resistance against microbial infection and tumor growth (23). The cytotoxic ability of NK cells may or may not represent the most physiologically significant function of these cells *in vivo*. NK cells, together with monocyte/macrophages, PMNs, platelets, etc., are an important effector cell type of nonadaptive immunity. In mediating these functions, the activity of NK cells is regulated by a complex network of cellular and humoral interactions with cell types of the adaptive and nonadaptive immune systems, nervous system, and others. Although many tesserae of this mosaic are still incomplete or missing, this review attempts to summarize the experimental evidence pointing to NK cells as a discrete cell subset that is highly regulated in its interaction with other systems of the organism.

II. Measurement of NK Cell-Mediated Cytotoxicity

A large variety of target cell types has been used to measure NK cytotoxicity, using unseparated lymphoid preparations from human donors and experimental animals. Cultured cell lines differ greatly in their sensitivity to NK cytotoxicity and, in general, cell lines from homologous species are lysed more efficiently than are heterologous cells. Tumor-derived cell lines are often used as NK target cells (11, 14), but NK cytotoxicity can also be demonstrated against normal target cells, including normal diploid fibroblast strains (34–36). The most sensitive and widely used target cell for human NK cells is K562 (11), a cell line derived from a patient with chronic myeloid leukemia in blastic crisis (37). These cells lack MHC class I and class II antigens and can be induced to differentiate *in vitro* to cells with myeloid, erythroid, or megakaryocytic characteristics (38, 39). The Moloney virus-induced lymphoma cell line YAC-1 is the most widely used target for the measurement of rodent NK cell cytotoxicity (40, 41).

The cytotoxic activity of NK cells can also be evaluated by the ability of these cells to lyse IgG antibody-coated target cells. In early studies ADCC activity of human lymphocytes was measured, using as target cells chicken erythrocytes (2), the Chang (HeLa) cell line (42), and T cell blasts (43) sensitized with hetero- or alloantisera. Antibody-sensitized nonnucleated erythrocytes are efficient target cells for ADCC mediated by monocytes and PMNs, but not by human NK/K cells (44). However, the use in ADCC of target cells that are sensitive to NK cell lysis in the absence of antibodies has complicated the interpretation of many studies. For this reason, the mouse mastocytoma cell line P815, which is almost completely resistant to both human and murine NK cell lysis, is now often used as the target cell for ADCC studies (32).

NK cell cytotoxicity is usually quantitated in the ^{51}Cr-release cytotoxicity assay, in which NK cell-containing cell preparations are mixed with a constant number of ^{51}Cr (sodium chromate)-labeled target cells at one or more effector-target (E:T) cell ratios, and cell lysis is evaluated, usually after 3–4 hours of incubation at 37°C, by measuring the amount of ^{51}Cr released into the supernatant fluid (45). In many studies NK cytotoxicity is expressed as the percentage of ^{51}Cr release at an arbitrarily chosen E:T ratio. However, the use of a single E:T ratio precludes a quantitative comparison of the relative cytotoxicity mediated by different donors or by the same lymphocyte preparations after different treatments. Figure 1 illustrates the great difference in relative NK activity of two donors, A and B, measured by using the percentages of ^{51}Cr release at different E:T ratios. Comparing the percentages of ^{51}Cr release at a given E:T ratio can yield the rank order of the cytotoxicity mediated by the cells of the two donors, but not a quantitative evaluation of the relative cytotoxicity. The use of several E:T ratios yields a quantitative evaluation of cytotoxicity by measuring lytic units (LU), defined as the number of effector cells required to lyse a given proportion (optimally 50%, but often 20 or 30% was used) of target cells in the assay period (3). This number can be extrapolated graphically or computed based on equations (43, 46, 47) that describe the relationship between effector cell concentration and percentage of ^{51}Cr release (Figs. 1 and 2). The use of LUs transforms a series of dose–response data to a single number (with standard errors, etc.) which is based on all of the data and which is directly proportional to NK cell lytic activity.

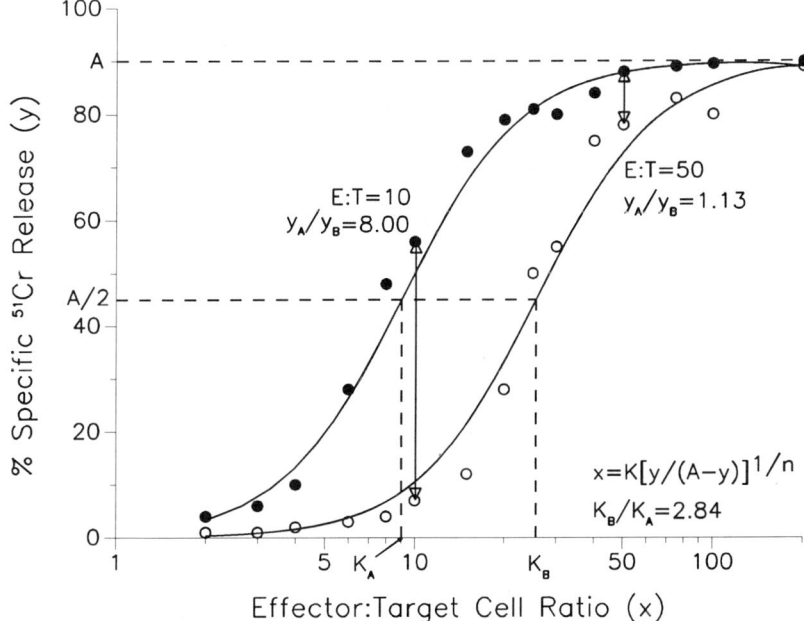

FIG. 1. Quantitation of NK cell-mediated cytotoxicity in a ^{51}Cr-release assay (4-hour incubation) using a constant number (10^4) of ^{51}Cr-labeled K562 target cells and a variable number of human PBLs as effector cells. ○, PBLs from donor A; ●, PBLs from donor B. Each symbol represents an experimental point. The relative cytotoxicity measured at the two arbitrarily chosen effector-target cell ratios (E : T) of 10 and 50 is indicated on the figure. Sigmoidal curves for the two donors were plotted using the modified von Krogh's equation (see text). When y is equal to $A/2$, K is equal to x, i.e., $K \times 10^4$ is equal to the number of effector cells required to lyse half of the target cells (5×10^3) and is defined as 1 LU. LUs calculated in this way can be used to quantitate the cytotoxicity of different effector cell preparations when the slopes (n) of the different sigmoidal curves are similar. The ratio K_B/K_A represents the relative cytotoxic efficiency of the two cell preparations calculated based on all of the experimental points.

Two equations are most commonly used to reduce ^{51}Cr release dose-response data to linearity: the simple exponential fit and a modified von Krogh equation. The exponential fit equation (46–48) may be written as

$$y = A(1 - e^{-kx}) \tag{1}$$

where y is the fractional ^{51}Cr release, A is a constant equal to the asymptote of the curve, x is the E : T ratio, and k is a constant which, for curves having the same asymptote, is directly proportional to the NK cell activity. If the assay is plotted as a target survival curve, i.e., as $\ln(A - y)$ versus x, the value k is the negative of the slope of the resulting straight line (Fig. 2, bottom right). The exponential fit equation defines a sigmoidal curve on a semilog plot (e.g., Fig. 2, top).

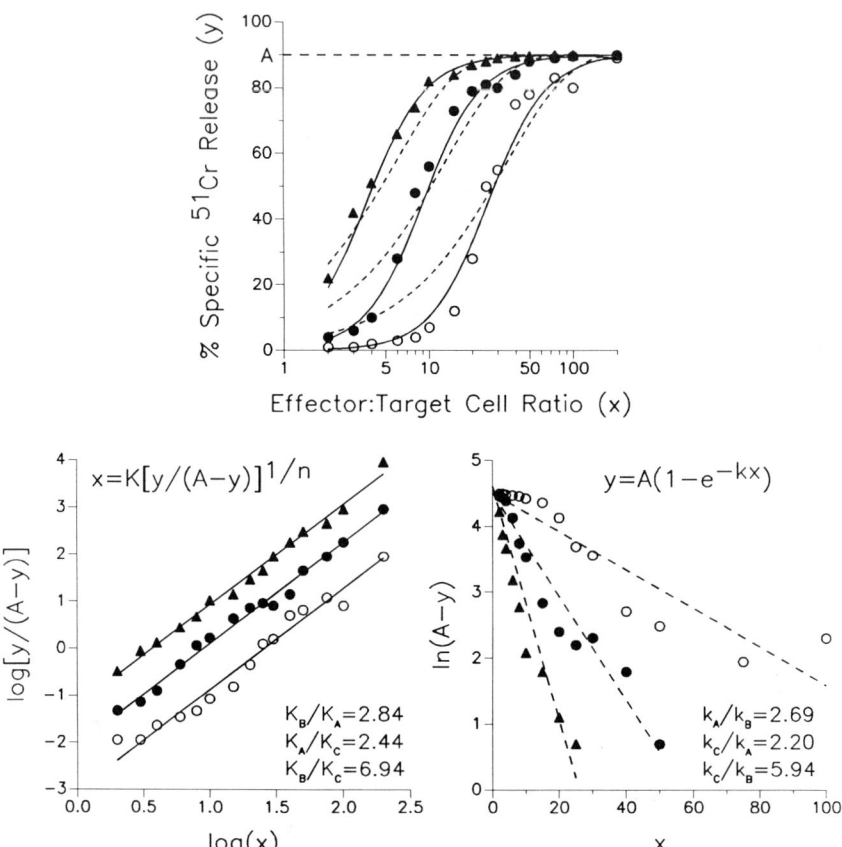

FIG. 2. Analysis of the cytotoxic activity of PBLs from donors A (●), B (○), and C (▲) using the von Krogh's equation or the exponential fit equation. The cytotoxic assay was performed as in Fig. 1. The top panel depicts the best-fit sigmoidal curves for the three donors using the modified von Krogh's equation (solid lines) or the exponential fit equation (broken lines). (Bottom left) Curves calculated according to the modified von Krogh's equation and expressed as $\log[y/(A - y)]$ versus $\log(x)$. (Bottom right) Curves calculated according to the exponential fit equation and expressed as $\ln(A - y)$ versus x. The relative cytotoxic efficiencies for the three preparations, calculated according to the two equations, are given in the bottom panels. Similar values were calculated with the two equations.

The von Krogh equation (49, 50) was originally described as an application of the Hill transformation (51) to the analysis of complement lysis and was modified for use in the analysis of ^{51}Cr-release data. Unlike complement lysis, where 100% hemolysis is obtainable, it is difficult to evaluate the maximum release of the isotope in the ^{51}Cr-release method. Complete release of incorporated ^{51}Cr is never observed, and most investigators use detergent lysis (usually 80-90% of incorporated isotope) as a measure of maximum release. However, the values observed for the maximum release upon cell-mediated cytotoxicity are usually lower than those obtained with detergent lysis and are variable among different target cells and experiments. Thus, the von Krogh equation had to be modified for analysis of ^{51}Cr-release data by the introduction of the constant A equal to the asymptote of the ^{51}Cr-release dose-response curve (43). The asymptote A has been estimated either by computer iteration (43) or experimentally (46). Like the exponential fit equation, the von Krogh equation also defines a sigmoid curve (Figs. 1 and 2, top panel), but contains a third variable which makes it possible to fit data in which there is a longer lag phase and a more abrupt rise in cytotoxicity in the exponential part of the curve. The modified von Krogh equation (43, 47) can be written as

$$y = \frac{A}{1 + (K/x)^n} \qquad (2)$$

where y, x, and A are as in the exponential fit equation, n is a constant which defines the shape of the curve on the semilog plot, and K (different from the k value in the exponential fit equation) is a constant equal to x at $y = A/2$, directly proportional to NK cell activity and equal to 1 LU (50%). The modified von Krogh equation can be linearized by log transformation as

$$\log x = \log k + 1/n \, \log[y/(A - y)] \qquad (3)$$

and a family of curves with the same n and A will therefore yield a series of parallel and straight lines when plotted $\log[y/(A - y)]$ versus $\log x$ (Fig. 2, bottom left).

Both equations have been found to result in a good correlation between the observed and calculated points (47, 48). However, the exponential fit equation is more sensitive to changes in the A value in calculating the LU. The von Krogh equation yields a better fit under these conditions, because it contains the slope of the line, $1/n$, as a third variable. However, because of this variable, a serious source of error is introduced in the LU calculation, and results of different effector cell preparations or of different target cells can be compared only when the slopes of the different curves are not significantly different.

The use of the cytotoxic assay to compare the NK cell activity of different normal donors or patients is complicated by a large variability of activity among normal donors and by day-to-day variation in sensitivity of the assay system. In sequential studies normalization of the assay is necessary in order to compare the results obtained in different experiments. The work of Pross and collaborators (48, 52–55), who studied this problem in detail, has generated several suggestions for the normalization of the NK cell assay. The rank of cytotoxic activity mediated by lymphocytes from normal donors remains relatively constant over an extended period, in the absence of situations such as infection or drug treatment that alter NK cell activity (52, 56). It is therefore possible to normalize the cytotoxic assay by using in each experiment a group of control donors with similar average activity, but not necessarily the same control donors in each experiment. However, because the repeated use of fresh normal controls is frequently impractical, cryopreserved lymphocytes are often used. NK cell functions are usually markedly reduced after cryopreservation (57), but are almost completely recovered if the lymphocytes are incubated for a few hours at 37°C after thawing (53). Although cryopreservation may reduce the absolute cytotoxic activity, the relative cytotoxicity of lymphocytes obtained from different donors is maintained, making the use of cryopreserved lymphocytes for normalization of the cytotoxic assay possible (53). Normalization in the cytotoxic assay is absolutely necessary in order to compare results within experiments or among different laboratories. Unfortunately, many of the published analyses of NK cell activity in patients completely lack any normalization.

Several factors that can affect *in vivo* or *in vitro* NK cell activity must be considered in analyses of NK cell cytotoxic activity of lymphocytes from patients. NK cell activity tends to increase with donor age and is, on average, higher in male than in female donors, making it important to use a control group that is age and gender matched (52). Alcohol, smoking, various common drugs (such as salicylates), stress, and concurrent diseases (such as infections) may also alter NK cell activity *in vivo*. *In vitro*, the presence of monocytes and PMNs can suppress NK cell cytotoxic activity, whereas the presence of erythrocytes in the assay determines a dose-dependent enhancement of cytotoxicity (58).

Other NK cell cytotoxic assays allow a direct microscopic observation of the effector–target cell interaction. In the single-cell cytotoxic assay in agarose, effector and target cells are allowed to form conjugates in a pellet for a few minutes, and the conjugates are then immobilized in smears of semisolid medium (agarose) (59, 60). The NK cells are prevented from recycling by the agarose. The smears, on petri dishes or on microscope slides, are incubated at 37°C for various periods, and the dead cells are evaluated by dye exclusion, using trypan blue. The slides can then be fixed and the conjugates and lytic conjugates can be counted. Different investigators have reported 15-40% human peripheral blood lymphocytes (PBLs) forming conjugates with K562 cells (48, 61-63). Although a large proportion of NK cells [up to 100% after interferon (IFN) stimulation] bind to target cells, not all conjugate-forming cells in human peripheral blood are NK cells. This has been clearly shown in several studies in which the phenotype of binding cells has been analyzed (63-66). As evaluated in the single-cell assay, the frequency of lytic NK cells in human peripheral blood has been reported to be 1-5% (61, 63). Combined use of the single-cell cytotoxic assay in agarose and estimation of the maximum NK cell cytotoxic potential by ^{51}Cr release to study recycling of effector cells indicated that, on average, an NK cell can lyse 2.3 target cells (62, 67).

Although laborious and difficult to quantitate, the single-cell assay allows an approximation of the number of active NK cells in cell preparation, and it has been extremely useful to study the mechanisms of cytotoxicity and their alteration in patients or upon *in vivo* or *in vitro* drug treatments. However, caution should be exercised in interpreting data, especially those concerning NK cell recycling that are based on the assumption that the single-cell assay has 100% efficiency in allowing conjugation and killing by active NK cells.

Under appropriate experimental conditions, cell-mediated cytotoxicity can be analyzed in a manner analogous to enzyme-catalyzed reactions. Initial studies of the kinetics of cellular cytotoxicity reactions generally applied the equation for simple enzyme kinetics originally developed by Michaelis and Menten (68-70). However, cellular cytotoxicity reactions do not follow simple Michaelian kinetics. The experimentally determined apparent Michaelis constant (K_m^{app}) varies in proportion to the number of lymphocytes present in the assay system (71). Because of the differences between enzyme-catalyzed reactions and cellular cytotoxicity reactions, more complex models were developed. Merrill (72) developed more general equations that took into account the possibility of noncytotoxic lymphocytes binding to target cells and inhibiting cytotoxicity. In this model V_{max}, the maximum velocity for a natural cytotoxicity reaction, is expressed as

$$V_{max} = k_2 \alpha f[L] \qquad (4)$$

where [L] is the lymphocyte concentration, f is the fraction of target-binding lymphocytes, α is the fraction of cytolytically active target-binding lymphocytes, and k_2 is the rate constant for target cell lysis. The expression of K_m^{app} that results from this model is very complex and takes into consideration the rate constants for programming for lysis (see Section V) and for target cell disintegration, the dissociation constant for target conjugates of nonlytic lymphocytes, and the fractions of lymphocytes that bind target cells and lyse target cells (72). However, for cytotoxicity mediated by human NK cells, Callewaert *et al.* (73, 74) determined that programming for lysis is the rate-limiting step and the value of K_m^{app} is directly related to the frequency of target-binding cells within the lymphocyte population. K_m^{app} can be approximated by the expression

$$K_m^{app} = f[L](K_m/K_I) \tag{5}$$

where K_m is the standard Michaelis–Menten constant and K_I is the dissociation constant for target-binding nonlytic lymphocytes.

V_{max} is a useful quantitative measure of the overall cytotoxic activity of a lymphocyte preparation. V_{max} values increase linearly with an increasing number of lymphocytes in the assay and are useful for the quantitative comparison of the relative cytotoxic activity of different lymphocyte preparations. V_{max} and LU values yield comparable estimates of relative cytotoxic activity (75). The physical significance of K_m^{app} is more difficult to interpret. For NK cell-mediated cytotoxicity, K_m^{app} is not constant but varies with the concentrations of lymphocytes tested, and it is approximately equal to the concentration of lytic lymphocytes (71). K_m^{app} therefore allows for the simultaneous determination both of the frequency of NK effector cells, according to the relationship

$$\% \text{ NK} = K_m^{app}/[L] \times 100 \tag{6}$$

and of the activity of NK effector cells, by determining the rate constant for target cells according to the relationship

$$k_2 = V_{max}/K_m^{app} \tag{7}$$

The initial rate of K562 cytolysis by human NK cells is maintained for 1–3 hours, followed by a stable plateau of cytotoxicity values (Fig. 3), reflecting the inability of NK cells to lyse additional target cells unless stimulated with IFN or IL-2 (76, 77). These results suggest that, although NK cells are able to lyse more than one target cell, their recycling ability, unlike that of CTLs, is extremely modest (76). The kinetics analysis of NK cell cytotoxicity is further complicated when target cell preparations are used that stimulate production of lymphokines, affecting NK cell cytotoxicity during the assay. For example, production of IFN-α or -γ, by NK cells or other cell types present in the lymphocyte preparation, is observed when target cells are sensitized with IgG antibodies (78) or infected with viruses (79, 80) or mycoplasmas (81, 82). A typical example is the lysis of virus-infected target cells in which V_{max} significantly increases after 4–6 hours of culture, because of IFN production or other stimuli for NK cells (56) (Fig. 3).

III. Phenotypic and Genotypic Characteristics of NK Cells

A. IDENTIFICATION OF NK CELLS

Identification of NK cells based solely on their ability to mediate spontaneous and antibody-dependent cytotoxicity, a function shared with other cell types, such as monocyte/macrophages and activated T cells,

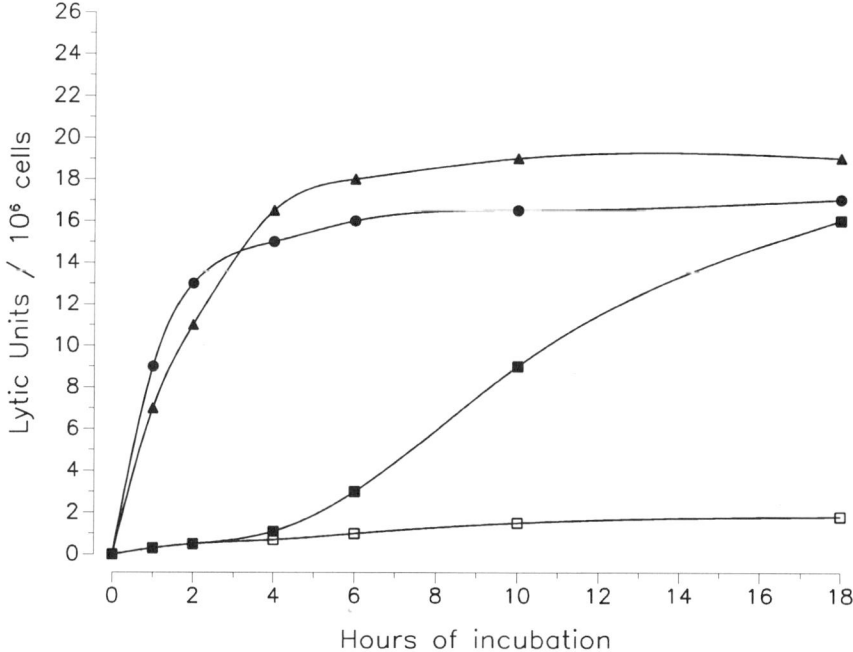

FIG. 3. Kinetics of NK cell-mediated cytotoxicity. PBLs from one donor were tested against 10^4 K562 cells (●—●), rabbit IgG-coated P815 cells (▲—▲), human fibroblasts (□—□), or human fibroblasts infected with the HK strain of influenza virus (■—■) in a ^{51}Cr-release cytotoxicity assay. Cytotoxicity was evaluated at different times and LUs were calculated from various effector-target cell ratios using the modified von Krogh's equation.

has represented a major limitation in the analysis of NK cells. One of the most significant contributions to the study of NK cells has been their identification as a relatively homogeneous cell type on the basis of physical and phenotypic characteristics and their LGL morphology (35). Human NK/K cells were originally described as nonadherent, nonphagocytic, FcγR-positive cells with lymphoid morphology. Although velocity sedimentation experiments demonstrated that human K cells were larger than the bulk of T lymphocytes (44), it was not until Saksela, Timonen, and collaborators (35, 83, 84) analyzed cytotoxic effector cells adsorbed-eluted from both fibroblast and cell line target cells that NK cells were identified as LGLs, i.e., large lymphocytes with a high cytoplasm-nuclear ratio and few discrete azurophilic granules. A separation technique involving a discontinuous Percoll gradient has been widely used for the enrichment of LGLs based on their light buoyant density (85). This technique has contributed much to the progress of studies of NK cells, allowing investigations utilizing semipurified preparations of NK cells. Such preparations have been used for the analysis of surface phenotype and morphology as well as functional characteristics of NK cells (86-90). However, the use of these semipurified preparations has also generated considerable artifact and confusion, due mostly to disregard of the following facts: (1) LGL morphology is not unique to NK cells, and not all NK cells may have typical LGL morphology at all times during differentiation and functional activation (91); (2) light-density Percoll fractions, although enriched for NK cells/LGLs, also contain monocytes, dendritic accessory cells, human leukocyte antigen (HLA)-DR$^+$ IFN-α-producing cells, T cell blasts, and memory T cells (92, 93), and even some of the most careful purification procedures could not completely eliminate all of these contaminant cell types; (3) whereas light-density Percoll fractions are enriched for accessory cells, enriched T cell preparations from high-density fractions are completely devoid of accessory cells; thus, some of the reported differential activity of NK and T cells might rest in the presence or absence of accessory cells in the cell preparations used.

The use of monoclonal antibodies to cell surface markers has greatly contributed to the progress in the identification of the NK cell subset. These studies are now being extended, with the use of molecular probes, to assay for gene transcript expression and genotypic organization of NK cells. Various methods of identification or purification of NK cells have been used for the phenotypic analysis of NK cells using monoclonal antibodies and molecular probes.

1. Elimination of antibody-positive cells with antibody and complement, or separation of cells by positive or negative selection using fluorescence-activated cell sorting or indirect antiglobulin rosetting methods, followed by analysis of the cytotoxic activity of the different cell preparations (66, 94-96), has been very successful, although in some cases not useful, in distinguishing between effector and accessory cells. A serious difficulty in the studies of positive selection stems from the possibility, now demonstrated for several cell surface markers, that the reaction of antibodies with surface receptors on NK cells alters the cytotoxicity and other functions of NK cells.

2. Analysis of surface markers of enriched preparations of LGLs from Percoll gradients has generated some confusion due to the presence of contaminant cells in the LGL preparations; however, they have also contributed to the identification of these contaminants and have provided means, using negative selection with appropriate monoclonal antibodies, to eliminate them (89).

3. Combined use of monoclonal antibody analysis, by fluorescence or complement cytotoxicity, and single-cell assay in semisolid medium has been used for a direct and accurate phenotypic analysis of both target

cell-binding lymphocytes and lytic effector NK cells (64, 66). Although powerful, these methods are technically difficult, laborious, and tedious to perform and have not been widely used.

4. Isolation of lymphocyte clones with NK cell activity, dependent on IL-2 for growth and usually with a limited *in vitro* life span, has been recently reviewed in another volume of this series (20). The availability of NK cell clones provides a unique opportunity to study NK cell functions and characteristics using homogeneous cell preparations. However, the ability to mediate non-MHC-restricted cytotoxicity is not a unique property of NK cells, and some T cells, especially after IL-2 activation, can also mediate non-MHC-restricted cytotoxicity (20, 97–99). Indeed, most of the NK clones described in early studies were of T cell origin (20). As in the case of Percoll separation of LGLs, the method of NK cell cloning has allowed some of the most significant progress in the study of NK cells, but has also generated artifactual information that underlies much of the current controversy and confusion in the NK cell field.

5. With bulk expansion of NK cells in short-term cultures using different methods (100, 101), large numbers of nearly pure NK cells can be obtained and used in biochemical and molecular studies that would be impossible to perform on the limited numbers of NK cells obtainable from fresh peripheral blood or spleen. However, as in the case of NK cell clones, the use of these preparations carries the possibility of selective expansion of NK cell subsets and the use of *in vitro* activated cells with functional and phenotypic characteristics different from those of resting NK cells obtained *ex vivo*.

6. The rat leukemia RNK-16 cell line, which has spontaneous cytolytic ability against YAC-1 cells and characteristics of NK cells (102), has been used for biochemical and functional analyses of NK cells and their cytotoxic mechanism. Human leukemias, chronic or acute, with expansion of cells with NK cell characteristics are also known, although rare, and have been used in some studies for the analysis of NK cell characteristics (103).

Except for the artifacts due to the use of contaminated or non-characterized NK cell preparations, the results obtained using all of these different approaches for the identification of NK cells have been, in general, consistent and serve to identify NK cells as a discrete lymphocyte subset with phenotypic and genotypic characteristics different from those of T and B cells.

B. SURFACE PHENOTYPE OF HUMAN NK CELLS

Early studies on human NK cells showed that virtually all of these cells express FcγR and about 50% of them form low-affinity rosettes with sheep erythrocytes at 4°C, but, unlike T cells, only a small proportion form high-affinity rosettes at 29°C (16, 104). The presence of complement receptors (CRs) on NK cells has been a controversial issue (11, 105–107). Most NK cells are now known to express the receptor for C3bi (CR3 or CD11b) but not those for either C3b (CR1 or CD35) or C3d (CR2 or CD21) (108–111). The use of monoclonal antibodies has revealed no surface antigen unique to NK cells, but rather a unique combination of antigens, each shared with other cell types, mainly T cells and myelomonocytic cells. Figure 4 summarizes the antigenic phenotype

Cluster	Mol wt (K)	Antibodies	B	T cells	NK/K	Monocytes	PMN
MHC-I	45,12	Class I MHC					
MHC-II	28,32	Class II MHC					
CD1	49	OKT6, Leu-6		(Thymocytes)			
CD2	45-50	OKT11, Leu-5b (E-R)					
CD3	22-28	OKT3, Leu-4					
CD4	55	OKT4, Leu-3					
CD5	67	OKT1, Leu-1					
CD6	120	T12					
CD7	40	3A1, Leu-9					
CD8	32,43	OKT8, Leu-2					
CD11a	180,90	LFA-1					
CD11b	170,90	OKM1 (CR3)					
CD11c	150,90	Leu-M5					
CD14	55	Mo2, B52.1					
CD15	(X-hapten)	My-1, B37.2					
CD16	50-70	3G8, B73.1, Leu-11 (FcR)					
CD18	90	(beta chain of CD11)					
CD20	32,37	B1					
CD21	145	THB-5 (CR2)					
CD24	42	BA1					
CD25	55	TAC (IL-2 R)					
CD28	44	Tp44, 9.3					
CD32	40	IV-3 (FcRII)					
CD35	160-250	(CR1)					
CD38	45	OKT10, Leu-17					
CD71	90,90	OKT9, 5E9 (Transf. R.)					
CD56	220	NKH-1, Leu-19 (NCAM)					
CD57	110	Leu-7, HNK-1					

FIG. 4. Surface markers of human NK/K cells as compared to B cells, T cells, monocytes, and polymorphonucleated neutrophilic cells (PMNs). The antigens are designated according to the clusters of differentiation (CD) defined for the leukocyte differentiation antigens. The molecular weights of the precipitated molecules (reduced form) and the prototype antibodies used for their identification are also indicated. The length of the filled bars within each cell population indicates the approximate proportion of cells expressing the antigens. However, the position of the bars within each cell population may not always be representative of the overlapping or exclusive expression of the antigens on different subsets. Solid bars, positive cells; stippled bars, low-density positive cells; hatched bars, activated cells only.

of NK cells in comparison to other leukocyte populations. Often, these cell surface markers are not present on all NK cells, suggesting some heterogeneity within the NK cell population. In general, human NK cells lack cell surface marker characterisrics of B cells, with the exception of the recently described CB02 antigen, present on B cells and a subset of NK cells (112). Most investigators agree that resting human NK cells do not significantly express class II MHC antigens (95, 113, 114), although Brooks and Moore (115) have reported the expression of HLA-DR, -DP, and -DQ antigens on a subset of NK cells.

1. FcR (CD16) Antigen

Various types of FcγR have been identified on human hematopoietic cells. Monocytes and macrophages express at least two types of FcγR: a high-affinity ($K_a \sim 10^8/M$) receptor (p72 or FcRI) able to bind monomeric IgG, and a low-affinity ($K_a \sim 10^6/M$) receptor (gp40, FcRII, or CDw32), also expressed on PMNs and B cells. PMNs also express a third type of FcγR (CD16 antigen) and, when activated by immune IFN (IFN-γ), FcRI. CD16 FcR is also expressed on the large majority of NK cells and on tissue macrophages as well as on monocyte-derived macrophages. B cells express only CDw32 FcR.

CD16 FcR is a low-affinity receptor that binds IgG in immune complexes with soluble or insoluble (e.g., antibody-coated cells) antigen but does not bind monomeric IgG. Several monoclonal antibodies produced against CD16 FcR (28, 95, 116–118) bind to few different antigenic determinants on the CD16 molecule and, as discussed below, might have different cellular specificity. During differentiation of PMNs, CD16 antigen appears at a late stage of myeloid differentiation in the bone marrow (metamyelocytes or later). In the peripheral blood, CD16 is expressed on virtually all neutrophils, but only on eosinophils with a more mature morphology. Basophils do not express CD16 FcR. Circulating monocytes express little, if any, CD16 FcR, but *in vitro* cultured monocytes express it at high density. Due to the limited information on NK cell differentiation, it remains unknown when CD16 FcR is first expressed on these cells.

The first anti-CD16 antibody, 3G8, was shown to react with PMNs and macrophages (116). Another anti-CD16 monoclonal antibody, B73.1 (95), reacts with the large majority of human NK cells. CD16+ lymphocytes contain virtually all of the lymphocytes able to mediate spontaneous cytotoxicity. Although not present exclusively on NK cells, the CD16 antigen still represents the best marker to identify and purify NK cells among peripheral blood mononuclear cells. Unlike 3G8, antibody B73.1 reacts with PMNs of only 50% of donors; both antibodies react with NK cells from all donors. Other antibodies that cross-compete with B73.1

but not with 3G8 for binding to NK cells also react with PMNs from only a proportion of donors. 3G8 and B73.1 (and other antibodies, such as anti-Leu-11a/b, CLB FcR-gran 1, and VEP-13) react with at least two different determinants on the CD16 molecule (28). Although the significance of this differential cellular reactivity of anti-CD16 antibodies to different determinants of the molecule is unknown, this observation points to a possible heterogeneity of the CD16 molecule on different cell types. The anti-CD16 antibody, CLB-gran 11, never reacts with NK cells and detects only PMNs of donors carrying the allele NA1 (phenotypic frequency, 46%) of the neutrophil-specific NA antigen biallelic system (119). These results show that PMN CD16 FcR, but not NK cell CD16 FcR, carries the NA antigenic determinants.

The antibody AB8.28 (120, 121) was originally described as specific for NK cell FcγR, based on its ability to block rosette formation with antibody-coated erythrocytes. However the antigen recognized by this antibody shows different molecular characteristics from those of CD16 antigen, is still present on the cells when the CD16 FcR is down-modulated by antibodies or immune complexes (122), and rapidly disappears from NK cells in culture when CD16 FcR is strongly expressed. The exact nature of the AB8.28 antigen remains to be established.

The CD16 molecules precipitated from the membrane of PMNs or NK cells appear on sodium dodecyl sulfate (SDS) gels as a broad band corresponding to a molecular weight between 50,000 and 70,000 (95, 116). The molecules are highly glycosylated and, after treatment with N-glycanase, resolve in small products as bands migrating at 23–28 and 32–36 kDa from PMNs and NK cells, respectively (123–126). From monocyte-derived macrophages, the anti-CD16 antibodies precipitate a 53 kDa species minimally altered, if at all, by treatment with N-glycanase (123). These results suggest that the CD16 antigen is expressed on different cell types on molecules with different levels of glycosylation and with a polypeptide backbone of different lengths.

Recently, a complementary DNA clone encoding CD16 determinants was isolated that gave rise to IgG-binding molecules with affinity and specificity expected for CD16 in transfected COS cells (124). The cDNA was isolated from an expression library of human placenta, and therefore the exact cellular origin is unknown.

CD16 cDNA-transfected COS cells bound human IgG_3 and IgG_1 and mouse IgG_{2a} and IgG_3 with a K_a of $\sim 10^6/M$ and murine IgG_1 with lower affinity, but did not bind human IgG_2 and IgG_4 or murine IgG_{2b} (124).

The cloned CD16 cDNA sequence spans 888 nucleotides and encodes a predicted peptide of 233 residues. The first 18 residues have the typical feature of a secretory signal sequence. The signal peptide is followed by two Ig-related segments with two intrachain disulfide bonds and significant homology to members of the constant-region C-2 set of the Ig superfamily. The predicted molecular mass of the expected polypeptide (~25 kDa) is consistent with that observed for CD16 molecules precipitated from PMNs and treated with N-glycanase. The polypeptide sequence ends with a short hydrophobic domain (residues 200–220), followed by four hydrophilic residues. A similar structure and hydropathicity profile is shared by membrane proteins bearing glycosyl phosphatidylinositol phospholipid (GPI-PL)-linked carboxy termini. Various groups (124, 127, 128) have provided evidence that the CD16 molecules are linked to the cell membrane through GPI-PL: (1) CD16 molecules are removed from the cell membrane and released into the supernatant when PMNs or CD16-transfected COS cells are treated with GPI-specific phospholipase C (GPI-PLC), and (2) PMNs from patients with paroxysmal nocturnal hemoglobinuria (PNH), an acquired abnormality affecting GPI tail biosynthesis or attachment, lack expression of CD16 FcR. However, the possibility remains that CD16 FcR in cell types other than PMNs (such as NK cells and macrophages) is at least in part a transmembrane molecule, as suggested by (1) heterogeneity in CD16 polypeptide molecular mass in different cell types, (2) normal expression of CD16 FcR on NK cells and cultured monocytes from PNH patients (127–129), and (3) an inability of GPI-PLC to remove CD16 FcR from human NK cells (124, 126). Both PMNs and NK cells spontaneously shed CD16 antigen in the absence of GPI-PLC treatment. After digestion with N-glycanase, the CD16 antigen shed from NK cells resolves in SDS gels in 23–28 kDa smaller fragments identical to those precipitated from both PMN supernatant and cells (126). Thus, the CD16 antigen on NK cells and PMNs might undergo spontaneous proteolytic cleavage at the same position, but, unlike in PMNs, the cleaved antigen from NK cells fails to remain on the membrane as a GPI-linked molecule and is released into the supernatant.

The CD16 sequence shares highest homology with the α gene of the murine FcRII, followed by the human CDw32 and the β gene of murine FcRII. Interestingly, murine NK cells express RNA transcripts of the α gene but not of the β gene of FcRII (130). The homology between CD16 FcR and murine FcRIIα genes extends through the putative transmembrane portion (17 identical nucleotides of 21 in that domain), but the α transcript, unlike the CD16 transcript, presents a long intracytoplasmatic domain, suggesting that the murine FcRIIα genes are transmembrane proteins. Analysis of FcγRIII (CD16) transcripts isolated from PMN and NK cells of single donors revealed multiple single nucleotide differences between these respective sequences (126). One of these differences converts an in-frame UGA termination codon to a CGA codon, resulting in an extended open reading frame encoding 21 additional amino acids (126). The CD16 FcR transcripts in NK cells therefore encode a 25-amino acid intracytoplasmatic domain that is highly homologous to that of murine FcRIIα (126). Recently, two nearly identical, linked genes have been cloned for Fcγ RIII (CD16). These genes are transcribed in a cell-type specific fashion to generate the alternatively anchored forms of this receptor (126). The close analogy between CD16 FcR and the murine FcRIIα indicates that CD16 is expressed on a molecule that represents the human equivalent of murine FcRIIα.

The functional relevance of the structural differences between CD16 FcR on NK cells and PMNs is indicated by the fact that NK cells, but not PMNs, are able to lyse anti-CD16 antibody-producing hybrid cells, indicating that CD16 antigen on NK cells functions as a signal-transducing structure in ADCC (125, 131). On the other hand, PMNs lyse anti-CDw32 FcRII-producing cells, indicating that in these cell types CDw32 FcRII, but not CD16 FcR, functions as signal-transducing structures in ADCC (131).

The surface expression of CD16 on human NK cells is highly regulated. Incubation of NK cells with anti-CD16 antibodies or immune complexes determines a rapid disappearance of the CD16 antigen from the cell surface (132). Treatment of NK cells with phorbol diesters also induces complete down-modulation of CD16 antigen expression in a few minutes (133). When anti-CD16 antibodies are cross-linked by a second anti-mouse Ig antibody on the NK cell surface, the CD16–antibody complex is internalized, as demonstrated by the disappearance of the antibody from the surface and by its release into the supernatant in the form of small proteolytic fragments (132, 134). However, CD16 antigen is spontaneously released from NK cells and PMNs, and release of CD16 from PMNs is increased by activation with chemotactic peptides (127). It is therefore possible that shedding of CD16 antigen plays some role in the down-modulation observed with antibodies and with phorbol diesters. In most healthy donors the CD16 antigen is expressed on an insignificant proportion of $CD3^+$ T cells. However, the presence of approximately 5–10% $CD3^+$, $CD16^+$ T cells has been described in two of 50 donors tested (135). These T cells express CD16 antigen at a much lower density than do $CD3^-$, $CD16^+$ NK cells. $CD3^+$ clones expressing CD16 antigen have also been described (136), and $CD3^+$, $CD16^+$ is a common phenotype of the cells from LGL lymphocytosis patients, as discussed later in this review.

CD16 FcR is the receptor used by NK cells for recognition of antibody-coated target cells, and in general only $CD16^+$ clones have ADCC activity. It was proposed that $Fc\gamma R^+$ and $Fc\gamma R^-$ subsets of NK cells mediate cytotoxicity against K562 cells and the Burkitt's lymphoma cell line, Daudi, respectively (137). However, these data have not been confirmed using anti-CD16 antibodies. CD16 antigen is expressed on more than 95% of the peripheral blood cells with cytotoxic activity for both K562 and Daudi target cells (95).

2. NKH-1/Leu-19 Antigen

A series of antibodies was produced that reacts with most NK cells and precipitates a molecule of molecular weight 200,000–220,000, often referred to as NKH-1 or Leu-19 antigen. The first antibody described, N901, was derived from mice immunized with cells from a chronic myeloid leukemia patient in blastic crisis (138). In addition to reacting with NK cells, antibody N901 recognizes an antigen expressed at high density on the immature myeloid cell line KG1a and on the majority of cells from some patients with acute myeloid leukemia (138). N901 also reacts with neurons, neuroblastoma cell lines, and human teratocarcinoma cells, especially after induced differentiation to neural cells (139; P. Andrews, personal communication). The NKH-1/Leu-19 antigen has been shown recently to be expressing the neural adhesion protein N-CAM (L. Lanier, personal communication). Two other antibodies, NKH-1A (140) and anti-Leu-19 (141), were shown to react with NK cells with the same specificity as N901 and to precipitate a protein of 200 kDa. Binding competition among different antibodies with this specificity is not usually observed, suggesting the existence of several antigenic sites on the molecule. The NKH-1/Leu-19 antigen is expressed at very low density on peripheral blood NK cells, but its density increases significantly following *in vitro* stimulation and growth of NK cells (100). The subset of PBLs expressing the NKH-1/Leu-19 antigen (on average, 15% of lymphocytes and 90% of LGLs) almost completely overlaps with that expressing the CD16 antigen (141). The $CD16^-$, $NKH-1^+$ cells, representing 2–3% of PBLs, can be subdivided into two subsets based on expression of the CD3 antigens (141). $CD3^-$, $NKH-1^+$, $CD16^-$ cells are probably NK cells that do not express the CD16 antigens because of differentiation or activation state. $CD3^+$, $NKH-1^+$, mostly $CD16^-$, cells represent a minor subset of T cells with low but significant non-MHC-restricted ability (141). Expansion *in vitro* of $CD3^+$, $NKH-1^+$ lymphocytes generates a high proportion of clones expressing the T cell receptor for antigen (TCR)-associated clonotype NKTa, which mediate non-MHC-restricted cytotoxicity by recognizing, via the TCR, the antigen TNK TAR detected by antibody 4F2 on proliferating target cells (142–144). NKH-1/Leu-19 antigen is almost invariably expressed on clones with non-MHC-restricted specificity, both $CD3^-$ and $CD3^+$ (20). However, the presence of NKH-1/Leu-19 antigen on some clones without cytotoxic activity excludes an association between the antigen and cytotoxicity (145).

Another monoclonal antibody, anti-NKH-2, also shows selective reactivity for LGLs (140) and precipitates a molecule of 60 kDa, distinct from NKH-1. About 7% of PBLs express NKH-2 antigens and partially overlap with the NKH-1$^+$, subsets. The NKH-1$^+$, NKH-2$^-$ cells in peripheral blood appear to have higher cytotoxic activity than do NKH-1$^+$, NKH-2$^+$ cells, although highly cytotoxic clones of either phenotype have been described (20, 140).

3. HNK-1/Leu-7 Antigen

The reactivity of antibody HNK-1 (anti-Leu-7), originally described as NK cell specific (146), is complex. This IgM antibody precipitates a 110-kDa antigen from PBLs and reacts with 30–70% of peripheral blood NK cells, with variability among donors (95, 96). Unlike the observation for CD16 and NKH-1/Leu-19 antigens, there is no correlation between the percentage of PBLs positive for HNK-1/Leu-7 antigen and NK cell cytotoxicity (95). The expression of HNK-1/Leu-7 is rapidly lost *in vitro*, and neither bulk cultures nor clones of NK cells express it (20, 100, 147). Cord blood NK cells, which normally express CD16 antigen and have reduced but significant NK cell activity, do not express HNK-1/Leu-7 antigen (95, 148). In addition to its reactivity with some NK cells, HNK-1 reacts with a variable proportion of CD3$^+$, CD8$^+$ and sometimes HLA-DR$^+$ T cells (149) and also with a rare population of CD4$^+$ T cells that is expanded in various pathological conditions (150–152). These CD4$^+$, HNK-1/Leu-7$^+$ cells are present in physiological conditions in germinal centers of lymphoid tissue and are granular lymphocytes with a lower ability to produce IL-2 and B cell-stimulating factor than HNK-1/Leu-7$^-$, CD4$^+$ helper T cells (153, 154). A morphology of LGLs or at least the presence of granules seems to characterize most HNK-1/Leu-7$^+$ lymphocytes with both T and NK cell markers (149).

The CD3$^+$, CD8$^+$, HNK-1$^+$ cells, which phenotypically resemble T cells but have a reduced response to mitogenic or allogeneic stimulation and are slightly larger and more granular than most T cells, have been proposed as the NK precursors (149, 155). However, transformation or maturation from one cell type to the other has never been demonstrated, and the presence of TCR gene rearrangement in CD3$^+$, HNK-1$^+$ but not in CD3$^-$, HNK-1$^+$ has definitively negated this hypothesis. Based on the present understanding of the specificity of HNK-1 antibody, most of the conclusions on NK cell biology and functions reached using this antibody as the only probe should be rejected and HNK-1 should not be used as an NK cell marker.

Four subsets of PBLs have been distinguished on the basis of reactivity of PBLs with HNK-1 and anti-CD16 antibody (96, 149): CD3$^-$, CD16$^+$, HNK-1$^-$ NK cells, with the highest cytotoxic activity; CD3$^-$, CD16$^+$, HNK-1$^+$ NK cells, with intermediate cytotoxic activity; CD3$^+$, CD16$^-$, HNK-1$^+$ T cells, with low (or null) cytotoxic activity; and CD3$^+$,

CD16⁻, HNK-1⁻ small T cells, with no cytotoxic activity. Interestingly, the T cells that can be induced to become cytotoxic by treatment with IL-2 are mostly included in the CD3⁺ HNK-1⁺ subset (156). Moreover, CD3⁺, CD4⁺, HNK-1⁺ PBLs bind but do not lyse NK cell-sensitive target cells (152).

Several cell types other than lymphocytes react with HNK-1/Leu-7 antibody. The antigen recognized by the antibody is present on myelin-associated glycoprotein (MAG) (157, 158), and several anti-MAG antibodies have the same specificity on lymphocytes as the HNK-1 antibody (159–162). Antibody HNK-1 reacts with peripheral nerves, spinal cord, small-cell carcinoma and adenocarcinoma of the lung, endocrine cells of the fetal bronchus, other neuroendocrine cells, and hypertrophic and malignant prostatic epithelium (163–168). HNK-1 also reacts with neural cell adhesion molecules (169). However, the possibility that antibody HNK-1 recognizes on NK cells an adhesion molecule involved in target cell recognition seems quite unlikely, since HNK-1⁻ NK cells are more cytotoxic than are HNK-1⁺ NK cells and expression of the antigen is rapidly lost on highly cytotoxic NK cell cultures and clones (20, 100). The reactivity of many different glycoproteins and cell types with HNK-1 antibody is explained by shared carbohydrate moieties (170, 171). The carbohydrate recognized by HNK-1 is present on both glycoproteins and glycolipids (170). The glycolipid recognized is an unusual glucuronic acid-containing sulfated glycosphingolipid with five sugars but without sialic acid (171).

Monoclonal IgM antibodies with the same reactivity as HNK-1 are present in the serum of patients with peripheral polyneuropathy, a benign chronic demyelinating disease of older patients (172–174). Although the monoclonal IgM from patients shows binding competition with HNK-1, suggesting an identical antigenic specificity, binding affinity is very low compared to HNK-1 and binding can be demonstrated at 4°C but not at 37°C (159). It is therefore unlikely that the human monoclonal antibodies bind *in vivo* to circulating NK cells. Neuropathy patients with monoclonal paraproteinemia usually have a normal number and activity of NK cells (175, 176), although a decreased number of HNK-1⁺ cells was reported in three patients (177).

4. CD11/CD18 Antigens and Myelomonocytic Antigens

CD11/CD18 is a family of three molecules composed of a common β subunit (CD18, 95 kDa) and different α subunits: CD11a or LFA-1, CD11b or CR3, and CD11c or p150 (178). All three molecules are expressed on human NK cells (179). CD11a or LFA-1 is expressed on all lymphocytes, whereas CD11b and CD11c tend to be expressed preferentially on NK cells/LGLs (110, 179). CD11b is strongly expressed on PMNs and monocytes (180). The reactivity of anti-CD11b antibody OKM1 with NK cells was first reported as evidence for the myeloid nature of NK cells (94, 110). However, CD11b is present at low intensity in the majority of, but not all, NK cells, is expressed on some T cells, and rapidly disappears from NK cells maintained in culture (100)

Two monoclonal antibodies, H25 and H366 (181, 182), generated against the human T cell line HSB-2 and precipitating polypeptide chains of 96 and 53 kDa, respectively, have been described to react with all NK cells and with few other PBLs. Antibodies H25 and H366 react with monocytes, myeloid and erythroid precursor cells, and myeloid blasts and promyelocytes, but not with more mature myeloid cells (181, 182).

With the exception of CD11b, CD16, NKH-1, H25, and H366, none of a series of other antigens present on myelomonocytic cells at various stages of differentiation is expressed on NK cells (183, 184).

5. T Cell-Associated Antigens and TCR

Human NK cells do not express the 69-kDa CD5 membrane antigen present on all T cells (95, 183, 185), although anti-CD5 antibodies react with a cytoplasmic antigen on permeabilized NK cells (186). CD4 antigen is not expressed on NK cells, whereas 30–50% of NK cells express the CD8 antigen at characteristic low density (66). The CD8 antigen precipitated by anti-CD8 antibodies from NK cells appears identical on SDS gels to that precipitated from T cells (132). CD8 antigen expression is maintained in bulk cultures of NK cells (100), but $CD3^-$ $CD8^+$ NK clones are rare (20). $CD8^+$ and $CD8^-$ NK cells have similar cytotoxic activity and no other different functional abilities have been identified in the two subsets (66). The CD7 and the D44 (187) antigens are also expressed on NK cells.

A proportion (~50%) of NK cells express a low-affinity receptor for sheep erythrocytes (E-R), forming rosettes at 4°C but not at 29°C. However, ~90% of NK cells react with anti-CD2 antibodies, which detect SRBCs. The expression of CD2 is more heterogeneous on NK cells than on T cells, and there is no correlation between CD2 expression and cytotoxic ability of NK cells.

Antibody NK9 (188, 189) against a distinct sialylated antigen of the T200 family was described to react specifically with NK cells, CTL precursor cells and both allospecific and non-MHC-restricted CTLs. However, antibody NK9 reacts with all leukocytes, at least at low intensity, and its specificity for cytotoxic cells appears to be more quantitative than qualitative (E. Säkselä and L. Lanier, personal communication).

The majority of NK cells express at low density the 46-kDa antigen CD38 recognized by antibody OKT10, whereas resting T cells are negative for this antigen (89). However, the antigen is strongly expressed on both T and NK cells activated *in vitro* to proliferate (190, 191). Like T cells (190), *in vitro* activated and proliferating NK cells express HLA-DR, transferrin receptor, 4F2 antigen, and IL-2 receptor TAC (CD25) (78, 191, 192). CD25 antigen and transferrin receptor are rapidly downmodulated when the cells revert to a resting state (78), whereas HLA-DR antigens are maintained for a longer time (100), possibly due to a longer half-life of these molecules at the cell surface.

Although minor subsets of $CD3^+$ cells have been reported to mediate very low levels of non-MHC-restricted cytotoxicity, virtually all natural cytotoxicity is mediated by $CD3^-$ lymphocytes (95, 117, 183, 185). No anti-CD3 antibodies, regardless of their specificity, have ever been described to react with NK cells, although the transcript of the $CD3\epsilon$ gene, encoding one of the four chains of the CD3 antigen, has been reproducibly detected in $CD3^-$ NK clones (193) and in bulk cultures of NK cells (194).

Analysis of TCRβ and γ genes showed no evidence of rearrangement in both fresh and cultured human NK cells (195-200), although, as expected, rearrangement was observed in $CD3^+$ T cell clones with non-MHC-restricted cytotoxic activity (195, 200). A germ-line organization of the TCRα genes in at least most NK cells is suggested by the lack of significant decrease of hybridization of NK cell DNA to the TCRδ cDNA probe in Southern blotting, contrary to what would be expected if the δ genes were deleted following TCRα rearrangement (194). No rearrangements were evident in the TCRδ region of NK cells (194, 201). T cell clones that rearrange the TCRγ and δ genes and express TCR$\gamma\delta$ at the cell surface have been originated from either adult or fetal blood and shown to mediate non-MHC-restricted cytotoxicity (202-205). However, fresh TCR$\gamma\delta^+$ PBLs do not mediate natural cytotoxicity (L. Lanier, personal communication).

NK cells do not have detectable TCR on the cell surface, as detected by antibodies to TCR$\alpha\beta$ or $\gamma\delta$, nor do these cells express TCR after *in vitro* culture (100). Whereas no transcripts for the TCRα and γ genes are detectable in NK cells, a nonfunctional 1.0-kb transcript of the TCRβ gene, containing no V region, is reproducibly detected in NK cells or $CD3^-$ NK cell clones (100, 195, 196). Whether the truncated message in NK cells is derived from a partial D-J rearrangement in the TCRβ gene or is due to transcription of a germ-line gene is not yet known. Interestingly, the TCRβ gene in NK cells is more methylated than in T cells, but less methylated than in B cells and monocytes, suggesting at least a partial activation of the gene (206). NK cells also express large amounts of truncated TCRδ transcripts of different sizes, containing J and C regions, but no V region (194, 201). A possible difference between

T cells and NK cells in the 3' untranslated region of TCRδ mRNA is suggested by the sequence data obtained by analyzing a limited number of transcripts cloned so far (194).

C. Surface Phenotype of NK Cells from Experimental Animals

Several antigens specifically expressed on mouse NK cells have been described. Alloantibodies different from anti-Lyt-2 and reacting specifically with NK cells were first described in anti-Ly-2 antisera generated by immunizing C3H mice with cells from the CE strain (207). A more specific antiserum (C3H × BALB/c) F_1 anti-CE, which lacks Ly-2 specificity, was prepared and used for the designation of a specific NK cell alloantigenic system, NK-1 (208). A monoclonal anti-NK-1 antibody, clone PK136, was also obtained (209). Sorting of spleen cells reactive or nonreactive with anti-NK-1 antibody from mouse strains expressing the NK-1.1 allele demonstrated that all the NK cytotoxic activity was present in the NK-1.1$^+$ subset (210). Anti-NK-1.1 antibody is specific for murine NK cells and reacts with a small population of spleen cells with granular lymphocyte morphology (210). Repeated weekly treatment *in vivo* of mice with anti-NK-1.1 antibody induces disappearance of mature NK cells, but not of NK cell precursors (211). NK cell-specific antibodies detected in CE anti-CBA alloantisera have been originally designated anti-NK-1.2 and considered to be specific for an allele of NK-1.1 (212). However, the existence of strains such as C57BL that react with both antibodies excluded the possibility that the two antigens were alleles (213). The strain specificity of the CE anti-CBA alloantiserum is similar, but not identical, to that of the NZB anti-BALB/c (anti-NK-2.1) sera (214). The two alloantisera are now considered to be directed against the same alloantigen, NK-2.1 (213). A third antigen, NK-3.1, which segregates independently of NK-1.1 and NK-2.1, was detected in several strains by a C3H anti-ST alloantiserum (215). When tested in the presence of complement against the appropriate strains of mice, these three antisera completely abolish the NK cell activity against YAC-1 and some other target cells. However, when other target cells, such as K562, were tested, the cytotoxic activity in C57BL spleens was eliminated by anti-NK-2.1 but not by anti-NK-1.1. Further, when RBL-5 and other target cells were used, neither antiserum affected NK cell activity. These results suggest a heterogeneity in the expression of the NK-1 and NK-2 antigens in murine NK cells (216).

The three antigens of the NK series are all alloantigens and therefore each is present only in a limited number of strains. Recently, a rat monoclonal antibody has been produced directed against an 87-kDa antigen, LGL-1, present on NK cells from all mouse strains tested (217), although some strains express it at a higher density than others (V. Kumar, personal communication). The LGL-1 antigen is specifically expressed on most or all NK cells, although a small subset of $CD3^+$ $LGL-1^+$ spleen cells was detected by immunofluorescence (217).

Heterologous anti-asialo-GM_1 antisera together with complement completely eliminate murine NK cell activity and partially abrogate CTL activity (218, 219). Flow-cytometric studies have shown that asialo-GM_1 is expressed on both NK cells and CTLs, but that NK cells are more sensitive than CTLs to treatment with anti-asialo-GM_1 and complement (220). Asialo-GM_1 is also present on activated and tumoricidal macrophages (221). However, even with these limitations of specificity, the anti-asialo-GM_1 reagents were an extremely useful tool for dissecting the role of NK cells *in vivo* and *in vitro* before monoclonal antibodies to more specific antigens became available (219, 220, 222). Also, on the basis of asialo-GM_1 expression, a possible heterogeneity of murine NK cells was detected, i.e., whereas all NK cells cytotoxic for YAC-1 cells are asialo-GM_1 positive, those lysing herpes simplex virus (HSV)-1-infected fibroblasts include both asialo-GM_1-positive and -negative subsets (223). The reduced specificity of the anti-asialo-GM_1 antisera might rest in their reactivity with other gangliosides, such as asialo-GM_2 and asialo-GM_3 (224). Monoclonal antibodies have been produced that are more specific for asialo-GM_1 than the antisera and can completely deplete NK cell activity: These monoclonal antibodies have a lower reactivity to T cells than the polyclonal antisera and could be more specific reagents for murine and rat NK cells (224, 225).

Another antigen that is shared by NK cells and a subset of T cells, including CTL precursors and some MHC-restricted CTLs, is the Qa-5 antigen (226, 227). An IgM monoclonal antibody, anti-Qa-5, produced by AKR mice immunized with C57BL/6 lymphocytes is a useful reagent, together with complement, to eliminate NK cell activity (228). However, the pattern of expression of Qa-5 on NK cells from different mouse strains was found to differ from that observed on lymph node cells but to match that observed for the strain distribution of the NK-1.1 antigen, raising the possibility that the Qa-5 antigenic determinant is an epitope of the NK-1 molecule on NK cells (229).

Ly-11, a cell surface marker present on 10–20% of the cells from various lymphoid organs, is also expressed on NK cells and prothymocytes, but not on mature B or T cells (230).

Thy-1 antigen has a variable distribution on NK cells, with some but not all monoclonal anti-Thy-1 antibodies reacting with up to 50% of the NK cells in normal mice and up to 90% of NK cells in nude mice (231–233). The Thy-1^+ subset of NK cells has higher cytotoxic activity and proliferative ability than the Thy-1⁻ subset (234). IL-2-activated NK cells are mostly Thy-1⁺, suggesting that either Thy-1 is an activation antigen on NK cells or that IL-2 induces preferential growth of Thy-1⁺ NK cells (234).

Ly-5 antigen, a polymorphic determinant of the T200 molecule, is expressed on all hematopoietic cells, including NK cells. Anti-Ly-5 and nonpolymorphic anti-T200 antibodies block NK cell activity even in the absence of complement (208, 235). The T cell antigens Qa-2, Qa-4, Ly-6, and Ly-10, but not Qa-1, Qa-3, or Ly-2, are also expressed on a proportion of NK cells (232). Ly-1 (CD5) antigen, present on thymocytes, T cells, and a subset of T cells, is usually not present on NK cells (235), although its expression on 25% of NK cells has been reported in Ly-1.1 congenic mice (232). B cell/macrophage antigen Ly-M and the Lyb-2 B cell-specific marker are not detected on NK cells (232). The antibody MAC-1, specific for the C3bi receptor on myelomonocytic cells, detects this antigen on NK cells obtained from the peritoneal exudate of *Listeria* monocytogene-infected mice (236, 237). However, only a minor subset of fresh, nonactivated NK cells was found to express the MAC-1 antigen (229).

Several cloned lines with NK cell characteristics have been generated from mouse lymphocytes (238–241). These cell lines have been shown to express both NK cell markers, such as NK-1.1 and NK-2.1, and T cell markers (239). Analysis of the rearrangement of TCR genes in these clones has definitively confirmed that most or all of these cell lines present functional rearrangements in the TCR genes, demonstrating that they are T cell clones with non-MHC-restricted cytotoxic ability (242, 243). The isolation of these T cell clones expressing NK cell markers may be due to the selective growth of the small subset of T cells expressing NK-1 and NK-2 antigens. The expression of these antigens is similar to that of the human NKH-1/Leu-19 antigen, which is usually found to be associated with T cell clones with non-MHC-restricted cytotoxicity. All studies performed on freshly isolated murine NK cells or on their short-term bulk cultures have confirmed that in mice, as in humans, NK cells neither functionally express nor rearrange any of the four TCR genes (234, 244, 245). Murine NK cells accumulate a nonfunctional 1.0-kb truncated TCRβ transcript but, unlike human NK cells, do not accumulate transcripts of any of the CD3 genes at detectable levels (244).

Murine NK cells, like human NK cells, can mediate ADCC, suggesting that at least a proportion of them bear FcγR (115, 246–248). The presence of FcγR on murine NK cells has also been suggested by data showing that absorption on monolayers of IgG-sensitized erythrocytes significantly reduces, but never completely abolishes, the NK cell activity of murine spleen cells (246) and that a relevant proportion of the murine splenic lymphocytes that form conjugates with YAC-1 belong to the subset that forms rosettes with IgG-sensitized erythrocytes (249). Recently, it has been shown that fresh and cultured murine NK cells react with the anti-FcγRII antibody 2.4G2 (250). Northern blot analysis has shown that *in vitro* propagated murine NK cells accumulate transcripts only for FcγRII-α, one of the two genes encoding the 2.4G2-reactive FcγRII in the mouse (130). Thus, murine NK cells, like human NK cells, express only one type of FcγR. FcγRII-α is highly homologous to the CD16 FcR expressed on human NK cells (124). FcγRII-α-encoded polypeptide is the receptor used by murine NK cells in ADCC, as shown by the ability of the 2.4G2 antibody to block the ADCC activity of murine NK cells (130).

Another type of spontaneously occurring cytotoxic cells has been described in the mouse and termed natural cytotoxic (NC) cells. NC cells are not active against NK-sensitive target cells such as YAC-1, but preferentially lyse another set of target cells, of which WEHI-164 is the prototype (251, 252). NC cells are present in animals lacking NK cells, such as neonatal or beige mice, and were reported originally not to express markers typically expressed on NK cells, such as NK-1, NK-2, Qa-5, or Thy-1 (252–255). However, these early studies were performed using negative selection with complement and were therefore unable to distinguish the contribution of distinct subsets of NC cells. Positive and negative selection experiments by fluorescence-activated cell sorter have shown that NC activity can be mediated by a variety of phenotypically distinct NC cell subsets, including Thy-1$^+$ and Qa-5$^+$ cells (256). WEHI-164 is a very sensitive target for tumor necrosis factor (TNF), and the cytotoxic activity of NC cells has been shown to be mediated by TNF (257, 258). Thus, NC cells are a heterogenous group of cells able to produce TNF and therefore may include macrophages; T, B, and NK lymphocytes; and basophils (78, 258–260).

In the rat, NK cells have a surface phenotype similar to that of human and murine NK cells. Rat NK cells are asialo-GM$_1$$^+$ and do not express the T cell-associated antigens CD4, CD5, and CD25 (IL-2 receptors) or class II MHC antigens (261, 262). However, all rat NK cells express CD8 (OX8) antigen, unlike murine NK cells, which are CD8 (Ly-2) negative, or human NK cells, which express CD8 at low density in only 30–50% of the cells. Rat NK cells, like human and murine NK cells, do not express or rearrange the genes encoding the TCR (263, 264). In the dog NK cells express some markers of T cells, including CD8 (265). Cells with NK cell activity and LGL morphology which are distinct from classical T cells have also been demonstrated in the horse, miniature swine, and other mammalian species (266-268). Cytotoxic cells possibly corresponding to NK cells have also been identified in birds (269), amphibians (270), and fish (271).

D. MORPHOLOGY AND CYTOCHEMISTRY OF NK CELLS

The morphological identification of most NK cells as LGLs was originally determined by analysis of lymphocytes binding to NK cell-sensitive target cells (35, 83, 84). The central role of LGLs as NK effector cells was suggested also by the positive correlation between the number of LGLs able to bind to K562 target cells and the level of cytotoxic activity among normal donors (84), and by the finding that both NK cell activity and LGLs are recovered in the same fractions when human PBLs are separated by centrifugation on discontinuous density Percoll gradients (85). At least 70% of the human peripheral blood LGLs have been shown to have NK cell activity (90). LGL morphology has also been shown in NK cells from experimental animals, including mice (272), rats (273), and horses (266).

Human peripheral blood cells with LGL morphology, i.e., with a high cytoplasm–nucleus ratio, indented nucleus, and azurophilic granules, were described in 1911 by Pappenheim and Ferrata (274) and termed monocytoid or leukocytoid lymphocytes. In transmission electron microscopy human LGLs appear as medium-sized lymphocytes with round or indented nuclei, condensed chromatin, and unusually prominent nucleoli (275-278) (Fig. 5). The cytoplasm is abundant and contains a variety of organelles. A well-developed Golgi apparatus with many smooth and coated vesicles is usually found in the nuclear notch. Prominent centrioles and associated microtubules are also detected in this area. The cytoplasm contains abundant mitochondria and a number of lysosomal organelles. Common among these are membrane-bound granules containing a homogeneous electron-dense matrix, but other structures, such as smooth vesicles, coated vesicles, and multivesicular bodies, are also normally present (275-278). The granules present typical internum and externum. In resting mature NK cells granules range in size from 50 to 800 nm in diameter, display a circular to elongated profile,

FIG. 5. Ultrastructural features of NK cells from a short-term (10-day) bulk culture of human PBLs. (A) ×9,100. (B) Details of the granules; ×26,000. (C) Details of the granules of NK cells treated for 20 minutes with anti-CD16 antibodies coupled with Sepharose. Most granules have lost their electron-dense core and present membrane formations, myelin figures, and multivesicular bodies, characteristic structures in activated and, sometimes, resting NK cells; ×26,000. (Electron-microscopic preparations were by C. Grossi and B. Perussia, modified from Ref. 100 with permission from Karger, Basel, Switzerland.)

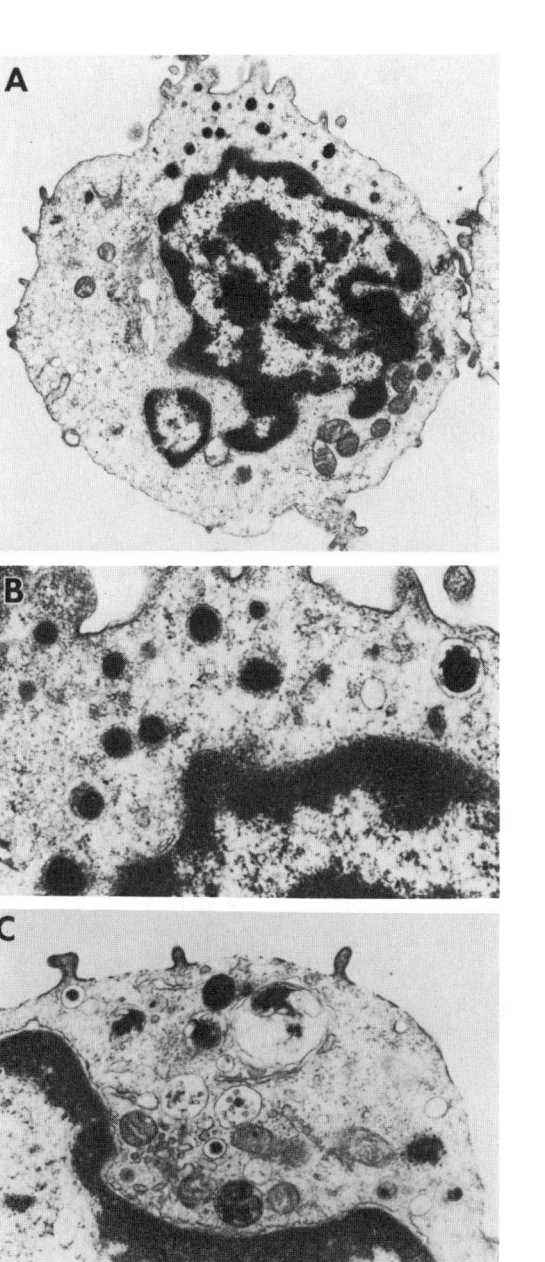

and contain an electron-dense core (internum) surrounded by a layer of less opacity (externum) (275, 276, 279, 280). The matrix of the granules is usually separated from the limiting trilaminar membrane by an electron-lucent space, within which electron-dense spikes can sometimes be seen radiating from the matrix to the membrane. The electron-dense core matrix is usually amorphous, except in cases in which a paracrystalline structure can be identified (279, 280). Various organelles which are probably a modification of the same granules are, however, observed in NK cells and have been attributed either to differentiation stages of the granules, similar to observations in granules of basophils, or to activation of the NK cells during lymphokine treatment or cytotoxic activity (275, 279, 281). Vesicles are observed, usually still containing a residual electron-dense matrix surrounded by small vesicles, to form multivesicular bodies, membrane myelin figures, and tubular structures. NK cells also contain numerous electron-lucent pinocytic vesicles and large vacuoles. The contents of the vacuoles are very heterogeneous, containing electron-dense particulate material and cellular debris. The endocytic nature of these structures was confirmed by the demonstration of Percoll beads in the vacuoles of LGLs incubated for 1–2 hours at 37°C in the presence of high concentrations of Percoll (276). Although NK cells and LGLs were originally described as nonphagocytic, being unable to phagocytize latex beads, opsonized RBCs, or immune complexes (275, 278, 282), several studies have demonstrated at least a limited ability of these cells to phagocytize 2-aminoethylisothiouronium bromide hydrobromide (AET)-treated SRBCs, opsonized *Staphylococcus aureus*, and complement-coated bacteria (277, 280, 283, 284).

Typical structures described in LGLs are the parallel tubular arrays (PTAs). These structures, originally described in PBLs (285, 286), were demonstrated to be a marker for FcγR-bearing lymphocytes (277, 278). The PTAs are quite variable in overall size, with some as large as 1.3 μm in diameter or 1.7 μm in length. Lymphocytes contain large PTAs, small PTAs, or both. All of the PTAs contain a tubular substructure formed by tubules packed in wall-to-wall contact and usually located in the notch region of the nucleus in close association with the centriole and the Golgi apparatus (276–278, 280, 287–290). Some of the PTAs are surrounded by a membrane, but, most often, distinct membranes are difficult to identify. Inclusions containing only tubules were termed type A PTAs, whereas other inclusions containing tubules and homogeneous electron-dense material were termed type B PTAs (287). Comparison of the diameters of the tubules in different reports reveals extreme heterogeneity, with measurements ranging from 13 to 44 nm. However, most papers report a diameter of either ~16 nm (276, 277, 287, 289) or ~40 nm

(280, 288, 290), suggesting the possibility of two classes of PTAs. Isolated reports of PTAs in only a very limited number of LGLs or in the complete absence of these structures (275, 279) have been attributed to the failure to use either ultrathin sections and high magnification or ammonium chloride for lysing RBCs in the cell preparation, which induces disappearance of the PTAs for a certain time after treatment (289, 291). However, the heterogeneity of the PTAs and the different proportions of LGLs containing PTAs reported by various authors may suggest that the PTA structure is unstable and may be affected by many different factors involved in the preparation of cells.

Recently Caulfield *et al.* (279) and Kang *et al.* (280) reported the presence of crystalline lattice or gratings in a proportion of granules from NK clones and peripheral blood LGLs, respectively. In stained sections crystalline structures were seen in about 10% of the densest granules, but in unstained sections all of the densest granules contained these structures (279). The lattices were composed of hexagonally packed points, each point equidistant from six other points. The gratings consisted of a set of parallel lines, usually straight, but occasionally in a whorled fingerprint pattern. The grating pattern also appeared to be superimposed on the lattice pattern, with the sets of parallel lines running in three directions that were at 120° with respect to one another. Lattice and gratings have been demonstrated to be simply different views of the same structures (279). The lattice spacings average 6.9 ± 0.3 nm, with a thickness of the electron-dense lines or points ranging from 2.5 to 3.6 nm. In addition to hexagonally packed lattices, cubic lattices were seen occasionally (279). In some granules the lattice appears smaller, with a looser packing, a microtubular appearance, and a diameter of 17 nm, similar to the PTA microtubules described by other authors. Frequently, the gratings or lattice unraveled and formed tubules and trilaminar strands of unit membrane that extended from the core of the granules (279). These laminar membranes, myelin figures, vesicles, and multivesicular bodies, in the presence or absence of residual crystalline dense material, are more frequently seen in activated NK cells (281) or in discharged granules during cytotoxic activity (279). These results strongly suggest that granules with PTAs, membranes, or lattices in NK cells may be in fact structural variants of a single granule type (279). The crystalline lattices most probably are formed by the phospholipids that give rise to the membranes and vesicles. Phospholipids in model lipid–water systems form either lamellar or nonbilayer arrangements (292). The phospholipids in nonbilayer arrangements form long rods, with the head groups and water in the center and acyl chains radiating outward, and the rods are then ordered in hexagonal or cubic arrays (Hex II phases), with center-to-center spacing of 4.5–7.0 nm (292). Alternatively, the rods may have the head groups on the outside (Hex I phase): In thin sections, this phase appears as an electron-dense honeycomb (279, 292), with a center-to-center distance of 16–17 nm, similar to the structure observed in some cases of PTA.

Because antibody HNK-1/Leu-7 has been shown to react with most of the PBLs with LGL morphology, although only a part of them represents NK cells, several studies have analyzed the morphology of the two subsets of Leu-7$^+$ cells: the Leu-7$^+$, CD3$^+$ T cells and the Leu-7$^+$ CD16$^+$ NK cells (280, 293–299). In most studies Leu-7$^+$, CD16$^+$ NK cells were shown to have the typical LGL morphology with numerous electron-dense granules, PTAs, and phagocytic ability for opsonized bacteria, whereas Leu-7$^+$, CD3$^+$ T cells have fewer granules than NK cells, no PTAs, and no phagocytic ability (280, 294–299). One study (293), however, reports that Leu-7$^+$, CD3$^+$ T cells have LGL morphology with PTAs, whereas most Leu-7$^+$, CD16$^+$ or CD11b$^+$ NK cells present a low number of granules and no PTAs.

The granules of NK cells stain for glycoproteins, acid phosphatase, trimetaphosphatase, arylsulfatase, and β-glucuronidase, indicating that they are primary lysosomes (275, 276, 280, 298, 300). The presence of endogenous peroxidase in LGLs has been reported in some (276, 280, 284) but not in many other (84, 275, 278, 301) studies. Babcock and Phillips (276) could detect peroxidase activity in only a few vacuoles and suggested that it could represent enzymatic activity of phagocytosed material and not endogenous peroxidase.

NK cells express various esterase activity, as detected by cytochemistry. Naphthol AS-D chloroacetate esterase, an enzyme characteristic of neutrophilic granulocytes, is also expressed at least in some granules of NK cells (87, 276). Nonspecific esterases, both α-naphthyl acetate (ANAE) and α-naphthyl butyrate (ANBE), are detectable in NK cells, although sometimes discordant results were obtained, depending on whether optical or electron microscopy was used in the analysis (84, 275, 276, 302). ANAE and ANBE are present in the granules of LGLs, giving a scattered staining often ignored in optical microscopy, and, as an ectoenzyme, in the membrane. Like monocyte esterase (303), the membrane activity but not the granule-associated activity is inhibitable by sodium fluoride (NaF) (275, 276). The staining pattern of LGLs is very different from that observed on most T cells, in which the esterase activity appears as a single discrete and NaF-noninhibitable cytoplasmic dot, corresponding ultrastructurally to the Gall body (a cluster of lysosomes adjacent to a lipid droplet) or to clustered dense bodies (303, 304).

IV. Origin and Differentiation of NK Cells

A. TISSUE DISTRIBUTION

Morphological evaluation of the peripheral blood of normal donors originally indicated that LGLs represent ~3.6% of the lymphocytes (90), and a similar proportion was detected when the number of cytotoxic NK cells was evaluated by single-cell cytotoxic assay (60). However, the use of monoclonal antibodies, such as anti-CD16 and NKH-1, has shown that these cells represent a much larger proportion of total PBLs. $CD16^+$ lymphocytes represent, on average, 15% of PBLs, with large variability among donors (ranging from 2 to 50%) (95, 114, 117, 118). The large majority of $CD16^+$ PBLs have LGL morphology and lack B or T cell markers (95, 114). More than 60% of $CD16^+$ PBLs freshly separated and more than 80% of IFN-treated $CD16^+$ PBLs bind to K562 cells (95) and the majority of these cells are cytotoxic in a single-cell assay in agarose (305). The spleen is one of the major sources of NK cells in both humans and experimental animals. $CD16^+$ cells in human spleen represent 3–4% of the total lymphocytes (95). LGLs localize in the spleen red pulp and not in the major areas of T cell recirculation, i.e., spleen white pulp and lymph nodes (95, 306, 307). $CD16^+$ cells and NK cell activity are absent from the lymph nodes of healthy individuals or animals (95, 308). NK cells are not present in recirculating thoracic duct lymphocytes, but treatment with IFN *in vivo* may induce the appearance of a small number of NK cells in the thoracic duct (309). In bone marrow, the number of $CD16^+$ lymphoid cells is very low, ~1% of the mononuclear cells, and the cytotoxic activity is also very low (95, 308, 310). $CD2^+$ lymphocytes sorted from bone marrow have an enriched NK activity, whereas $Fc\gamma R^+$ cells are inactive, perhaps suggesting the presence of immature $CD16^+$ NK cells in the bone marrow (310). The low activity of NK cells in the bone marrow might also rest in the presence of NK cell-sensitive target cells in the bone marrow that determine a functional inactivation of the NK cells (76). In the mouse, $NK1.1^+$ bone marrow cells can be purified by fluorescence cell sorting and shown to have cytotoxic activity comparable to that of spleen $NK1.1^+$ cells (229).

In the human tonsilla palatina, the number of $CD16^+$ lymphocytes and NK cell activity is reduced (95, 311, 312). $Leu-7^+$ cells are present in the tonsils, some with small lymphocyte and some with LGL morphology (311). The $Leu-7^+$ cells with LGL morphology are found in the crypt epithelium, whereas the small $Leu-7^+$ are located in the germinal center (311). The contribution of Leu-7$^+$ LGLs to cytotoxicity from tonsil cells is, however, not clear, and macrophages might account for some of the observed cytotoxicity (312). Germinal center Leu-7$^+$ cells, in tonsils and lymph nodes, belong to the CD3$^+$, CD4$^+$, Leu-7$^+$ subset of noncytotoxic T cells (154).

NK cell activity has been detected, at least in long-term assays, in both the airspace and the interstitial compartments of the lung (313). However, analysis using anti-CD16 monoclonal antibodies suggests that typical LGLs or NK cells are present primarily in the lung interstitium (314). The NK cell population in the lung is responsive to locally derived regulatory factors (e.g., intratracheal virus infection or IL-2 administration), but relatively unresponsive when systematic routes of administration of lymphokines or viruses are used (315).

LGLs and NK cells have been demonstrated in the intestinal mucosa of mice (316) and rats (317). In the rat large intestine, LGLs represent up to 25% of the intraepithelial lymphocytes (318). The murine LGLs from intestinal epithelium have the same surface phenotype as spleen NK cells (319). Although the number of mucosal NK cells is low, their participation in the local defense against murine enteric coronavirus has been demonstrated (320). Peritoneal exudate cells are also a good source of NK cells. However, several studies of humans have failed to show elevated NK cell activity or CD16$^+$ cells in intestinal mucosa lymphocytes (321–326). Shanahan *et al.* (326) demonstrated that human mucosa NK cells are NKH-1/Leu-19$^+$ but CD16$^-$, and that CD3$^-$ non-MHC-restricted cytotoxic cells can be generated from CD2$^+$, CD8$^+$, CD16$^-$, NKH-1$^-$ cells, possibly representing pre-NK cells.

Nonparenchymal cells from murine and rat liver kill both the NK cell-sensitive target cell YAC-1 and the NK cell-resistant P815 cell (327–332). The killing of both target cells was attributed to asialo-GM$_1$-positive cells with characteristics (e.g., density, half-life, kinetics of killing, age dependence, and nonadherence) typical of NK cells (327, 330). The pattern of target cell specificity of these liver NK cells suggests that they, unlike peripheral blood and spleen NK cells, might be in an activated state (328, 331). Macrophages (Kupffer cells) were usually cytotoxic only after activation *in vivo* by stimulants such as *Corynebacterium parvum* (328, 329, 332). In the rat, the LGLs or NK cells in the liver have been found to be identical to the previously described liver "Pit cells" (333–335). These cells are CD8$^+$, CD5$^-$, mostly asialo-GM$_1$-positive cells with the morphology of LGLs and typical electron-dense acid phosphatase-positive granules (335). Pit cells are contained in the liver sinusoid, where they are in close interaction with endothelial cells and present fingerlike extensions that penetrate through the sinusoid endothelial cells (334). In liver cell suspensions obtained by enzymatic dissociation, LGLs represent 5.3% of the cells, but their proportion in cell preparations obtained by high-pressure liver perfusion is up to 30% (334).

Treatment of mice with biological response modifiers such as maleic anhydride divinyl ether (MVE-2) or *C. parvum* induces a dramatic augmentation of liver NK cell activity 3–5 days after treatment (327). The increase in NK cell cytotoxicity corresponded to a ten- to 50-fold increase in the number of lymphoid cells with LGL characteristics that were isolated from enzymatically digested suspensions of perfused liver (327). The phenotype of the isolated LGLs is the one typical of NK cells, i.e., asialo-GM_1^+, Thy-1^+, Ly-5^+, Qa-5^+, MAC-1^+, Ly-1^-, Ly-2^-, L3T4^- (327).

The migratory pattern of NK cells has been studied by adoptive cell transfer studies, using purified radiolabeled rat LGLs from blood or spleen (306, 313). Following intravenous injection, more LGLs than T cells localized in the capillary bed of the lung, but fewer LGLs migrated to the spleen, where, unlike T cells, they localized in the red pulp (306). The adoptively transferred LGLs did not appear in the thoracic lymph. While NK cells do not appear to recirculate, levels of NK cell activity can be dramatically altered in various organ sites following administration of immunostimulants (327, 336). The mechanisms responsible for these alterations could be increased activity or proliferation of preexisting NK cells, localization of blood-borne NK cells or NK cell precursors, or redistribution of mature NK cells from one site to another. In the case of increased NK cell activity and numbers in the liver following MVE-2 or *C. parvum* treatment, it was shown that the accumulation of LGLs in the liver is not affected by splenectomy, but is prevented by ^{89}Sr-induced destruction of the bone marrow environment, suggesting that the accumulation is due to migration in the liver of NK cells recently derived from bone marrow progenitors (336).

The pattern of migration of NK cells suggests specific interaction with endothelial cells. Some T cells interact with high endothelial venules in the lymphoid tissue by expressing a homing receptor recognized by antibody MEL 14 (235). NK cells from normal mice do not express MEL 14 antigen, but up to 10% of IL-2-propagated NK cells from *scid* (severe combined immunodeficiency) mice express it (229). NK cells also express LFA-1 antigen, which has as a putative ligand intercellular adhesion molecule (ICAM-1) found on endothelial cells (178). The epitope recognized by HNK-1/Leu-7 antibody has also been involved in various systems of intercellular interaction and might play some role in LGL migration (169).

B. AGE, GENDER, AND GENETIC CONTROL OF NK CELLS

Information on human NK cells during fetal development is very fragmentary. Marginal cytotoxic activity against K562 cells was observed in fetal liver cells at 8–11 weeks of gestational age, and higher cytotoxicity was observed with liver cells from an 18-week fetus, especially after stimulation in mixed-leukocyte culture (337). At no time was cytotoxic activity mediated by fetal thymus cells (337). In peripheral blood, no activity was observed in 20-week fetuses, even after boosting with IFN-γ (338). However, induction of cytotoxic cells was observed with IL-2 treatment (338). In premature infants at 27 weeks of gestation, NK cell activity was constitutive in peripheral blood and was augmented by IFN-γ or IL-2 treatment (338). At birth, cord blood lymphocytes usually have normal ADCC activity, but NK cell activity against K562 target cells ranges from severely depressed to normal (95, 339–341). However, cytotoxic activity mediated by cord blood lymphocytes against another NK cell-sensitive target cell line, MOLT-4, was found to be comparable to that of adult PBLs (340). In cord blood, about 19% of the lymphocytes are $CD16^+$, similar to the proportion observed in adult PBLs (95). However, the HNK-1/Leu-7 antigen was not expressed on $CD16^+$ cord blood lymphocytes (95, 342). The number of LGLs in cord blood is also comparable to that of adult peripheral blood (341); therefore, NK cells are present in normal number in cord blood and their low cytotoxic efficiency may depend on immaturity (339) or the presence of suppressor cells (341). In the miniature swine, as in humans, at birth lymphocytes mediate ADCC but not NK cell cytotoxicity (267). If the piglets are hysterectomy derived and maintained germ free, NK cell activity appears only after 4 weeks of age, whereas piglets maintained in the standard specific pathogen-free animal colony develop NK cell activity at 2–3 weeks, suggesting that stimulation by the microbial flora and environment plays some role in the maturation of NK cells (343). In humans the proportion of $CD16^+$ cells in PBLs remains relatively constant after birth, whereas the number of $Leu-7^+$ cells increases almost linearly with age (148). A modest increase in NK cell cytotoxicity was observed in individuals more than 80 years old (344–349). The $Leu-7^-$ $CD16^+$ subset, with the highest cytotoxic activity was not increased in these subjects, whereas a significant increase was observed in the $Leu-7^+$ $CD16^+$ NK cell and $Leu-7^+$ $CD16^-$ T cell subsets (345–347, 349, 350). This increase in NK cell activity in older individuals may reflect a normal maturation of the NK cell system, or a preferential survival of subjects with elevated NK cell activity. In the age group between 20 and 60 years, male donors have a higher proportion of both CD16$^+$ lymphocytes and NK cell activity than do female donors (56, 95, 344, 345, 351).

Although the relative cytotoxic ability of healthy donors is relatively constant when tested at different times (52), circadian and circannual rhythms of NK cell activity have been demonstrated for both human and murine NK cells (352–355). The maximum of activity for human donors occurs early in the morning and with a second minor peak in the afternoon, with a peak-to-trough difference of 50% or more of the average activity (352). These data point to the importance of collecting control donors and patients' blood at similar times during the day when sequential studies are performed.

Accurate genetic studies are lacking in humans, but a partial correlation between NK cell activity and the presence of certain HLA alloantigens has been reported (56, 356–358).

In mice spleen cells at birth are devoid of NK cell activity, and this activity cannot be detected during the first 11 days of life (359, 360). A small fraction of mice develop marginal splenic NK cell activity between 12 and 21 days, and all mice show NK cell activity at 26–28 days, although lower than observed at its peak at 6–10 weeks of age and afterward continuously declining with age in most strains of mice (359–361). However, SM/J (362) and AKR (363) strains do not show this decline, and the decrease is less rapid in the peripheral blood of all strains (364). IL-2 and IFN can induce NK cytotoxic cells in cultures of spleen cells from old mice, suggesting that asialo-GM_1-positive pre-NK cells are present in the spleen (365–367). The failure of NK cells in old mice to mediate cytotoxicity has been variably attributed to the presence of suppressor cells (367, 368), a loss of competence to lyse target cells (369, 370), or a change in the regulatory interaction between NK cells and other cell types (371).

Mouse NK cell activity is under polygenic control, with at least two controlling genes associatad with the D locus of the H-2 region, and high responsiveness is usually dominant over low responsiveness (372–375). Analysis of the participation of non-H-2-linked genes in determining NK cell activity in H-2^s congenic mice (376) revealed not only the dominance of the high NK cell activity phenotype over the low-activity phenotype in F_1 hybrid offspring, but also that crosses between two low NK cell strains were complementary in generating F_1 offspring with high or intermediate NK cell activity. Such genetic complementation between the low-activity NK cell pairs indicates that the low-activity NK cell phenotype in the various strains have different genetic bases. In the

SJL strain, three different non-MHC-linked genes were found to account for the poor responsiveness of NK cells to IFN (376).

C. CONGENITAL DEFECTS OF NK CELLS

Complete absence of NK cells is rare and has been described in only a few patients. Two of these patients, one male and one female, belong to a group of four siblings with recurrent viral infections (375). All four siblings developed infectious mononucleosis (IM) as young adults. A boy who had respiratory infections and progressive bronchiectasis since the age of 7 died at the age of 16 of complications of IM. All immunological parameters tested were normal, but NK cell activity was not tested. A sister and a brother also had recurrent viral infections and pneumonia and the sister had progressive bronchiectasis starting at age 7–10, before any evidence of Epstein-Barr virus (EBV) infection, as shown by the absence of anti-EBV antibody before developing IM. Both patients lacked NK cell activity against both K562 cells and HSV-1-infected target cells (375). No NK cells could be detected in peripheral blood of the sister 4 and 9 years after IM, using various monoclonal antibodies, including anti-NKH 1/Leu-19 and anti-CD16. All other immunological parameters tested were normal. A fourth brother developed IM at 21 years of age, but he was otherwise healthy. He had a somewhat reduced level of NK cell activity, which was augmented by *in vitro* treatment with IFN (375). Both parents were healthy and had normal NK cell activity (375). Biron *et al.* (377) have described another young female with severe viral infections, including varicella and cytomegalovirus, and complete absence of both NK cell activity and NKH-1/Leu-19$^+$ and CD16$^+$ lymphocytes. In all of these patients CD16 and CD11b antigens were normally expressed on neutrophils and on monocyte/macrophages.

NK cell activity is also deficient in patients with defective expression of the CD11/CD18 group of surface receptors (378); however, in these patients the clinical pathology is dominated by the defect in phagocytic cells and severe bacterial infections, and it is difficult to evaluate the role of the NK cell defect in the pathogenesis of the disease.

Depressed, but not absent, NK cell activity has been observed in patients with X chromosome-linked lymphoproliferative disorder (X-LPD) (379, 380). However, NK cell activity is normal in males at risk (i.e., sons of X-LPD heterozygous mothers with 50% risk of developing X-LPD after EBV infection). Thus, the defect in NK cell activity, apparently due to a lack of recycling ability rather than to a decrease in NK cell number, is acquired after EBV infection (379).

A specific NK cell hyporesponsiveness is observed in patients with Chediak-Higashi syndrome (CHS), a rare autosomal recessive disease associated with cellular dysfunction, including fusion of cytoplasmic granules and defective degranulation of neutrophil lysosomes. Granules of the neutrophils are abnormally large, and clinical manifestations of the disease include defective pigmentation and increased susceptibility to infection (381). Humoral immunity and delayed-type hypersensitivity are normal, but children usually die of pyogenic infection, presumably resulting from their neutrophil abnormality. Survivors generally succumb to an LPD that may be malignant (382). NK cell activity in CHS patients is ten to 100 times lower than in normal controls (383–386): The number of NK cells is normal, as judged by the number of target binding cells and of cells positive with anti-NK monoclonal antibodies, but the number of cytotoxic cells is decreased, and the kinetics of lysis is slower than in normal NK cells (387–389). IFN increases the activity of CHS patients' NK cells (383, 387, 388). The NK cells in CHS patients characteristically contain a single, large granule in the cytoplasm (390): The decreased cytotoxic activity of these cells is probably due to a defect of the ability to secrete factors involved in cytotoxicity. Other lymphocyte-mediated functions in CHS patients appear to be normal, but the lysosomal defects can also be observed in granular Leu-7$^+$ T cells and in activated B cells (391).

In mice the functional activity of NK cells has been found to be modulated by several point mutations associated with coat color. The most commonly studied gene is *Bg*, which determines beige coat color (392). Mice carrying the *Bg* gene have been regarded as animal models for CHS. Homozygosity at the *Bg* gene determines defects in lysosomal membrane functions, resulting in granulocytes with giant lysosomes and abnormal functions and in altered melanosomal functions, leading to beige coat color (392). Beige mice have strongly depressed NK cell activity; the NK cell defect is post-target cell recognition and is only partially reversed by IFN (393, 394). Other B and T lymphocyte functions are almost normal. Beige mice have also been widely used as experimental models to analyze the role of NK cells *in vivo*. Of other color mutations in the mouse, leaden, fuzzy, and pale ears have no effect on NK cell activity, whereas satin (*Sa*) is also suppressive (395). When *Sa* and *Bg* are present in the same animal, their suppressive effect on NK cells is synergistic, but allospecific CTLs are also affected (395).

In various types of congenital B cell immunodeficiency (X chromosome-linked agammaglobulinemia, transient hypogammaglobulinemia, and most cases of ataxia telangiectasia and common varied immunodeficiency), NK cell activity is normal (396–405). Normal NK cell activity is also observed in patients with DiGeorge's syndrome, showing that functional thymus is not required for NK cell differentiation (398, 401, 406). The thymic independence of NK cells is also supported by the fact that athymic nude mice and rats have stronger NK cell activity than do their euthymic littermates (360, 407). About half of the patients with Wiskott-Aldrich syndrome have normal NK cell activity against K562 target cells, but all of these patients have severely depressed NK cell activity against virus-infected target cells, despite normal IFN-α titers (405). Some patients with SCID show a depressed NK cell activity and some display normal or augmented activity (95, 399, 404, 405, 408–411). In SCID patients with elevated NK cell activity, most circulating lymphocytes have the characteristics of Cl1b$^+$ LGLs (409–411). These LGLs are probably in an activated state, as suggested by the presence of activation antigens and the resistance of their cytotoxic ability to functional inactivation by *in vivo* irradiation (409–411). Some of the interesting findings in SCID patients are the dissociation among NK cell activity against K562 cells, cytotoxicity against virus-infected cells, and ability to produce IFN (405).

In *scid* mice that lack both T and B cells, NK cell activity is normal (412, 413) and NK-2.1$^+$ NK cells comprise the large majority of spleen lymphocytes (229). Unlike the thymus of normal mice, that of *scid* mice contains cytotoxic NK cells that express typical NK cell markers, at least after short culture in the presence of IL-2 (229).

Microphthalmic (*mi/mi*) mice are congenitally osteopetrotic, with reduced marrow and a deficiency in natural killing (414). Experimentally, osteopetrosis and loss of NK cell activity can be observed by treating mice with 17β-estradiol for 6 weeks (414, 415). Estradiol-treated mice possess nonlytic, IFN-nonresponsive immature cells which express the NK cell-specific antigen NK-1.1, presumably arrested prior to a bone marrow-dependent stage of NK cell differentiation (210, 415).

D. MALIGNANT EXPANSION OF NK CELLS

Acute leukemia with an NK cell phenotype has been described in only a few cases. Komiyama *et al.* (416, 417) described three cases in children with an acute course. The patients presented with lymphoadenopathy, splenomegaly, hepatomegaly, and 300,000–400,000 lymphocytes per cubic millimeter of peripheral blood. The circulating cells were CD3$^-$, CD4$^-$, CD8$^-$, CD16$^+$, CD11b$^+$, HNK-1/Leu-7 and mediated strong cytotoxicity against K562 target cells (416, 417). The cell morphology was lymphoblastic, without evident granules. Two continuous cell lines were generated from one of the patients, and these maintained cytotoxic activity and cell surface markers of NK cells. Another case of aggressive NK cell leukemia was described in an adult. The cells of this patient bore the typical LGL morphology and were CD3$^-$, CD4$^-$, CD8$^-$, CD16$^+$, HNK-1/Leu-7$^-$, with strong cytotoxic activity against K562 target cells (418). An IL-2-dependent cell line derived from this patient was maintained for several months. All of these cases of acute NK cell leukemia were clonal in origin, as shown by analysis of chromosomal aberrations (416–418).

Cells from about half of the patients with chronic T cell lymphocytosis have LGL morphology and some of the markers or functions of NK cells. LGL lymphocytosis is usually manifested by granulocytopenia or RBC aplasia, thrombocytopenia, hypo- or hypergammaglobulinemia, and a relative or absolute increase in cells displaying LGL morphology (103). Since the first description of LGL lymphocytosis 10 years ago (419, 420), the number of reported cases of this disease, initially considered very rare, has increased and a large number of patients have now been described. In most cases of LGL lymphocytosis the phenotype of LGLs is rather homogeneous and these cells express CD3 and CD8 antigens. CD2 is expressed in cells from most patients, but the CD5 antigen present on all normal T cells and some B cells is usually absent or expressed at very low density on the LGLs. All cases of LGL lymphocytosis that express the CD3 antigen have rearranged TCR genes and express either TCR$\alpha\beta$ or TCR$\gamma\delta$, indicating the T cell origin of these cells (421–428). The heterogeneity of the LGLs in the patients, the frequent spontaneous remission observed, as well as the chronic and relatively benign course of the disease have led to the hypothesis that LGL lymphocytosis is not a malignancy, but a reactive process (429, 430). Although reactive LGL lymphocytosis can probably occur, for example, in B cell chronic lymphatic leukemia or EBV infections, cells in all tested patients with $CD3^+$, $CD8^+$ LGL lymphocytosis have unique rearrangements of the TCR genes, demonstrating the monoclonality of the disease (421–429).

The $CD3^+$ LGLs usually mediate efficient ADCC but low spontaneous cytotoxicity, if any (103). Surface antigens preferentially expressed on NK cells, such as CD11b, HNK-1/Leu-7, and NKH-1/Leu-19, are expressed on the cells from some patients. Cells from almost all patients express FcγR, as shown by rosette formation with IgG-sensitized RBCs or binding of immune complexes, and the FcγR is usually functionally active in mediating ADCC. Relatively few studies have tested anti-CD16 FcR antibodies, but among these, some (431, 432) reported reactivity of cells from most patients with anti-CD16 antibodies such as B73.1 or Leu-11, whereas in another study (433) cells from only a few patients reacted with antibody B73.1; instead, a more consistent reactivity was observed with AB8.28, an antibody reacting with a surface molecule different from CD16 antigen, but perhaps functionally related to the FcγR on NK cells and neutrophils (120). In another study, anti-Leu-11 antibodies were negative, but consistent reactivity was observed with the anti-CD16 CLB FcR-gran 1 antibody (434). The same phenotype

(CLB FcR-gran 1$^+$, Leu-11$^-$) was previously reported for CD3$^+$ clones with ADCC activity derived from healthy individuals (136). Unlike other anti-CD16 antibodies, the CLB FcR-gran 1 antibody reacts at low intensity with a proportion of T cells in peripheral blood, in addition to NK cells (G. Trinchieri, unpublished observations). Different types of FcγR (e.g., CD16 and CDw32) are highly homologous in their extracellular portions (124). In the mouse, antibody 2.4G2 reacts with both the product of FcRII-α, expressed on NK cells and macrophages, and the product of FcRII-β, expressed on B and T cells and macrophages (130, 250). It is possible that some of the anti-CD16 antibodies have similar specificity in humans. Thus, although CD3$^+$ cells from some patients probably express CD16 FcγR, in other patients a different type of FcγR might be used in mediating ADCC. The CD3$^+$ CD16$^+$ phenotype expressed by some patients might be an aberrant antigenic expression (lineage infidelity) by the malignant cells, as observed in many cases of leukemias from various cell lineages. Alternatively, monoclonal LGLs could originate from the T cell subset characterized by high CD3 and low CD16 antigen expression, and constituting a measurable subset in about 4% of healthy donors (135). The spontaneous cytotoxicity of CD3$^+$ LGLs is usually low and can be augmented by treatment with IL-2 or anti-CD3 antibodies (432, 434). The rare cases of LGL lymphocytosis with TCR$\gamma\delta$ have spontaneous cytotoxic activity that is blocked by anti-CD3 antibodies, analogous to observations of TCR$\gamma\delta^+$ clones with non-MHC-restricted cytotoxic activity (203, 205). Thus the TCR$\gamma\delta^+$ cells, unlike TCR$\alpha\beta^+$ cells, might use their TCR for non-MHC-restricted cytotoxicity in this form of LGL lymphocytosis (434).

Only about 10% of the patients with LGL lymphocytosis have cells with an NK cell phenotype (CD3$^-$, CD16$^+$, CD2$^+$, CD8$^+$ or CD8$^-$) which usually have high spontaneous cytotoxic activity and show no TCR gene rearrangements (423, 431, 432, 435, 436). However, evidence for monoclonality is given in several cases by chromosomal aberrations (435, 436). LGL lymphocytosis with an NK cell phenotype has been described in some cases to have a more benign course than does CD3$^+$ lymphocytosis, but other cases present the same hematopoietic, immunological and rheumatoid disorders present in the CD3$^+$ cases (436-438).

LGL lymphocytosis in some cases presents mostly in the form of T lymphomas (439-441). However, the organ localization of these lymphomas is not that typical of T lymphomas, even if the few cases analyzed for cell surface phenotype were CD3$^+$ LGLs of T cell origin (440). LGL infiltrates are observed in the red pulp only of the spleen and in the liver sinusoids, with minimal involvement of lymph nodes and no involvement of the thymus, i.e., following the typical localization of NK cells in healthy individuals (439-441).

A possible retroviral etiopathogenesis has been suggested in some cases of LGL lymphocytosis, because of the presence of high-titer antibodies to either human T lymphotropic virus type I (HTLV-I) or HTLV-II (441).

E. *In Vivo* DIFFERENTIATION OF NK CELLS

In experimental animals there is evidence that NK cells originate and, at least in part, differentiate in the bone marrow. Treatment of mice with ^{89}Sr (a bone-seeking isotope) depresses splenic NK cell activity, but leaves CTL generation and macrophage-mediated cytotoxicity intact (442–444). Moreover, bone marrow reconstitution of radiation chimeras produced between pairs of histocompatible high and low NK cell-reactive mouse strains resulted in restoration of NK cell activity in the spleen. The chimeras were high or low NK cell reactive, depending on the bone marrow donor strain, and were independent of host environment (445). Similar experiments have been performed using the beige mouse strain presenting defective NK cell activity (446, 447). Radiation chimeras were used to demonstrate that NK cell activity was determined by the phenotype of the marrow donor and not by the genotype of the irradiated recipient (448), confirming that the generation of NK cells is an inborn and autonomous function of the bone marrow.

The role of the bone marrow as a necessary microenvironment for NK cell differentiation is further suggested by the failure of NK cell differentiation in congenital or 17β-estradiol-induced osteopetrotic mice (210, 414, 415). However, data obtained using osteopetrotic *mi/mi* mice must be interpreted cautiously: Heterozygous $^+$/*mi* animals, which have no defect in the final bone formation, present a level of NK cell activity that is 50% of that of +/+ animals, suggesting the possibility of an effect of the *mi* locus on NK cells not mediated through osteopetrosis (449). In the estradiol-treated mice, NK1.1$^+$ target-binding lymphocytes, which are noncytotoxic and not IFN inducible, are detectable. These cells might represent NK precursor cells preceding the marrow-dependent stage of NK cell differentiation (210). This NK-1.1 target-binding, nonlytic NK cell precursor was also observed in 8- to 9-day-old mice, before functional mature NK cells appear (210).

Data from irradiated patients and experimental animals suggest that mature NK cells might be relatively short-lived and radiation resistant (450–456). In mice sublethal total body irradiation induces a decrease in NK cell activity, beginning on day 14 after irradiation; the activity is fully restored, however, after 6–8 weeks (454). These data suggest that murine mature NK cells are relatively radioresistant, renewable cells with a life span of up to 2 weeks and that their direct progenitors are radiosensitive. Leukemogenic split-dose irradiation determines a more persistent depression of NK cell activity (453, 457). Similarly, in most irradiated patients depression of NK cell activity is observed, with subsequent recovery after 3-4 months (450). The lack of recovery in some patients could be attributed either to the irradiation or the immunosuppressive protocol used or to the effect of the underlying malignant disease that prompted irradiation.

A different and probably more accurate evaluation of the life span of NK cells has been obtained by Miller (455), using the cell cycle-specific cytotoxic agent hydroxyurea (HU). Total NK cell activity of murine femoral marrow was unchanged for 10.5 hours after the first HU injection, indicative of the transition time for the DNA-synthesizing NK cell precursor to become an active NK cell. This was followed by an exponential decline with a half-time of 7.9 hours, reflecting the rapid exponential renewal of NK cells in the marrow. In the spleen total NK cell activity was unchanged for 20.5 hours, indicating the transit time from the last DNA synthesis of the precursor cells in the bone marrow to the appearance of the functional NK cells in the spleen, and then declined exponentially, with a half-time of 24.15 hours, suggesting a half-life of NK cells in the spleen of, on average, 1 day (455). These results have been extended by Pollack and Rosse (458), using [^{3}H]thymidine pulse-chase techniques *in vivo*. In these experiments, NK cells were identified by their ability to bind YAC-1 cells, after elimination of B cells. Two NK cell populations could be distinguished in the bone marrow: large proliferating target-binding cells (TBCs) (25% in S phase) and small postmitotic TBCs, probably derived from the large TBCs which, in turn, were derived from a more rapidly proliferating precursor population. Migration of labeled NK cells from the bone marrow to the spleen required at least 2 days; some of these cells in the spleen survived 2 months or longer, and little or no proliferation of NK cells occurred in the periphery of unstimulated mice (458).

The persistence of NK cells observed in the spleen in this study was much longer than that reported in the study by Miller (455). This discrepancy might reflect an underestimation of long-lived NK cells in the spleen in the latter study, since cells with reduced NK cell activity, which might characterize older NK cells, would not necessarily be detected in experiments based on measurement of residual cytotoxic activity. Analysis of renewal of NK cells using HU depletion experiments also showed that nude mice, with increased NK cell activity, have increased cell dynamics, involving proliferating precursor NK cells (459).

After bone marrow transplantation NK cells are the first lymphocyte population to reconstitute the recipient (460, 461). The pretransplant irradiation therapy does not immediately abrogate NK cell activity in the patients, but the ability of their cells to maintain cytotoxic activity against K562 cells or to generate activity against tumor cells during culture in the presence of IL-2 is completely suppressed, suggesting a complete block in the proliferative ability of both NK cells and their precursors (462). After transplantation NK cells and LGLs appear, in both humans (463) and experimental animals (464), already at 1 week, and their number and activity increase to a peak at 30–50 days, slightly declining thereafter to normal or slightly subnormal levels (461,463). The appearance of NK cells precedes that of any other lymphocyte type, and at 20 30 days NK cells may represent 50–90% of all peripheral lymphocytes (465). The appearance of cytotoxic NK cells parallels that of IL-2-inducible cytotoxic cells: Both precursor and effector LAK cells in the patients are $CD3^-$ cells with an NK phenotype (462). The spontaneously cytotoxic NK cells in the recipient are activated, as suggested by their lymphoblastic appearance and by their ability to lyse efficiently not only K562 cells but also Daudi cells, tumor cells, and fresh leukemia cells (462, 464, 466). The $CD3^-$ NK cells obtained from transplanted leukemia patients and able to lyse leukemia cells have been cloned and shown by chromosomal analysis to derive from the donor bone marrow (466). Graft-versus-host disease (GVHD) in some cases has been associated with an accelerated appearance of cytotoxic NK cells following transplantation (467). The level of NK cell activity posttransplantion correlates inversely with the probability of CMV active infection (468). The establishment of active CMV infection has been shown to be followed by either a decrease (467) or an increase (463) in NK cell activity. These data confirm that NK cell precursors are contained in bone marrow and can rapidly proliferate and reconstitute the organisms.

The requirement for cell division during the maturation of NK cells after injection of bone marrow cells in irradiated mice was shown by the ability of irradiation or treatment with HU 7 days after bone marrow cell inoculation to prevent the appearance of normal NK cell levels (469). The replicating NK cells freshly derived from the bone marrow are $Thy-1^+$ but rapidly differentiate to $Thy-1^-$ cells, except in thymectomized mice, in which they remain $Thy-1^+$ (470, 471). The suppressor effect of the thymus on NK cell differentiation has also been shown in the low-NK cell activity mouse strain SJL; thymectomy of SJL mice as late as 25 days after birth increases the NK cell activity from low to intermediate levels (472).

The transplantable precursor cells for murine NK cells have been analyzed in detail by Hackett *et al.* (210, 412, 473). The bone marrow NK cell precursors were analyzed by transplantation in anti-asialo GM_1 antibody-injected mice and by detection of NK cell activity as the ability of the animals to clear intravenously injected labeled YAC-1 cells from the lung (473). The bone marrow precursor cells were found to be $NK\text{-}2.1^-$, asialo-GM_1^-, $Thy\text{-}1.2^-$, $Qa\text{-}5^-$, $Qa\text{-}2^+$, and $H\text{-}2^+$ (473). Differentiation of the NK precursor cells *in vivo* requires an intact marrow microenvironment, because 17β-estradiol-treated mice fail to sustain NK cell differentiation (473). Bone marrow cells from *W/Wv* anemic mice and marrow from *scid* mice contain a normal frequency of NK cell precursors, indicating that the NK precursor cells are distinct from those of myeloid cells and of T and B lymphocytes, respectively (412, 473). In a similar system, i.e., transplantation of NK precursor cells in aged syngeneic mice with low splenic NK cell activity, if any, Miller (474) demonstrated that spleen cells but not fetal thymocytes, rich in prethymocytes, contain NK precursor cells. Thus, fetal thymic pre-T cells neither demonstrate nor develop NK cell activity. IL-1, IL-2, and IFN-α/β accelerate the reconstitution of irradiated mice by NK precursor cells (475-477). However, IFN at 14 days after transplantation induces a significant suppression of NK cell activity due to the induction of suppressor cells (476). Treatment of recipient animals with IL-3 determined a reduced appearance of NK cell activity and cells with NK cell phenotypic markers (477).

F. *In Vitro* MODELS OF NK CELL DIFFERENTIATION

The availability of culture systems for the analysis of NK cell differentiation could allow a more precise identification of the precursor cells and of the cellular and humoral interactions that are required for differentiation-maturation. As discussed in detail in Section V, one of the difficulties of these studies is that most mature terminally differentiated NK cells can be rapidly induced into the cell cycle and can continue proliferating *in vitro* in the presence of IL-2 for several weeks. Any system that analyzes *in vitro* differentiation of NK cells should clearly distinguish between the differentiation of NK cell precursors and the induced proliferation of mature resting NK cells. Recently, various experimental systems have been described that strongly suggest the *in vitro* differentiation of NK cell precursor cells from bone marrow and peripheral blood. Unlike bone marrow and peripheral blood, cultures of thymocytes seem to generate mostly non-MHC-restricted CTLs.

1. Bone Marrow

The original studies of NK cell differentiation *in vitro* using murine bone marrow and other organs were difficult due to the lack of well-characterized and monospecific reagents. Using alloantisera against NK-1.1 antigen, Koo *et al.* (478, 479) identified $NK\text{-}1.1^-$ and $NK\text{-}1.1^+$ NK cell precursors devoid of cytotoxic activity, but their observation was weakened by the reactivity of the alloantisera with a large proportion of immature hematopoietic cells. The availability of better reagents, including monoclonal antibodies against NK-1.1 (209), and of purified or recombinant lymphokines now allows a more detailed analysis of NK cell differentiation *in vitro*. IL-2 or IL-2-containing conditioned medium allows the generation of cytotoxic NK cells from murine bone marrow cultures depleted of mature NK cells by treatment with antibodies or with 5-fluorouracil, which is selectively toxic for differentiated cells (480–483). The cytotoxic cells generated in these culture systems have, at least in part, the phenotype of mature NK cells, including expression of asialo-GM_1 and, often, Thy-1 and NK-1.1 (481–483). The precursor cells are asialo-GM_1^- but usually Thy-1^+ (482, 483). The NK precursor cells detected in these *in vitro* systems might therefore be more mature than the NK progenitor cells detected by adoptive transfer *in vivo*, which are asialo-GM_1^-, Thy-1^-. In the absence of IL-2, differentiation of NK cells from bone marrow cells was not induced by IL-1, IL-3, or IFN-α/β (481). However, IFN and IL-1 (or hemopoietin 1) are able to synergize with IL-2 in inducing differentiation (483–486). A similar effect was observed with TNF and lymphotoxin (486). On the contrary, IL-3 (487), transforming growth factor-β (TGF-β), IL-4 and granulocyte-macrophage colony-stimulating factor (GM-CSF) (486) significantly inhibit NK cell differentiation. Epidermal growth factor and fibroblast growth factor have no effect (486).

Functionally active NK cells are no longer detectable by 1 week of culture in cultured murine bone marrow harvested from Dexter-type long-term marrow cultures (488). IFN does not induce cytotoxic NK cells in these cultures. However, up to 9 weeks of culture, cells cytotoxic for YAC-1 target cells could be generated after 1 week in secondary cultures in the presence of IL-2-containing conditioned medium (488). Like NK cells, the cytotoxic cells were asialo-GM_1^+, Thy-1^+, Ly-5^+, NK-1^+, Ly-1^-, but, unlike NK cells, $\sim 30\%$ of the cells expressed Ly-2 antigen (488).

Studies using human bone marrow (489, 490) have shown that IL-2 induces a proliferation-dependent generation of cells cytotoxic for K562 targets that are $CD3^-$ NKH-1/Leu-19^+ and, in part, $CD16^+$ cells. A detailed analysis of the precursor cells in these cultures has not yet been presented.

2. Peripheral Blood

Numerous studies have analyzed the activation of peripheral blood NK cells and the induction of their proliferation by biological response modifiers such as IL-2 or IFN. However, few attempts have been made to distinguish the differentiation of precursor cells from the proliferation of mature resting NK cells. PBLs treated with the lysosomotropic agent L-leucine methyl ester (LeuOMe) are specifically depleted of $CD16^+$, $CD11b^+$, $HNK-1/Leu-7^+$ cells. LeuOMe-treated PBLs were not responsive to IFN, but regenerated NK cell activity after treatment with IL-2 or stimulation in mixed-leukocyte culture (491). The precursor cells of the cytotoxic NK cells are not granular, but are of the same low density as mature NK cells (large agranular lymphocytes). Generation of NK cells with LGL morphology from high-density small lymphocytes of $CD3^-$, $CD2^+$, $CD11b^+$ phenotype has been demonstrated by culturing the lymphocytes in the presence of mitomycin C-treated autologous T blasts and IL-2-containing conditioned medium (492, 493).

3. Thymus

Early studies showed that IL-2 induces human thymocytes to bind and lyse K562 target cells (494, 495). Cytotoxic activity is not present in fresh thymocytes, appears after 3-day culture in the presence of IL-2, and reaches a maximum at day 7 (496). All of the cytotoxic cells are $NKH-1/Leu-19^+$ (496–498) and granular, as shown by staining with the lysosomotropic vital dye quinacrine (498). Although one of the original studies reported the presence of FcγR on the effector cells (494), the presence of CD16 antigens has never been detected in the thymocyte cultures (498). The majority of $NKH-1/Leu-19^+$ cells in cultured thymocytes are also $CD3^+$, but a significant proportion of $NKH-1/Leu-19^+$, $CD3^-$ cytotoxic cells is always present (496, 498). Because both $CD3^+$ and $CD3^-$ thymus-derived, non-MHC-restricted cytotoxic cells do not express CD16, and because NKH-1 and CD3 are often coexpressed in non-MHC-restricted T cell clones, it is difficult to identify whether the $CD3^-$ cells are T or NK cells. Because the thymus has been shown not to contain NK cell progenitors in adoptive transfer experiments, the possibility should be considered that the $CD3^-$ cells represent expansion/activation of T cells at an immature stage of development, before functional expression of the TCR on these cells.

V. Activation and Effector Mechanisms of NK Cells

When NK cells leave the bone marrow, they revert to a resting state and all or most circulating or tissue NK cells are noncycling. NK cells are short-lived in the peripheral blood and in spleen, but it is as yet unknown how long tissue-associated NK cells persist. The most striking characteristic of NK cells is that resting circulating NK cells, present at all times in all healthy individuals, are "natural" functionally active cells, i.e., they can be triggered to lyse a target cell within minutes when confronted with the appropriate target structure or with an antibody-coated target cell. Other NK cell functions, such as lymphokine production and the regulation of hematopoietic and adaptive immune cells, are also mediated by resting NK cells. This ability of NK cells to respond to a triggering stimulus without the need for preactivation enables them to participate in the first line of defense against various pathogens. In this respect NK cells resemble other effector cell types of nonadaptive immunity such as granulocytes and monocyte/macrophages. Moreover, the functional activity of NK cells, like that of other nonadaptive effector cells, is rapidly enhanced by cytokines such as IFN and IL-2. This modulation of NK cell functional activity does not require cell division. *In vivo*, however, conditions such as virus infection or a strong antigenic stimulus induce both the activation of NK cells and an increase in NK cell number, due to increased proliferation, probably mostly at the bone marrow level. This *in vivo* response is maximal at 3–4 days, before adaptive immune responses become effective, and is reminiscent of the myelopoietic reaction to bacterial infection. Unlike myelomonocytic cells, differentiated resting NK cells and also resting T and B lymphocytes can be rapidly induced into the cell cycle and maintained *in vitro* in a proliferative state, for 30 or more cell divisions in a 2- to 3-month period. The *in vivo* proliferative response of NK cells is likely to be contributed by both the centralized proliferation of NK progenitor cells in the bone marrow and the induction of circulating NK cells into the cell cycle.

As illustrated in Fig. 6 and detailed in this chapter, the response of NK cells to an external stimulus can be divided into three sequential phases. In the first phase interaction of NK cells with target cells or with immune complexes induces a rapid response (1–10 minutes) associated with cytotoxicity and the release of granule contents. These same interactions and also stimulation by IL-2 induce (10 minutes to 2 hours), independently and synergistically, the second phase, in which genes encoding lymphokines and surface activation antigens, including the p55 chain of the IL-2 receptor (CD25 antigen), are transcribed and expressed. In the presence of IL-2, the NK cells proceed into the third phase (1–3 days) of the response, with blast formation, DNA synthesis, and proliferation. The various stimuli and modulating factors affect these three phases of the NK cell response differently, and the role of each phase in the various *in vivo* and *in vitro* functions of NK cells differs.

A. Sensitivity of Target Cells to NK Cell-Mediated Killing

There is considerable variability in the sensitivity of different cell lines and fresh tumor or normal cells to the cytotoxicity mediated by NK cells. The recognition structure on NK cells has not been identified, but the studies described below suggest the possibility that more than one single

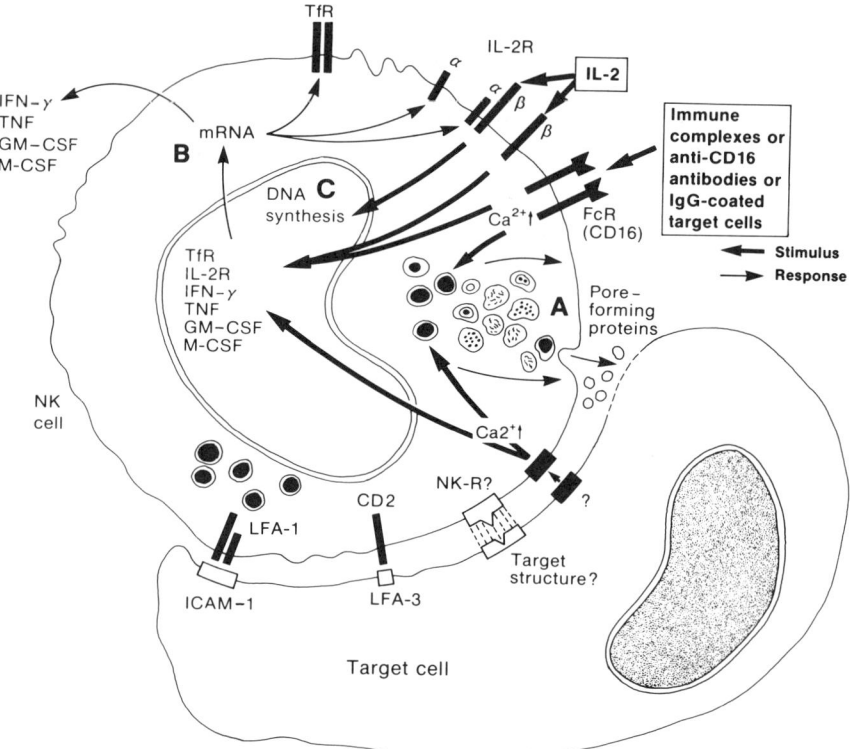

FIG. 6. Model of NK cell activation following interaction with target cells or immune complexes. The interaction of NK cells with target cells involves unknown receptor(s) responsible for binding and NK cell activation (signal transduction). Signal transduction involves enhanced phosphoinositide turnover and increase of $[Ca^{2+}]_i$, due to release of Ca^{2+} from intracellular stores and influx of extracellular Ca^{2+}, observed upon interaction of NK cells with NK cell-sensitive target cells. Similar signal transduction mechanisms are activated during interaction of CD16 FcR with ligands, i.e., with anti-CD16 antibodies, immune complexes, or IgG-coated target cells. Three types of response are observed: (A) activation of the cytotoxic mechanism, with morphological alteration and secretion of the content of granules, including cytotoxic molecules such as pore-forming proteins, NKCF, and others; (B) transcription of lymphokine and cell surface receptor genes and expression of their products, with a synergistic induction mediated by IL-2; (C) proliferation of NK cells, mostly induced by IL-2 interaction with the high-affinity IL-2 receptor (IL-2R) [p75 (β) and p55 (α) chain dimer] or with the p75 chain (β) of the IL-2 receptor, but modulated by the regulatory effect of NK-target cell or FcR (CD16)-ligand interactions on the expression of the IL-2 receptor [p55 chain (α) or CD25 antigen] gene. These mechanisms are discussed in detail in the text.

structure is involved and that different target cells might be recognized through different structures. One general characteristic of NK cell-mediated killing is that cells from the homologous species are usually killed more efficiently than are heterologous cells; however, this phenomenon has been rarely studied and remains unexplained (499–501).

The prototype target cell lines used in each species, the K562 cell line for human NK cells and the YAC-1 cell line for mouse and rat NK cells, are among the most sensitive cell lines in each system. However, almost any cell is sensitive to a certain extent to NK cells, if the concentration of effector cells is sufficiently high or if the NK cells are activated by IFN or IL-2. When evaluating the sensitivity of target cells to lysis, it should be considered that several different factors play a role in determining cell lysis. The ability of a cell line to bind to NK cells is necessary but not sufficient to render it sensitive to lysis (502). In order to activate the cytotoxic mechanism in the NK cells, a structure on the target cells, possibly distinct from the one responsible for cell binding, must trigger the effector cells (503, 504). This second requirement can be circumvented if the target cells present molecules that can interact directly with functional receptors on the NK cell surface, such as: (1) IgG antibodies, binding to CD16 (ADCC); (2) C3, presumably binding to CD11b (C3bi receptor) (505, 506); (3) antibodies to CD16 or CD2 antigens on NK cells and binding with the Fc fragment to the FcR on target cells (reverse ADCC) (507); and (4) heterocross-linked antibodies that recognize an NK cell receptor (e.g., CD16) and an antigen on the target cells (508, 509). When target cells are bound to NK cells and the lytic mechanism is activated, lysis of the target cells still depends on the intrinsic sensitivity of the target cells to the lytic mechanism. Certain types of target cells may activate the cytotoxic ability of NK cells and therefore might appear to be very sensitive to NK cells. For example, NK cell activation is observed with target cells infected with viruses or mycoplasmas (79–82), but may require the participation of accessory cells and IFN (510), and is characterized by an increase of the rate of lysis during the cytotoxic assay (see Fig. 3).

The intrinsic susceptibility of target cells to NK cell lysis appears to be dependent on components of the cell membrane. Glycoproteins isolated from the target cell membrane and inserted into artificial membranes were able to inhibit conjugate formation between human or rat NK cells with their target cells in a species-specific manner (500). However, cytotoxicity was not inhibited in these experiments (500), raising the possibility that lytic factors acting at short range but not requiring cell contact might play a role in NK cell-mediated cytotoxicity. The species specificity of the inhibition suggests that the species specificity of the NK cell cytotoxicity is at the level of NK-target cell conjugate formation. If liposomes containing membrane components from sensitive target cells are fused with resistant target cells, the resistant target cells become sensitive to NK cell-mediated lysis (501). In this experimental system (501) NK cells did not bind to or lyse heterologous target cells even when fused with liposomes containing membrane components from homologous, sensitive target cells. Moreover, liposomes containing membrane components from heterologous NK cell-sensitive target cells could not confer NK cell sensitivity to homologous NK cell-resistant target cells. These results suggest that species restriction might be at both the recognition (binding) and triggering levels.

Although NK cell lysis is often defined as specific for tumor and virus-infected targets, these cytotoxic cells can also lyse normal cells, and often it is difficult to demonstrate lysis of malignant cells. In most cases, virus-infected cells are no more sensitive than uninfected cells but are lysed through mechanisms that involve activation of NK cells (79, 511-513). Lysis of freshly obtained tumor target cells can be demonstrated using both autologous and allogeneic NK cells, but often procedures such as enrichment or stimulation with IFN or IL-2 must be used before significant killing is observed (514-517). In some cases tumor cells freshly obtained from the patients are insensitive to NK cell-mediated lysis; however, brief (24-hour) incubation *in vitro* in the case of acute myeloid leukemia blasts (518) or treatment with anti-Ig antibodies in the case of B cell chronic leukemia cells (519) render these cells sensitive to NK cell lysis. YAC-1 cells, when grown *in vivo* and directly obtained from the animals, are also resistant to lysis unless cultured for a few days (520). In this case the NK cell sensitivity increases during *in vitro* culture concomitant with a decrease of H-2 antigen expression, suggesting that an effect of IFN *in vivo*, as discussed below, might be responsible for NK cell resistance (521). Experiments using IL-2-activated NK cells against autologous endometrial carcinoma cells and normal endometrial epithelium cells have shown that the carcinoma cells were lysed more efficiently than were the normal cells, suggesting that activated NK cells might, at least for this type of tumor, selectively lyse the malignant cells (522). In several studies, transfection with the *ras* oncogenes has been shown to render cells sensitive to NK cell lysis (523-525), although the lack of correlation of sensitivity to lysis with transformation (525) makes it difficult to conclude from these observations that NK cell sensitivity arises during the early stages of cellular transformation. However, Nabi *et al.* (526) showed that suppression of some characteristics of transformed cells, such as lack of contact inhibition, renders human malignant target cells resistant to NK cell lysis.

The possibility that the sensitivity of transformed cells to NK cell lysis is determined by their high proliferation rate and by structures expressed at particular stages of the cell cycle was excluded by studies showing that susceptibility to lysis is independent of the cell cycle stage (527, 528).

Kiessling and Wigzell (529) proposed that the function of NK cells was the surveillance of primitive cells, since embryonic thymus and bone marrow contain NK-sensitive cells (36), NK cells lyse undifferentiated but not differentiated embryonic carcinoma cells (530), and induction of differentiation of the K562 (531, 532) and U937 (529) cell lines reduces their sensitivity to NK cells. Evidence against this theory comes from the observation that NK-deficient beige mice are no more susceptible than are normal mice to the growth of experimental embryo-induced teratoma and teratocarcinoma (533). Also, phorbol diester treatment of K562 cells, which was originally shown to induce differentiation and decrease sensitivity to NK cell lysis (531, 532), was subsequently reported to increase sensitivity (534) or to have opposite effects on different subclones of K562 (535). Phorbol diesters induce NK cell sensitivity in many cell lines (534, 536), possibly by inducing a decrease in cell surface sialic acid content (534, 537). That autologous or allogeneic NK cells or activated NK cells can lyse normal differentiated cells is supported by the relative sensitivity of normal fibroblast strains (34, 35) and normal fresh monocytes to NK cell lysis (538, 539).

Several experimental observations suggest an inverse correlation between expression of class I MHC antigen on target cells and sensitivity to NK cell lysis. Differentiation of teratocarcinoma cells and of normal thymocytes results in increased H-2 expression and decreased sensitivity to lysis (530, 540). In the YAC-1 and other cell lines, low expression of class I antigens correlates with high sensitivity to NK cells and limited growth potential *in vivo*, whereas variants with high class I expression are resistant to NK cells and highly metastatic *in vivo* (541–546). IFN treatment of target cells determines both resistance to NK cell lysis and increased expression of class I MHC antigens (543, 544, 546). However, other studies failed to demonstrate an absolute correlation between class I MHC expression and sensitivity to NK cell lysis (547, 548), including two studies (549, 550) in which transfection and expression of H-2D or H-2K genes in target cells were shown to have no influence on NK cell susceptibility.

Another example of dissociation between class I MHC antigen expression and NK cell sensitivity comes from adenovirus-transformed cells: When the *E1A* gene from adenovirus 5 was present, transformed cells had little or no class I MHC antigen expression and were resistant to NK cell lysis and tumorigenic, whereas when the *E1A* gene from adenovirus 12 was present, transformed cells expressed high levels of class I MHC antigens and were sensitive to NK cells and poorly tumorigenic (551). Overall studies suggest that in some cases class I MHC antigen expression prevents the triggering of NK cells and, as suggested in one study (545), the formation of NK-target cell conjugates; however, in other cases this negative control is ineffective, possibly because other structures are present on the target cell membrane and are recognized by NK cells.

Several antigens present on target cell membranes have been proposed as possible NK cell target structures. The data are largely contrasting, and evidence in favor of the role of a single molecule has not been confirmed in other systems. It is possible that NK cells recognize different molecules that either play a primary role as target molecules responsible for conjugate formation and/or triggering or exert an accessory but not essential role in increasing the binding affinity between NK and target cells. The transferrin receptor (TfR) has received much attention as a possible target antigen on the basis of inhibition by anti-TfR antibodies and correlation between TfR expression on target cells and sensitivity to NK cells or ability of the cells to compete (552–554). However, in several other studies (533, 555, 556) these results could not be reproduced, indicating that the role, if any, of the TfR as a target cell antigen is not unique. One study (557) suggested that the presence of either TfR or CDw32 FcγRII on cell lines could be sufficient for NK cell recognition, on the basis of antibody inhibition analysis. Expression of the CD15 antigen (3-fucosyl-N-acetyl-lactosamine hapten or X-hapten) on cell lines has been correlated with binding to and lysis by NK cells (558). Those findings, together with the ability of anti-CD15 antibody to inhibit NK cell-mediated lysis (559), suggested a role for the CD15 hapten in NK cell killing. Other investigators (143) identified the 140-kDa heterodimer detected by antibody 4F2 as the target cell structure recognized by several non-MHC-restricted cytotoxic T cell clones that express an identical TCR idiotype and recognize target cells through the TCR in an antigen-specific fashion; however, no role for 4F2 antigen was found in the killing mediated by human peripheral blood $CD3^-$, TCR^- NK cells (554, 560). Recently, it was found that monoclonal antibodies directed against a 42-kDa molecule, possibly existing as a homodimer on target cells, efficiently inhibit NK cell binding to and lysis of all human and mouse target cell lines tested and of the fish parasite *Tetrahymena pyriformis*, suggesting that the antigen is a primitive recognition structure present on the target cells (561).

Several reports have described the ability of simple or complex sugars to inhibit NK cell-mediated lysis (562–564). The inhibition was observed only at high sugar concentrations (>50 mM), but hexose phosphates at less than 25 mM were inhibitory (562) and hexose 6-O-sulfate esters such as mannose-6-sulfate or galactose-6-sulfate were inhibitory at 1-2 mM concentrations (564). Although it is known that sugars act at a postbinding stage (after the Ca^{2+}-requiring step) to inhibit lysis, the mechanism of this inhibition remains unclear (563, 564). The ability of certain glycopeptides from the target cell membrane to inhibit NK cell-mediated lysis suggests the requirement for target cell expression of certain carbohydrate structures (565). However, several lines of experimental evidence have excluded a role for the mannose-6-phosphate receptor on either the effector or target cell surface in NK cell-mediated lysis (566, 567). A possible role for lectinlike substances has been proposed on the basis of inhibition of pig NK cells by lectin-specific antibodies (568).

IFN, a potent activator of NK cell cytotoxic activity, antagonistically protects target cells from NK cell lysis (34, 503, 569, 570). These antagonistic effects of IFN may play a major regulatory role in *in vivo* NK cell activity, as discussed further in Section IX. Treatment of several cell lines for a few hours with IFN-α, -β, or -γ induces a dose-dependent inhibition of target cell sensitivity to NK cell lysis (34, 503, 569, 571). Lysis by complement, ADCC, or CTLs is not affected (503, 569, 570, 572). The induction of resistance requires active RNA and protein synthesis in the target cells (34). After 24-48 hours' incubation in the absence of IFN, target cells regain their sensitivity to NK cell lysis (503). The inhibition of NK cell lysis by IFN treatment of target cells is at a postbinding stage, as indicated by the observations that IFN-treated target cells are able to form conjugates with NK cells (503, 570) but not to induce NK cell cytotoxic factor (NKCF) release (573, 574) or Ca^{2+} influx in the effector cells (575). However, IFN-treated cold target cells fail to compete for the lysis of untreated ^{51}Cr-labeled target cells (503, 570), showing that competition experiments measure the functional interaction of NK cells with target cells and not only target cell recognition (76). IFN-treated target cells are still sensitive to NK cell lysis triggered by IgG antibodies in ADCC (503, 569), and to the lysis mediated by NKCF (573, 574). Surprisingly, however, sensitivity of IFN-treated K562 cells to the lysis mediated by purified granule material was reduced (575). These contrasting results might reflect the use of different target cell types, i.e., normal fibroblast strains or K562 cells, in the various studies.

Different cell lines differ greatly in their sensitivity to the NK cell-protecting effect of IFN, and a correlation has been found between the abilities of IFN to induce antiviral activity and to protect the target cells from NK cell lysis (34, 569). A few units of IFN-α completely protected fibroblasts from lysis, whereas even very high concentrations of IFN-α or -γ induced only partial protection of K562 cells (34, 576). Transformed or tumor-derived cell lines, on average, are more sensitive than are normal fibroblasts to IFN, although individual tumor-derived cell lines display high or intermediate sensitivity to the protective effect of IFN (569). Infection of target cells with most viruses completely prevents the ability of IFN to protect target cells, probably because lytic infection by these viruses suppresses host cell RNA and protein synthesis (34). However, viruses such as lymphocyte choriomeningitis virus that do not suppress RNA and protein synthesis do not prevent the protective effect of IFN on target cells (511). In addition to fibroblasts, other normal cells are protected by IFN against NK cells, including normal thymocytes (521) and monocytes (577). The IFN-induced increase in sialic acid expression on target cells has been inversely correlated with sensitivity to NK cell lysis (578). The abilities of IFN to increase class I MHC expression and to decrease sensitivity to NK cells have been considered as evidence for the preferential NK cell lysis of target cells with low class I MHC expression (543, 544, 546); however, the demonstration that IFN can protect target cells without inducing class I expression (579) has shown that this is not the major mechanism by which IFN protects target cells. Normal and tumor target cells are rendered resistant to NK cell lysis by *in vivo* exposure to IFN (521, 570), and IFN-treated B16 melanoma cells become NK cell resistant *in vitro*, with increased metastatic potential *in vivo* (580). The antagonistic effects of IFN on NK cells and their target cells *in vivo* may render NK cells selective against virus-infected target cells or IFN-resistant malignant cells by protecting normal cells from NK cell lysis and from competition with sensitive target cells. However, malignant cells that maintain IFN sensitivity or viruses that do not induce IFN resistance in the host cells might be able to escape the surveillance mechanism of NK cells.

B. Receptors Involved in NK Effector–Target Cell Interaction and Signal Transduction Mechanisms

With the exception of the CD16 FcγR used in ADCC, there is no definitive information yet on the type of receptor used by NK cells for target cell recognition and killing. TCR genes are not rearranged and TCR proteins are not expressed on peripheral blood CD3$^-$ NK cells, although TCRαβ$^+$ and possibly most TCRγδ$^+$, non-MHC-restricted CTLs may use their TCR for target cell recognition (142, 202–204).

Experiments of target cell cross-competition served to define several cross-competing target cell groups (13, 581, 582), suggesting some selectivity in the specificity of NK cells. Studies of the specificity of IL-2-grown

NK cells have indicated heterogeneity in the range of target cells lysed by the clones but have not demonstrated a clonally distributed specificity of NK cells (20, 583, 584). Recently, TCR$^-$, CD3$^-$ NK cell clones, originated from mixed-leukocyte cultures with lymphocytes from some but not all donors, were shown to specifically lyse allogeneic cells bearing the stimulating alloantigens (585). The molecular basis of this phenomenon is not known and may involve preferential growth in the mixed cultures of NK cells with a single receptor or a combination of receptors that preferentially recognize non-MHC-encoded polymorphic structures on the stimulator cells.

It was hypothesized that, at least in some experimental systems, NK cell activity depends on the presence of natural cytophilic antibodies bound *in vivo* to the FcγR and directed against target cell surface antigens (586–588). Although this mechanism may play a role in some systems, it is clearly not a general mechanism for NK cell-mediated cytotoxicity, as shown by several lines of evidence: (1) anti-IgG or anti-CD16 FcγR antibodies inhibit ADCC but not NK cell killing (79, 114, 132, 589–591), (2) phorbol diesters induce down-modulation of CD16 FcγR and inhibition of ADCC but not of NK cell killing (133), and (3) NK cells from *scid* mice and from several SCID patients are cytotoxic both *in vitro* and *in vivo* even if the animals and the patients do not produce IgG (400, 401, 410, 412, 413). However, interaction of CD16 FcγR with aggregated IgG, immune complexes, or cross-linked monoclonal anti-CD16 antibodies at 37°C induces inhibition of both ADCC and spontaneous cytotoxic activity (32, 132, 592–594). These data suggest that CD16 FcγR are not directly involved in the mechanism of NK cell-mediated spontaneous cytotoxicity, but that aggregation of the FcγR, e.g., by interaction with IgG-sensitized target cells or with immune complexes, may trigger and eventually exhaust the same cytotoxic mechanism involved in spontaneous cytotoxicity.

Like the inactivation of NK cells upon interaction with IgG-coated target cells, the interaction with NK cell-sensitive target cells also induces inactivity of NK cells, resulting in a decrease in cytotoxic rate with time of incubation (76). When PBLs containing NK cells were incubated at 37°C, but not at 4°C, with K562 target cells, NK cells were completely unable to lyse freshly added target cells after 4 hours of incubation (76). This inactivation was not seen with target cells, such as mycoplasma- or virus-infected cells, that were able to induce IFN production (76, 595), and IFN (76) and IL-2 (596) restored cytotoxic ability in NK cells that were separated from the target cells. The inactivation of NK cells was not target cell specific, and NK cells also showed abrogated or reduced cytotoxicity against target cells unrelated to those used for inactivation or against IgG-coated target cells (76, 597). IFN-treated target cells, which were resistant to NK cell lysis, were unable to induce NK cell inactivation (503, 595). These data were originally interpreted by assuming that after one or a few lytic interactions with the target cells, NK cells exhausted preformed lytic mediators required for both ADCC and spontaneous cytotoxicity and therefore became unable to mediate additional cytotoxicity unless stimulated by IFN or IL-2 (76). However, Brahmi et al. (598) demonstrated that the target cell-induced NK cell inactivation also occurs in the absence of Ca^{2+}, suggesting that it affects an early calcium-independent event in the activation of the human NK cell cytolytic mechanism.

Many studies have shown that interaction of NK cells with NK cell-sensitive target cells stimulate phosphoinositide turnover with production of the Ca^{2+}-mobilizing messengers inositol trisphosphate (IP3) and IP4 (599–602; M. Cassatella and G. Trinchieri, unpublished observations). Ca^{2+} influx in the effector cells has been suggested on the basis of ^{45}Ca uptake data (575, 603), although uptake by effector and target cells could not be distinguished by those experimental procedures. Recently, Windebank et al. (604), using liquorin-loaded NK cells, and we (M. Cassatella and G. Trinchieri, unpublished observations), using Fura-2-loaded NK cells, have shown that interaction of NK cells with target cells induces an increase in intracellular Ca^{2+} concentration ($[Ca^{2+}]_i$) that is approximately proportional to the sensitivity of the target cell to lysis. The increase in $[Ca^{2+}]_i$ upon interaction with the target cell depends on both the release of Ca^{2+} from intracellular stores and the uptake of extracellular Ca^{2+} (M. Cassatella and G. Trinchieri, unpublished observations). The stimulation of NK cell phosphoinositide metabolism by target cells has been shown to require extracellular Ca^{2+} in one study (602) but not in others (601; M. Cassatella and G. Trinchieri, unpublished observations). These contrasting results are not surprising because chelation of extracellular Ca^{2+}, depending on the experimental conditions, may result in a slower depletion of $[Ca^{2+}]_i$, which eventually blocks phosphoinositide metabolism by preventing activation of the Ca^{2+}-dependent phospholipase C. Cross-linking of the CD16 FcγR by antibodies, immune complexes, or IgG-coated target cells also induces formation of IP3 and IP4 that does not depend on the presence of extracellular Ca^{2+} (601; M. Cassatella and G. Trinchieri, unpublished observations) and an increase in $[Ca^{2+}]_i$ (601).

In analogy with the data on activation of T cells through the CD3 complex (605, 606), it is possible to postulate that activation of NK cells through either CD16 FcγR or the receptor(s) for target cells induces activation of the same G protein, with subsequent induction of IP3 and

IP4 and increased $[Ca^{2+}]_i$. Following this activation, again by analogy with T cells (605, 606), the G protein may remain in a refractory state, thereby preventing activation of NK cells by either IgG-coated or sensitive target cells. The independence from extracellular Ca^{2+} of the stimulation of phosphoinositide metabolism in NK cells suggests that inactivation of the G protein, like the inactivation of the cytotoxic mechanism by target cells (598), should also not require extracellular Ca^{2+}.

The surface molecules of the CD11/CD18 family appear to play important functional roles in NK cell killing. Patients with severe deficiency of the common CD18 chain and therefore lacking all three molecules are deficient in NK cell activity (378, 607). Antibodies to the CD18 chain efficiently block NK cell-mediated cytotoxicity by preventing binding of NK cells to target cells (179, 608, 609). Patients with selective deficiency in CD11a (LFA-1) expression are also deficient in NK cell-mediated cytotoxicity (608). A series of antibodies directed against various epitopes of the CD11a molecule inhibited both NK cell-mediated and CTL-mediated cytotoxicity; these antibodies had different efficiency in inhibiting cytotoxicity, but the same hierarchy of functionally relevant CD11a epitopes was shown for NK cells and CTLs (608). The antibodies inhibited lysis at the effector cell level by preventing NK-target cell conjugate formation (608). When peripheral blood NK cells were tested, inhibition by anti-CD11a antibodies was observed with several different target cell lines (610); with one NK cell clone used as effector cells, lysis of K562 cells but not that of other target cells was inhibited (610), whereas with other clones, the opposite result was observed (611). CD11a (LFA-1) is therefore an important adhesion molecule in the interaction of cytotoxic cells, both NK cells and CTLs, with target cells; the variable requirements for the CD11a molecules in binding of different target cells from different clones suggest that that either CD11a is one of several receptors that NK cells can use for binding or it has only an accessory function, essential only when other receptors responsible for the specificity of the binding do not ensure a binding of sufficient affinity. No evidence has been provided that CD11a is a functional receptor capable of signal transduction and triggering of NK cells.

A possible role for the CD11b molecules, or receptor for the C3bi fragment (CR3), in NK cell-mediated cytotoxicity is suggested by the increased efficiency of NK cell lysis of Raji target cells when these cells bind C3 through their CR2 (505, 506). Expression of CD11b on the NK cells is required for the enhancing effect (612); however, it is possible that this phenomenon reflects only a bridging effect that enhances NK-target cell contact, without triggering of the NK cells through the CD11b molecule. Antibodies to CD11b or CD11c did not directly affect

NK cell-mediated cytotoxicity against a variety of target cells, including the Raji cell line, in the absence of complement (179), although the lysis of Raji cells with bound C3 was inhibited by anti-CDllb antibodies (612).

Antibodies against non-lineage-restricted epitopes of the T200 molecule (CD45) inhibit NK cell-mediated lysis but not CTL-mediated lysis, acting at the effector cell level at a postbinding stage (613, 614). Some antibodies blocked lysis of a wide range of target cells (614), but antibody 13.1 blocked lysis of K562 cells but not of T cell lines, even when clones able to lyse both types of target cells were used as effector cells (613). Antibody 9.1C3, which binds a protein dimer of 66 and 76 kDa that is associated with the T200 molecule, also blocked NK cell-mediated lysis at the effector cell level and at a postbinding phase (615). A rabbit antiidiotypic antiserum generated against antibody 9.1C3 was highly reactive with K562 cells, precipitating two molecules of 94 and 79 kDa, and inhibited NK-mediated lysis of K562 cells at a postbinding stage (616). Thus, T200, or molecules associated with it, appear to interact with cell surface molecules on at least some target cell types, creating a secondary postbinding NK-target cell interaction; however, the functional significance of this secondary interaction is unknown.

Laminin or its receptor represents another adherence system that plays a major role in NK cell killing (617). Rodent and human NK cells, more than other lymphocyte types, express a lamininlike structure (48 kDa on rat cells and 38 kDa on human cells) that is recognized by antilaminin antibodies (618-620). The 48-kDa molecule on rat NK cells is translated from a 2.4-kb mRNA homologous to part of the 8-kb mRNA encoding the β_2 subunit of laminin (617). Laminin and F(ab')$_2$ antilaminin antibodies block cytotoxicity at a postbinding stage, without inhibiting NK-target cell interaction (619, 620). The sensitivity of murine target cells to NK cell-mediated lysis has been correlated with the ability of NK cells to bind laminin (618). Expression of lamininlike molecules on the NK cell surface increases upon stimulation with IL-2 (620). Thus, it is possible that a lamininlike molecule on the NK cell after conjugate formation acts in continuing the lytic mechanism by binding to the target cells either through laminin receptors or to matrix laminin expressed by the target cells (620).

C-reactive protein (CRP) is expressed on a proportion of PBLs (621). The CRP present on PBLs is not bound to the CRP receptor; it is present in monomeric form and not in the pentameric native form, and is presumably produced by the lymphocytes (622). Earlier studies using antibodies against native CRP detected expression of CRP on 3-4% of the PBLs, and all of the positive cells had the phenotype of NK cells (621); however, using antibodies specific for determinants expressed only in the monomeric form, 20-30% of PBLs expressed CRP, suggesting that cells other than NK cells might express it (622). Anti-CRP F(ab')$_2$ antibodies reduced NK cell function at a postbinding stage (623), suggesting that CRP might be another of the molecules involved in the secondary interaction between NK and target cells, or that anti-CRP antibodies act directly on effector cells by preventing NK cell triggering.

The CD2 E-R antigen expresses at least three distinct epitopes: Tll$_1$, the erythrocyte binding site; Tll$_2$, an epitope unrelated to the binding site but with the same cellular distribution of Tll$_1$; and Tll$_3$, an epitope expressed only in activated cells or in cells treated with anti-Tll$_2$ antibodies (624). CD2 is an antigen-independent pathway of T cell activation, and treatment of T cells with anti-Tll$_2$ plus anti-Tll$_3$ antibodies induces expression of IL-2 receptor, secretion of IL-2, and proliferation of T cells (624). Treatment of peripheral blood NK cells with anti-Tll$_2$ and anti-Tll$_3$ does not induce cell proliferation (625). This lack of a proliferative effect of anti-CD2 antibodies is probably due to a lack of IL-2 production (626), because anti-CD2 antibodies stimulated expression of the IL-2 receptor in NK cell clones (627) and increased the cytotoxic activity of both fresh NK cells (628) and NK cell clones (629, 630). Anti-CD2-treated NK cells showed increased adhesion to the target cells and oriented discharge of granules on the area of contact with the target cells (630); simultaneous treatment with anti-CD11a antibodies blocked NK–target cell adhesion and induced NK cells to secrete their intracellular granules, as measured by release of proteoglycans, without reorientation of the granules (630). This activation by anti-CD2 antibodies was induced when F(ab')$_2$ fragments were used, excluding the involvement of FcγR (630). However, when a single anti-CD2 antibody was used, signal transduction, as shown by increased $[Ca^{2+}]_i$ and cytotoxicity, was induced by interaction of the Fc portion of the anti-CD2 antibody with the CD16 FcR, since the F(ab')$_2$ fragment of the anti-CD2 antibody did not induce signal transduction and anti-CD16 antibodies partially blocked signal transduction induced by the intact anti-CD2 IgG antibody (631).

Monoclonal antibodies that block cytotoxicity mediated by NK cells from the catfish *Ictalurus panctatus* have been generated by immunization with enriched fish cytotoxic lymphocytes (271). These antibodies also react with human NK cells and inhibit the cytotoxicity of human NK cells and non-MHC-restricted CTLs against a variety of target cells (632, 633). The antibodies precipitate a heterodimer of 41 and 38 kDa from fish cells and of 43 and 38 kDa from human cells (271, 632, 633). These results, together with the studies (561) suggesting common target molecules on the fish parasite *Tetrahymena pyriformis* and NK cell-sensitive target cells, suggest that NK cells recognize target cells as using a receptor–ligand system that is highly conserved during evolution.

Preliminary reports have described other possible NK cell receptors. Ortaldo et al. (634) showed that antiidiotypic antibodies directed against an antibody specific for a glycoprotein of K562 cells react with an 80-kDa molecule on NK cells, block target binding and lysis by NK cells, and, when used to pretreat NK cells, enhance cytotoxicity and induce IFN production. Timonen et al. (635) have shown that certain antibodies to the F(ab')$_2$ of IgG specifically stain LGLs, precipitate predominantly a 60-kDa molecule from them, and block lysis by preventing postbinding reorientation of the effector cells. Interestingly, an antibody that reacts with the p48 lamininlike molecules on LGLs cross-reacts with the Ig light chain (636).

Of the different molecules for which a role has been proposed in NK-target cell binding or in postbinding events during NK cell-mediated cytotoxicity, only CD16 and CD2 have been shown to act directly in the signal transduction and activation of the cytotoxic mechanisms (630, 637). Only in the case of CD16 molecules has activation of NK cell cytotoxic and other functions been shown to be induced by their natural ligand, immune-complexed IgG (637). The large number of molecules that have been proposed to be NK cell receptors for target cells or to play some role in NK cell-mediated cytotoxicity is reminiscent of the confusion in the T cell receptor field before the TCR was identified. It is possible to speculate that most of the molecules described so far do not represent real receptors and that some of the results are artifacts due to a direct effect of the antibodies used on the NK cells, independent of any role of the recognized molecules in the cytotoxic process. However, unlike CTLs, NK cells do not appear to have antigenic specificity or clonally distributed receptors. Yet heterogeneity of NK cell and selectivity for target cells have been shown by competition experiments and by analysis of the selectivity of NK cell clones. Thus, the selectivity of NK cells might be determined by the relative expression of several cell surface molecules and receptors, and all of the molecules discussed above might play some role in either the recognition or the postbinding phases, with no single molecule playing a unique and essential role. Different sets of molecules might be involved in each combination of NK-target cells and a heterogeneity in the functional role of the various molecules might exist at both the NK and target cell levels.

C. Mechanisms of Cytotoxicity

The studies on the mechanism involved in T and NK cell-mediated cytotoxicity have been recently reviewed by Young and Cohn (638) and by Carpén and Säkselä (639). In this review, therefore, these studies are briefly summarized, and only those aspects particularly relevant to the understanding of NK cell biology are emphasized.

Binding of NK cells to target cells occurs rapidly at both 4°C and 37°C (640, 641) and requires Mg^{2+} but not Ca^{2+} (641-644). After binding to the target cells, the NK cell undergoes a series of events known as activation and programming of the target cell to lysis. These events are temperature dependent (optimal temperature, 37°C), Ca^{2+} dependent, and sensitive to Ca^{2+} channel blockers and calmodulin inhibitors (406, 643-648). As previously discussed, initiation of NK cell activation might depend on an enhancement of phosphoinositide metabolism that is independent of extracellular Ca^{2+}, and it is triggered by interaction of CD16 FcγR with antibody-coated target cells or of other unknown NK cell membrane structures with NK cell-sensitive target cells. The formation of IP3 and IP4 induces an increase in $[Ca^{2+}]_i$, first by release of Ca^{2+} from intracellular stores and then by the influx of extracellular Ca^{2+}, which is required for maintenance of increased levels. Chelation of extracellular Ca^{2+} probably prevents continuation of the lytic mechanism at this stage. An increase in cAMP has been shown to inhibit NK cell-mediated cytotoxicity; although inhibition of NK-target cell conjugates has been observed when cAMP levels in NK cells are increased (649), the major effect of increased cAMP is probably inhibition of the increased phosphoinositide metabolism (601, 604). Inhibition of NK cell activity by interaction with monomeric IgG is also primarily mediated by elevation of cAMP (650). Following the enhancement of phosphoinositide metabolism, activation of protein kinase C is probably involved in the cytotoxic mechanism, as indicated by inhibition of cytotoxicity by specific inhibitors (602).

The morphological analysis of NK-target cell interation showed broad cell to-cell adhesion of NK cells with the target cells, evidence of activation and degranulation in the NK cells with membrane material of probable granule origin present in the space between the two cells (284, 651). NK cells are often deeply invaginated and in some cases have been observed within the cytoplasm of the target cells, in a vesicle completely surrounded by a membrane and without communication with the extracellular medium. This phenomenon is defined as emperipolesis (284, 652).

Several observations indicate that the activation of lysis may require the release of fatty acids from the cell membrane. Exposure of PBLs to NK cell-sensitive target cells increases phospholipid methylation, and natural killing is reduced by the inhibition of methyltransferases as well as by inhibitors of phospholipase A_2 (576, 653), although some caution should be exerted in interpreting the specificity of phospholipase A_2

inhibitors (654). These findings suggest that metabolism of arachidonic acid is required for NK cell activity. However, inhibition of cyclooxygenase and prostaglandin synthesis does not affect NK cell activity, and various prostaglandins inhibit NK cell activity at binding and postbinding stages by increasing cAMP levels in the NK cells (655, 656). IFN and IL-2 activation of NK cells reduces the sensitivity to inhibition by prostaglandin and cAMP-elevating agents (655, 657). Inhibition of lipooxygenase decreases NK cell cytotoxicity, suggesting a role for endogenous lipooxygenase metabolites (leukotrienes) in NK cell activity (654, 658, 659). Recently, it has been shown that specific inhibitors of leukotriene C_4 (LTC_4) synthesis inhibit NK cell cytotoxicity and that addition of LTC_4 prevents the inhibition, suggesting an essential although unknown role of this arachidonic acid metabolite in cytotoxicity (659).

The lymphocyte-dependent events in NK cell-mediated cytotoxicity are followed by cytolysis of the target cells during the killer cell-independent lysis (KCIL) (642). This latter phase requires neither Ca^{2+} nor Mg^{2+}, but it is relatively sensitive to reduced temperature, prostaglandin E_2, heterologous anti-LGL antibody, and proteolytic enzymes (406, 642, 645). Recent studies have shown a rapid initial phase of Ca^{2+}-independent KCIL with a calculated half-life of less than 3 minutes (660). This rapid phase, which is independent of temperature over the range $10-37°C$, is followed by a very slow, Ca^{2+}-independent disintegration of additional target cells (660). This second slow phase is temperature dependent and probably mediated by soluble factors released into the supernatant during effector-target cell interaction in the presence of Ca^{2+} (660).

Several morphological and metabolic inhibitor studies suggest that lysis is mediated by a vesicular secretory mechanism, involving polarization of granules to the part of the effector cell in contact with the target, followed by discharge of the granular content (see Ref. 639 for a complete review of directed exocytosis). Drugs that block vesicular secretion in other cell types inhibit NK cell killing without affecting the ability of the effector cells to bind the target cells (661). Degranulating agents both deplete the granules from LGLs and inhibit killing (643). The programming phase has been shown to involve transfer of a protease-sensitive material from the effector cells to the target cells (662, 663).

Wright and Bonavida (664-666) demonstrated that a soluble lytic factor is secreted by NK cells following lectin stimulation or NK-target cell interaction. This NK cell cytotoxic factor (NKCF) is lytic for NK cell-sensitive target cells, but not for most NK cell-resistant target cells (664, 665, 667). Detailed studies have shown that successful NK cell-mediated lysis requires that the target cells: (1) be recognized by NK cells, allowing conjugate formation, (2) be able to induce release of NKCF (or other lytic mediators) from NK cells, and (3) be sensitive to the effect of the lytic mediators (573, 667). IFN-treated cells form conjugates with NK cells and are sensitive to NKCF but fail to induce release of the factor (573). These findings might explain the failure of IFN to protect target cells from ADCC mediated by NK cells (503): The interaction of the antibodies with FcγR on NK cells may induce release of lytic mediators, circumventing the step blocked by IFN treatment of the target cells.

NKCF is probably composed of more than one cytotoxic factor, and different factors can be active on different target cells. When the U937 cell line is used as a target for measuring NKCF activity, most of the activity is mediated by TNF, indicating that TNF is one component of NKCF and is produced by NK cells upon interaction with target cells (668, 669). When TNF-resistant cell lines such as K562 are used, the presence in NKCF of lytic factors different from TNF can be clearly demonstrated (669–672). However, these lytic molecules have not yet been purified, and molecular weights between 5,000 and 50,000 have been reported (668, 671, 672). A 50-kDa lytic molecule that cross-reacts with both TNF and lymphotoxin has been demonstrated in the granules and the cytoplasm of CTLs (673). Whether this lytic molecule is also present in NK cells and is related to NKCF remains to be determined. The characteristics of the lysis mediated by NKCF, especially the slow kinetics of lysis, make it unlikely that NKCF is the only mediator of lysis and participates in the rapid phase of disintegration of the target cells (660), although it is possible that faster kinetics of lysis is induced when high local concentrations of NKCF are reached in the contact area between effector and target cells. However, the slow second phase of target cell disintegration has been shown to be mediated by soluble factors produced by NK cells in the supernatant fluid and probably is induced by the lytic effect of NKCF (660).

Work from several laboratories has established that during NK cell-mediated lysis tubular lesions with an average internal diameter of 150–170 Å are observed on the target cell membrane and that isolated granules are able to mediate the formation of similar lesions (reviewed in Ref. 638). The granule molecule able to form the pores is a 70-kDa protein called pore-forming protein (PFP), or perforin (638). PFP requires Ca^{2+} for pore formation in membranes and it is rapidly aggregated and inactivated by the presence of Ca^{2+} in the medium; thus, PFP cannot represent a lytic factor present in the supernatant fluid, such as NKCF. Both human and murine perforins cross-react with antibodies to the C9 component of complement, another molecule able to polymerize to form pore structures in membranes in the presence of

Zn^{2+} (638). Human PFP was cloned and the high homology with C9 was confirmed by the nucleotide sequence (674). Whereas resting CTL precursor cells do not contain PFP and accumulate it only after stimulation, a low level of PFP can be isolated from the granules of human resting NK cells (675). NK cells are the only resting lymphocytes expressing detectable amounts of PFP constitutively (675).

It was initially reported that PFP isolated from freshly obtained human NK cells was able to form functional pores in liposome membranes but that it lacked efficient hemolytic activity, as measured on SRBCs (675, 676). It was also observed that NK cells are resistant to the lysis mediated by PFP, suggesting that they are protected from autolysis during cell-mediated cytotoxicity (677, 678). C9-mediated lysis is inefficient on homologous RBCs and nucleated target cells; therefore, lysis of autologous cells is probably prevented when complement is activated *in vivo* (678, 679). This homologous restriction is mediated by a 65-kDa protein called homologous restriction factor (HRF), related to C8 and C9 and present on RBCs (679) and nucleated cells (678, 679). By complexing rapidly with attacking C8 and C9 molecules, HRF is thought to interrupt the C polymerization process that leads to channel formation, and it has also been shown, in high concentrations, to prevent lysis of RBCs by the C9-related PFP and by NK cells in ADCC (679). It was postulated that the resistance of NK cells and CTLs to PFP was mediated by membrane and granule-associated soluble HRF (679, 680). However, human PFP from NK cells shows a species preference (i.e., it is unable to lyse RBCs from sheep and other species) but not an homologous restriction (i.e., it lyses human and mouse RBCs) (674, 678). These data explain the previously described lack of hemolytic activity of human PFP when tested on SRBCs, and exclude that the resistance of NK cells to PFP is mediated by HRF (674, 678). NK cells and CTLs, like other nucleated targets, are resistant to lysis by homologous but not heterologous complement; however, these cell types are resistant to both homologous and heterologous PFP (678). The resistance of NK cells to PFP is a property of resting NK cells and it is increased by stimulation with IL-2 (678). The mechanism of protection of cytotoxic cells against PFP is unknown and could be mediated by a protein with similar functional characteristics but distinct from HRF.

The rapid phase of target cell lysis mediated by NK cells is consistent with the type of cytotoxic mechanism mediated by PFP, and PFP is always present in NK cells, both freshly obtained from peripheral blood or activated. However, PFP-mediated lysis is not a universal mechanism of cell-mediated lysis, and much controversy exists about whether it is the major mechanism of lysis, mediated by CTLs (681). *In vitro* grown,

IL-2-dependent CTLs have LGL morphology and contain PFP in their granules. However, highly efficient CTLs freshly obtained from alloimmunized animals do not have LGL morphology, do not contain detectable PFP, and no channels are demonstrable on the lysed target cells (681). Also, CTLs can kill certain target cells in the absence of Ca^{2+} in the medium, contradicting the granule exocytosis model (682). Thus, these CTLs probably use a different mechanism of lysis, and it has been proposed that direct interaction between CTL receptors and target cell antigens may irreversibly damage target cell membranes, activating an endogenous mechanism of cell lysis (681). There is indeed a major difference in the KCIL following NK cell or CTL interaction which has received little attention but may reflect fundamentally different mechanisms of lysis: If Ca^{2+} is chelated during lysis mediated by noncultured CTLs, the release of ^{51}Cr continues for 1-2 hours, showing a slow lysis of the programmed target cells (683), whereas in the case of ADCC (684) or spontaneous lysis mediated by NK cells (73) an almost immediate arrest of ^{51}Cr release is observed upon chelation of Ca^{2+}.

The mechanism of cell-mediated lysis following channel insertion in the membrane is referred to as colloid osmosis (685). The lethal hit initiates with a progressive series of cytoplasmic convulsive movements in the target cells accompanied by nuclear and plasma membrane blebbing, termed zeiosis, which precedes an increase of transmembrane fluxes and loss of cytoplasmic contents (685).

Russell (686) has proposed an alternative model of "internal disintegration" to explain the mechanism of cell-mediated lysis, according to which lymphocytes trigger an autocatalytic cascade within the target, which results in nuclear membrane damage and DNA fragmentation. DNA fragmentation has also been demonstrated during NK cell-mediated lysis, although the kinetics is slower than that observed with CTLs, suggesting that in addition to cell-to-cell contact, a soluble factor such as NKCF is involved in inducing the intracellular damage (687). Human target cells present little or no DNA degradation when lysed by either human or murine cytotoxic cells (688, 689); because the difference in DNA degradation depends on the species of the target cells, not the effector cells, the degradation is probably due to activation of target cell endogenous endonucleases.

Proteases have been implicated in the mechanism of cell-mediated lysis. ADCC (690) and spontaneous cytotoxicity (691, 692) mediated by NK cells have been shown to be inhibited by various synthetic and naturally occurring protease inhibitors, especially chymotrypsin-specific inhibitors. Protease inhibitors blocked NK cell-mediated lysis at or after the postbinding Ca^{2+}-requiring step (690). However, these original observations were difficult to interpret because the studies were performed with intact cells, and the most effective protease inhibitors used, the single-amino acid chloromethylketones, also induced nonspecific alkylation.

Human NK cells contain a urokinase-type plasminogen activator in vesicles that polarize during conjugate formation with target cells (693). Serine esterases 1 and 2 (or granzymes A and B), with no plasminogen activator activity, have been identified in murine CTLs (694); equivalent esterases have been cloned from human cells, and their mRNAs have been demonstrated on fresh peripheral blood NK cells (695-697). Serine esterases are secreted from lymphocytes stimulated by calcium ionophores or by interaction with target cells and might be involved in cytotoxicity (638, 694, 697). Using various protease inhibitors and measuring the ability to degrade serum amyloid A, Zucker-Franklin et al. (698) showed that NK cells, but not other PBLs, carry several enzymes with different substrate specificities, some of which may be involved in cytotoxicity.

Hudig et al. (699) and Zunino et al. (700) analyzed the requirement for proteases in the lysis mediated by granules obtained from RNK-16 cytotoxic rat lymphocytes. The chloromethylketone Z-Gly-Leu-Phe-CH_2Cl and the irreversible mechanism-based inhibitors 7-amino-4-chloro-3-(2-phenylethoxy)-isocoumarin and dichloroisocoumarin completely blocked RNK-16 granule-mediated cytolysis, demonstrating a requirement for trypsin- and chymotrypsinlike proteases in the lysis mediated by the granules. Although the mechanism of action of the proteases is unknown, it is possible that lytic molecules, e.g., PFP, are present in the granules in an inactive form and that proteolysis is required for activation. A potential substrate could be an inhibitory PFP-binding protein similar to HRF (680).

The granules of NK cells contain proteoglycans of the chondroitin sulfate A type which are released during cytotoxicity or activation by anti-CD2 antibodies (701-703). A role for proteoglycans in the mechanism of cytotoxicity or in the protection of effector cells has been proposed (701-703), although it was shown that a significant decrease of proteoglycan synthesis induced by culturing NK cells in β-D-xyloside neither decreased NK cell cytotoxic activity nor increased autolysis (704).

D. Regulation of NK Cell Cytotoxic Activity and Proliferation

Infection of mice with viruses, certain microorganisms, and their products has been shown to result in enhanced NK cell cytotoxicity (17, 705), and IFN, a potent NK cell activator, was found to be produced under most of the *in vivo* or *in vitro* conditions in which augmentation of NK cell activity has been observed (34, 80, 104, 591, 706).

IFN efficiently enhances the cytotoxic activity of NK cells (34, 591). This effect can be readily demonstrated and quantitated by preincubating lymphocytes in the presence of IFN and then testing their cytotoxic ability against target cells unable to induce IFN production (34). All three known types of IFN, fibroblast (β), different species of leukocyte type I (α), and leukocyte type II or immune (γ) are able to enhance human NK cell cytotoxicity (272, 408, 707). However, IFN-γ is not effective with cells from all donors and always enhances NK cell cytotoxicity at a lower extent and with a slower kinetics than does IFN-α or IFN-β (708–711). Human NK cells, as well as other lymphocytes, express high affinity receptors for IFN-α/β and IFN-γ (712). IFN treatment of NK cells induces 2′,5′-oligoadenylate (2′,5′A) synthetase and, under appropriate experimental conditions, 2′,5′A augments NK cell cytotoxicity, suggesting that, as in the case of IFN antiviral activity, the pathway of IFN-mediated augmentation of NK cell cytotoxicity may involve 2′,5′A (713, 714). However, although most species of recombinant IFN-α enhance NK cell cytotoxicity, recombinant IFN-α J, with potent antiviral and antiproliferative activity, fails to do so (715). IFN-α J binds to the same receptors as the other IFN-α and blocks the NK cell-activating effect of the other species of IFN-α (716). These results indicate possible differences in the mechanisms of action of IFN in inducing antiviral activity or augmenting NK cell cytotoxicity.

In addition to IFN and IFN-inducing cells (such as virus- or mycoplasma-infected cells), other IFN inducers, such as viruses and polyinosinic–polycytidylic acid (poly I:C), also enhance NK cell activity by inducing IFN production by cells present in the cell preparations used as a source of NK cells (34, 591). The IFN-dependent enhancement of the cytotoxic activity of NK cells is very rapid and requires *de novo* protein synthesis but not cell proliferation (34). Although NK cells show increased cytotoxic activity after IFN treatment, they do not show a pattern of target cell specificity different from that of untreated ones. However, they can very efficiently kill target cells that are not very sensitive to the killing by untreated NK cells (34). The increase in killing ability as a result of IFN stimulation is proportionally greater against these less susceptible target cells than against very susceptible target cells; the number of cells lysed increases up to 20-fold in the former situation, whereas that of cells lysed when the NK-susceptible cell line K562 is used, for example, increases only 1.5- to twofold (591). IFN-treated NK cells are also able to lyse fresh tumor target cells, which are relatively resistant to lysis by nonstimulated NK cells (717). IFNs stimulate the cytotoxic activity of NK cells only and do not endow T or B cells with non-MHC-restricted cytotoxic activity (95, 272).

IFNs have been shown to affect NK cell cytotoxicity through at least three different mechanisms: (1) by increasing both the number of NK cells able to bind to their targets and the proportion of cytotoxic cells within the NK cell population (59, 95, 502, 718–721), (2) by accelerating the kinetics of lysis (720, 721), and (3) by increasing the recycling ability of active NK cells (76, 502).

The major changes in NK cell morphology after IFN treatment are observed in the structure of the granules. Cytoplasmic granules containing an electron-dense matrix or PTA become virtually undetectable and are replaced by large vesicular structures with, often, a residual electron-dense matrix surrounded by aggregates of round vesicles or membranous myelin figures (281).

The effect of IFN on the ability of NK cells to mediate ADCC is more controversial (34, 591, 722–725). In many of the reports that claim enhanced NK cell ADCC activity, the researchers have disregarded the confounding effect of (1) increased spontaneous (antibody-independent) background killing of the target cells mediated by NK cells and (2) the possibility that the high concentrations of antibodies used to sensitize the target cells trigger both monocyte and NK cell cytotoxicity. However, experimental conditions have been reported that rigorously demonstrated an enhancing effect, although modest, of IFN on NK cell ADCC activity (724). Spontaneous cytotoxicity and ADCC are two functions mediated by the same NK cell type. These functions may depend on discrete mechanisms of target cell recognition that activate the same or two different lytic processes. Although the differential effect of IFN on spontaneous cytotoxicity and ADCC might be considered evidence for separate mechanisms, it is more likely that the enhancing effect of IFN on ADCC activity of NK cells is difficult to demonstrate because the interaction of IgG on target cells with CD16 FcR on NK cells determines optimal stimulation of NK cells and maximal killing that cannot be further increased by IFN. The inefficiency of IFN in enhancing ADCC activity is therefore analogous to its inefficiency in enhancing the lysis of target cells very sensitive to NK cell-mediated lysis, as discussed above. In support of this interpretation, it was reported that the enhancing effect of IFN on ADCC activity of NK cells is observed only when suboptimal concentrations of antibodies are used (726, 727).

In vivo IFN treatment of patients determined in most cases an increase in NK cell activity that is, however, often transient and in some cases followed by depression (728–733). IFNs *in vitro* do not induce NK cell proliferation, but *in vivo*, in the mouse, IFNs were shown to induce blast formation, DNA synthesis, and probably proliferation of NK cells (734).

Suppressor cells have been described by several investigators in the murine system and appear to be responsible for the depressed NK cell activity observed in animals treated with IFN (735) or with carrageenan (736). Murine suppressor cells for NK cell activity have been shown to be both macrophages (735-740) and T cells (741, 742). Prostaglandins (PGs), which inhibit spontaneous cytotoxicity *in vitro*, are probably the soluble mediators of the suppression mediated by macrophages (743). In humans normal granulocytes (104) and, to a lesser extent, peripheral blood monocytes (104, 744, 745) have suppressor activity on NK cells. Tumor-associated lymphocytes and macrophages from patients with different types of malignancies have been found to inhibit NK cell cytotoxicity (746-750). Indomethacin, in some cases, reverses the inhibition, suggesting that PGs are also involved in the suppressive effect mediated by human macrophages (748, 751). PGs of the E series suppress human NK cell activity (751-754); however, IFN treatment of NK cells decreases their sensitivity to this suppressive effect (755). Activation of human lymphocytes in culture induces the generation of suppressor cells for NK cell activity (756, 757). In one study these suppressor cells were identified as HNK-1$^+$, FcμR$^+$ but FcγR$^-$, CD16$^-$ non-T cells (756). On the basis of this phenotype, it was suggested that NK cells themselves can function as immunoregulators, controlling their own cytotoxic activity. Suppressor cells for NK cell activity have also been found in normal human cord blood (341); these suppressor cells are probably in part responsible for the reduced NK cell activity mediated by human cord blood lymphocytes, notwithstanding a normal proportion of both LGLs (341) and CD16$^+$ cells (95). The cord blood suppressor cells have been identified as medium-sized CD3$^+$, FcγR$^+$ T cells. IFN treatment of these cells abolishes their suppressive activity (341).

TGF-β and platelet-derived growth factor have inhibitory effects on NK cell-mediated cytotoxicity (758, 759). TGF-β prevents the enhancement of NK cell cytotoxicity induced by IFN, but not that induced by IL-2 (758).

T cell growth factor or IL-2 is a potent enhancer of NK cell activity *in vitro* and *in vivo* (708, 760-764). The optimal doses of IL-2 able to enhance NK cell-mediated cytotoxicity are 100- to 1000-fold higher than those required for maintaining proliferation of activated T lymphocytes, and antibodies against the p55 chain (TAC or CD25 antigen) of the IL-2 receptor are unable to prevent NK cell enhancement of cell cytotoxicity (708, 763). These data suggested the existence on NK cells of an IL-2 receptor different from the high-affinity IL-2 receptor associated with the TAC antigen and became interpretable when it was discovered that the high-affinity IL-2 receptor is composed of the p55 chain (TAC antigen) and a second p70 chain (765). Resting NK cells express higher levels of the p70 chain than do other lymphocytes (766). The p70 chain, when not associated with the p55 chain, binds IL-2 with an affinity approximately one hundredth that of the complete receptor and is responsible for the response of resting NK cells to IL-2 (766, 767). The same high concentrations of IL-2 induce a modest production of IFN-γ from resting NK cells (708). It was originally reported that the enhancement of NK cell cytotoxicity by IL-2 was mediated by endogenously produced IFN-γ (761, 763). However, the use of impure anti-IFN-γ antibody preparations was shown to be responsible for some of the results originally reported (768), and there is now general agreement that the effect of IL-2 is direct and not mediated by IFN-γ, because (1) anti-IFN-γ monoclonal antibodies do not prevent the enhancement of NK cell cytotoxicity mediated by IL-2 (708, 768–770), (2) the enhancement of cytotoxicity mediated by IL-2 precedes by several hours the appearance of detectable IFN-γ in the supernatant fluids (708, 770), and (3) the production of IFN-γ by NK cells requires the participation of class II MHC-positive accessory cells, whereas the enhancement of cytotoxicity is independent of accessory cells. The morphological aspect of IL-2-activated NK cells is different from that of IFN-activated NK cells: The morphology of the IL-2-activated cells is altered, with expansion of the Golgi apparatus and increase in the number of electron-dense granules and vesicles; the granules, however, do not show the deaggregation of the electron-dense matrix observed in IFN-treated NK cells (281). IFN and IL-2 synergize in their enhancing effect on NK cell cytotoxicity (770, 771). Short-term treatment with IL-2 (up to 24 hours) enhances the cytotoxicity of purified $CD3^-$, $CD16^+$ NK cells and does not endow freshly obtained $CD3^+$ cells with non-MHC-restricted cytotoxicity when tested against NK cell-sensitive or -resistant target cells (156, 708).

The enhancement of cytotoxic activity of NK cells is demonstrable after 3–6 hours of incubation and does not require proliferation (708). Incubation of PBLs with IL-2 in the absence of other stimuli, however, induces moderate cellular proliferation after 3–4 days of incubation (708). Analysis of the proliferating cells by autoradiography after treatment of PBLs with IL-2 has shown that a proportion of both NK and T cells is induced into the cell cycle (708). However, limiting dilution experiments (93, 772) and colchicine blockage experiments (93) showed that the majority of mature peripheral blood NK cells can be induced into the cell cycle by IL-2 alone, whereas only a minor proportion of low-density T cells is induced to proliferate. The effect of endogenously produced IFN-γ on the IL-2-induced proliferation of NK cells is controversial, but inhibition of proliferation by anti-IFN-γ antibodies was shown in cultures of both human (773) and murine (774) NK cells. Induction of proliferation of NK cells requires the same high concentrations of IL-2 as the enhancement of cytotoxic activity or production of IFN-γ and does not depend on expression of the TAC antigen on NK cells (93). It is therefore likely that induction of proliferation is also mediated through the p70 chain of IL-2 receptor, with intermediate affinity for IL-2. However, IL-2 induces expression of TAC (CD25) antigen on purified NK cells after 2–4 days of culture (191) and anti-TAC antibodies suppress proliferation (93), suggesting that expression of the high-affinity IL-2 receptor is required for maintenance of proliferation. In addition to TAC (CD25) antigen, other activation antigens such as TfR, CD38, and class II MHC antigens become strongly expressed on proliferating NK cells (191). When NK cells revert to a resting state, cell surface expression of CD25, CD38, and TfR decreases or ceases, whereas NK cells remain class II MHC positive (100). Recently, cell surface expression Leu-23, an antigen present as a 60-kDa heterodimer composed of two chains of 32 and 28 kDa, has been shown to be induced and phosphorylated on the large majority of NK cells after a few hours of stimulation with IL-2 (775), confirming that the majority of resting NK cells respond to IL-2.

Culture of PBLs with IL-2 for a few days induces the generation of non-MHC-restricted cytotoxic cells, termed LAK cells, that are able to efficiently lyse NK cell-resistant target cells, including fresh tumor cells (776–778). Infusion of autologous *in vitro* generated LAK cells in patients, together with recombinant IL-2, has resulted in at least partial regression of solid tumors in a low but significant proportion of patients (27). Although LAK cells have been originally described as $CD3^+$ cytotoxic cells originated from $CD3^-$ precursors (777), studies from many groups have clearly shown that most of the cytotoxicity mediated by LAK cells is due to IL-2-activated $CD3^-$ NK cells, although a minor component could be due to non-MHC-restricted cytotoxic $CD3^+$ T cells (156, 708, 764, 779–781). The cytotoxic cells present in the peripheral blood of patients receiving IL-2 have also been shown to be mostly or exclusively $CD3^-$ NK cells (764). The identification of NK cells as the major mediators of LAK cell cytotoxic activity, as measured by *in vitro* assays, does not, however, provide information on the cell type responsible for tumor regression *in vivo* in patients treated with unfractionated, IL-2-treated PBLs, composed, in large proportion, of T cells. The definition of LAK cells does not identify a single or novel cell type, but rather identifies a phenomenon, i.e., the ability of IL-2 to enhance the cytotoxicity of NK cells and to endow certain T cells with non-MHC-restricted cytotoxic ability. The analysis of the LAK cell phenomenon has generated little original information on the biology of NK cells, and its description is beyond the scope of the present review.

The LAK cell phenomenon appears in part to be similar to the generation of "anomalous" killer cells in mixed-lymphocyte cultures (782–786), although it remains unclear, in this latter system, whether the progenitor cells are NK cells, T cells, or both (784, 785).

NK cells, but not T cells, have been shown to be capable of chemokinesis and chemotaxis when exposed to C5a, N-formyl-methionyl-leucyl-phenylalanine, and casein (787, 788), suggesting that NK cells have receptors for these typical stimulants of PMNs and monocytes. IFN and IL-2 increase the locomotor ability of NK cells, without increasing their ability to respond to chemoattractants (789). The migration of NK cells can be demonstrated by using nitrocellulose filters, but not polycarbonate filters, which require the migrating cells to behave as adherent cells (790). Treatment of NK cells with phorbol diesters, however, activates NK cells, enhancing their cytotoxic ability (133, 791) and making them able to adhere to various substrates (792). Phorbol diester-activated NK cells migrate through polycarbonate filters as adherent cells (791). These data, together with the ability of IL-2 to induce adherence of NK cells, but not T cells, to endothelial cells (793, 794), suggest that the change of adherence capability and migratory behavior of NK cells following activation may be determinant to induce activated NK cells to adhere to vascular lining and localize in tissues.

The ability of IL-2-activated NK cells to adhere to plastic has been utilized for obtaining enriched preparations of activated NK cells in both humans and experimental animals (795, 796). PBLs or spleen cells are cultured for 24 hours in the presence of high doses of IL-2, then the nonadherent cells are further cultured in the presence of IL-2; after 14 days of culture a several hundredfold proliferation of the adherent cells is observed and the majority of the collected cells have the phenotype of NK cells with potent cytotoxic activity (795, 796). This method has been proposed as a relatively simple technique to obtain activated NK effector cells for antitumor adoptive immunotherapy (796).

Irradiated B lymphoblastoid cell lines, in the presence of a source of IL-2, augment proliferation of mature NK cells, enhance NK cell clonal efficiency, and facilitate the growth of IL-2-dependent NK cell clones (93, 99, 191, 797). Although the exact mechanism of action of the cell line is unknown, it has been shown that they do not increase the frequency of NK cells entering the cell cycle in response to IL-2, but rather facilitate the continuous proliferation of the NK cells (93). During culture of total PBLs with irradiated B lymphoblastoid cell lines, cell surface activation antigens are rapidly induced (100, 192). NK target cell structures present on the cell lines used as a stimulator may play a direct role in inducing NK cell activation because the MHC-negative, NK-sensitive K562 cell line has been reported to induce proliferation of NK cells but not T cells (798).

Certain irradiated B lymphoblastoid cell lines, such as Daudi and RPMI 8866 cells, but not various T or myeloid cell lines induce preferential proliferation of $CD16^+$, $NKH-1^+$, $CD3^-$ human NK cells when cocultured with total PBLs (100). After 10 days of cultures, an average fourfold increase in total cell number is observed, with NK cells representing between 50 and 90% of the total cells recovered (100). NK cells can be easily purified from these cultures. This represents a technically simple method for obtaining large quantities of pure NK cells without the need of adding IL-2 to the culture and has been instrumental in obtaining large numbers of human NK cells for molecular and biochemical studies (78, 637, 675, 799). The preferential NK cell proliferation is not observed when PBLs are stimulated by irradiated allogeneic PBLs in a classical mixed-lymphocyte culture or when PBLs are cultured in the pressnce of IL-2 alone (100). NK cell proliferation occurs in the absence of exogenously added IL-2, but is blocked by anti-IL-2 antibodies and requires the presence of $CD4^+$ T cells in the starting PBL preparation, suggesting that the $CD4^+$ T cells stimulated by the allogeneic lymphoblastoid cell lines produce IL-2 that, together with irradiated cell line, induce the preferential proliferation of NK cells (100). An alternative, or additional, interpretation may be suggested by the observation (492, 493) that mitomycin C-treated autologous T cell blasts are able to induce generation of NK-like cells from $CD3^-$ small-lymphocyte precursors. It is possible that $CD4^+$ blasts, generated by allogeneic stimulation with the irradiated B cell lines, similarly induce proliferation/differentiation of NK cells and/or NK precursor cells.

Mitogenic lectins are unable to induce proliferation of purified human NK cells (191), although they can enhance phosphoinositide turnover and increase $[Ca^{2+}]_i$ in both NK and T cells (M. Cassatella, personal communication). The inefficiency of NK cells to produce growth factor such as IL-2 might be responsible for the failure of lectins to induce NK cell proliferation. Phorbol diesters and calcium ionophores together have been shown to induce proliferation of Percoll-enriched preparations of NK cells (800); however, using the same stimuli, we (L. London and G. Trinchieri, unpublished observations) have been unable to obtain proliferation of NK cells purified by positive selection of $CD16^+$ cells, raising the possibility that contaminant accessory or suppressor cells may regulate NK cell proliferation in these experimental conditions.

The effect of IL-4 on NK cell cytotoxicity and proliferation is controversial, with opposite results reported with human and murine NK cells. IL-4 has no effect on the cytotoxic ability of human resting NK cells, but it inhibits in a dose-dependent manner the IL-2-induced cytolytic activation of NK cells, but not the IFN-induced activation (801, 802). IL-4 acts directly on purified NK cells and does not require accessory cells (802). In the murine system, however, IL-4 alone was shown to induce non-MHC-restricted cytotoxic cells against fresh tumor cells and to augment the effect of IL-2 on the generation of cytotoxic cells (803, 804), although, unlike IL-2-induced cytotoxic cells, T cells, not NK cells, represent the major component of the IL-4-induced cytotoxic cells (804). Indeed, IL-4 was shown to have a modest effect, if any, on the cytotoxicity and proliferation of purified murine NK cells or on spleen cells from *scid* mice, lacking T cells (229).

The possible effect of IL-1 on NK cell cytotoxicity and activation has not been extensively studied. IL-1 does not affect directly the cytotoxicity of NK cells, but might act synergistically with IL-2 or IFN in enhancing cytotoxicity of NK cells against certain tumor cells (805). This effect of IL-1 is possibly dependent on the ability of IL-1 to induce CD25 (p55 chain of IL-2 receptor) antigen on a proportion of human NK cells (806). The cytotoxicity of human NK cells is enhanced by treatment with high doses of TNF (807). TNF also acts synergistically with IL-2 in enhancing the cytotoxicity of human NK cells (807) and inducing generation of non-MHC-restricted cytotoxic cells (808).

E. Production of Lymphokines by NK Cells

NK cells have been described to be able to produce a large number of lymphokines. However, in many early studies contaminant cell types were present in the enriched NK cell preparation, and definitive identification of NK cells as the lymphokine producer cells was not provided.

Various factors and other substances might be preformed in the granules of NK cells and be secreted during interaction of NK cells with target cells or immune complexes. NKCF, PFP, esterases, proteoglycans, and various enzymes are included in this group of substances. A series of three probably distinct factors with activity on macrophages and other cell types have been found to be associated with cytoplasmic granules, obtained from both human NK cells and rat LGL leukemia RNK cells, and are released upon interaction with target cells or treatment with substances inducing degranulation such as Sr^{2+} (809–811).

Activation of intracellular microbicidal activity in rat and human alveolar macrophages was shown to be mediated by one of these preformed NK cell cytokines, a protein of 10-20 kDa, heat and pH labile (809). Another NK granule-associated factor, released during granule secretion, was a leukocyte chemotactic factor inducing chemokinesis and chemotaxis of LGLs, neutrophils, and macrophages (810). A third factor, NK cell granule–macrophage activating factor, is a small protein (less than 10 kDa), heat stable and able to activate the tumoridical activity of bone marrow-derived macrophages in the presence of lipopolysaccharide (811). The optimal release of these factors from the granules requires ionic solubilization in 2 M NaCl, suggesting that they are tightly bound to an internal granule matrix. Because these factors are released in active form during degranulation, physiological mechanisms equivalent to this ionic solubilization should take place, and granule proteases may act to digest an internal matrix to liberate some molecules stored in an inactive form (810, 811). The granule-associated factors with activity on phagocytic cells might play role in the effect of NK cells *in vivo* against bacterial infections, as discussed in Section IX.

Factor(s) present in the supernatant fluid of NK cells activated by interaction with target cells stimulate a strong luminol-dependent chemiluminescence (CL) response in monocytes (812). This activation of CL in monocytes mediated by NK cells was found to be responsible for the CL response attributed directly to NK cells in previous studies (813, 814). The CL response described in NK cells after interaction with target cells was shown to be due to the presence of few contaminant monocytes stimulated by NK cells or NK products (812). NK cells are incapable of oxidative burst and do not produce superoxide anion during interaction with target cells (812, 815-817). NK cell cytotoxic activity does not require oxygen-dependent mechanisms, as shown by intact NK cell cytotoxic activity in chronic granulomatous disease patients (818). Because several hydroxyl radical (OH) scavengers inhibit cytotoxicity, it was proposed that OH is critical for NK cell cytotoxicity (815, 819, 2186). Because NK cells do not have NADPH oxidase acrivity, as was also confirmed by the impossibility to demonstrate in purified NK cells mRNA for the heavy chain of cytochrome b_{245}, an integral part of the NADPH oxidase system (M. Cassatella and G. Trinchieri, unpublished observations), it was hypothesized that OH scavengers are formed by the lipooxygenase pathway of arachidonic acid metabolism (819). However, the observations that OH scavengers inhibit NK cell cytotoxicity only when used at concentrations higher than those required to inhibit CL in monocytes (816) and that electron spin resonance spectroscopy does not reveal OH radical production in activated NK cells (820) strongly argue against the hypothesis that OH radical production plays a role in the early event of NK cell activation.

The possibility that NK cells might be able to secrete factors with NK-enhancing activity, such as IFN and IL-2, and thus be capable of self-regulation has generated much interest (34, 79, 821). In the early studies of NK cell cytotoxicity against cell lines able to induce IFN-α production, e.g., virus-infected target cells, it was not possible with the reagents available to unambiguously distinguish between NK cells and IFN-α-producing cells, although the fact that IFN-α-producing cells were all E-rosette negative—whereas about 50% of NK cell cytotoxic activity was recovered in the E-rosette-positive cell fraction—excluded a complete identity between the two cell types (34, 569, 706, 822). Several reports have, however, subsequently appeared, suggesting that the major IFN-α producer cells in peripheral blood were NK cells, based on results showing that the cells were found in the light-density fractions of a Percoll gradient and that they adhered to NK target cells (821, 823–826). Recently, however, several groups have shown that the IFN-α-producing cells in response to viruses, virus-infected cells, and other stimuli are HLA-DR$^+$ nonadherent cells, distinct from monocytes, dendritic cells, or T, B, or NK cells (92, 510, 827–829). Resting NK cells have null or very low ability to produce IFN-α (92, 510). The role of this IFN-α-producing cell type in the cytotoxicity of NK cells against virus-infected target cells will be discussed in Section IX.

NK cells are powerful producers of IFN-γ when stimulated with IL-2 (78, 708, 763, 830). The IFN-γ induced in total PBL preparations by IL-2 treatment is produced predominantly by NK cells and in part by T cells (708, 830). The production of IFN-γ by resting NK cells, as well as by resting T cells, requires, however, the participation of HLA-DR$^+$ accessory cells, with a mechanism still unclear (831). Because the majority of NK calls are rapidly induced by IL-2 to produce IFN-γ, it is likely that *in vivo* during an immune response the few antigen-specific T cells that may respond to antigen with production of IL-2 secondarily recruit NK cells as the major producers of IFN-γ; the role of NK cell-produced IFN-γ in B cell response is discussed in Section X.

The ability of NK cells to produce IL-2 is controversial. Although NK cell preparations have been reported to produce IL-2 (824, 832), the phenotype of the IL-2-producing cells was ambiguous and never corresponded to that of the majority of NK cells (824). IL-2 production has never been conclusively demonstrated using highly purified preparations of NK cells and the bulk of evidence, showing that NK cells cannot be induced to proliferate by a variety of mitogenic stimuli in the absence of IL-2-producing cells or an exogenous source of IL-2, suggests that NK cells are unable to produce IL-2 or are very poor producers. A comparison of T and NK cell clones, showing non-MHC-restricted cytotoxic activity, showed that the majority of the T cell clones produced high levels of IL-2, whereas only two of 11 NK cell clones produced small levels of IL-2 (833).

NK cells have been shown to produce B cell growth factors (834, 835) and various types of colony-stimulating factors, as discussed in detail in Section VIII. During the study of the effect of human NK cells on bone marrow colony formation, it was found that NK cells, when cultured with bone marrow cells or NK-sensitive target cells, release low levels of TNF (668). This result was surprising because TNF was considered a macrophage product, but production of TNF by both NK and T lymphocytes was subsequently confirmed at both the protein (78, 260, 836, 837) and molecular (78, 260) levels.

Recently, study of the ability of human NK cells to produce various lymphokines was facilitated by the ability to obtain large numbers of highly purified NK cells from the cultures of PBLs and irradiated lymphoblastoid cell lines (100) and by the specific stimulation of NK cells through CD16 FcR ligands, i.e., Sepharose linked anti-CD16 antibodies or immune complexes (IgG antibody-coated RBCs or target cells) (78). Cross-linking of CD16 FcR or IL-2 treatment of highly purified NK cells induces low levels of IFN-γ and TNF production; the two stimuli, however, strongly synergize and high levels of both cytokines are released when NK cells are stimulated by the two stimuli together (78). Both stimuli induce transcription of the lymphokine genes and accumulation of mRNA transcripts in the cytoplasm; however, the synergistic effect of the two stimuli is observed at the mRNA accumulation level but not at the transcription level, suggesting that both stimuli induce lymphokine expression by acting at the transcriptional level, but that the synergistic effect is mostly posttranscriptional (78). The induction of transcription of lymphokine genes by CD16 ligands or IL-2 takes place in less than 20 minutes and mRNA accumulation does not require protein synthesis, suggesting a direct effect without other *de novo* produced proteins acting as intermediate messengers (78). CD16 ligands but not IL-2 induce phosphoinositide turnover and an increase of $[Ca^{2+}]_i$, originated from intracellular stores and from extracellular Ca^{2+} (637). The accumulation of mRNA and the induction of transcription by CD16 ligands but not by IL-2 require extracellular Ca^{2+}, indicating the importance of the increased $[Ca^{2+}]_i$ in the induction of transcription by CD16 ligands and the different signal transduction mechanisms used by the two stimuli (637).

Stimulation of purified NK cells with CD16 ligands and IL-2 induces high levels of mRNA accumulation and release of IFN-γ, TNF, GM-CSF, and CSF-1 (78, 799). Nonspecific stimulation with phorbol diesters and calcium ionophore induces IFN-γ, TNF, GM-CSF, and IL-3 (799). In neither case was accumulation of transcripts for G-CSF, IL-1α, or IL-1β observed (799). The lack of detection of IL-1α or β mRNA was surprising, because previous studies have shown that NK cells are powerful producers of IL-1 in response to endotoxin (838, 839). However, NK cells, unlike monocyte/macrophages, are not stimulated to produce TNF by endotoxin (799), and it is possible that the IL-1 production in the NK cell preparation previously reported was due to contamination with a small number of monocytes, activated by NK cells as shown for the CL response, or that the IL-1 activity reported was due to a cytokine different from IL-1α or IL-1β.

VI. Interaction between NK Cells and the Central Nervous System

Bidirectional communication between the immune and central nervous systems provides the opportunity for coordinate mobilization of the specialized capacities of each system to sense and respond to environmental and autologous challenges (804). The study of neuroimmunology has been focused mostly on the neuroanatomy of lymphoid organs and shared or interdependent biochemical, functional, developmental characteristics of the two systems, with only limited emphasis on the effect of behavior on neuroimmunological communication (840). The NK cell system has been shown in many studies to be profoundly affected by neuro-immunological interactions, although the mechanisms of these interactions and their physiological significance are still unclear.

Several antigens present on NK cells are also expressed on cells of the central nervous system. The distributions of the HNK-1/Leu-7 and NKH-1/Leu-19 antigens in nervous tissues have already been discussed. In addition, the Thy-1 antigen is present on both murine T and NK cells and neurons.

The control of NK cell activity by the central nervous system is suggested by a decrease in NK cell activity *in vivo* following electrolytic lesions of the hypothalamus. Lesions in the anterior hypothalamus in the rat (841) and the median region of the hypothalamus in the mouse (842) were effective in inducing a decrease in NK cell activity lasting 1–2 weeks.

A series of clinical and experimental observations associates behavioral depression and stress with suppression of NK cell activity. A clinical syndrome characterized by general symptoms of remittent fever and persistent uncomfortable fatigue, often with severe depression, has been significantly associated with decreased NK cell activity in peripheral blood (843, 844). This syndrome has been called chronic fatigue syndrome, low NK cell syndrome, or chronic active EBV infection, although many patients have a negative or normal anti-EBV titer. In many patients the $CD16^+$, $CD3^-$, NKH-1/Leu-19$^+$ NK cell subset is significantly reduced, whereas the $CD3^+$, NKH-1/Leu-19$^+$ one is present in normal proportions ($\sim 3\%$) and is responsible for most of the low NK cell cytotoxic activity mediated by the PBLs of these patients (844).

NK cell cytotoxicity was found to be significantly lower in a group of hospitalized depressed men than in matched controls (845). In patients with breast cancer, the level of NK cell activity was associated with various pathological parameters, such as nodal status; however, more than half of the baseline NK cell activity variance could be accounted for by factors such as patient adjustment, lack of social support, and fatigue/depression symptoms (846). NK cell activity is reduced in women undergoing conjugal bereavement (847, 848). Bereaved women showed reduced NK cell activity and increased plasma cortisol levels as compared to controls; however, anticipatory bereaved women also showed significantly reduced NK cell activity, although levels of plasma cortisol were comparable to those of controls; thus, the reduction of NK cell activity could not be explained on the basis of increased cortisol secretion (848). The importance of depression associated with commonplace stressful events was shown by a study of medical students during academic examinations: PBLs from blood samples collected at the time of the examination produced significantly less IFN and mediated significantly lower NK cell cytotoxicity than did PBLs from samples taken 6 weeks earlier (849). That the depression symptoms are more important than the stressful event per se in determining NK cell activity was shown in a study of 114 healthy undergraduate volunteers undergoing life change stress (850). The group of students reacting to the stress with psychiatric symptoms of depression (poor copers) had significantly lower NK cell activity than the group without symptoms (good copers) (850).

A clinically relevant cause of NK cell depression is surgical stress. A significant reduction of NK cell activity persists for 1-2 weeks after surgical operation (851-853). Studies in animal models showed that the surgical procedure and not the anesthesia was the cause of the NK cell suppression (853). Suppressor cells for NK cell activity after surgical stress have been demonstrated in both humans and mice (851, 853). The depressed NK cell activity after surgery could facilitate tumor metastasis spread (853).

In experimental animals depressed NK cell activity was observed in old rats subjected to isolation stress (854) and in mice subjected to restraint stress (855) or to rotation-induced stress (856). Transportation stress in mice was sufficient to induce a significant decrease in NK cell activity lasting 24 hours and correlating with an increased plasma corticosterone level (857).

To test the hypothesis that opioid peptides released upon stress mediate the effect of the stress on the immune system, Shavit *et al.* (858–860) investigated the effect on NK cells of two types of inescapable foot-shock stress: (1) applied intermittently, causing analgesia that appears to be mediated by opioid peptides and learned helplessness, considered to be a model for human psychological depression and (2) applied continuously, inducing equally potent analgesia not involving opioids. The opioid but not the nonopioid form of stress suppresses the cytotoxic activity of NK cells in rats. The decrease in NK cell cytotoxicity by opioid stress is blocked by the opioid receptor antagonist naltrexone and is mimicked by systemic administration of morphine (858, 860). Morphine injected into the lateral ventricle of the brain suppresses NK cell activity to the same degree as a systemic dose three orders of magnitude higher, and this effect is also blocked by naltrexone (861). NK cell activity was unaffected by a morphine analog that does not cross the blood–brain barrier (861). These data implicate brain opiate receptors in the morphine-induced suppression of NK cell cytotoxicity. Morphine induces tolerance, i.e., repeated injections of morphine no longer result in suppression of NK cell activity, whereas foot-shock stress does not induce tolerance and is not prevented by the morphine-induced tolerance (859). The lack of tolerance and cross-tolerance with morphine might mean that the two effects on NK cells are mediated by different mechanisms or use different opiate receptors (859).

Corticotropin-releasing factor (CRF) administered as a single dose intraventricularly produced a dose-dependent suppression of rat splenic NK cell activity (862); however, neither systemic CRF nor CRF *in vitro* significantly altered NK cell activity. The NK cell-suppressive effect of CRF was antagonized by intraventricular, but not systemic, preadministration of a CRF antagonist (862). These data suggest that CRF released in the brain following stressful stimuli may have a role in controlling the modulation of NK cell cytotoxicity. The observed effect of CRF might be mediated by increased sympathoadrenal activity and/or activation of the pituitary–adrenal axis. Intraventricular administration of CRF produces an activation of sympathetic outflow and an acute increase in plasma concentrations of norepinephrine and epinephrine. Release of norepinephrine from sympathetic nerve endings innervating the spleen might then inhibit NK cell cytotoxicity (863). CRF might also act in part by stimulating the release of adrenocorticotropic hormone (ACTH) and β-endorphin from the anterior pituitary. However, the systemic administration of CRF, which does not affect NK cell cytotoxicity, is able to induce ACTH and β-endorphin release from the pituitary gland. Furthermore, the suppression of NK cells is not blocked by the peripheral administration of CRF analogs, which prevent the effect on the pituitary mediated by the centrally administered CRF. ACTH and β-endorphin therefore do not appear to play a major role in the effect of CRF on NK cells *in vivo* (862).

Tail electrode shock, as well as foot shock, induces a transient depression of NK cell activity that is prevented by the opioid antagonists naloxone or naltrexone (864). However, β-endorphin injected *in vivo* increased NK cell activity, raising some doubt about the role of endogenous opioids in the suppression of NK cell activity in this system and about the specificity of naloxone and naltrexone as opioid antagonists (864). Indeed, in several *in vitro* studies, β-endorphin, Leu-enkephalin, and Met-enkephalin actually enhanced NK cell cytotoxicity and production of IFN-γ (865–869). However, Williamson *et al.* (870) have demonstrated activation of NK cells by β-endorphin in the range 10^{-11}–$10^{-8}M$, but inhibition of NK cell activity by this opioid in the range 10^{-17}–$10^{-13}M$. Thus, it is possible that β-endorphin is present *in vivo* after stress at the low concentration that induces suppression of NK cell cytotoxicity and is responsible for the inhibition. N-acetyl-β-endorphin, which has no opioid activity, does not affect NK cell activity (870). However, nonopioid fragments of β-endorphin enhance NK cell cytotoxicity, and the effect is blocked by naloxone (871). These data raise the possibility that the enhancement of NK cell cytotoxicity by endorphin fragments is not mediated through opioid receptors. The increase in cytotoxic activity of NK cells treated with β-endorphin is due to the increased number of target-binding cells and of cytotoxic cells among binders and to increased recycling capacity (872).

The evidence to date clearly shows that the activity of NK cells, as well as other cells of the immune system, is under the control of the central nervous system and is sensitive to various neuropeptides. There is little information as to whether NK cells, like other immune cells, can produce neuropeptides. The interaction between the nervous system and the NK cells is likely to have physiological and clinical relevance, although very little is known about the mechanisms of such interactions.

VII. NK Cells and Reproduction

The hormonal control of NK cell activity is suggested by alteration in NK cell cytotoxicity during the menstrual cycle and pregnancy. One study (873) reported a significant fall in human NK cell activity during the periovulatory period, although another study (217) found no significant difference. In the mouse highest NK cell activity, corresponding to the time of the lowest metastatic potential of surgically removed mammary adenocarcinoma, occurs during the proestrus and estrus stages (874). During pregnancy, an NK cell depression is present from the first trimester to the postpartum period (875, 876). The mechanism of this depression is not clear, and both normal and decreased levels in the numbers of NK cells, in the NK cell cytotoxic potential, and in the recycling ability have been reported (877-880). The depression of NK cell cytotoxic activity in pregnancy correlates inversely with the level of 17β-estradiol in the sera of pregnant women. Treatment of mice with 17β-estradiol or diethylstilbestrol decreases NK cell cytotoxicity by decreasing the number of NK cells at the bone marrow level (881-883). Eventually, these hormones induce a condition of osteopetrosis, with destruction of the bone marrow environment and complete suppression of NK cell maturation (415). In some experimental conditions, however, 17β-estradiol treatment induced an activation of NK cells for the first 30 days, followed by NK cell depression (884). This early NK cell-stimulating effect of 17β-estradiol correlates with an estrogen-induced resistance to metastasis formation by B16 melanoma, an effect thought to be mediated by NK cells (884). *In vitro*, 17β-estradiol and diethylstilbestrol treatment of PBLs has been reported by some authors (885-887) to inhibit NK cell-mediated cytotoxicity, but not by others (888, 889).

Human, murine, and porcine embryos have been shown to recruit NK cells to the uterus (890-892). A modest increase of NK cell activity in the uterus was also observed in 17β-estradiol-induced pseudopregnancy, showing that hormonal regulation may play a role but not completely account for the sustained increase of NK cell activity in the decidua, which requires the presence of an embryo (891). In the human early pregnancy decidua 75% of the cells obtained by enzymatic digestion are of bone marrow origin (893). Immunohistological analysis showed that macrophages and $CD3^+$, $HLA-DR^+$ activated T cells predominate in the region, with prominent infiltration of the decidua by the trophoblast (894). In the area of the endometrium in which trophoblast invasion is not prominent or where it is still associated with endometrial glands or spiral arteries, the predominant cell type is that previously defined as endometrial granulocytes (895) and consisting of $CD2^+$, $CD3^-$, $CD5^-$, $CD38^+$, $NKH-1/Leu-19^+$, partly $HLA-DR^+$ cells (890, 894). These leukocytes tend to aggregate adjacent to degenerated endometrial glands or to spiral arteries (894). These granular lymphocytes are absent from term decidua. Flow-cytometric analysis of enzymatically dissociated decidua cells showed that less than 10% of the cells were $CD3^+$, on average 40% were $NKH-1/Leu-19^+$, 30% were $CD2^+$, 10% were $CD16^+$, and over 50% were $CD38^+$ (893). Two-color analysis showed that the two major cell populations were $NKH-1^+$, $CD2^+$ and $NKH-1^+$, $CD2^-$, followed by $CD16^+$ cells (mostly expressing NKH-1/Leu-19 antigen at low density) and $CD3^+$ T cells (893). Most of these cells have an LGL morphology. Thus, it appears that more than 50% of the decidua cells in the first trimester of pregnancy have a phenotype compatible with that of NK cells. Similar results have been reported in the mouse system, although the phenotype of the cell was not extensively characterized (892, 896).

NK cells are unlikely to cause damage to the embryos because blastocysts or freshly dissociated 9.5-, 11.5-, and 14-day murine embryonic cells resist NK cell lysis as well as ADCC (892, 897). Human placental trophoblast cells are almost completely resistant to NK cell-mediated cytotoxicity, but are sensitive to ADCC (873). Lytic NK cells are absent from the decidua of beige mice and are reduced in the decidua of mice treated with anti-asialo-GM_1 serum (892), although pregnancy progresses normally in these animals, suggesting that NK cells do not play an essential role for a successful pregnancy. However, those data do not exclude the presence of NK cells defective in cytotoxic potential in the decidua which could mediate noncytotoxic functions of NK cells. It is possible that NK cells affect placentation by modulating the maternal immune response in the decidua or by producing lymphokines, such as IFN-γ, which have been shown to stimulate placental growth (898). Alternatively, decidual NK cells, through cytotoxic effects or by releasing cytolytic factors such as TNF, could participate in the necrosis of endometrial tissue, facilitating the trophoblast invasion. The striking predominance of NK cells in the decidual cellular infiltrate and the activated characteristics of these cells suggested by the expression of HLA-DR and CD38 antigens cannot be easily discounted as findings with little relevance for successful implantation. The absence of CD16 antigen from most of the cells with NK cell phenotype in the decidua might also mean that these NK cells are highly activated. CD16 antigen is known to be down-modulated following interaction of NK cells with immune complexes (132) or under conditions in which protein kinase C is activated (133). The high level expression of NKH-1/Leu-19 antigen on these cells is also an indicator of activation (100). Alternatively, the $NKH-1/Leu-19^+$, $CD16^-$ NK cells may represent relatively immature NK cells that are generated by rapid proliferation of NK progenitor cells in the decidua or that have recently migrated from the bone marrow. Although there is no information on whether the NK cells in the decidua are cycling, the data suggest that the presence of an embryo induces an activation and localization of NK cells analogous to the localization observed at the site of virus infection (899). However, unlike during virus infection, systemic NK cell cytotoxic activity in early pregnancy is depressed and not stimulated.

The recruitment of NK cells may be mediated by products of the activated T cells observed in the decidua (894) or by soluble products from the endometrial cells or from the trophoblast. An alternative possible role of NK cells in the decidua is to suppress the immune response of the mother against the embryo. Decidua cells, especially at times of gestation later than those corresponding to the peak of NK cell activity, strongly suppress NK cell cytotoxic activity, as well as that of CTLs and ADCC effector cells (900, 901). Suppressor cells in the decidua also inhibit CTL generation. The suppressor cells have been identified as FcγR$^+$ non-T cell type, that can, however, be distinguished from classical NK cells because of lack of reactivity with anti-asialo-GM$_1$ serum, slower sedimentation rate, and presence in the decidua of beige mice (902). However, it is possible that the suppressor cells are NK cells at a stage of maturation or activation in which cytotoxic activity is low, and some of their antigenic and physical characteristics are different from those of resting mature NK cells with cytotoxic activity.

Although the studies described above have suggested a relative resistance of trophoblastic cells to the lytic effect of NK cells, other studies have shown that embryonal carcinoma cells are sensitive to NK cell-mediated cytotoxicity *in vitro* (530). It is therefore conceivable that if NK cell cytotoxic activity in the decidua is abnormally high, the trophoblast could be damaged. Indeed, some studies have suggested a direct correlation between NK cell activity and abortion rate. The NK cell activity of 50 women with threatened preterm delivery was found to be significantly higher than in 50 healthy pregnant women (903). In a murine model (CBA females × DBA/2J males) with a high spontaneous abortion rate, a significant correlation was found between NK cell infiltrates at 6–9 days and embryo abortion (904). In the same mouse model, poly I:C treatment was found to increase and anti-asialo-GM$_1$ serum treatment to decrease, the abortion rate in parallel with NK cell activity (905).

VIII. NK Cells and Hematopoiesis

Lymphocytes, mostly T cells, represent a small but significant proportion of bone marrow cells from healthy donors. Although NK cells originate and differentiate in the bone marrow (442), active mature

NK cells are almost entirely absent from the bone marrow of healthy donors (95). Alterations of T and NK cells in the bone marrow can be quantitative (increased number or change in the proportion of different subsets) or qualitative (activation of the cells). Although T and NK cells can produce both stimulating and inhibiting factors, bone marrow failure in one or more lineages is the hematopoietic condition most often associated with lymphocyte activation (906). The presence of inhibitory lymphocytes may represent a primary autoimmune mechanism, or they may be generated as a reaction to a pathogenic stimulus, e.g., infection or malignancy, with a secondary effect on hematopoietic cells. In some patients, the clonal or malignant expansion of a lymphocyte population with inhibitory activity is responsible for the failure of other hematopoietic cells. Lymphocytes may act directly on progenitor or stem cells or affect other accessory cell types required for growth factor production. Inhibition by lymphocytes may require direct cellular contact or be mediated via soluble factors.

A. Experimental and Clinical *in Vivo* Evidence for a Role of NK Cells in Regulation of Hematopoiesis

A role for NK cells in hematopoietic homeostasis was originally suggested by the pioneering studies by Cudkowicz and collaborators (361, 907, 908) on hybrid resistance to parental bone marrow transplantation in irradiated mice. Parental hematopoietic or lymphoid grafts do not survive in lethally irradiated F_1 hybrids, even though these animals are universal recipients of grafts of other types of parental tissue (907). The genetic control of hybrid resistance contrasts with the classical transplantation studies which show that graft compatibility rests predominantly on multiple genetic determinants of cellular antigens inherited codominantly: the histocompatibility (H) antigens. The F_1 hybrid anti-parent reaction has been explained by assuming the existence of a class of noncodominant genes, designated Hh for hematopoietic (or hybrid) histocompatibility, with tissue distribution restricted to hematopoietic cells (907). By transplanting across allogeneic and xenogeneic barriers, using recipients in which the T cell response has been abrogated by irradiation, it was possible to demonstrate an Hh-controlled allogeneic and xenogeneic resistance to hematopoietic cells that shares most of the properties of hybrid resistance (909). The characteristics of the effector cells mediating hybrid resistance (e.g., radioresistance, age of maturation, bone marrow dependence, thymus independence, sensitivity to split-dose irradiation, and lack of immunological memory) suggested their identity with NK cells (361, 908). In the mouse both hybrid resistance and NK cell activity are under similar genetic control (374) and are abrogated *in vivo* by treatment with antisera recognizing NK cells (910, 911); hybrid resistance is reduced in NK-deficient beige mice (912), and the ability to reject bone marrow in a genetically restricted way is adoptively transferred by clones with NK cell activity (913). However, the list of properties shared between the cells responsible for hybrid resistance and NK cells does not include the single most pertinent property of hematopoietic resistance, i.e., its immunogenetic specificity. The genetic restriction of natural hybrid resistance has been reproduced in an *in vitro* system in which purified murine F_1 NK cells inhibit parental granulocyte–macrophage colony-forming units (CFU-GMs) (914), although a lower but significant suppression was also observed against syngeneic progenitor cells (914, 915). The genetic specificity has been shown by *in vivo* experiments of competitive inhibition to reside at the effector cell level (916). A possible role of regulatory radioresistant T cells or of natural antibodies in determining genetic specificity of hybrid resistance has been proposed, but these models do not account for all properties of hybrid resistance (917).

In vivo NK cells suppress hematopoietic progenitors in mice experimentally infected with lymphocyte choriomeningitis virus (LCMV) (918). Adult mice injected intraperitoneally with LCMV undergo a relatively mild disease followed by marked immunological and hematological dysfunction (919, 920). During the first week of infection, there is a profound suppression of spleen CFUs (CFU-Ss) and CFU-GMs (919, 920). Erythropoiesis, as measured by ^{59}Fe uptake into hematopoietic tissue, is also markedly suppressed. After day 10 of infection, CFU-S and erythropoiesis return to levels higher than normal in spleen, whereas hematopoiesis remains depressed for over 3 weeks in bone marrow. The *in vivo* infection of mice with LCMV results in IFN production and increased NK cell activity in spleen and bone marrow (921), accompanied by the appearance of NK blasts and proliferation of NK cells (922). In the infected mice, NK cell activity and tissue distribution in the animals correlate with hematopoietic dysfunction (918) although the long-lasting bone marrow defect cannot be completely explained by the effect of NK cells. NK cell activity is detected in the bone marrow during LCMV infection, suggesting that the depression of hematopoiesis at early times during infection might be attributed to NK cells (918). The NK cells in bone marrow have the antigenic phenotype of immature NK cells, suggesting that either increased local production or delayed migration of NK cells from bone marrow accounts for the increased cytotoxic activity (918). An adoptive transfer system was used to show that irradiated LCMV-infected mice reject syngeneic bone marrow and that this resistance is almost completely abolished by treatment with anti-asialo-GM_1

antiserum, which abolishes NK cell activity (918). These experimental observations in LCMV-infected mice demonstrated that *in vivo* activated NK cells can suppress growth and proliferation of syngeneic hematopoietic progenitor cells and that this suppression can occur in organs, such as the bone marrow, in which NK cell-mediated cytotoxicity is normally low.

The possibility that NK cells play an important regulatory role in physiological hematopoiesis, at least in extramedullary sites, is strongly suggested by data showing that CFU-GM precursors in the spleen but not in the bone marrow are increased severalfold in normal mice depleted of endogenous NK cells by chronic treatment with antibody NK-1.1 (923).

In humans several clinical situations of bone marrow depression are associated with the presence of activated lymphocytes (906). In many cases the activated lymphocytes capable of hematopoietic suppression are T cells, mostly of the suppressor/cytotoxic $CD8^+$ subset (924), that express HLA-DR and CD25 activation antigens (925). The identification of NK cells as responsible for bone marrow suppression in human pathology has been difficult because of the ambiguity of distinctive characteristics between NK cells and activated T cells. The LGL morphology, typical of resting NK cells, is often presented by activated T cells, especially $CD8^+$ T cells. In several early studies antibody HNK-1/Leu-7 was used as a reagent for NK cells (146). The Leu-7 antigen is present in normal PBLs on a proportion of NK cells and in a small subset of T cells (95), and in patients with activated T cells a large proportion of $Leu-7^+$ T cells is often observed. The low-affinity FcγR recognized by anti-CD16 antibodies (95) is also expressed on T cells from some patients. Cells bearing the receptor for SRBCs (CD2 antigen) and FcγR, often referred to as Tγ cells, in normal peripheral blood correspond to the NK cell subset (95). However, in several patients with bone marrow failure (e.g., EBV infection, pure RBC aplasia during chronic lymphocytic leukemia, and LGL lymphocytosis), $CD2^+$ cells expressing FcγR and/or CD16 antigens have characteristics of T cells, i.e., they express the TCR and the TCR-associated CD3 antigen. Approximately 10% of the patients with LGL lymphocytosis present cells with $CD3^-$, $CD16^+$, $CD2^+$, $CD8^+$ or $CD8^-$, high spontaneous cytotoxic activity, and no rearrangements in the TCR genes (423, 430–432). These cells have phenotypic and functional characteristics identical to those of peripheral blood NK cells. Chan *et al.* (437) observed that nine patients with $CD3^+$ LGL lymphocytosis presented neutropenia, whereas two patients with $CD3^-$ LGL presented no abnormalities in granulopoiesis. However, other recent studies described patients with $CD3^-$, $CD16^+$ LGL lymphocytosis associated with neutropenia and anemia (438, 926, 927). Cells from two of these patients were studied *in vitro* and were shown to inhibit proliferation/differentiation of progenitor cells (926, 927).

Expansion of Leu-7$^+$ LGLs was also reported in patients with Felty's syndrome (neutropenia, arthritis, splenomegaly) and with adult-onset cyclic neutropenia (928, 929). In the patients with Felty's syndrome the Leu-7$^+$ LGLs are CD3$^+$ and of T cell origin, but, unlike in LGL lymphocytosis, the CD3$^+$ cells express the CD5 antigen and show polyclonality of TCR gene rearrangement (928, 930). On the other hand, two of three patients with cyclic neutropenia described by Loughran *et al.* (929) showed expansion of LGLs with the typical phenotype of NK cells.

B. Inhibition of *in Vitro* Hematopoiesis by Human NK Cells

It has been hypothesized that the *in vivo* role of NK cells might be surveillance of primitive cells (529). The proportion of NK cells is high in blood, spleen, and liver, but low in bone marrow and thymus. Normal primitive cell types with significant susceptibility to NK cell lysis *in vitro* can be found in bone marrow and thymus (36, 931-933).

Because progenitor cells represent only a very small proportion of bone marrow cells and their purification has presented serious technical difficulties, it has been very difficult to directly analyze a cytotoxic effect of NK cells on progenitor cells. Most of the *in vitro* evidence for a role of NK cells in inhibiting hematopoiesis comes from experiments testing the ability of purified NK cell preparations to suppress proliferation and differentiation of CFUs. Several early studies suggested that human lymphocytes with some characteristics of NK cells (e.g., light density and expression of FcγR and E receptor) inhibit both autologous and allogeneic bone marrow CFUs, that the inhibition was enhanced by pretreatment of NK cells with IFN, and that NK cell-sensitive target cells competed for the inhibition (934-937). The inhibitor cells were resistant to 10 Gy irradiation but required several hours of contact with the bone marrow cells before plating in semisolid medium, in order to mediate maximum inhibition (936). Bone marrow-derived CFU-GMs and erythrocyte CFUs (CFU-Es) are maximally inhibited by NK cells (668, 934-939), whereas inhibition of erythrocyte burst-forming units (BFU-Es) was observed in only one study (939) using HNK-1/Leu-7$^+$ cells. Two studies have shown that peripheral blood-derived CFU-GMs are not inhibited, but rather are stimulated by NK cells (122, 940).

A possible role for NK cells in inhibiting not only normal hematopoietic progenitor cells but also clonogenic growth of leukemia cells was suggested by Beran *et al.* (941), who found that allogeneic Percoll-purified NK cells prevented colony formation by the blasts of three patients with acute myeloid leukemia. The anti-leukemia cell effect of NK cells was boosted by pretreatment of effector cells with IFN. Interestingly, as observed for NK cell-mediated killing of target cell lines (34, 503), IFN treatment of the leukemic cells rendered them resistant to the suppressive effect of NK cells (941).

Degliantoni et al. (668, 938) showed that the peripheral blood cells that spontaneously suppress bone marrow hematopoietic colonies have the exact phenotype of NK cells (i.e., $CD16^+$, $NKH-1^+$, $CD3^-$, $CD5^-$, $CD4^-$, $HLA-DR^-$, mostly $CD2^+$, and, in part, $CD8^+$ and $HNK-1^+$). The suppressive effect of these cells was increased by pretreatment with IFN-α. Herrmann et al. (942) have recently analyzed the ability of human NK cell clones and $CD3^+$ T cell clones with NK cell-like cytotoxic activity to suppress in vitro hematopoiesis. The NK cell clones did not promote hematopoietic colony growth, and individual NK cell clones suppressed subpopulations of progenitor cells in a heterogeneous but clonally stable manner. The generation of the inhibitory effect required cell-to-cell contact, and maximum inhibition was observed after 8–18 hours of preincubation.

The possibility that NK cells residing in the bone marrow have an inhibitory effect on colony formation was suggested by studies showing a significant increase in the number of CFUs when NK cells were removed from bone marrow preparations using anti-CD16 antibodies and complement (943). However, in most studies the bone marrow used as the source of CFUs is obtained by aspiration and is likely to be contaminated by peripheral blood, making it difficult to establish the origin of the NK cells.

The in vivo relevance of the observed reactivity of NK cells in vitro against syngeneic progenitor cells is suggested by studies of cells from a patient with aplastic anemia that twice failed to reconstitute after engraftment with bone marrow of an identical twin (944). The patient's peripheral blood cells, with characteristics of NK cells (e.g., LGLs, $CD4^-$, $CD8^-$, cytotoxic for K562 cells) caused marked inhibition of syngeneic CFU-GM colonies (944), suggesting that NK cells might be involved in both the pathogenesis of the anemia and the rejection of the graft.

C. Role of Soluble Factors in the Modulation of Hematopoiesis by Lymphocytes

NK cells produce various types of factors, including growth factors, which affect hematopoiesis. Stimulated highly purified NK cells have been shown to produce high levels of GM-CSF and, in certain conditions, M-CSF and IL-3 (799). GM-CSF and/or IL-3 could account for the burst-promoting activity produced by NK cells (945). NK cells have also been shown to support megakaryocyte colony formation by producing a soluble CSF (945, 946); because IL-3 has the same activity, it is not clear whether IL-3 accounts for the activity produced by NK cells, or instead, whether NK cells produce a separate factor.

Inhibitory factors released by activated T cells and NK cells have also been shown to be responsible for hematopoietic suppression *in vitro* and possibly *in vivo* (947, 948). The effect of NK cell supernatant fluids on *in vitro* colony formation is a balance between these inhibitory and stimulatory activities. However, most assays of colony formation in the presence of optimal concentrations of exogenously added CSF preferentially detect inhibitory activities, whereas, in the absence of added CSF, stimulatory activity can be observed (949).

Degliantoni *et al.* (668, 938) showed that purified NK cells produce colony-inhibiting activity (NK-CIA) when cocultured for several hours with NK-sensitive cells (such as K562 cells) or with allogeneic or autologous bone marrow cells, but not with NK-insensitive cells (such as Raji cells). HLA-DR$^+$ bone marrow cells, highly enriched for hematopoietic progenitor cells, induce NK-CIA production, whereas HLA-DR$^-$ cells, depleted of precursor cells, fail to do so, suggesting that NK cells produce NK-CIA following direct interaction with the progenitor cells. The specificity of inhibition of hematopoietic colonies by NK-CIA and by NK cells was almost identical: Both inhibited CFU-GEMMs, CFU-Es, and CFU-GMs on day 14, but not BFU-Es or CFU-GMs day 7 (938). NK-CIA was synergistic with IFN-γ in inhibiting CFU-GMs on day 14; NK-CIA and IFN-γ together but not separately, also inhibited CFU-GMs on day 7 (668). The NK-CIA concentration in the supernatant fluid was sufficient to account for the inhibition of colony formation observed when NK cells were added directly to the bone marrow cells used for colony formation, although the contribution of a direct cytotoxic effect of NK cells on progenitor cells to the observed inhibitory effect cannot be ruled out. NK-CIA-containing supernatants did not contain significant amounts of IFN-α or -γ, and the NK-CIA activity was not inhibited by antibodies to IFN (668). NK-CIA inhibition of colony formation was efficiently abolished by monoclonal antibodies to TNF but not lymphotoxin (LT) (668). The NK-CIA-containing supernatants have low (0.1–10 U/ml) TNF activity, as evaluated by biological assay (cytotoxicity on actinomycin D-treated mouse L cells) or by radioimmunoassay (260). Such levels of TNF were sufficient to account for the observed inhibition of colony formation, as determined by using recombinant TNF (668, 950, 951).

Purified recombinant TNF as well as LT inhibit CFU-GEMMs, BFU-Es, and CFU-Es with similar efficiency ($\sim 50\%$ inhibition with

1 U/ml), and the inhibition is augmented by IFN-γ (951). The fact that homogeneous TNF but not supernatants from NK cells containing TNF inhibited BFU-E colonies is probably due to the fact that NK cells produce burst-promoting activity, masking the inhibition by TNF (945). Both TNF and LT poorly inhibit CFU-GMs but strongly synergize with IFN-γ in inhibiting this colony type (951). When NK and T cells simultaneously produce IFN-γ and TNF or LT, the ability of the supernatants to inhibit CFUs, because of this synergistic effect, might be almost completely abolished by anti-IFN-γ, leading to the mistaken conclusion that IFN-γ alone is responsible for the inhibition. In the study by Herrmann *et al.* (942) NK cell clones that produced both IFN-γ and NK-CIA activity inhibited erythroid and myeloid colonies, including CFU-GMs on day 7. Anti-IFN-γ monoclonal antibodies prevented the inhibition of CFU-GMs on day 7, but not of other colony types, suggesting that the inhibition was mediated by a factor (possibly TNF) acting synergistically with IFN-γ. Cells from several LGL lymphocytosis patients have been shown to produce IFN-γ (432, 438). In one case of $CD3^-$, $CD16^+$ LGL lymphocytosis, IL-2-stimulated LGL produced both IFN-γ and a CIA that was only partially abolished by anti-IFN-γ antibodies, also suggesting a synergistic effect between IFN-γ and other factors, possibly cytotoxins (438).

Because progenitor cells in peripheral blood and in bone marrow are not qualitatively different, it is difficult to interpret the data showing that bone marrow CFUs but not peripheral blood CFUs are inhibited (122, 940). However, it was recently shown that removal of NK cells from the peripheral blood of patients with β-thalassemia results in increased CFUs but that the effect of NK cell removal is abolished if adherent cells are removed (952). These data suggest that the inhibition of CFUs mediated by NK cells in the peripheral blood of the patients requires interaction with adherent cells. It is possible that the $HLA-DR^+$ cell population in bone marrow shown to induce NK-CIA/TNF formation by NK cells (938) contains a stromal or hematopoietic cell population in addition to precursor cells. This stromal/hematopoietic cell type, but not the precursor cells, could interact with NK cells and induce NK-CIA/TNF production. The absence of this accessory cell type from nonadherent preparations of peripheral blood mononuclear cells might explain the inability of NK cells to suppress CFUs from peripheral blood.

Both experimental and clinical observations support the possibility that NK cells are the cellular mediators of certain types of pathological dysregulation of hematopoiesis. *In vitro* models have offered insights into the mechanisms of interaction of NK cells with hematopoietic progenitor cells. NK cells probably directly interact with progenitor cells, with a mechanism of specificity still unknown, and are triggered to produce various soluble mediators. NK cells can produce factors with both enhancing and inhibiting activity on hematopoiesis. The activity of NK cells and their ability to produce cytotoxins are also regulated by other cell types through factors such as IL-2 and IFN-α.

The evidence for a role of NK cells in maintaining physiological hematopoietic homeostasis is much less compelling. However, if, as in many other systems, the pathological aspects of NK cell functions are interpreted to be an exaggeration of the physiological functions of this cell type, a role of NK cells in hematopoietic homeostasis can be assumed. The observation that depletion of NK cells *in vivo* does not affect bone marrow hematopoiesis, but determines a significant increase in the number of progenitor cells in the spleen (923), suggests the possibility that NK cells are mostly involved in the regulation of extramedullary hematopoiesis. This possibility is also compatible with observations in the hybrid resistance system (912), with NK cell organ distribution, and with the localization of their effect against metastatic diffusion of tumors or parasite infection (23).

D. NK Cells and Graft-versus-Host Reaction

The pathogenesis of acute graft-versus-host disease (GVHD), a major complication of allogeneic bone marrow transplantation, remains obscure. The identity of the effector cells involved in acute GVHD is still controversial, and CTLs, NK cells, and a decreased activity of suppressor T cells have all been implicated, but none of these cell types has been definitively incriminated in the production of target cell injury *in vivo*.

In humans Lopez *et al.* (953–955) found an association between high pretransplantation NK cell activity in the recipient against HSV-1-infected target cells and incidence of GVHD after bone marrow transplantation. However, in other studies, no correlation was found with NK cell cytotoxic activity against K562 target cells (953, 956, 957) or, in one study (957), against HSV-1-infected target cells. The failure to reproduce the original finding of an association between NK cell activity in the recipient and GVHD is probably due to the number of different factors that affect measurement of NK cell activity *in vitro*, making it impossible to use this activity as a clinical prognostic indicator of GVHD. However, the data of Lopez *et al.* (953–955) are in agreement with observations in experimental animals, as detailed below, and represent suggestive important evidence of a role for NK cells in both the inductive and effector phases of GVHD.

Dokhelar *et al.* (467) reported further evidence supporting a role for NK cells in human GVHD by showing that the occurrence of acute

GVHD was associated with an early appearance of maximal NK cell activity within 2-4 weeks of transplantation, whereas in patients without acute GVHD NK cell activity was restored later. More direct evidence of NK cell participation is represented by *in situ* analysis during GVHD of human rectal mucosa (958) and skin (959), in which cells with immunohistochemical features of NK cells were detected. In the murine model of GVHD induced by bone marrow transplantation between strains differing only in the minor histocompatibility antigens, Guillen *et al.* (960) demonstrated that the prepondcrant mononuclear cells in GVHD lesional skin have phenotypic characteristics of NK cells. These cells have the morphology and ultrastructure of LGLs with typical vesicles and PTAs, express asialo-GM_1, Thy-1, and CD11b (MAC-1) antigens, but are mostly Ly-1 and Ly-2 negative. Membrane association was observed between LGLs and degenerating keratinocytes, including apposition of cell membranes and invagination of elongated microvilli of mononuclear cells into adjacent degenerating keratinocytes (960). On the basis of this association and a granule morphology suggesting discharge or dissolution of the granule contents, it has been postulated that the NK cells are directly cytotoxic for the keratinocytes (960). However, it has recently been reported in a similar mouse model that anti-TNF antibodies *in vivo* completely prevent acute GVHD (961). Because activated NK cells are powerful producers of TNF (78), it is possible that the tissue necrosis observed is mediated by TNF and not by NK cell-mediated cytotoxicity. Alternatively, TNF may act as an immune potentiating cytokine that enhances the cytotoxic/necrotic effect of NK cells and, possibly, of macrophages and neutrophils.

Although the data presented above provide compelling evidence for a major role of NK cells in the effector phase of GVHD, the role of NK cells in the inductive phase and their host or donor origin remain controversial. In experimental animals (962) and possibly in humans (963) elimination of mature T cells from the bone marrow graft prevents GVHD. A role for transplantation antigen-specific T cells in the initiation of most cases of GVHD is certain. NK cells might be recruited by the products of T cells as effector cells, but they might also participate in the induction phase, providing necessary help for the T cell response (see Section X). Various experimental systems have been utilized to demonstrate the requirement of host or donor NK cells in GVHD. When +/*bg* (normal NK cell activity) or *bg*/*bg* (deficient NK cell activity) mice were used as the host or donor of bone marrow cells, early splenomegaly and moderate B cell suppression were observed in all of the combinations. However, +/*bg* but not *bg*/*bg* bone marrow cells were able to induce severe GVHD with histopathological lesions and profound B and T cell suppression in either *bg*/*bg* or +/*bg* recipients (964). These results suggest that donor NK cells rather than host NK cells play an active role in GVHD-associated tissue damage and long-term immune suppression. Elimination of either asialo-GM_1^+ (965) or NK-1.1^+ (966) cells from transplanted bone marrow did not prevent GVHD, indicating that mature donor NK cells were not required. However, when donor mice were stimulated with *in vivo* allogeneic immunization, maturation of a proportion of lymphocytes, possibly NK progenitors, from asialo-GM_1^- to asialo-GM_1^+ was observed (965). When bone marrow from these immunized animals was used for transplantation, treatment of the animals with anti-asialo-GM_1 serum before marrow harvest prevented GVHD in the recipients (965). Thus, both mature and precursor NK cells in the bone marrow graft might generate GVHD.

Other studies have shown that treatment of the recipient with anti-asialo-GM_1 serum prevents GVHD following semiallogeneic bone marrow transplantation in irradiated (967) or unirradiated (968) animals. In animals treated with anti-asialo-GM_1 serum the anti-host CTL response (967) and the enhancement of NK cell activity (968) found in the control grafted animals were suppressed.

The most likely interpretation of these apparently contradictory results is that radioresistant NK cells are required in the host to provide necessary helper function for the generation of alloantigen-specific CTLs. This helper function of NK cells might be present in the noncytotoxic NK cells from beige mice, as suggested by the development of GVHD in *bg/bg* mice transplanted with +/*bg* bone marrow (964). Probably secondary to CTL activation, donor NK cells or NK progenitor cells are activated and induced to proliferate, generating the early and elevated reconstitution of NK cell activity after transplantation. These activated NK cells probably represent the effector cells of GVHD without antigenic specificity. The lack of antigenic specificity of this phase of the GVHD is elegantly demonstrated by experiments in which a graft of fetal intestine syngeneic with the bone marrow donor was implantad under the kidney capsule of mice undergoing GVHD (969). Although the intestine should not have been recognized by the anti-host CTLs, it was nonetheless rapidly infiltrated by lymphocytes and presented the same pathological aspects (e.g., villus atrophy and crypt hyperplasia) observed in the recipient intestine.

IX. Antimicrobial Activity of NK Cells

A. ANTIVIRAL ACTIVITY OF NK CELLS

A central role for NK cells in the defense against virus infection in humans is strongly suggested by the prevalently viral pathology in the few patients who have a selective absolute deficiency of NK cells (375, 377). These patients show frequent infections with varicella zoster, CMV, EBV, and other viruses. Unlike patients with X-LPD, in whom the NK cell defect is subsequent to EBV infection and might be induced by the virus (339), the NK cell-deficient patients had a history of repeated viral infection before EBV infection (375).

NK cells, together with IFN and other natural resistance mechanisms, represent the first line of defense of the organism against infection by certain viruses, before humoral and cellular effectors of adaptive immunity are activated. During virus infection, an NK cell response, which usually peaks at 3 days postinfection, is followed by a CTL response, which peaks at 7-9 days postinfection (921). Mice acutely infected with LCMV are characterized by high levels of virus-induced IFN and NK cell activity in spleen, peritoneum, liver, lung, bone marrow, and peripheral blood (17, 899, 918, 921, 970, 971). The increase in NK cell activity is due to an absolute increase in the number of NK cells, originating *de novo* from the bone marrow, as indicated by the prevention of activation of NK cells by HU treatment (922, 972). NK cells in the infected mice have blast morphology, are of lighter density than are those in control mice, and are replicating, as shown by experiments combining single-cell cytotoxic assay and autoradiography using NK cells pulsed with[^{3}H]thymidine (972). Similar *in vivo* activation and proliferation of NK cells are observed when mice are treated with IFN or with IFN-inducers such as poly I:C (734), suggesting that the effect of virus infection on NK cell blastogenesis *in vivo* is mediated through IFN induction.

Although virus-infected mice show systemic activation of NK cells, there is also a preferential localization of NK cells in the infected organs, as shown by higher peritoneal accumulation of LGLs when viruses are injected intraperitoneally rather than intravenously and by higher liver accumulation of NK cells observed with infection by hepatotropic viruses than by nonhepatotropic viruses (899, 973). Production of chemotactic factors at sites of virus replication is at least partially responsible for NK cell or LGL accumulation at these sites, as suggested by the presence of *in vitro* chemotactic activity for NK cells and other cell types in the washout fluid from the peritoneal cavity of virus-infected animals (922).

LCMV infection is very efficient in inducing NK cell activation *in vivo*. However, experimental evidence suggests that NK cells do not play a primary role in protecting the mice against this virus (974–976). The inflammatory exudate found in the cerebrospinal fluid of mice after intracerebral infection with LCMV contains a substantial population of NK cells in addition to CTLs; however, various experimental protocols, including adoptive cell transfer, suggest that NK cells, even if they participate in the inflammatory process, are not uniquely required for the induction of neurological symptoms (977). On the other hand, the severity of the encephalopathy induced in mice by intracerebral injection of influenza virus is significantly reduced by elimination of NK cells *in vivo* using anti-asialo-GM_1 serum (978). Thus it appears that under conditions in which NK cells are unable to prevent the virus infection, they might participate in the pathogenic process itself.

CMV infection of the mouse is presently the system with the most convincing evidence that NK cells play a role in resistance to virus infection *in vivo*. This was shown by correlative experiments in different mouse strains, by altering NK cell activity *in vivo* with stimulators and inhibitors, including treatment with anti-asialo-GM_1 antiserum, and by adoptive transfer experiments (976, 979, 980). Injection of anti-asialo-GM_1 antiserum up to the third day of infection increases the virus titer up to 1000-fold (980). However, systemic treatment with anti-asialo-GM_1 serum does not exacerbate infection by mouse CMV administered intranasally (980). This phenomenon, originally interpreted as evidence against a role for NK cells in protection against viral infection in the lung, is now known to be due to a compartmentalization of lung NK cells, which respond poorly to systemic stimuli but can be efficiently activated in their antiviral function by local stimulation (315, 981).

It is possible to speculate why NK cells are very efficient against certain viruses but not others. IFN production is a constant feature of virus infection and IFN renders tissue cells resistant to the lysis mediated by both resting and activated NK cells (34, 503, 570). Because cells infected by most viruses are not protected against NK cells by IFN, due to the inhibition of host RNA and protein synthesis, IFN protection of normal but not infected target cells was proposed as a major mechanism by which NK cell cytotoxicity is directed toward virus-infected cells and spare uninfected cells (34, 569). This theory predicted that NK cells would not be effective *in vivo* against viruses that do not shut off host RNA and protein synthesis during cell infection. Cells infected by such viruses would be protected by IFN and therefore not lysed by NK cells. The work of Welsh and collaborators (511, 570, 976, 982) has provided supportive evidence for this hypothesis by showing that (1) normal cells such as thymocytes are protected *in vivo* by IFN against NK cell cytotoxicity during LCMV infection and (2) infection of target cells with viruses sensitive to NK cells *in vivo*, such as mouse CMV, prevents the protective effect of IFN, whereas LCMV does not.

The role of NK cells in the defense against infection by HSV-1 in mice is controversial. Original data that anti-asialo-GM_1 serum suppresses resistance to HSV-1 infection (983) were challenged by the observation that the antiserum suppresses both NK cell activity and IFN production

(984). The use of lower concentrations of anti-asialo-GM_1 serum that were able to block NK cell activity but not IFN production failed to confirm a role of NK cells against HSV-1, and adoptive transfer experiments were also inconclusive in supporting a role for NK cells (984). More recently, however, adoptive transfer of purified NK-1.1^+, asialo-GM_1^+ NK cells in cyclophosphamide-treated mice has been shown to induce protection against HSV-1 infection, providing direct evidence for a role of NK cells in protection against development of fatal infection in mice (985). These data also point to the need for caution in interpreting studies that fail to demonstrate a role for NK cells against other viruses. Several adaptive and nonadaptive mechanisms of resistance to virus infection are simultaneously active in the organism. When one mechanism fails or is suppressed, it seems reasonable to expect that other mechanisms might compensate, making it difficult to dissect the role of a particular mechanism. In this respect, it is interesting that the IFN titer *in vivo* in mouse CMV-infected mice is higher when NK cells are ablated by anti-asialo-GM_1 serum treatment (976). Experimental evidence, even if not always conclusive, suggests a role for NK cells in the defense against infection by mouse hepatitis virus, vesicular stomatitis virus, influenza virus, togaviruses, retroviruses, poxviruses, and also non-enveloped viruses such as coxsackie B and encephalomyocarditis viruses (982).

Studies of NK cell activity during virus infection in patients are rare, and in most cases the available information is not based on sufficiently standardized assays. Enhanced NK and K cell activity has been observed during several acute virus infections (986-992). An increase in NK cell activity was observed in renal transplant patients during CMV infection (986), and a significant correlation was found between fatal CMV infection and failure to develop NK cell activity in immunosuppressed bone marrow transplant recipients (993). A correlation has also been observed between susceptibility to HSV-1 infection and low NK cell activity against HSV-1-infected target cells in newborns and in patients with acquired immunodeficiency syndrome (AIDS) (992, 994).

In vitro, human NK cells efficiently lyse virus-infected cells. Cytotoxicity against HSV-1-infected target cells was originally shown to be due either to an ADCC mechanism induced by minimal concentrations of antibodies produced *in vitro* (995) or to cross-linking mediated by immune complexes or aggregated Igs between FcγR$^+$ effector cells and the FcR induced by HSV-1 infection on the target cells (996). However, antibody-independent natural cytotoxicity was demonstrated on mumps-infected target cells (997), an observation subsequently extended to target cells infected by a variety of viruses (34, 998, 999), demonstrating that

(1) sensitivity of virus-infected target cells to NK cell cytotoxicity was not significantly different from that of noninfected target cells, but infected cells induced activation of NK cells, resulting in increased killing of the infected (and uninfected bystander) target cells starting after 3-4 hours of culture, (2) activation of NK cell cytotoxicity was concomitant with the production of IFN-α by the PBL preparations used as a source of NK cells, and (3) the IFN-α released into the supernatant was able to stimulate the cytotoxic activity of fresh PBLs. These data served to identify IFN-α as the major factor responsible for the enhanced NK cell cytotoxicity against virus-infected target cells.

An IFN-independent cytotoxic mechanism was described particularly for target cells infected with paramyxovirus and myxoviruses. Lysis against these target cells can be blocked by antibodies to viral glycoproteins, specifically hemagglutinin, and purified glycoproteins can activate the effector cells (999-1002). Antibodies to the glycoproteins do not block the cytotoxicity if added after the glycoproteins have activated the effector cells. This type of cytotoxicity has been defined as virus-dependent cellular cytotoxicity (VDCC) (1003) and has characteristics quite different from those of the NK cell-mediated lysis of virus-infected target cells. The increase in cytotoxicity is observed within 3-4 hours after the treatment of PBLs with glycoproteins, at a time in which NK cell-mediated killing of virus-infected target cells is usually not observed (1001). This type of killing is reminiscent of lectin-dependent cytotoxicity and both NK cells and CD3$^+$ T cells are able to mediate VDCC and lectin-dependent killing (1004-1008). In other experimental models target cells infected by herpesviruses have been shown to be lysed mostly or exclusively by NK cells (510, 1009, 1010). Interestingly, the nature of the infected target cells seems to indicate which type of effector cells is involved: mumps virus-infected Chang target cells were lysed only by CD3$^-$ effector cells, whereas mumps virus-infected T24 cells were lysed by both CD3$^-$ and CD3$^+$ effector cells (1007). This observation may indicate different mechanisms of lysis that may or may not involve IFN. In the murine system HSV-1-infected YAC-1 cells are lysed by NK cells activated by a mechanism involving exclusively IFN activation, whereas HSV-1-infected WEHI-164 cells are lysed by NC cells that are not stimulated by IFN (1011). The possible involvement of NC cells is interesting because the cytotoxicity of NC cells is mostly mediated by TNF, and it was recently shown that NK cell clones can also lyse vesicular stomatitis virus (VSV)-infected target cells through the release of TNF (1012).

It is difficult to evaluate the relative participation of VDCC and IFN-mediated activation of NK cells in the cytotoxicity of PBLs against virus-infected target cells. Casali and Oldstone (1013) have shown that lysis of measles-infected target cells occurs in two phases. The first phase occurs within 4 hours and is blocked by antibody to the hemagglutinin glycoprotein but is not blocked by antibody to IFN; the second phase of lysis occurs betwen 8 and 16 hours and is inhibited by antibody to IFN. Because enhanced lysis of virus-infected target cells in most experimental systems is not detectable until 4 hours (Fig. 3), it is possible that VDCC requires a very high density of viral glycoproteins on the target cell surface and does not play a major role in most *in vitro* systems.

Activation of human NK cells has also been shown with influenza hemagglutinin in an IFN-independent system (1014). Those results were confirmed using recombinant influenza virus proteins (nonstructural protein 1, alone or fused with the hemagglutinin or matrix protein) but in this case, the activation of NK cells was shown to be mediated entirely by IFN-α induced by the virus proteins (1015).

The hypothesis that IFN is a major inducer of NK cell activation against virus-infected target cells has been challenged by several authors (512, 513, 1016–1019) on the basis that (1) antibodies against IFN do not block cytotoxicity, (2) IFN-activated NK cells are able to lyse virus-infected target cells more efficiently than uninfected ones, and (3) using as effector cells PBLs from normal donors or immunodeficient patients, there is no correlation between IFN titer in the supernatant fluid and cytotoxicity. Although the third observation can be easily explained by factors such as the variable response of PBLs of different donors to IFN stimulation, the characteristics of the dose–response curve for IFN-mediated NK cell activation, and the possibility of other mechanisms operating together with IFN, the underpinnings of the first two points are less obvious. The inability of anti-IFN antibodies to inhibit cytotoxicity might rest in the use of the antibodies at concentrations too low to efficiently inhibit, before NK cell activation, the high concentrations of IFN expected to be present in the intercellular space in the cell pellet. Also, both the antiviral and the NK cell-activating activities of IFN can be transferred directly from cell to cell, without secretion of IFN into medium containing anti-IFN antibodies (1020, 1021). The ability of IFN-stimulated NK cells to lyse virus-infected cells more efficiently than uninfected cells suggests that virus-infected target cells are intrinsically more sensitive to NK cells. These results have been reported by some laboratories (1016, 1018), whereas others found a similar or lower lysis of infected versus uninfected target cells when optimally stimulated NK cells were used (79, 511–513). The interpretation of these results is complicated by the facts that maximal activation of NK cells may not always be obtained, that IFN produced during an 18-hour cytotoxic assay further increases or at least maintains the cytotoxic activity of the IFN-treated PBLs, and that IFN, when added to the assay, protects the uninfected but not the infected target cells from lysis, mimicking the higher sensitivity of the virus-infected target cells.

Because the cells that produce IFN-α in cultures of PBLs and virus-infected target cells share some characteristics with NK cells, e.g., similar density on a Percoll gradient, it was proposed that NK cells produce IFN-α and therefore stimulate themselves with an autocrine mechanism (821). However, it was found that the major type of IFN-α-producing cells in response to CMV, HSV-1, and influenza virus infection is a light-density, nonadherent, HLA-DR$^+$, non-NK, non-B, non-T cell type that represents no more than 1–2% of PBLs (92, 510, 827, 828). The lineage of this cell type is not known, but it can be clearly distinguished from monocyte/macrophages and from dendritic cells on the basis of antigenic and adherence characteristics (92; S. Bandyopadhyay, personal communication). The killing of virus-infected target cells, but not of K562 target cells, by CD16$^+$, HLA-DR$^-$ NK cells has an absolute requirement for the IFN-α-producing HLA-DR$^+$ cells (510, 1022, 1023). The HLA-DR$^+$ cells in contact with virus-infected target cells produce a factor that activates NK cells, as shown by supernatant fluid transfer or by separating the HLA-DR$^+$ cells and CD16$^+$ NK cells by filters (510). In both cases the NK cell-activating activity is completely blocked by anti-IFN-α antibodies (510). The same antibodies do not prevent lysis of virus-infected cells by total PBLs (510), as was also described in other studies (1016, 1018). However, anti-IFN-α antibodies efficiently inhibit cytotoxicity on virus-infected target cells when the cultures are rocked to reduce cellular interactions or when the number of HLA-DR$^+$ cells in the culture, normally in large excess, is reduced to the minimal concentration required for efficient cytotoxicity (S. Bandyopadhyay, personal communication). These results strongly support the original hypothesis that activation of NK cells by IFN-α is the major and most efficient mechanism responsible for the enhanced lysis of virus-infected target cells by PBLs *in vitro*. However, other mechanisms, such as the direct interaction of NK cells with IFN-α-producing cells or with viral glycoproteins on the target cell surface are likely to play a role in the activation of NK cells.

B. NK Cells in Bacterial and Parasitic Infection

A role for microbial infection in the maturation and activity of NK cells is supported by data showing earlier maturation and increased NK cell activity in newborn mice or piglets maintained in normal colony conditions versus germ-free animals (276, 1024).

Infection of mice with various bacterial strains such as *Listeria monocytogenes* or *Chlamydia trachomatis* induces a systemic increase of NK cell activity, which peaks at day 3 and returns to normal levels at day 7 in the bone marrow and spleen, but remains increased for more than 10 days in the peripheral blood and peritoneal exudate (1025, 1026). However, no direct role in the resistance to *L. monocytogenes* infection could be attributed to NK cells, because the increase in NK cell cytotoxicity was observed in strains of mice genetically resistant or sensitive to *L. monocytogenes* infection (1025, 1027) and treatment of mice with ^{89}Sr to suppress NK cell activity had no effect on this infection (1028).

It is possible that the major role of NK cells against bacterial infection is the production of lymphokines such as IFN-γ, GM-CSF, TNF, and macrophage-chemotactic factor that activate other effector cells of nonadaptive resistance. However, in some experimental conditions *in vitro* NK cells have been shown to be able to directly lyse extracellular bacteria (1029, 1030) or cells infected with intracellular bacteria, such as *Shigella flexneri*-infected HeLa cells (1031), or monocytes infected with *Legionella pneumophila* (1032) or *Mycobacterium avium* (1033). Recently, purified CD16$^+$, NKH-1/Leu-19$^+$ NK cells have been shown to kill both gram-positive and -negative bacteria. This bactericidal activity is mediated at least in part by an extracellular mechanism involving soluble factors (1034). Treatment of human lymphocytes *in vitro* with fixed *Shigella* or *Salmonella* bacteria induces activation of NK cells and production of both IFN-α and -γ (1035–1037). The cytotoxic NK cells generated have been shown to be Leu-19$^+$ cells, most of which bear the CD16 antigen but not T cell antigens (1036, 1037). The activation of NK cells is also observed using bacteria concentrations too low to induce IFN production, suggesting the possibility that the enhancement of cytotoxicity is due to a direct effect of the bacteria on NK cells and that it is not mediated by IFN (1036). Elimination of CD16$^+$ NK cells from the lymphocyte preparation almost completely eliminates the production of IFN (1037), suggesting that at least the IFN-γ induced in PBL preparations by bacteria is produced by NK cells. Similar results indicating the production of IFN-γ by NK cells have been obtained with murine NK cells induced by *L. pneumophila* (1038). Bacterial lipopolysaccharide (LPS) from *Salmonella* fails to induce IFN production or NK cell activation and inhibits NK cell stimulation by the fixed bacteria (1035, 1037). However, LPS from *Escherichia coli*, *Pseudomonas aeruginosa*, or human periodontal pathogens plays a central role in the activation of NK cells by these bacteria (1039, 1040). LPS is internalized in NK cells and induces an increase in cytotoxic as well as phagocytic activities for opsonized bacteria. This functional effect is accompanied by morphological changes (e.g., dilatation of the intracellular membrane compartment, formation of tubuloreticular inclusions, and increase in acid phosphatase activity) that are reminiscent of those induced by IFN (1040).

Soluble streptococcal products also activate NK cells and induce IFN-γ production (1041). The increase in cytotoxicity induced by these products is mostly mediated by the IFN-γ (1041). Streptococcal preparation OK432, often used in therapeutic trials, also has strong IFN-inducing and NK cell-enhancing activity (1042, 1043). *In vivo*, OK432 stimulates an increase in NK cell generation in the bone marrow and the appearance of proliferating NK cells in spleen (1043).

Murine and human NK cells can bind and inhibit growth of fungi such as *Cryptococcus neoformans*, *Paracoccidioides brasiliensis*, and *Coccidioides immitis* (1044–1046). There is some evidence that NK cells play a role in controlling cryptococcal infection. Beige mice are less resistant to *C. neoformans* infection than are their normal heterozygous littermates (1047), and the ability of cyclophosphamide-treated mice to clear the fungus is restored by adoptive transfer of normal spleen cells but not by that of spleen cells treated with anti-asialo-GM_1 serum (1048). *In vivo* treatment with anti-asialo-GM_1 serum or anti-NK-1.1 monoclonal antibodies reduces the lung clearance of intravenously injected *C. neoformans*, but has no effect on long-term survival of the mice (1049). The colonization of *C. neoformans* to lung, spleen, and brain after infection via the respiratory route is also not affected by *in vivo* depletion of NK cells (1049). Thus, NK cells have activity against *C. neoformans* but do not appear to play an essential role in the defense against infection in the normal host, although their activity might be required in the immune-compromised host.

Candida albicans enhances NK cell activity (1050) and induces production of TNF from NK cells and monocytes (1051). However, NK cells do not kill *C. albicans*, although an excess of *C. albicans* blocks NK cell lysis of K562 cells (1052). NK cells may participate in the defense against *C. albicans* infection by secreting TNF, IFN-γ, or other lymphokines that activate the fungicidal activity of neutrophils and macrophages (1053).

Few studies have been published on the possible role of NK cells in the defense against protozoa. *In vivo* infection with *Toxoplasma* or *Plasmodium* is associated with increased NK cell activity (1054, 1055). A role for NK cells in the defense against these pathogens is suggested by the shorter survival time of *Plasmodium berghei*-infected beige mice than normal mice (1056), and by the ability of murine NK cells to lyse *Toxoplasma gondii in vitro* (1057). NK cell activation in acute infection and depression in chronic infection has been demonstrated in mice infected with

Leishmania (1058). Studies employing beige mice, split-dose irradiation, and adoptive transfer of an NK cell clone have suggested a possible role for NK cells in the clearance of *Leishmania* from spleen and liver (1059). NK cells show little spontaneous cytotoxicity for trypanosomes, but efficient ADCC (1060). Trypanosomes are not efficiently lysed by NK cell granular pore-forming proteins, but are sensitive to a Ca^{2+}-independent granule lytic protein (1060).

X. NK Cells and Adaptive Immunity

A. Immunoregulatory Role of NK Cells on B Cell Response

Moretta *et al.* (1061) originally showed that E-rosetting $Fc\gamma R^+$ lymphocytes, after interaction with immune complexes, suppress the polyclonal B cell differentiation induced by pokeweed mitogen (PWM). E-rosetting $Fc\gamma R^+$ cells are now known to be almost exclusively $CD2^+$, $CD16^+$ NK cells. Lobo (1062) showed that non-E-rosetting $Fc\gamma R^+$ cells, probably corresponding to the $CD2^-$ subset of NK cells, spontaneously enhanced PWM-induced B cell differentiation but suppressed it after interaction with immune complexes, providing the first experimental evidence that NK cells might have both enhancing and suppressive effects on B cell response. The effect of NK cells on PWM-induced B cell differentiation was attributed to an indirect effect of NK cells on helper T cells rather than to a direct effect on B cells (1061, 1063). A murine NK cell clone was shown to inhibit B cell response both *in vivo* and *in vitro* (1064). Although some studies have shown that B cells at different stages of activation are sensitive to the lytic effect of NK cells (1064–1066), this sensitivity has not always been confirmed (1067) and most evidence from different experimental systems suggests that B cell lysis by NK cells during an immune response is not a major mechanism by which NK cells modulate B cell response.

The human suppressor cells activated by immune complexes were further identified as NK cells by reactivity with antibody HNK-1/Leu-7: the ER^-, HNK-1/Leu-7^+ cells were more suppressive than were ER^+, HNK-1/Leu-7^+ cells, suggesting a role for NK cells rather than for HNK-1/Leu-7^+ T cells (1068). Suppressor ability of NK cells [identified by HNK-1/Leu-7 (1069) or CD16 (1070) expression] was shown to be activated by IFN-α, whereas a subset of suppressor T cells was activated by PWM (1069). Within the $CD8^+$ cells, $CD8^+$, $CD11b^-$ T cells required the presence of $CD4^+$, $2H4^+$ suppressor/inducer cells to suppress PWM-induced B cell differentiation, whereas $CD8^+$, $CD11b^+$ cells (mostly NK cells) did not require the inducer cell population and, unlike suppressor T cells, were enhanced in their suppressor effect by IL-2 (1071). In addition to their suppressive action on PWM-induced B cell differentiation, human NK cells suppress ongoing Ig synthesis by *in vivo* activated B lymphoblasts secreting anti-tetanus toxoid antibodies (1069), by EBV-induced B cells (1070), and by certain lymphoblastoid cell lines (1072), although they enhance Ig synthesis by other cell lines (1072). These results suggest that NK cells can interact directly with B cells and modulate their activity. The possible involvement of at least some of the mechanisms of the lytic process in suppression of the B cell response by NK cells is suggested by the competitive effect of a low number of K562 target cells (1069), by the ability of antibody 13.1 (anti-gp200) to inhibit both NK cell-mediated cytotoxicity and Ig synthesis suppression (1073), and by the possible involvement in both mechanisms of the B cell TfR, as indicated by the reversal of the inhibitory effect in the presence of iron ions (1074).

Normal human and murine bone marrow contains potent natural suppressor cells. The human natural suppressor cells are HNK-1/Leu-7$^+$ and devoid of T cell markers, and possibly include mature or immature NK cells (1075). In murine bone marrow natural suppressor cells are radiation-sensitive Qa-2$^+$ cells that express markers of mature NK cells only after stimulation with IL-2-containing conditioned medium, suggesting that they might be proliferating pre-NK cells (1076). The same cells appear to be responsible for "veto" activity, i.e., they are able to specifically prevent the generation of CTLs directed against their own MHC antigens (1076).

The presence of HNK-1/Leu-7$^+$ cells in the germinal center of lymphoid follicles was originally considered as morphological evidence for the involvement of NK cells in the immune response, but these cells have now been identified as CD4$^+$ T cells without NK cell cytotoxic activity (154, 1077).

Treatment of mice with anti-NK-1.1 serum before or at the time of immunization with either T cell-dependent or -independent antigens induces a severalfold increase in the number of antibody-forming cells in the spleen (1066, 1078). Injection of antiserum 8 hours after immunization has no effect, suggesting that the suppressive effect of NK cells is mostly at the induction phase of the B cell response (1066, 1078). *In vivo* treatment with anti-asialo-GM$_1$ serum enhances the IgM response to different types of pneumococcal polysaccharides, in both adult and weanling mice (1079). Because weanling mice do not have cytotoxic NK cells but do have a normal number of cells with phenotypic characteristics of NK cells, it is possible that NK cells are able to suppress the B cell response even when their cytotoxic activity is absent, because of either immaturity or suppression (1079). In all of these experimental systems, in which depletion of NK cells enhances the B cell response, *in vivo* activation of NK cells with poly I:C is accompanied by inhibition of the B cell response (1066, 1079).

In contrast with the studies showing an effect of NK cells mostly on the induction phase of the B cell response, Abruzzo and Rowley (1080) proposed that NK cells have an homeostatic effect on the antibody response by both inhibiting induction and promoting termination of the primary IgM response *in vivo* when administered in animals up to 3 days after immunization. Poly I:C or IFN treatments resulted in inhibition or termination of the IgM response (1081) and in activation of NK cells able to suppress B cell responses *in vitro*. The involvement of NK cells in the normal homeostasis of immunity was suggested by the fact that immunization itself induced NK cell activation with a peak at 2-3 days using T cell-independent antigens and at 4-5 days using T cell-dependent antigens (1081). The suppressive effect of NK cells is not antigen specific and the immunized mice showed a generalized IgM hyporesponsiveness to unrelated antigens, corresponding to the peaks of NK cell activation induced by the primary immunization (1081). This hyporesponsiveness was abolished in mice in which NK cell activity was depressed by treatment with pristane, by growth of a transplantable fibrosarcoma, or by repeated injection of poly I:C (1081). The NK cells in this experimental model have been shown to act by suppressing the accessory capacity of dendritic cells exposed to antigens (1080). This effect on dendritic cells and the suppressive effect of NK cells on the B cell response was shown to be mediated by Thy-1$^-$ NK cells but not by Thy-1$^+$ NK cells (1082).

Evidence for an enhancing effect of NK cells on the B cell response was provided by studies showing that NK cells, in the absence of T cells, support the *in vitro* antigen-specific murine B cell response in T cell-replacing, factor-dependent systems or upon *in vitro* stimulation with T cell-independent antigens (1083, 1084). In these systems, the enhancing effect of NK cells was mediated by the production of IFN-γ (1083, 1084).

The supernatant of unstimulated purified NKH-1/Leu-19$^+$ human NK cells was found to enhance ongoing IgE, IgG, and IgA syntheses from appropriate B cell lines, without increasing cell proliferation (1085). This late-acting B cell differentiation activity was produced by CD3$^-$, but not CD3$^+$, NKH-1/Leu-19$^+$ cells and was found to be different from that of other known lymphokines with partially overlapping activities (1085). PBLs from patients after T cell-depleted allogeneic bone marrow transplantation contain an expanded and activated NK cell population; these PBLs spontaneously produce IL-2, IFN-γ, and B cell differentiation factor and provide non-antigen-specific help for Ig production by autologous B cells, more consistently observed after treatment of the cells with anti-CD2 antibodies (1086, 1087). Anti-CD2 antibodies, which moderately inhibit NK cell cytotoxicity, might prevent a suppressive or toxic effect of NK cells on B cells, although anti-CD18 antibodies, which suppress cytotoxicity of K562 target cells more efficiently than do anti-CD2 antibodies, have no effect on B cell response (1086).

Purified human $CD3^-$, NKH-1/Leu-19$^+$ NK cells are induced to express FcεR or FcαR on 10–20% of the cells, when exposed to IgE–anti-IgE or IgA–anti-IgA immune complexes, respectively. Supernatant fluids enhanced IgE or IgA syntheses from Ig-secreting B cell lines in an isotype-specific fashion without increasing proliferation (1088). Thus, NK cells, but not $CD3^+$ T cells, express isotype-specific FcR and produce differentiation factors for that isotype after interaction with specific Ig isotypes in complexes (1088). NK cells incubated with IgE complexes react with antibody anti-CD23, specific for the low-affinity FcεR; fragments of the FcεR are able to become soluble IgE-binding factors able to regulate IgE synthesis (1089)

Human NK cell clones can produce B cell differentiation factors that induce Ig production from B cell lines and can induce Ig synthesis from purified B cells only when the NK cell clones are cocultured with the B cells (1090). TNF and IFN-γ are among the factors produced by NK cell clones and by non-MHC-restricted CTL clones that enhance *in vitro* antibody formation (R. F. Schmidt, personal communication).

B. Immunoregulatory Role of NK Cells on T Cell Response

Treatment of mice with anti-asialo-GM_1 serum prevents the induction of alloantigen-specific CTLs *in vivo* by immunization with allogeneic spleen cells (1091, 1092). The same requirement for asialo-GM_1^+ cells in the generation *in vitro* of alloantigen-specific CTLs was shown in one study (1092), whereas many other studies (1091, 1093–1095) have shown that asialo-GM_1^+ murine NK cells or $CD16^+$ human NK cells suppress *in vitro* T lymphocyte proliferation or generation of CTLs and that this suppressive effect is enhanced by IFN-α.

NK cells suppress CTL generation and T cell proliferation in allogeneic or autologous mixed-leukocyte culture by suppressing or eliminating dendritic cells that have interacted with antigen (1094, 1096). In secondary mixed-leukocyte cultures, which are efficiently stimulated by either dendritic cells or macrophages, NK cells suppress only the stimulation by dendritic cells (1097). On the other hand, studies using Percoll-purified LGL preparations have suggested that subsets of human LGLs provide accessory cell functions for T cell proliferation in autologous and allogeneic mixed-leukocyte cultures (1098) and for *in vitro* generation of virus-specific CTLs (1099). However, those studies did not exclude contamination of the LGL preparation with accessory cells such as dendritic cells or the HLA-DR$^+$ IFN-α-producing cells that copurify with LGLs in Percoll gradient. Purified human NK cells are unable to function as antigen processing cells, although they can present alloantigens after *in vitro* activation with phytohemagglutinin and IL-2 (115). Purified CD16$^+$ human NK cells are also unable to function as accessory cells in various types of T cell-proliferative responses (1100, 1101), although they did support phytohemagglutinin-induced T cell proliferation to a very low extent (1100) and, in the presence of a source of accessory cells, enhanced a mixed-leukocyte reaction (1101).

XI. Anti-Tumor Activity of NK Cells

A. STUDIES OF EXPERIMENTAL ANIMALS

In order for NK cells to play a role in the control of tumor growth, they require the ability to interact with and destroy syngeneic tumor cells or to indirectly activate other adaptive and nonadaptive mechanisms of antitumor resistance. The ability of NK cells to lyse syngeneic cells was proven using transformed cell lines as the target (56), but fresh tumor cells are almost insensitive to NK cell lysis. Studies in which NK cells were enriched and/or activated with IFN or IL-2 showed that allogeneic and autologous fresh tumor cells are sensitive to NK cell-mediated cytotoxicity (37, 79, 776). However, NK cells are not specifically cytotoxic for tumor or transformed cells, and normal cells, e.g., fibroblasts, may be as sensitive or more sensitive to NK cell lysis than are tumor cells (34, 56). The *in vivo* existence of NK cytotoxic cells with a possible function in the surveillance against tumors suggests the importance of *in vivo* regulatory mechanisms to recruit and activate NK cells locally, in analogy with other nonadaptive mechanisms of defense of the organism (34).

In experimental animals the *in vivo* effect of NK cells against tumors was investigated by evaluating long-term growth of tumors (1102), metastasis formation (1103), and short-term elimination of radiolabeled tumor cells from the whole animal or from certain organs (e.g., lungs) (1104, 1105). The experimental protocols used involved analysis of the correlation of NK cell activity and tumor resistance (373, 1106), the use of NK cell-deficient mice (e.g., beige mice) (1107, 1108), or the use of experimental procedures able to enhance (e.g., treatment with IFN or IFN-inducing substances) (1109–1111) or depress NK cell activity. The latter was achieved by the use of ^{89}Sr (442), split-dose irradiation (453), anti-asialo-GM$_1$ antiserum (222, 1112), anti-NK cell alloantisera (1113, 1114), anti-NK-1.1 monoclonal antibodies (1115), and anti-IFN antisera (1116). Altogether, these experiments have clearly shown that NK cells are effective *in vivo* and can destroy tumor cells. Transplanted NK cell-sensitive tumors and experimental tumor metastasis can be inhibited by NK cells. The direct role of NK cells in the prevention of metastasis formation was confirmed by reconstitution experiments in which formation of metastasis in NK cell-depleted animals was prevented by adoptive transfer of purified NK cells (1103, 1117) or cloned cell lines with NK activity (1118). However, the evidence for an effective role of NK cells in resistance to spontaneously arising neoplastic cells is much less compelling (1119).

Metastasis often advances by hematogenous spread; the presence, in the blood, of NK cells with cytotoxic activity that can be up-regulated may allow them to lyse tumor cells present in the circulation before these cells colonize to form metastasis. The experiments of *in vivo* clearance of intravenously injected tumor cells, especially when clearance from the lung is measured, mostly measure intravasal destruction of tumor cells, because NK cell-mediated effects are observed before appreciable extravasation of the tumor cells occurs starting at 4 hours (1120). The demonstration that NK cells can eliminate tumor cells in the circulation does not exclude, however, the possibility that prevention of metastasis takes place also at the tissue level. An extravasal antimetastatic effect of NK cells in the lung and the liver was demonstrated using mice treated sequentially with MVE-2 and anti-asialo-GM$_1$ antiserum, which have increased NK cell activity in both the lung and the liver but depressed circulating NK cells. In these mice metastasis formation was suppressed, suggesting that organ-associated extravasal NK cell activity is a possible mechanism for the antimetastatic therapeutic effects of *in vivo* treatment with NK cell-activating substances (1121).

IL-2-activated lymphocytes (i.e., LAK cells) suppress metastasis formation. The role of NK cells in this activity was determined (1122) by comparing the effect of unfractionated rat LAK cells with that of enriched IL-2-stimulated NK cells obtained by the plastic adherence method (101). The enriched NK cell preparation in combination with IL-2, compared to unfractionated LAK cells, demonstrated a dramatic and superior antimetastatic effect both at liver and lung levels and significantly prolonged survival of the host after treatment (1122).

B. Studies of Cancer Patients

The role of NK cells in the defense against tumors in humans has been the subject of hundreds of papers, but a relationship between NK cell activity and tumor progression has been difficult to establish (1123). The major obstacle to these studies has been the high variability of NK cell number and activity among control healthy donors and the difficulty of a careful quantitation of the results. The difficulties in the quantitative evaluation of NK cell activity and the criteria to be used in order to obtain statistically interpretable data have been reviewed in Section II. The data presented in most studies are the result of experiments that have been performed in a limited number of patients, lack appropriate healthy controls, and do not apply acceptable criteria of quantitation and standardization. The studies in which the phenotype of NK cells has been analyzed often failed to use appropriate reagents and, in most cases, the number of NK cells was expressed only as a proportion of total lymphocytes and not as an absolute concentration of cells. Many reports should therefore be considered anecdotal and do not add much to our knowledge of NK cell functions *in vivo*.

In patients with advanced cancer NK cell cytotoxic activity is usually depressed (1124–1128); this depression appears to be secondary to tumor invasion and due either to interaction of NK cells with tumor cells or to the presence of suppressor cells (746–749). Pross and Baines (1123) reported the analysis of data from the first 307 patients in a study of a total of 1600 randomly chosen cancer patients. The study was performed using monocyte-depleted PBLs in an overnight assay using K562 target cells and applying careful criteria of quantitation and standardization of the assay (53). Each donor was tested in repeated assays (median, 3). Randomly chosen control healthy donors, patients with no evidence of disease, and patients with local disease had comparable cytotoxic activity; patients with metastatic disease and, more so, patients with advanced metastases, displayed significantly lowered NK cell cytotoxic activity (1123). However, the actual differences (0.82 ± 0.09 for advanced metastases versus 1.05 ± 0.07 for patients with no evidence of disease) were not marked, and certainly were not as high as those reported by the same authors (1127) for patients with liver metastases or by others using, in most cases, unfractionated mononuclear cells (1124, 1125, 1128).

The depression of NK cell activity in cancer patients is probably due to several different mechanisms, reflecting the complexity of NK cell regulation *in vivo*. Competition or inactivation by tumor cells, reduced number of NK cells, reduced responsiveness to IFN or IL-2, ability to produce IFN or IL-2, presence of suppressor cells (including monocyte/macrophages acting through release of prostaglandins), presence of inhibitory substances such as glycoproteins and glycolipids, and other mechanisms have been described as responsible for NK cell depression in cancer patients (reviewed in Ref. 1123).

Most of the studies of NK cell cytotoxic activity in cancer patients have been performed using cells from peripheral blood. It is therefore possible that the decrease in NK cell function or number is in part due to altered circulation of the cells or their sequestration at tumor sites or in draining lymph nodes. However, virtually no NK cell activity is found in malignant effusions or among tumor-infiltrating lymphocytes (747, 1129–1131). The lack of NK cell activity at tumor sites could be due in part to an *in situ* inhibition of NK cell activity, because in some studies (1132–1135) functional cytotoxic NK cells have been enriched from ascites fluid and tumor-infiltrating lymphocytes using Percoll gradient fractionation. Highly cytotoxic $CD2^+$, $CD3^-$, $CD16^+$ cells have been grown in IL-2-containing medium from the ascitic fluid or pleural effusions of patients with advanced ovarian or metastatic breast cancer (1136). NK cell activity was demonstrated in breast tumor draining lymph nodes, whereas it was almost absent in normal lymph nodes (572); however, NK cell activity was suppressed in the lymph nodes more proximal to the tumor and/or with tumor infiltration (572), indicating that both alteration of NK cell localization and *in situ* suppression takes place in cancer patients.

The regulation of NK cell activity in patients with hematopoietic tumors is somewhat different from that observed in patients with solid tumors. Patients with preleukemia or myelodysplastic syndrome have generally reduced NK cell activity (1137–1141). The number of phenotypically identifiable NK cells is, however, normal in most patients and defects in the ability of patients' cells to produce IFN-α or to respond to IFN-α have been reported (1138, 1140). The alteration in the bone marrow environment in these patients is probably responsible for deficient production/differentiation of NK cells, analogously to the situation in 17β-estradiol-treated mice in which noncytotoxic NK-1.1$^+$ NK precursor cells are found (210). A depression of NK cell activity is also observed in patients with acute or chronic leukemia; B cell and myeloid chronic leukemia patients often present a significant proportion of cells with the $CD3^+$, $CD16^+$ phenotype and non-MHC-restricted cytotoxicity (1142, 1143). Cells with this phenotype are rare or absent in healthy donors (135). In patients with pure RBC aplasia associated with B cell chronic lymphocytic leukemia, $CD3^+$, $CD16^+$ cells have been shown to suppress

RBC colony formation *in vitro* and have been proposed to be responsible for the *in vivo* erythropoietic defect (1142, 1144; reviewed in Ref. 1145).

If NK cells play a role in surveillance against malignancies, low NK cell activity should have a prognostic value in determining the risk of developing tumors. Patients with genetic diseases such as CHS or X-LPD, with a primary and secondary depression of NK cell activity, respectively, have a high probability of developing an LPD. In these cases, the etiology of the disorder is probably viral and the role of NK cells may reflect their antiviral, rather than their antitumor, activity (C. Lopez, as quoted in Ref. 1146). In familial melanoma, relatives of the patients, who have an increased risk of developing the tumors, also showed a depressed NK cell cytotoxic activity, suggesting a possible role of NK cells resistance to tumor growth (1147). Unlike patients with other solid tumors, those with primary noninvasive melanoma have low NK cell activity (1147, 1148). Strayer *et al.* (1149) reported NK cell cytotoxicity lower than controls in family members of patients with a higher incidence of tumors and observed that NK cell activity varied inversely with the number of family members with cancer. However, in another study of 155 women at high relative risk for breast cancer (1150), no difference in NK cell activity was found compared to normal controls, with the exception of women with benign breast syndrome, who had slightly elevated NK cell cytotoxicity, possibly because of systemic hormonal changes. Because NK cell activity in healthy donors is variable and the disease itself affects NK cell activity, it is still unknown whether NK cells really have any role in tumor surveillance despite many years of investigation for a possible relationship between low versus high NK cell activity and the probability of developing primary tumors (1151). Only when studies of an extremely large number of patients have been performed, using quantitative and standardized methods, will a possible significant correlation (or lack of correlation) between NK cell cytotoxic activity and tumor development be obtained.

Some information is, however, available on the prognostic value of NK cell cytotoxic activity for the probability of developing metastasis in patients with primary tumors. The recurrence of distant melanoma metastases has been found to be significantly lower in patients with high NK cell cytotoxicity than in those with low activity (1148). Schantz *et al.* (1152) indicated a strong inverse correlation between high NK cell activity and formation of metastasis in patients with head and neck cancer. Pross (1146, 1153), in a 14-year ongoing comparative study of NK cell activity and clinical course in patients with solid tumors, reported a definitive trend correlating high NK cell activity with increased survival time, but this did not quite reach significance ($p < 0.06$; $n = 430$). In those patients who have been tested multiple times while metastasis free and who subsequently develop metastasis, the correlation between average NK cell activity and time from diagnosis to metastasis was significant ($p < 0.029$; $n = 91$). By contrast, in patients who were disease free (as opposed to metastasis free) at the time of NK cell testing, NK cell activity had no prognostic significance (1147).

XII. Alterations of Human NK Cell Number and Function in Other Pathological Conditions

Numerous studies have been published evaluating the cytotoxic activity or, more rarely, the number of human NK cells in almost any pathological condition. Alterations of NK cell activity, most often a decrease in cytotoxicity, have been reported in patients with different types of disease. Unfortunately, as discussed in the case of cancer patients, most of these studies are performed on a limited number of patients, lack adequate controls, and do not use standardized quantitative methods for NK cell analysis. In the previous sections many of these studies, relevant for the understanding of regulation and function of NK cells, have been reviewed. In this section, other pathological conditions in which NK cells might play a role or in which NK cells are functionally altered will be briefly reviewed. In the interpretation of these studies it is important to consider that, with few exceptions, it is not possible to determine whether the alteration in NK cell activity is primary or secondary to the pathological condition or to the therapy used.

Decreased NK cell-mediated cytotoxicity is generally observed in connective tissue disorders, particularly in systemic lupus erythematosus (SLE), rheumatoid arthritis, and Sjögren's syndrome (reviewed in Ref. 1154). Peripheral blood mononuclear cells from a high percentage of SLE patients have a reduced ability to produce IFN-α *in vitro*, but most patients have measurable circulating IFN-α, suggesting that the defect of NK cell activity might be secondary to continuous exposure to IFN-α *in vivo* (1155). Because of the predominantly suppressive effect of NK cells on B cell activation, the defect in NK cell activity in these patients could favor the activation of B cells producing autoreactive antibodies. This possibility is supported by the observations in mice carrying the autosomal recessive *lpr* gene. These mice spontaneously develop an SLE-like syndrome, accompanied by profoundly decreased NK cell activity in spleen and peripheral blood (1156) but by elevated hepatic NK cell activity (1157). The spontaneous decrease in NK cell activity in *lpr* mice was observed to be associated with an increased autologous plaque-forming B cell

(APFC) response (1156). The APFC response was diminished when NK cell activity was increased with poly I:C treatment, whereas ablation of NK cells with anti-asialo-GM_1 antisera before poly I:C treatment increased the APFC response (1156). The massive T cell proliferation associated with autoimmune disease in *lpr* mice was shown to be similarly regulated by NK cell activity. Neonatal thymectomy increased NK cell activity and retarded the development of lymphoproliferation and autoantibody formation, whereas thymectomized mice treated with anti-asialo-GM_1 antisera developed LPD and splenomegaly (1158). (NZB × NZW)F_1 mice also spontaneously develop an autoimmune disease resembling SLE. In these animals, however, progression of the autoimmune disease is accompanied by development of a high level of natural killing (1159). Suppression of NK cells *in vivo* using ^{89}Sr reduces both the autoimmunity and the pathologic lesions of SLE, suggesting that in (NZB × NZW)F_1 mice, unlike in *lpr* mice, NK cells play a role in the acceleration of autoimmunity (1159).

In diabetic *BB/W* rats a role for NK cells in the destruction of islet cells has been suggested on the basis of (1) increased NK cell activity in diabetic or diabetes-prone rats in comparison to diabetes-resistant rats, (2) ability of NK cells from *BB/W* rats to lyse *in vitro* dispersed islet cells, and (3) prevention of diabetes when NK cells are eliminated by *in vivo* treatment with anti-CD8 (OX8) antibodies (1160–1162). In Type I diabetes patients, however, NK cell-mediated cytotoxic activity against K562 cells is lower than in normal controls (1163–1165). The low NK cell activity in these patients is probably genetically determined because nondiabetic identical twins of the patients have been reported to have low NK cell activity (1165). The cytotoxicity of PBLs from active diabetic patients against dispersed islets was, however, higher than that of PBLs from healthy individuals or patients in remission, suggesting the possibility that subsets of NK cells might be differentially regulated in diabetes (1164). The exact nature of the cells cytotoxic for the islets and the mechanism of cytotoxicity remain, however, to be determined.

Multiple sclerosis patients with acute remitting or chronic progressive disease have been shown by numerous investigators to have reduced NK cell-mediated cytotoxicity and ability to produce both IFN-α and IFN-γ (reviewed in Ref. 1166), although in other studies a normal NK cell activity has been reported (56, 1167). Because a similar MHC-linked genetic control has been suggested for both low NK cell activity and multiple sclerosis (56, 356), it is possible that the NK cell defect in the patients is genetically determined and has relevance in the etiopathogenesis of multiple sclerosis, a disease of probable viral origin.

However, the association of low NK cell activity with an active status of the disease (1166) may suggest that the defect in NK cell activity is secondary and irrelevant for the etiopathogenesis of multiple sclerosis.

Alteration of NK cell activity has been described following organ (e.g., kidney) transplantation. In general, a depression of circulating NK cell activity was observed for up to 2 years following transplantation, but an increase in NK cell cytotoxicity was reported during rejection episodes (1168, 1169). These alterations of NK cell cytotoxicity are probably secondary to the immunosuppressive therapy and to the response of the host adaptive immune system against the graft. In experimental animals cytotoxic NK cells have been shown to infiltrate sponge matrix grafts or kidney graft at an early time of rejection (peak at day 4) and to disappear at a later time, when CTLs appear (1170, 1171). *In vivo* treatment with anti-asialo-GM_1 antisera abrogated NK cell activity and delayed appearance of CTLs (1170): these results suggest that NK cells might directly participate in graft rejection and may act as accessory cells for CTL generation. There is, however, no evidence that NK cells are involved as effector cells in organ rejection following clinical transplantation (1172).

Depressed NK cell cytotoxicity is one of the many immunological defects observed in patients with AIDS, AIDS-related complex, or lymphoadenopathy syndrome (1173–1176). NK cells from these patients are characterized by a defect at the postbinding stage of lysis (1173–1176). After binding to target cells, they fail to polarize tubulin (1176) and to release NKCF (1174). In addition to the defect in the lytic mechanism, a selective depletion of lymphocytes with the phenotype of NK cells was observed among human immunodeficiency virus (HIV)-positive infected patients (1177). The decrease in NK cells was both relative and absolute; the $CD8^+$, $CD16^+$, NKH-1/Leu-19$^+$ subset of NK cells was much more decreased than was the $CD8^-$, $CD16^+$, NKH-1$^+$ subset (1177). Because no functional differences between the $CD8^+$ and $CD8^-$ subsets of NK cells have been described, the significance of the selective depletion of one subset only is difficult to interpret.

Cytolytic activity of human mononuclear PBLs from healthy donors cultured in IL-2 was abrogated after 3 days of cultures by *in vitro* infection with HIV (1178). HIV antigens were expressed on infected cells after only 14 days of culture. At this time all $CD4^+$ cells and most $CD16^+$ cells expressed HIV antigens, suggesting that HIV might also have a tropism for NK cells (1178). The possibility that HIV might infect NK cells directly is an interesting finding that deserves further investigation. PBLs from AIDS patients have a reduced expression of IFN-α, but not IFN-γ, receptors (1179). The down-modulation of the IFN-α receptor may be due to the continuous exposure to the circulating serum acid-labile IFN-α observed in the patients; continuous exposure to IFN-α

might also be responsible for the inactivation of NK cell cytotoxicity. The peripheral blood mononuclear cells from AIDS patients are severely deficient, compared to cells from healthy individuals, in their ability to produce IFN-α in response to HSV-1-infected fibroblasts (1180). The defect in IFN-α production has been reported to correlate with susceptibility to opportunistic infection better than the decrease in NK cell cytotoxicity (1180). Thesa data suggest absence or a functional deficiency of the IFN-α-producing HLA-DR$^+$ cells, which are necessary accessory cells for NK cell cytotoxicity against virus-infected cells.

HIV proteins, or fragments of them, might be responsible for the NK cell defect as well as for other immunological defects in AIDS patients. Two synthetic peptides constructed on the basis of two sequences of the HIV transmembrane gp41 (1181), and one peptide with homology to a region of p15E conserved among numerous retroviruses (1182), are potent suppressors of several immunological responses, including NK cell-mediated cytotoxicity. These peptides inhibit lysis by interfering with postbinding lytic mechanisms (1181, 1182). It is interesting to note that NK cells, treated with these peptides, are able to bind to target cells, but fail to polarize the Golgi apparatus toward the target cells, thus appearing to be blocked at the same postbinding stage described as the NK cells from AIDS patients with defective cytotoxic ability.

AIDS patients have very complex immunological and hematological defects, and it is difficult at this time to define the role of decreased NK cell activity in the pathogenesis of the disease. However, because NK cells have antimicrobial and antitumor activities and are able to affect hematopoiesis, it is of theoretical and practical importance to determine whether NK cells in AIDS patients play roles in preventing opportunistic infections or sarcoma development and in determining the hematopoietic dysfunctions observed in these patients.

Acknowledgments

I would like to thank the numerous colleagues who, by providing me with reprints, manuscripts, and, in some cases, their unpublished data, have greatly contributed to the preparation of this review. I also thank Marion Kaplan for typing and Marina Hoffman for editing the manuscript. The author's experimental data described here were obtained through support, in part, by U.S. Public Health Service Grants CA 10815, CA 20833, CA 32898, and CA 40256.

References

1. Govaerts, H. (1960). Cellular antibodies in kidney homotransplantation. *J. Immunol.* **85**, 516.
2. Perlmann, P., and Holm, G. (1969). Cytotoxic effect of lymphoid cells in vitro. *Adv. Immunol.* **11**, 117.
3. Cerottini, J. C., and Brunner, K. T. (1974). Cell mediated cytotoxicity, allograft rejection and tumor immunity. *Adv. Immunol.* **18**, 67.

4. Rosenau, W., and Moon, H. D. (1964). The specificity of the cytolytic effect of sensitized lymphoid cells in vitro. *J. Immunol.* **93**, 910.
5. Trinchieri, G., Bernoco, D., Curtoni, S. E., Miggiano, V. C., and Ceppellini, R. (1973). Cell-mediated lympholysis in man: Relevance of HL-A antigens and antibodies. *In* "Histocompatibility Testing—1972" (J. Dausset, ed.), p. 509. Munksgaard, Copenhagen.
6. Eijsvoogel, V. P., Koring, L., De Groot-Koo, Y. L., Huismans, L., Van Rood, J. J., Van Leenmen, A., and Dutoit, E. D. (1972). Mixed lymphocyte culture and HL-A. *Transplant. Proc.* **4**, 199.
7. Nabholz, M., Vives, J., Young, H. M., Meo, T., Miggiano, V., Rijnbeek, A., and Schreffler, D. C. (1974). Cell-mediated cell lysis *in vitro*: Genetic control of killer cell production and target specificities in the mouse. *Eur. J. Immunol.* **4**, 378.
8. Hellström, I., Hellström, K. E., Pierce, G. E., and Yang, J. P. S. (1968). Cellular and humoral immunity to different types of human neoplasms. *Nature (London)* **220**, 1352.
9. Zinkernagel, R. M., and Doherty, P. (1974). Immunological surveillance against altered self components by sensitized T lymphocytes in lymphochoriomeningitis. *Nature (London)* **251**, 547.
10. Trinchieri, G., Aden, D., and Knowles, B. B. (1976). Cell-mediated cytotoxicity to SV40-specific tumor-associated antigens. *Nature (London)* **261**, 312.
11. Jondal, M., and Pross, H. (1975). Surface markers on human B and T lymphocytes. VI. Cytotoxicity against cell lines as a functional marker for lymphocyte subpopulations. *Int. J. Cancer* **15**, 596.
12. Matthews, N., MacLaurin, B. P., and Clarke, G. N. (1975). Characterization of the normal lymphocyte population cytolytic to Burkitt's lymphoma cells of the EB2 cell line. *J. Exp. Biol. Med. Sci.* **53**, 389.
13. Ortaldo, J. R., Oldham, R. K., Cannon, G. C., and Herberman, R. B. (1977). Specificity of natural cytotoxic reactivity of normal human lymphocytes against a myeloid leukemia cell line. *J. Natl. Cancer Inst. (U.S.)* **59**, 77.
14. Peter, H. H., Pavie-Fischer, J., Fridman, W. H., Aubert, C., Cesarini, J. P., Roubin, R., and Kourilsky, F. M. (1975). Cell-mediated cytotoxicity in vitro of human lymphocytes against a tissue culture melanoma cell line (IGR3). *J. Immunol.* **115**, 539.
15. Takasugi, M., Mickey, M. R., and Terasaki, P. I. (1973). Reactivity of lymphocytes from normal persons on cultured tumor cells. *Cancer Res.* **33**, 2898.
16. West, W. H., Cannon, G. B., Kay, H. D., Bonnard, G. D., and Herberman, R. B. (1977). Natural cytotoxic reactivity of human lymphocytes against a myeloid cell line: Characterization of the effector cells. *J. Immunol.* **118**, 355.
17. Herberman, R. B., Nunn, M. E., Holden, H. T., Staal, S., and Djeu, J. Y. (1977). Augmentation of natural cytotoxic reactivity of mouse lymphoid cells against syngeneic and allogeneic target cells. *Int. J. Cancer* **19**, 555.
18. Bloom, B. R. (1982). Natural killers to rescue immune surveillance? *Nature (London)* **300**, 214.
19. Patek, P. Q., and Collins, J. L. (1988). Tumor surveillance revisited: Natural cytotoxic (NC) activity deters tumorigenesis. *Cell. Immunol.* **116**, 240.
20. Ritz, J., Schmidt, R. E., Michon, J., Hercend, T., and Schlossman, S. F. (1988). Characterization of functional surface structures on human natural killer cells. *Adv. Immunol.* **42**, 181.
21. Reynolds, C. W., and Ortaldo, J. R. (1987). Natural killer activity: The definition of a function rather than a cell type. *Immunol. Today* **8**, 172.

22. Lanier, L. L., Phillips, J., Hackett, J., Tutt, M., and Kumar, V. (1986). Natural killer cells: Definition of a cell type rather than a function. *J. Immunol.* **137**, 2735.
23. Trinchieri, G., and Perussia, B. (1984). Human natural killer cells: Biologic and pathologic aspects. *Lab. Invest.* **50**, 489.
24. Trinchieri, G., Degliantoni, G., Kobayashi, M., London, L., and Perussia, B. (1985). Surface phenotype and functions of human natural killer cells. *In* "Mechanisms of Cytotoxicity by NK Cells" (R. B. Herberman and D. M. Callewaert, eds.), p. 29. Academic Press, Orlando, Florida.
25. Lanier, L. L., and Phillips, J. H. (1988). What are natural killer cells? *ISI Atlas of Sci.: Immunol.* p. 15.
26. Fitzgerald-Bocarsly, P., Herberman, R., Hercend, T., Hiserodt, J., Kumar, V., Lanier, L., Ortaldo, J., Pross, H., Reynolds, C., Welsh, R., and Wigzell, H. (1988). A definition of natural killer cells. *Immunol. Today* **9**, 292.
27. Rosenberg, S. (1985). Lymphokine-activated killer cells: A new approach to immunotherapy of cancer. *JNCI, J. Natl. Cancer Inst.* **75**, 595.
28. Perussia, B., Trinchieri, G., Jackson, A., Warner, N. L., Faust, J., Rumpold, H., Kraft, D., and Lanier, L. L. (1984). The Fc receptor for IgG on human natural killer cells: Phenotypic, functional and comparative studies using monoclonal antibodies. *J. Immunol.* **133**, 180.
29. Kay, H. D., Bonnard, G. D., West, W. H., and Herberman, R. B. (1977). A functional comparison of human Fc-receptor-bearing lymphocytes active in natural cytotoxicity and antibody-dependent cellular cytotoxicity. *J. Immunol.* **118**, 2058.
30. Nelson, D. B., Bundy, B. M., and Strober, W. (1977). Spontaneous cell-mediated cytotoxicity by human peripheral blood lymphocytes *in vitro*. *J. Immunol.* **119**, 1401.
31. Ozer, H., Strelkauskas, A. J., Callery, R. T., and Schlossman, R. T. (1979). The functional dissection of human peripheral null cells with respect to antibody-dependent cellular cytotoxicity and natural killing. *Eur. J. Immunol.* **9**, 112.
32. Perussia, B., Trinchieri, G., and Cerottini, J. C. (1979). Functional studies of Fc receptor-bearing human lymphocytes: Effect of treatment with proteolytic enzymes. *J. Immunol.* **123**, 681.
33. Perussia, B., Santoli, D., and Trinchieri, G. (1980). Are spontaneous and antibody-dependent lysis two different mechanisms of cytotoxicity mediated by the same cells? *In* "Natural Cell-Mediated Immunity against Tumors" (R. B. Herberman, ed.), p. 365. Academic Press, New York.
34. Trinchieri, G., and Santoli, D. (1978). Antiviral activity induced by culturing lymphocytes with tumor-derived or virus-transformed cells. Enhancement of human natural killer cell activity by interferon and antagonistic inhibition of susceptibility of target cells to lysis. *J. Exp. Med.* **147**, 1314.
35. Saksela, E., Timonen, T., Ranki, A., and Häyry, P. (1979). Morphological and functional characterization of isolated effector cells responsible for human natural killer activity to fetal fibroblasts and to cultured cell line targets. *Immunol. Rev.* **44**, 71.
36. Hansson, M., Kiessling, R., and Andersson, B. (1981). Human fetal thymus and bone marrow contain target cells for natural killer cells. *Eur. J. Immunol.* **11**, 8.
37. Lozzio, B. B., Lozzio, C. B., and Machado, E. (1976). Human myelogenous (Ph_1^+) leukemia cell line: Transplantation into athymic mice. *J. Natl. Cancer Inst. (U.S.)* **56**, 627.
38. Andersson, L., Jokinen, M., and Gahmberg, C. G. (1979). Induction of erythroid differentiation in the human leukemia cell line K562. *Nature (London)* **278**, 364.
39. Huberman, E., and Callaham, M. F. (1979). Induction of terminal differentiation

in human promyelocytic leukemia cells by tumor-promoting agents. *Proc. Natl. Acad. Sci. U.S.A.* **76**, 1293.
40. Kiessling, R., Klein, E., and Wigzell, H. (1975). "Natural" killer cells in the mouse. I. Cytotoxic cells with specificity for mouse Moloney leukemia cells. Specificity and distribution according to genotype. *Eur. J. Immunol.* **5**, 112.
41. Nunn, M. E., and Herberman, R. B. (1979). Natural cytotoxicity of mouse, rat, and human lymphocytes against heterologous target cells. *JNCI, J. Natl. Cancer Inst.* **62**, 765.
42. MacLennan, I. C. M., and Loewi, G. (1965). Effect of specific antibody to target cells on their specific and non-specific interactions with lymphocytes. *Nature (London)* **205**, 887.
43. Trinchieri, G., De Marchi, M., Mayr, W., Savi, M., and Ceppellini, R. (1973). Lymphocyte antibody lymphocytolytic interaction (LALI) with special emphasis on HLA. *Transplant. Proc.* **5**, 1631.
44. Trinchieri, G., Bauman, P., De Marchi, M., and Tokes, Z. (1975). Antibody-dependent cell-mediated cytotoxicity in humans. I. Characterization of the effector cell. *J. Immunol.* **115**, 249.
45. Brunner, K. T., Manuel, J., Cerottini, J. C., and Chapuis, B. (1968). Quantitative assay of the lytic action of immune lymphoid cells on ^{51}Cr-labeled allogeneic target cells *in vitro*: Inhibition by isoantibody and by drugs. *Immunology* **14**, 181.
46. Miller, R. G., and Dunkley, M. (1974). Quantitative analysis of the ^{51}Cr release cytotoxic assay for cytotoxic lymphocytes. *Cell. Immunol.* **14**, 284.
47. Pross, H. F., Baines, M. G., Rubin, P., Shragge, P., and Patterson, M. S. (1981). Spontaneous human lymphocyte-mediated cytotoxicity against tumor target cells. IX. The quantitation of natural killer cell activity. *J. Clin. Immunol.* **1**, 51.
48. Pross, H. F., Callewaert, D., and Rubin, P. (1986). Assays for NK cell cytotoxicity—Their values and pitfalls. *In* "Immunobiology of Natural Killer Cells" (E. Lotzova and R. B. Herberman, eds.), Vol. 1, p. 1. CRC Press, Boca Raton, Florida.
49. von Krogh, M. (1916). Colloidal chemistry and immunology. *J. Infect. Dis.* **19**, 452.
50. Kabat, E. A., and Mayer, M. M. (1967). "Experimental Immunochemistry," 2nd ed. Thomas, Springfield, Illinois.
51. Hill, A. V. (1910). The possible effect of the aggregation of the molecules of hemoglobin on its dissociation curves. *J. Physiol. (London)* **4**, 40.
52. Pross, H. F., and Baines, M. G. (1982). Studies of human natural killer cells. I. In vivo parameters affecting normal cytotoxic function. *Int. J. Cancer* **29**, 383.
53. Pross, H. F., and Maroun, J. A. (1984). The standardization of NK cell assays for use in studies of biological responses modifiers. *J. Immunol. Methods* **68**, 235.
54. Pross, H. F. (1986). The involvement of natural killer cells in human malignant disease. *In* "Immunobiology of Natural Killer Cells" (E. Lotzova and R. B. Herberman, eds.), Vol. 2, p. 11. CRC Press, Boca Raton, Florida.
55. Pross, H. F. (1986). Natural killer cell activity in human malignant disease. The prognostic value of repetitive natural killer testing. *In* "Natural Immunity, Cancer and Biological Response Modification" (E. Lotzova and R. B. Herberman, eds.), p. 196. Karger, Basel.
56. Santoli, D., Trinchieri, G., Zmijewski, C. M., and Koprowski, H. (1976). HLA-related control of spontaneous and antibody-dependent cell-mediated cytotoxic activity in humans. *J. Immunol.* **117**, 765.
57. Oldham, R., Dean, J. H., Cannon, G. B., Ortaldo, J. R., Dunston, G., Applebaum, F., McCoy, J. L., Djeu, J., and Herberman, R. B. (1976). Cryopreservation of human lymphocyte function as measured by *in vitro* assay. *Int. J. Cancer* **18**, 145.

58. Shau, H., and Golub, S. H. (1988). Modulation of natural killer-mediated lysis by red blood cells. *Cell. Immunol.* **116**, 60.
59. Grimm, E., and Bonavida, B. (1979). Mechanism of cell-mediated cytotoxicity at the single cell level. I. Estimation of cytotoxic T lymphocyte frequency relative lytic efficiency. *J. Immunol.* **123**, 2861.
60. Neville, M. E., Grimm, E., and Bonavida, B. (1980). Frequency determination of K cells by a single cell cytotoxic assay. *J. Immunol. Methods* **36**, 255.
61. Targan, S. (1980). A single cell marker of active NK cytotoxicity: Only a fraction of target binding lymphocytes are killer cells. *J. Clin. Lab. Immunol.* **4**, 165.
62. Ullberg, M., and Jondal, M. (1981). Recycling and target binding capacity of human natural killer cells. *J. Exp. Med.* **153**, 615.
63. Rubin, P., Pross, H. F., and Roder, J. C. (1982). Studies on human natural killer cells. II. Analysis at the single cell level. *J. Immunol.* **128**, 2553.
64. Varcas-Cortes, V., Hellström, U., and Perlmann, P. (1983). Surface markers of human natural killer cells as analyzed in a modified single cell cytotoxicity assay on poly-L-lysine coated cover slip. *J. Immunol. Methods* **62**, 87.
65. Salata, R. A., Schaeter, B. Z., and Ellner, J. J. (1983). Recruitment of OKM1 staining lymphocytes with selective binding of K562 tumour targets by interferon. *Clin. Exp. Immunol.* **52**, 185.
66. Perussia, B., Fanning, V., and Trinchieri, G. (1983). A human NK and K cell subset shares with cytotoxic T cell expression of the antigen recognized by antibody OKT8. *J. Immunol.* **131**, 223.
67. Ullberg, M., Merrill, J., and Jondal, M. (1981). Interferon-induced NK augmentation in humans. An analysis of target recognition, effector cell recruitment and effector cell recycling. *Scand. J. Immunol.* **14**, 285.
68. Michaelis, L., and Menten, M. L. (1913). Kinetics of invertase action. *Biochemistry* **49**, 333.
69. Thorn, R. M., and Henney, C. S. (1976). Kinetic analysis of target cell destruction by effector T cells. I. Delineation of parameters related to the frequency and lytic efficiency of killer cells. *J. Immunol.* **117**, 2213.
70. Callewaert, D. M., Johnson, D. F., and Kearney, J. (1978). Spontaneous cytotoxicity of cultured cell lines mediated by normal peripheral blood lymphocytes. III. Kinetic parameters. *J. Immunol.* **121**, 710.
71. Callewaert, D. M., Genyea, J., Mahle, N. H., Dayner, S., Korzeniewski, C., and Schult, S. (1983). Simultaneous determination of the concentration and lytic activity of effector cells that mediate natural and antibody-dependent cytotoxicity. *Scand. J. Immunol.* **17**, 479.
72. Merrill, S. J. (1982). Foundations of the use of an enzyme—Kinetic analogy in cell-mediated cytotoxicity. *Math. Biosci.* **62**, 219.
73. Callewaert, D. M., Mahle, N. H., Genyea, J., Wilusz, J. R., Chores, J. B., Baker, S., Thomas, R., and Ruedisveli, E. (1984). Experimental application of a multistep kinetic model for natural cytotoxicity: Determination of rate constants for lytic programming and killer cell-independent lysis. *Nat. Immun. Cell Growth Regul.* **3**, 310.
74. Callewaert, D. M., and Mahle, N. H. (1985). Kinetic models for natural cytotoxicity and their use for studying activated NK cells. *In* "Mechanisms of Cytotoxicity by NK Cells" (R. B. Herberman and D. M. Callewaert, eds.), p. 381. Academic Press, Orlando, Florida.
75. Callewaert, D. M., Smeekens, S. P., and Mahle, N. H. (1982). Improved quantification of cellular cytotoxicity reactions: Determination of kinetic parameters

for natural cytotoxicity by a distribution-free procedure. *J. Immunol. Methods* **49**, 25.

76. Perussia, B., and Trinchieri, G. (1981). Inactivation of natural killer cell cytotoxic activity after interaction with target cells. *J. Immunol.* **126**, 754.
77. Brahmi, Z., Bray, R. A., and Abrams, S. I. (1985). Evidence for an early calcium-independent event in the activation of the human natural killer cell cytolytic mechanism. *J. Immunol.* **135**, 4108.
78. Anegón, I., Cuturi, M. C., Trinchieri, G., and Perussia, B. (1988). Interaction of Fc receptor (CD16) with ligands induces transcription of IL-2 receptor (CD25) and lymphokine genes and expression of their products in human natural killer cells. *J. Exp. Med.* **167**, 452.
79. Santoli, D., Trinchieri, G., and Koprowski, H. (1978). Cell-mediated cytotoxicity in humans against virus-infected target cells. II. Interferon induction and activation of natural killer cells. *J. Immunol.* **121**, 532.
80. Trinchieri, G., Santoli, D., Dee, R., and Knowles, B. B. (1978). Anti-viral activity induced by culturing lymphocytes with tumor-derived or virus-transformed cells. Identification of the anti-viral activity as interferon and characterization of the human effector lymphocyte subpopulation. *J. Exp. Med.* **147**, 1299.
81. Beck, J., Engler, H., Brunner, H., and Kirchner, H. (1980). Interferon production in cocultures between mouse spleen cells and tumor cells. Possible role of mycoplasmas in interferon induction. *J. Immunol. Methods* **38**, 63.
82. Birke, C., Peter, H. H., Langenberg, U., Müller-Hermes, W. J., Peters, J. H., Heitmann, J., Leibold, W., Dallugge, H., Krapf, E., and Kirchner, H. (1981). Mycoplasma contamination in human tumor cell lines: Effect on interferon induction and susceptibility to natural killing. *J. Immunol.* **127**, 94.
83. Timonen, T., Ranki, A., Säkselä, E., and Häyry, P. (1979). Human natural cell-mediated cytotoxicity against fetal fibroblasts. III. Morphological and functional characterization of the effector cells. *Cell. Immunol.* **48**, 121.
84. Timonen, T., Säkselä, E., Ranki, A., and Häyry, P. (1979). Fractionation, morphological and functional characterization of effector cells responsible for human natural killer activity against cell line targets. *Cell. Immunol.* **48**, 133.
85. Timonen, T., and Säkselä, E. (1980). Isolation of human natural killer cells by density gradient centrifugation. *J. Immunol. Methods* **36**, 285.
86. Bloom, E. T. (1981). Density gradient fractionation of effector cells in human natural cell-mediated cytotoxicity. *Cell. Immunol.* **61**, 231.
87. Heumann, D., Colombatti, M., and Mach, J. P. (1983). Human large granular lymphocytes contain an esterase activity usually considered as specific for the myeloid series. *Eur. J. Immunol.* **13**, 254.
88. Neighbour, P. A., Huberman, H. S., and Kress, Y. (1982). Human large granular lymphocytes and natural killing: Ultrastructural studies of strontium induced degranulation. *Eur. J. Immunol.* **12**, 588.
89. Ortaldo, J. R., Sharrow, S. O., Timonen, T., and Herberman, R. B. (1981). Determination of surface antigens on highly purified human NK cells by flow cytometry with monoclonal antibodies. *J. Immunol.* **127**, 2401.
90. Timonen, T., Ortaldo, J. R., and Herberman, R. B. (1981). Characteristics of human large granular lymphocytes and relationship to natural killer and K cells. *J. Exp. Med.* **153**, 569.
91. Dvorak, A. M., Galli, S. J., Marcum, J. A., Nabel, G., Der Simonian, H., Goldin, J., Monahan, R. A., Pyne, K., Cantor, H., Rosenberg, R. D., and Dvorak, H. F. (1983). Cloned mouse cells with natural killer function and cloned suppressor

T cells express ultrastructural and biochemical features not shared by cloned inducer T cells. *J. Exp. Med.* **157**, 843.

92. Perussia, B., Fanning, V., and Trinchieri, G. (1985). A leukocyte subset bearing HLA-DR antigens is responsible for in vitro interferon production upon infection with viruses. *Nat. Immun. Cell Growth Regul.* **4**, 120.
93. London, L., Perussia, B., and Trinchieri, G. (1986). Induction of proliferation *in vitro* of resting human natural killer cells: IL-2 induces into cell cycle most peripheral blood NK cells, but only a minor subset of low density T cells. *J. Immunol.* **137**, 3845.
94. Zarling, J. M., Clouse, K. A., Biddison, W. E., and Kung, P. C. (1981). Phenotypes of human natural killer cell populations detected with monoclonal antibodies. *J. Immunol.* **127**, 2575.
95. Perussia, B., Starr, S., Abraham, S., Fanning, V., and Trinchieri, G. (1983). Human natural killer cells analyzed by B73.1, a monoclonal antibody blocking Fc receptor functions. I. Characterization of the lymphocyte subset reactive with B73.1. *J. Immunol.* **130**, 2133.
96. Lanier, L. L., Le, A. M., Phillips, J. H., Warner, N. L., and Babcock, G. F. (1983). Subpopulations of human natural killer cells defined by expression of the Leu7 (HNK-1) and Leu11 (NK-15) antigens. *J. Immunol.* **131**, 1789.
97. Brooks, C. G. (1983). Reversible induction of natural killer cell activity in cloned murine cytotoxic T lymphocytes. *Nature (London)* **305**, 155.
98. Brooks, C. G., Urdal, D. L., and Henney, C. S. (1983). Lymphokine-driven "differentiation" of cytotoxic T-cell clones into cells with NK-like specificity: Correlations with display of membrane macromolecules. *Immunol. Rev.* **72**, 43.
99. Van De Griend, R. J., Krimpen, B. A., Ranfeltap, C. P. M., and Bolhuis, R. H. (1984). Rapidly expanded activated human killer clones have strong antitumor cell activity and have the surface phenotype of either T, non-T, or null cells. *J. Immunol.* **132**, 3185.
100. Perussia, B., Ramoni, C., Anegon, I., Cuturi, M. C., Faust, J., and Trinchieri, G. (1987). Preferential proliferation of natural killer cells among peripheral blood mononuclear cells cocultured with B lymphoblastoid cell lines. *Nat. Immun. Cell Growth Regul.* **6**, 171.
101. Vujanovic, N. L., Herberman, R. B., Maghazachi, A. A., and Hiserodt, J. C. (1988). Lymphokine activated killer cells in rats. III. A simple method for the purification of large granular lymphocytes and their rapid expansion and conversion into lymphokine-activated killer cells. *J. Exp. Med.* **167**, 15.
102. Ward, J. M., and Reynolds, C. W. (1983). Large granular leukemia in F344 rats. *Am. J. Pathol.* **111**, 1.
103. Reynolds, C. W., and Foon, K. A. (1984). T_γ-lymphoproliferative disease and related disorders in humans and experimental animals: A review of the clinical, cellular, and functional characteristics. *Blood* **64**, 1146.
104. Santoli, D., Trinchieri, G., Moretta, L., Zmijewski, C. M., and Koprowski, H. (1978). Spontaneous cell-mediated cytotoxicity in humans. Distribution and characterization of the effector cells. *Clin. Exp. Immunol.* **33**, 309.
105. Nocera, A., Cadoni, A., Zicca, A., Diprimio, R., Leprini, A., and Ferrarini, M. (1982). Receptors for the third complement component on a proportion of large granular lymphocytes from human peripheral blood. *Scand. J. Immunol.* **15**, 573.
106. Pross, H. F., Baines, M. G., and Jondal, M. (1977). Spontaneous human lymphocyte-mediated cytotoxicity against tumor target cells. II. Is the complement receptor necessarily present on the killer cells? *Int. J. Cancer* **20**, 353.

107. Vierling, J. M., Steer, C. J., Bundy, B. M., Strober, W., Jones, E. A., Hague, N. E., and Nelson, D. L. (1978). Studies of complement receptor on cytotoxic effector cells in human peripheral blood. *Cell. Immunol.* **35**, 403.
108. Ault, K. A., and Springer, T. A. (1981). Cross-reaction of a rat-anti-mouse phagocyte specific monoclonal antibody (anti-MAC-1) with human monocytes and natural killer cells. *J. Immunol.* **126**, 359.
109. Beller, D. L., Springer, T. A., and Schreiber, R. D. (1982). Anti-Mac-1 selectively inhibits the mouse and human type three complement receptor. *J. Exp. Med.* **156**, 1000.
110. Kay, H. D., and Horwitz, D. A. (1980). Evidence by reactivity with hybridoma antibodies for a probable myeloid origin of peripheral blood cells active in natural cytotoxicity and antibody-dependent cell-mediated cytotoxicity. *J. Clin. Invest.* **66**, 847.
111. Perussia, B., Trinchieri, G., Lebman, D., Jankiewicz, J., Lange, B., and Rovera, G. (1982). Monoclonal antibodies that detect differentiation surface antigens on human myelomonocytic cells. *Blood* **59**, 382.
112. Funaro, A., Bellone, G., Alessio, M., De Monte, L., Palestro, G., Matera, L., Caligaris-Cappio, F., and Malavasi, F. (1988). Recognition by monoclonal antibody CB02 of a surface molecule shared by B lymphocytes and a discrete large granular lymphocyte subset with cytotoxic activity. *Nat. Immun. Cell Growth Regul.* **7**, 106.
113. Ng, A. K., Indiveri, F., Pellegrino, M. A., Molinaro, G. A., Quaranta, V., and Ferrone, S. (1980). Natural cytotoxicity and antibody-dependent cellular cytotoxicity of human lymphocytes depleted of HLA-DR bearing cells with monoclonal HLA-DR antibodies. *J. Immunol.* **124**, 2336.
114. Perussia, B., and Trinchieri, G. (1984). Antibody 3G8, specific for the human neutrophil Fc receptor, reacts with natural killer cells. *J. Immunol.* **132**, 1410.
115. Brooks, C. F., and Moore, M. (1986). Presentation of a soluble bacterial antigen and cell-surface alloantigens by large granular lymphocytes (LGL) in comparison with monocytes. *Immunology* **58**, 343.
116. Fleit, H. G., Wright, S. D., and Unkeless, J. C. (1982). Human neutrophil Fc receptor distribution and structure. *Proc. Natl. Acad. Sci. U.S.A.* **79**, 3275.
117. Rumpold, H., Kraft, D., Obexer, G., Bock, G., and Gebhart, W. (1982). A monoclonal antibody against a surface antigen shared by human large granular lymphocytes and granulocytes. *J. Immunol.* **129**, 1458.
118. Phillips, J. H., and Babcock, G. F. (1983). NKP-15: A monoclonal antibody reactive against purified human natural killer cells and granulocytes. *Immunol. Lett.* **6**, 143.
119. Werner, G., Von Dem Borne, A. E. G. K., Bos, M. J. E., Tromp, J. F., Van Der Plas-Van Dalen, C. M., Visser, F. J., Engelfriet, C. P., and Tetteroo, P. A. T. (1986). Localization of the human NA1 alloantigen on neutrophil-Fc receptors. *In* "Leukocyte Typing II" (E. L. Reinherz, L. M. Haynes, L. M. Nadler, and I. D. Bernstein, eds.), Vol. 3, p. 109. Springer-Verlag, New York.
120. Malavasi, F., Bellone, G., Matera, L., Milanese, C., Ferrero, E., Funaro, A., Demaria, S., Caligaris-Cappio, F., Camussi, G., and Dellabona, P. (1985). Murine monoclonal antibodies as probes for the phenotypical, functional and molecular analysis of a discrete peripheral blood lymphocyte population exerting natural killer activity *in vitro. Hum. Immunol.* **14**, 87.
121. Malavasi, F., Tetta, C., Funaro, A., Bellone, G., Ferrero, E., Collifranzone, A., Dellabona, P., Rusci, R., Matera, L., Camussi, G., and Caligaris-Cappio, F. (1986). Fc receptor triggering induces expression of surface-activation antigens and release

of platelet-activating factor in large granular lymphocytes. *Proc. Natl. Acad. Sci. U.S.A.* **83**, 2443.
122. Matera, L., Santoli, D., Garbarino, G., Pegoraro, L., Bellone, G., and Pagliardi, G. (1986). Modulation of *in vitro* myelopoiesis by LGL: Different effects on early and late progenitor cells. *J. Immunol.* **136**, 1260.
123. Clarkson, S. B., and Ory, P. A. (1988). CD16. Developmentally regulated IgG Fc receptors on cultured human monocytes. *J. Exp. Med.* **167**, 408.
124. Simmons, D., and Seed, B. (1988). The Fc receptor of natural killer cells is a phospholipid-linked membrane protein. *Nature (London)* **333**, 568.
125. Lanier, L. L., Ruitenberg, J. J., and Phillips, J. H. (1988). Functional and biochemical analysis of CD16 antigen on natural killer cells and granulocytes. *J. Immunol.* **141**, 3478.
126. Ravetch, J. V., and Perussia, B. (1989). Alternative membrane form of FcγRIII (CD16) on human NK cells and neutrophils: Cell-type specific expression of two genes which differ in single nucleotide substitutions. *J. Exp.Med.* (in press).
127. Huizinga, T. W. J., Van Der Schoot, C. E., Jost, C., Klaassen, R., Kleijer, M., von dem Borne, A. E. G. K., Ross, D., and Tetteroo, P. A. T. (1988). The PI-linked receptor FcRIII is released on stimulation of neutrophils. *Nature (London)* **333**, 667.
128. Selvaraj, P., Rosse, F., Silber, R., and Springer, T. A. (1988). The major Fc receptor in blood has a phosphatidylinositol anchor and is deficient in paroxysmal nocturnal haemoglobinuria. *Nature (London)* **333**, 565.
129. Yoda, Y., and Abe, R. (1985). Deficient natural killer (NK) cells in paroxysmal nocturnal haemoglobinuria (PNH): Studies of lymphoid cells fractionated by discontinuous density gradient centrifugation. *Br. J. Haematol.* **60**, 669.
130. Perussia, B., Tutt, M. M., Qiu, W. Q., Kuziel, W. A., Tucker, P. W., Trinchieri, G., Bennett, M., Ravetch, J. V., and Kumar, V. (1989). Murine natural killer cells express functional Fc receptor II encoded by the FcγRα gene. *J. Exp. Med.* (in press).
131. Graziano, R. F., Looney, R. S., Shen, L., and Fanger, M. W. (1989). FcγR-mediated killing by eosinophils. *J. Immunol.* **142**, 230.
132. Perussia, B., Acuto, O., Terhorst, C., Faust, J., Lazarus, R., Fanning, V., and Trinchieri, G. (1983). Human natural killer cells analyzed by B73.1, a monoclonal antibody blocking FcR functions. II. Studies of B73.1 antibody–antigen interaction on the lymphocyte membrane. *J. Immunol.* **130**, 2142.
133. Trinchieri, G., O'Brien, T., Shade, M., and Perussia, B. (1984). Phorbol esters enhance spontaneous cytotoxicity of human lymphocytes, abrogate Fc receptor expression and inhibit antibody-dependent lymphocyte-mediated cytotoxicity. *J. Immunol.* **133**, 1869.
134. Perussia, B., and Trinchieri, G. (1988). Structure and functions of NK cell Fc receptor. *EOS—J. Immunol. Immunopharmacol.* **8**, 147.
135. Lanier, L. L., Kipps, T. J., and Phillips, J. H. (1985). Functional properties of a unique subset of cytotoxic CD3$^+$ T lymphocytes that express Fc receptors for IgG (CD16/Leu11 antigen). *J. Exp. Med.* **162**, 2089.
136. Van De Griend, R. J., Bolhuis, R. L. H., Stoter, G., and roozemond, R. C. (1987). Regulation of cytolytic activity in CD3$^-$ and CD3$^+$ killer cell clones by monoclonal antibodies (anti-CD16, anti-CD2, anti-CD3) depends on subclass specificity of target cell IgG-FcR. *J. Immunol.* **138**, 3137.
137. Masucci, M. G., Masucci, G., Klein, E., and Berthold, W. (1980). Target selectivity

of interferon-induced human killer lymphocytes related to their Fc receptor expression. *Proc. Natl. Acad. Sci. U.S.A.* **77**, 3620.

138. Griffin, J. D., Hercend, T., Beveridge, R., and Schlossman, S. F. (1983). Characterization of an antigen expressed on human natural killer cells. *J. Immunol.* **130**, 2947.

139. McGarry, R. C., Pinto, A., Hammersley-Straw, D. R., and Trevenen, C. L. (1988). Expression of markers shared between human natural killer cells and neuroblastoma lines. *Cancer Immunol. Immunother.* **27**, 47.

140. Hercend, T., Griffin, J. D., Bensussan, A., Schmidt, R. E., Edson, M. A., Brennan, A., Murray, C., Daley, J. F., Schlossman, S. F., and Ritz, J. (1985). Generation of monoclonal antibodies to a human natural killer clone. Characterization of two natural killer-associated antigens, NKH1A and NKH2, expressed on a subset of large granular lymphocytes. *J. Clin. Invest.* **75**, 932.

141. Lanier, L. L., Le, A. M., Civin, C. I., Loken, M. R., and Phillips, J. H. (1986). The relationship of CD16 (Leu-11) and Leu-19 (NKH-1) antigen expression on human peripheral blood NK cells and cytotoxic T lymphocytes. *J. Immunol.* **136**, 4480.

142. Hercend, T., Meuer, S., Brennan, A., Edson, M. A., Acuto, O., Reinherz, E. L., Schlossman, S. F., and Ritz, J. (1983). Identification of a clonally restricted 90KD heterodimer on two human cloned natural killer cell lines. Its role in cytotoxic effector function. *J. Exp. Med.* **158**, 1547.

143. Hercend, T., Schmidt, R., Brennan, A., Edson, M. A., Reinherz, E. L., Schlossman, S. F., and Ritz, J. (1984). Identification of a 140 kDa activation antigen as a target structure for a series of human cloned natural killer cell lines. *Eur. J. Immunol.* **14**, 844.

144. Schmidt, R. C., Murray, J. F., Daley, S. F., Schlossman, S. F., and Ritz, J. (1986). A subset of natural killer cells in peripheral blood displays a mature T cell phenotype. *J. Exp. Med.* **164**, 351.

145. Lanier, L. L., Le, A. M., Ding, A., Evans, E. L., Krensky, A. M., Clayberger, C., and Philips, J. H. (1987). Expression of Leu-19 (NKH-1) antigen on IL-2-dependent cytotoxic and non-cytotoxic T cell lines. *J. Immunol.* **138**, 2019.

146. Abo, T., and Balch, C. M. (1981). A differentiation antigen of human NK and K cells identified by a monoclonal antibody (HNK-1). *J. Immunol.* **127**, 1024.

147. Abo, T., and Balch, C. M. (1983). *In vitro* propagation of cultured human natural killer cells expressing the HNK-1 differentiation antigen and spontaneous cytotoxic function. *Eur. J. Immunol.* **13**, 383.

148. Abo, T., Cooper, M. D., and Balch, C. M. (1982). Postnatal expansion of the natural killer and killer cell population in humans identified by the monoclonal HNK-1 antibody. *J. Exp. Med.* **155**, 321.

149. Abo, T., Cooper, M. D., and Balch, C. M. (1982). Characterization of HNK-1(+) (Leu-7) human lymphocytes. I. Two distinct phenotypes of human NK cells with different cytotoxic capability. *J. Immunol.* **129**, 1752.

150. Velardi, A., Prchal, J. T., Prasthofer, E. F., and Grossi, C. E. (1985). Expression of NK-lineage markers on peripheral blood lymphocytes with T-helper (Leu 3^+/T4$^+$) phenotype in B cell chronic lymphocytic leukemia. *Blood* **65**, 149.

151. Velardi, A., Clement, L. T., and Grossi, C. E. (1985). Quantitative and functional analysis of a human lymphocyte subset with the T-helper (Leu 3/T4+) phenotype and natural killer (NK)-cell characteristics in patients with malignancy. *J. Clin. Immunol.* **5**, 329.

152. Velardi, A., Grossi, C. E., and Cooper, M. D. (1985). A large subpopulation of

lymphocytes with T helper phenotype (Leu-3/T4+) exhibits the property of binding to NK cell targets and granular lymphocyte morphology. *J. Immunol.* **134**, 58.

153. Pizzolo, G., Semenzato, G., Chilosi, M., Morittu, L., Abrosetti, A., Warner, N., Bofill, M., and Janossy, G. (1984). Distribution and heterogeneity of cells detected by HNK-1 monoclonal antibody in blood and tissues in normal, reactive and neoplastic conditions. *Clin. Exp. Immunol.* **57**, 195.

154. Velardi, A., Mingari, M. C., Moretta, L., and Grossi, C. E. (1986). Functional analysis of cloned germinal center CD4+ cells with natural killer cell-related features. Divergence from typical T helper cells. *J. Immunol.* **137**, 2808.

155. Abo, T., Miller, C. A., Gartland, G. L., and Balch, C. M. (1983). Differentiation stages of human natural killer cells in lymphoid tissues from fetal to adult life. *J. Exp. Med.* **157**, 273.

156. Phillips, J. H., and Lanier, L. L. (1986). Dissection of the lymphokine-activated killer phenomenon. Relative contribution of peripheral blood natural killer cells and T lymphocytes to cytolysis. *J. Exp. Med.* **164**, 814.

157. McGarry, R. G., Helfand, S. L., Quarles, R. H., and Roder, J. C. (1983). Recognition of myelin-associated glycoprotein by the monoclonal antibody HNK-1. *Nature (London)* **306**, 376.

158. Sato, S., Tanaka, M., Miyatani, N., Baba, H., and Miyatake, T. (1985). Shared antigen between the myelin-associated glycoprotein (MAG) and a cell line from human T cell leukemia (HSB-2). *J. Neuroimmunol.* **7**, 287.

159. Miller, S., Trinchieri, G., Perussia, B., and Kahn, S. (1987). Murine and human monoclonal IgM antibodies with specificity for myelin-associated glycoprotein: Comparative binding to myelin and to lymphocytes. *J. Neuroimmunol.* **15**, 229.

160. Tanaka, M., Nishizawa, M., Inuzuka, T., Baba, H., Sato, S., and Miyatake, T. (1985). Human natural killer cell activity is reduced by treatment of anti-myelin-associated glycoprotein (MAG) monoclonal mouse IgM antibody and complement. *J. Neuroimmunol.* **10**, 115.

161. Tanaka, M., Sato, S., Yanagisawa, K., and Miyatake, T. (1984). Myelin-associated glycoprotein (MAG): Expression on the surface of human natural killer cells. *Biomed. Res.* **5**, 71.

162. Dobersen, M. J., Gascon, P., Trost, S., Hammer, J. A., Goodman, S., Noronha, A. B., O'Shannessy, D. J., Brady, R. O., and Quarles, R. H. (1985). Murine monoclonal antibodies to the myelin-associated glycoprotein react with large granular lymphocytes of human blood. *Proc. Natl. Acad. Sci. U.S.A.* **82**, 552.

163. Ando, I., and Tamaki, K. (1985). HNK-I antibody reacts with peripheral nerves and sweat glands in the skin. *Br. J. Dermatol.* **113**, 175.

164. Stoll, G., Schwendemann, G., Heininger, K., Steck, A. J., and Toyka, K. V. (1985). Human monoclonal anti-MAG antibody and anti-Leu 7 recognize shared antigenic determinants in peripheral nerve and spinal cord. *J. Neurol., Neurosurg. Psychiatry* **48**, 635.

165. Hozumi, I., Sato, S., Tunoda, H., Inuzuka, T., Tanaka, M., Nishizawa, M., Baba, H., and Miyatake, T. (1987). Shared carbohydrate antigenic determinant between the myelin-associated glycoprotein (MAG) and lung cancers. An immuno-histochemical study by an anti-MAG IgM monoclonal antibody. *J. Neuroimmunol.* **15**, 147.

166. Ball, E. D., Sorenson, G. D., and Pettengill, O. S. (1986). Expression of myeloid and major histocompatibility antigens on small cell carcinoma of the lung cell lines analyzed by cytofluorography: Modulation by gamma-interferon. *Cancer Res.* **46**, 2335.

167. Bunn, P. A., Jr., Linnoila, I., Minna, J. D., Carney, D., and Gazdar, A. F. (1985). Small cell lung cancer, endocrine cells of the fetal bronchus, and other neuroendocrine cells express the Leu-7 antigenic determinant present on natural killer cells. *Blood* **65**, 764.
168. Rusthoven, J. J., Robinson, J. B., Kolin, A., and Pinkerton, P. H. (1985). The natural-killer-cell-associated HNK-1 (Leu-7) antibody reacts with hypertrophic and malignant prostatic epithelium. *Cancer (Philadelphia)* **56**, 289.
169. Kruse, J., Mailhammer, R., Wernecke, H., Faissner, A., Sommer, I., Goridis, C., and Schacher, M. (1984). Neural cell adhesion molecules and myelin-associated glycoprotein share a common carbohydrate moiety recognized by monoclonal antibodies L2 and HNK-1. *Nature (London)* **311**, 153.
170. Ilyas, A. A., Quarles, R. H., MacIntosh, T. D., Dobersen, M. J., Trapp, B. D., Dalakas, M. C., and Brady, R. O. (1984). IgM in a human neuropathy related to paraproteinemia binds to a carbohydrate determinant in the myelin-associated glycoprotein and to a ganglioside. *Proc. Natl. Acad. Sci. U.S.A.* **81**, 1225.
171. Chou, K. H., Ilyas, A. A., Evans, J. E., Quarles, R. H., and Jungalwala, F. B. (1985). Structure of a glycolipid reacting with monoclonal IgM in neuropathy and with HNK-1. *Biochem. Biophys. Res. Commun.* **128**, 383.
172. Braun, P. E., Frail, D. E., and Latov, N. (1982). Myelin-associated glycoprotein is the antigen for a monoclonal IgM in polyneuropathy. *J. Neurochem.* **39**, 1261.
173. Steck, A. J., Murray, N., Meier, C., Page, N., and Perruisseau, G. (1983). Demyelinating neuropathy and monoclonal IgM antibody to myelin-associated glycoprotein. *Neurology* **33**, 19.
174. Leibowitz, S., Gregson, N. A., Kennedy, M., and Kahn, S. N. (1983). IgM paraproteins with immunological specificity for a Schwann cell component and peripheral nerve myelin in patients with polyneuropathy. *J. Neurol. Sci.* **59**, 153.
175. Sriram, S., and Lanier, L. (1986). NK cell function in a patient with IgM monoclonal antibody against myelin-associated glycoprotein. *Neurology* **36**, 566.
176. Della-Casa-Alberighi, O., Nobile-Orazio, E., Bonara, P., Hu, C., Spagnol, G., Radelli, L., and Scorza-Smeraldi, R. (1988). NK cells in patients with peripheral neuropathy and IgM monoclonal protein reacting with the myelin-associated glycoprotein (MAG). *J. Neuroimmunol.* **18**, 207.
177. Murray, N., and Steck, A. J. (1984). Indication of a possible role in a demyelinating neuropathy for an antigen shared between myelin and NK cells. *Lancet* **1**, 711.
178. Springer, T. A., Dustin, M. L., Kishimoto, T. K., and Marlin, S. D. (1987). The lymphocyte function-associated LFA-1, CD2, and LFA-3 molecules: Cell adhesion receptors of the immune system. *Annu. Rev. Immunol.* **5**, 223.
179. Timonen, T., Patarroyo, M., and Gahmberg, C. G. (1988). CD11a-c/CD18 and GP84 (LB-2) adhesion molecules on human large granular lymphocytes and their participation in natural killing. *J. Immunol.* **141**, 1041.
180. Breard, J. E., Reinherz, L., Kung, P. C., Goldstein, G., and Schlossman, S. F. (1980). A monoclonal antibody reactive with human peripheral blood monocytes. *J. Immunol.* **124**, 1943.
181. Bai, Y., Beverley, P. C. L., Knowles, R. W., and Bodmer, W. F. (1983). Two monoclonal antibodies identifying a subset of human peripheral mononuclear cells with natural killer cell activity. *Eur. J. Immunol.* **13**, 521.
182. Wisniewski, D., Knowles, R., Wachter, M., Strife, A., and Clarkson, B. (1987). Expression of two natural killer cell antigens, H-25 and H-366, by human immature myeloid cells and by erythroid and granulocytic/monocytic colony-forming units. *Blood* **69**, 419.

183. Perussia, B., Fanning, V., and Trinchieri, G. (1982). Phenotypic characterization of human natural killer and antibody-dependent killer cells as an homogeneous and discrete cell subset. In "NK Cells and Other Natural Effector Cells" (R. B. Herberman, ed.), p. 39. Academic Press, New York.
184. Rumpold, H., Obexer, G., and Kraft, D. (1982). Analysis of human NK cells by monoclonal antibodies against myelomonocytic and lymphocytic antigens. In "NK Cells and Other Natural Effector Cells" (R. B. Herberman, ed.), p. 47. Academic Press, New York.
185. Zarling, J. M., and Kung, P. C. (1980). Monoclonal antibodies which distinguish between human NK cells and cytotoxic T lymphocytes. *Nature (London)* **288**, 394.
186. Morgan, A. C., Jr., Schroff, R. W., Klein, R. A., McIntyre, R. F., Mason, A., Herberman, R. B., and Ortaldo, J. (1987). Occult (non-surface expression) of T, B and monocyte markers in human large granular lymphocytes. *Mol. Immunol.* **24**, 117.
187. Calvo, C. F., Boumsell, L., Kolb, J. P., Laffy, B., Bernard, A., and Senik, A. (1984). Preferential elimination of NK and CTL functions by anti-D44 monoclonal antibody. *J. Immunol.* **132**, 2345.
188. Nieminen, P., and Säkselä, E. (1984). A shared antigenic specificity of human large granular lymphocytes and precursors of NK-like and allospecific cytotoxic effector cells. *J. Immunol.* **133**, 702.
189. Nieminen, P., and Säkselä, E. (1986). NK-9, a distinct sialylated antigen of the T200 family. *Eur. J. Immunol.* **16**, 513.
190. Hercend, T., Ritz, S., Schlossman, S. F., and Reinherz, E. L. (1981). Comparative expression of T9, T10 and Ia antigens on activated human T cell subsets. *Hum. Immunol.* **3**, 247.
191. London, L., Perussia, B., and Trinchieri, G. (1985). Induction of proliferation *in vitro* of resting human natural killer cells: Expression of surface activation antigens. *J. Immunol.* **134**, 718.
192. Phillips, J. H., Le, A. M., and Lanier, L. L. (1984). Natural killer cells activated in a human mixed lymphocyte response culture identified by expression of Leu-11 and class II histocompatibility antigens. *J. Exp. Med.* **159**, 993.
193. Biassoni, R., Ferrini, S., Prigione, I., Moretta, A., and Long, E. O. (1988). CD3-negative lymphokine-activated cytotoxic cells express the CD3 epsilon gene. *J. Immunol.* **140**, 1685.
194. Isobe, M., Russo, G., Cuturi, M. C., Jiang, M., Kozbor, D., Sherman, F., Loudon, R., Croce, C., Perussia, B., and Trinchieri, G. (1989). Human natural killer cells transcribe unrearranged T cell receptor δ gene: Analysis and cloning of the transcripts. Submitted for publication.
195. Ritz, J., Campen, T. J., Schmidt, R. E., Royer, H. D., Hercend, T., Hussey, R. E., and Reinherz, E. L. (1985). Analysis of T-cell receptor gene rearrangement and expression in human natural killer cell clones. *Science* **228**, 1540.
196. Lanier, L. L., Cwirla, S., Federspiel, N., and Phillips, J. H. (1986). Human natural killer cells isolated from peripheral blood do not rearrange T cell antigen receptor chain genes. *J. Exp. Med.* **163**, 209.
197. Lanier, L. L., Cwirla, S., and Phillips, J. H. (1986). Genomic organization of the T cell genes in human peripheral blood natural killer cells. *J. Immunol.* **137**, 3375.
198. Triebel, F., Graziani, M., Faure, F., Jitsukawa, S., and Hercend, T. (1987). Cloned human CD3− lymphocytes with natural killer-like activity do not express nor rearrange T cell receptor gamma genes. *Eur. J. Immunol.* **17**, 1209.
199. Pelicci, P. G., Allavena, P., Subar, M., Rambaldi, A., Pirelli, A., Di Bello, M.,

Barbui, T., Knowles, D. M., Dalla-Favera, R., and Mantovani, A. (1987). T cell receptor (alpha, beta, gamma) gene rearrangements and expression in normal and leukemic large granular lymphocytes/natural killer cells. *Blood* **70**, 1500.

200. Leiden, J. M., Gottesdiener, K. M., Quertermous, T., Coury, L., Bray, R. A., Gottschalk, L., Gebel, H., Seidman, J. G., Strominger, J. L., and Landay, A. L. E. A. (1988). T-cell receptor gene rearrangement and expression in human natural killer cells: Natural killer activity is not dependent on the rearrangement and expression of T-cell receptor alpha, beta, or gamma genes. *Immunogenetics* **27**, 231.

201. Biondi, A., Allavena, P., Rossi, V., Rambaldi, A., and Mantovani, A. (1989). Expression of the T cell receptor delta gene in natural killer cells. *J. Immunol. Res.* **1**, 7.

202. Nowill, A., Moingeon, P., Ythier, A., Graziani, M., Faure, F., Delmon, L., Rainaut, M., Forrestier, F., Bohuon, C., and Hercend, T. (1986). Natural killer clones derived from fetal (25 wk) blood. Probing the human T cell receptor with WT31 monoclonal antibody. *J. Exp. Med.* **163**, 1601.

203. Alarcon, B., De Vries, J., Pettey, C., Boylston, A., Yssel, H., Terhorst, C., and Spits, H. (1987). The T-cell receptor gamma chain-CD3 complex: Implication in the cytotoxic activity of a CD3+ CD4− CD8− human natural killer clone. *Proc. Natl. Acad. Sci. U.S.A.* **84**, 3861.

204. Ang, S. L., Seidman, J. G., Peterman, G. M., Duby, A. D., Benjamin, D., Lee, S. J., and Hafler, D. A. (1987). Functional gamma chain-associated T cell receptors on cerebrospinal fluid-derived natural killer-like T cell clones. *J. Exp. Med.* **165**, 1453.

205. Moingeon, P., Jitsukawa, S., Faure, F., Troalen, F., Triebel, F., Graziani, M., Forrestier, F., Bellet, D., Bohuon, C., and Hercend, T. (1987). A gamma-chain complex forms a functional receptor on cloned human lymphocytes with natural killer-like activity. *Nature (London)* **325**, 723.

206. Sakamoto, S., Ortaldo, J. R., and Young, H. A. (1988). Methylation patterns of the T cell receptor beta-chain gene in T cells, large granular lymphocytes, B cells, and monocytes. *J. Immunol.* **140**, 654.

207. Glimcher, L., Shen, F. W., and Cantor, H. (1977). Identification of a cell surface antigen selectively expressed on the natural killer cell. *J. Exp. Med.* **145**, 1.

208. Cantor, H., Masai, M., Shen, F. W., Leclerc, J. C., and Glimcher, L. (1979). Immunogenetic analysis of "natural killer" activity in the mouse. *Immunol. Rev.* **44**, 3.

209. Koo, G. C., and Peppard, J. R. (1984). Establishment of monoclonal anti-NK-1.1 antibody. *Hybridoma* **3**, 301.

210. Hackett, J., Tutt, M., Lipscomb, M., Bennett, M., Koo, G., and Kumar, V. (1986). Origin and differentiation of natural killer cells. II. Functional and morphologic studies of purified NK1.1+ cells. *J. Immunol.* **136**, 3124.

211. Koo, G. C., Durmont, F. J., Tutt, M., Hackett, J., and Kumar, V. (1986). The NK-1.1(−) mouse: A model to study differentiation of murine NK cells. *J. Immunol.* **37**, 3742.

212. Burton, R. C., and Winn, H. J. (1981). Studies on natural killer (NK) cells. I. NK cell specific antibodies in CE anti-CBA serum. *J. Immunol.* **126**, 1985.

213. Pollack, S. B., and Emmons, S. L. (1982). NK-2.1: An NK-associated antigen detected with NZB anti-BALB/c serum. *J. Immunol.* **129**, 2277.

214. Pollack, S. B., and Emmons, S. L. (1982). Anti-NK 2.1: An activity of NZB anti-

BALB/c serum. *In* "NK Cells and Other Natural Effector Cells" (R. B. Herberman, ed.), p. 113. Academic Press, New York.
215. Burton, R. C., Koo, G. C., Smart, Y. C., Clark, D. A., and Winn, H. J. (1988). Surface antigens of murine natural killer cells. *Int. Rev. Cytol.* **3**, 185.
216. Emmons, S. L., and Pollack, S. B. (1985). Murine NK cell heterogeneity: A subpopulation of C37BL/6 splenic NK cells detected by NK-1.1 and NK-2.1 antisera. *Nat. Immun. Cell Growth Regul.* **4**, 169.
217. Mason, L., Giardina, S. L., Hecht, T., Ortaldo, J., and Mathieson, B. J. (1988). LGL-1: A non-polymorphic antigen expressed on a major population of mouse natural killer cells. *J. Immunol.* **140**, 4403.
218. Kasai, M., Iwamori, M., Nagai, Y., Okumura, K., and Tada, T. (1980). A glycolipid on the surface of mouse natural killer cells. *Eur. J. Immunol.* **10**, 175.
219. Young, W. W., Jr., Hakomori, S.-I., Durdik, J. M., and Henney, C. S. (1980). Identification of ganglio-N-tetraosylceramide as a new cell surface marker for murine natural killer (NK) cells. *J. Immunol.* **124**, 199.
220. Suttles, J., Schwarting, G. A., Hougland, M. W., and Stout, R. D. (1987). Expression of asialo Gm1 on a subset of adult murine thymocytes: Histological localization and demonstration that the asialo Gm1-positive subset contains both the functionally mature and the proliferating thymocyte subpopulations. *J. Immunol.* **138**, 364.
221. Mercurio, A. M., Schwarting, G. A., and Robbins, P. W. (1984). Glycolipids of the mouse peritoneal macrophage. Alterations in amount and surface exposure of specific glycolipid species occur in response to inflammation and tumoricidal activation. *J. Exp. Med.* **160**, 1114.
222. Kasai, M., Yoneda, T., Habu, S., Maruyama, T., Okumura, K., and Tokunaga, T. (1981). In vivo effect of anti-asialo Gm1 antibody on natural killer activity. *Nature (London)* **291**, 334.
223. Tang, J., De Long, D. C., Marder, P., Butler, L. D., and Ades, E. W. (1985). Identification of functional subpopulations of murine natural killer cells based on their cell surface asialo GM_1 phenotype. *Cell. Immunol.* **96**, 386.
224. Solomon, F. R., and Higgins, T. J. (1987). A monoclonal antibody with reactivity to asialo GM_1 and murine natural killer cells. *Mol. Immunol.* **24**, 57.
225. Miller, V. E., Legarde, A. E., Longenecker, B. M., and Greenberg, A. H. (1986). A phenyl-beta-galactoside (phi-beta-gal)-specific monoclonal antibody reactive with murine and rat NK cells. *J. Immunol.* **136**, 2968.
226. Weyand, C., Hammerling, G. J., and Hammerling, U. (1980). The murine T-cell antigens Qa4 and Qa5-surface markers on natural killer cells. *Immunobiology* **157**, 298.
227. Chun, M., Fernandes, G., and Hoffmann, M. K. (1981). Mechanism of NK cell activation: Relationship between Qa5+ NK cells and lymphocytes. *J. Immunol.* **126**, 331.
228. Hammerling, G. J., Hammerling, U., and Flaherty, L. (1979). Qat-4 and Qat-5, new murine T-cell antigens governed by the Tla region and identified by monoclonal antibodies. *J. Exp. Med.* **150**, 108.
229. Tutt, M. M. (1988). Regulation and differentiation of murine natural killer cells. Ph.D. Thesis. pp. 219-231. University of Texas Southwestern Medical Center, Dallas.
230. Meruelo, D., Paolino, A., Flieger, N., and Offer, M. (1980). Definition of a new T lymphocyte cell surface antigen: Ly 11.2. *J. Immunol.* **125**, 2713.
231. Mattes, M. J., Sharrow, S. O., Herberman, R. B., and Holden, H. T. (1979). Identification and separation of THY-1 positive mouse spleen cells active in natural

cytotoxicity and antibody-dependent cell-mediated cytotoxicity. *J. Immunol.* 123, 2851.
232. Koo, G. C., Jacobson, J. B., Hammerling, G. J., and Hammerling, U. (1980). Antigenic profile of murine natural killer cells. *J. Immunol.* 125, 1003.
233. Minato, N., Reid, L., and Bloom, B. R. (1981). On the heterogeneity of murine natural killer cells. *J. Exp. Med.* 154, 750.
234. Tutt, M. M., Kuziel, W. A., Hackett, J. J., Bennett, M., Tucker, P. W., and Kumar, V. (1986). Murine natural killer cells do not express functional transcript of the α, β, or γ chain genes of the T cell receptor. *J. Immunol.* 137, 2998.
235. Pollack, S. B., Tam, M. R., Nowinski, R. C., and Emmons, S. L. (1979). Presence of T cell-associated surface antigens on murine NK cells. *J. Immunol.* 123, 1818.
236. Holmberg, L. A., Springer, T. A., and Ault, K. A. (1981). Natural killer activity in the peritoneal exudates of mice injected with listeria monocytogenes: Characterization of the natural killer cells by using a monoclonal rat anti-murine macrophage antibody (M1/70). *J. Immunol.* 127, 1792.
237. Holmberg, L. A., and Ault, K. A. (1984). Characterization of natural killer cells induced in the peritoneal exudates of mice infected with Listeria monocytogenes: A study of their tumor target specificity and their expression of murine differentiation antigens and human NK-associated antigens. *Cell. Immunol.* 89, 151.
238. Dennert, G. (1980). Cloned lines of natural killer cells. *Nature (London)* 287, 47.
239. Dennert, G., Yogeeswaran, G., and Ymagata, S. (1981). Cloned cell lines with natural killer activity. Specificity, function, and cell surface markers. *J. Exp. Med.* 153, 545.
240. Brooks, C. G. (1983). Reversible induction of natural killer cell activity in cloned murine cytotoxic T lymphocytes. *Nature (London)* 305, 155.
241. Brooks, C. G., Urdal, D. L., and Henney, C. S. (1983). Lymphokine-driven "differentiation" of cytotoxic T-cell clones into cells with NK-like specificity: Correlations with display of membrane macromolecules. *Immunol. Rev.* 72, 43.
242. Yanagi, Y., Caccia, N., Kronenberg, M., Chin, B., Roder, J., Rohel, J., Rohel, P., Kiyohara, T., Lauzon, B., Toyonaga, B., Rosenthal, K., Dennert, G., Acha-Orbea, H., Hengartner, H., Hood, L., and Mac, T. W. (1985). Gene rearrangement in cells with natural killer activity and expression of the chain of the T-cell antigen receptor. *Nature (London)* 314, 631.
243. Ikuta, K., Hattori, M., Wake, K., Kano, S., Honjo, T., Yodo, I. J., and Minato, N. (1986). Expression and rearrangement of the alpha, beta, and gamma chain genes of the T cell receptor in cloned murine large granular lymphocyte lines. No correlation with the cytotoxic spectrum. *J. Exp. Med.* 164, 428.
244. Biron, C. A., Van Den Elsen, P., Tutt, M. M., Medveczky, P., Kumar, V., and Terhorst, C. (1987). Murine natural killer cells stimulated in vivo do not express the T cell receptor α, β, γ, T3δ or T3ϵ genes. *J. Immunol.* 139, 1704.
245. Tutt, M. M., Schuler, W., Kuziel, W. A., Tucker, P. W., Bennett, M., Bosma, M. J., and Kumar, V. (1987). T cell receptor genes do not rearrange or express functional transcripts in natural killer cells of SCID mice. *J. Immunol.* 138, 2338.
246. Herberman, R. B., Bartram, S., Haskill, J. S., Nunn, M., Holden, H. T., and West, W. H. (1977). Fc receptor on mouse effector cells mediating natural cytotoxicity against tumor cells. *J. Immunol.* 119, 322.
247. Ojo, E., and Wigzell, H. (1978). Natural killer cells may be the only cells in normal mouse lymphoid cell populations endowed with cytolytic ability for antibody-coated tumor target cells. *Scand. J. Immunol.* 7, 297.

248. Santoni, A., Herberman, R. B., and Holden, H. T. (1979). Correlation between natural and antibody-dependent cell-mediated cytotoxicity against tumor targets in the mouse. I. Distribution of the reactivity. *JNCI, J. Natl. Cancer Inst.* **62**, 109.
249. Beaumont, T. J., Roder, J. C., Elliott, B. E., Kerbel, R. S., Dennis, J. W., Kasai, M., and Okumura, K. (1982). A comparative analysis of cell surface markers on murine NK cells and CTL target-effector conjugates. *Scand. J. Immunol.* **16**, 123.
250. Unkeless, J. C. (1979). Characterization of a monoclonal antibody directed against mouse macrophage and lymphocyte Fc receptors. *J. Exp. Med.* **150**, 580.
251. Stutman, O., Paige, C. J., and Figarella, E. R. (1978). Natural cytotoxic cells against solid tumors in mice. I. Strain and age distribution and target cell susceptibility. *J. Immunol.* **121**, 1819.
252. Stutman, O., Lattime, E. C., and Figarella, E. F. (1981). Natural cytotoxic cells against solid tumors in mice: A comparison with natural killer cells. *Fed. Proc., Fed. Am. Soc. Exp. Biol.* **40**, 2699.
253. Burton, R. P., Bartlett, S. P., Kumar, V., and Winn, H. J. (1981). Studies on natural killer (NK) cells. II. Serologic evidence for heterogeneity of murine NK cells. *J. Immunol.* **127**, 1864.
254. Lust, J. A., Kumar, V., Burton, R. C., Bartlett, S. P., and Bennett, M. (1981). Heterogeneity of natural killer cells in the mouse. *J. Exp. Med.* **154**, 306.
255. Lattime, E. C., Pecoraro, G. A., and Stutman, O. (1981). Natural cytotoxic cells against solid tumors in mice. III. A comparison of effector cell antigenic phenotype and target cell recognition structures with those of NK cells. *J. Immunol.* **126**, 2011.
256. Bykowski, M. J., and Stutman, O. (1986). The cells responsible for murine natural cytotoxic (NC) activity: A multi-lineage system. *J. Immunol.* **137**, 1120.
257. Ortaldo, J. R., Mason, L. H., Mathieson, B. J., Liang, S., Flick, D. A., and Herberman, R. B. (1986). Mediation of mouse natural cytotoxic activity by tumor necrosis factor. *Nature (London)* **321**, 700.
258. Richards, A. L., Okuno, T., Takagaki, Y., and Djeu, J. Y. (1988). Natural cytotoxic cell-specific cytotoxic factor produced by IL-3-dependent basophilic/mast cells. Relationship to TNF. *J. Immunol.* **141**, 3061.
259. Richards, A. L., Dennert, G., Pluznik, D. H., Tagakaki, Y., and Djeu, J. (1989). Natural cytotoxic (NC) activity in a cloned natural killer (NK) cell line is mediated by tumor necrosis factor (TNF). *Nat. Immun. Cell Growth Regul.* (in press).
260. Cuturi, M. C., Murphy, M., Costa-Giomi, M. P., Weinmann, R., Perussia, B., and Trinchieri, G. (1987). Independent regulation of tumor necrosis factor and lymphotoxin production by human peripheral blood lymphocytes. *J. Exp. Med.* **165**, 1581.
261. Reynolds, C. W., Shannon, S. O., Ortaldo, J. R., and Herberman, R. B. (1981). Natural killer cell activity in the rat. II. Analysis of surface antigens on LGL by flow cytometry. *J. Immunol.* **127**, 2204.
262. Woda, B. A., McFadden, M. L., Welsh, R. M., and Bain, K. M. (1984). Separation and isolation of rat natural killer cells from T cells with monoclonal antibodies. *J. Immunol.* **137**, 2183.
263. Young, H. A., Ortaldo, J. R., Herberman, R. B., and Reynolds, C. W. (1986). Analysis of T cell receptors in highly purified rat and human large granular lymphocytes (LGL): Lack of functional 1.3 kb beta-chain mRNA. *J. Immunol.* **130**, 2701.
264. Reynolds, C. W., Bonyhadi, M., Herberman, R. B., Young, H. A., and Hedrick, S. M. (1985). Lack of gene rearrangement and mRNA expression of the beta chain of the T cell receptor in spontaneous rat large granular lymphocyte leukemia lines. *J. Exp. Med.* **161**, 1249.

265. Loughran, T. P., Jr., Deeg, H. J., and Storb, R. (1985). Morphologic and phenotypic analysis of canine natural killer cells: Evidence for a T-cell lineage. *Cell. Immunol.* **95**, 207.
266. Magnuson, N. S., Perryman, L. E., Wyatt, C. R., Mason, P. H., and Talmadge, J. E. (1987). Large granular lymphocytes from SCID horses develop potent cytotoxic activity after treatment with human recombinant interleukin 2. *J. Immunol.* **139**, 61.
267. Kim, Y. B., Huh, N. D., Koren, H. S., and Amos, D. B. (1980). Natural killing (NK) and antibody-dependent cellular cytotoxicity (ADCC) in specific pathogen-free (SPF) miniature swine and germfree piglets. I. Comparison of NK and ADCC. *J. Immunol.* **125**, 755.
268. Bielefeldt-Ohmann, H., Davis, W. C., and Babiuk, L. A. (1985). Functional and phenotypic characteristics of bovine natural cytotoxic cells. *Immunobiology* **169**, 503.
269. Ding, A. H., and Lam, K. M. (1986). Enhancement by interferon of chicken splenocyte natural killer cell activity against Marek's disease tumor cells. *Vet. Immunol. Immunopathol.* **11**, 65.
270. Klempau, A. E., and Cooper, E. L. (1984). T-lymphocyte and B-lymphocyte dichotomy in anuran amphibians: III. Assessment and identification of inducible killer T-lymphocytes (IKTL) and spontaneous killer T-lymphocytes (SKTL). *Dev. Comp. Immunol.* **8**, 649.
271. Evans, D. L., Jaso-Friedmann, L., Smith, E. E., Jr., St. John, A., Koren, H. S., and Harris, D. T. (1988). Identification of a putative antigen receptor on fish nonspecific cytotoxic cells with monoclonal antibodies. *J. Immunol.* **141**, 324.
272. Lucero, M. A., Fridman, W. H., Provost, M. A., Billardon, C., Pouillart, P., Dumont, J., and Falcoff, E. (1981). Effect of various interferons on the spontaneous cytotoxicity exerted by lymphocytes from normal and tumor-bearing patients. *Cancer Res.* **41**, 294.
273. Reynolds, C. W., Timonen, T. T., and Herberman, R. B. (1981). Natural killer (NK) cell activity in the rat. I. Isolation and characterization of the effector cells. *J. Immunol.* **127**, 282.
274. Pappenheim, A., and Ferrata, A. (1911). Uber die verschiedenen lymphoiden Zellformen des normalen und pathologischen Blutes. *Folia Haemat.* **10**, 78.
275. Grossi, C. E., Cadoni, A., Zicca, A., Leprini, A., and Ferrarini, M. (1982). Large granular lymphocytes in human peripheral blood: Ultrastructural and cytochemical characterization of the granules. *Blood* **59**, 277.
276. Babcock, G. F., and Phillips, J. H. (1983). Human NK cells: Light and electron microscopic characteristics. *Surv. Immunol. Res.* **2**, 88.
277. Payne, C. M., and Glasser, L. (1981). Evaluation of surface markers on normal human lymphocytes containing parallel tubular arrays: A quantitative ultrastructural study. *Blood* **57**, 567.
278. Huhn, D., Huber, C., and Gastl, G. (1982). Large granular lymphocytes: Morphological studies. *Eur. J. Immunol.* **12**, 985.
279. Caulfield, J. P., Hein, A., Schmidt, R. E., and Ritz, J. (1987). Ultrastructural evidence that the granules of human natural killer cell clones store membrane in a nonbilayer phase. *Am. J. Pathol.* **127**, 305.
280. Kang, Y.-H., Carl, M., Grimley, P. M., Serrate, S., and Yaffe, L. (1987). Immunoultrastructural studies of human NK cells. I. Ultracytochemistry and comparison with T cell subsets. *Anat. Rec.* **217**, 274.
281. Zarcone, D., Prasthofer, E. F., Malavasi, F., Pistoia, V., LoBuglio, A. F., and

Grossi, C. (1987). Ultrastructural analysis of human natural killer cell activation. *Blood* **69**, 1725.
282. Grossi, C. E., and Ferrarini, M. (1982). Morphology and cytochemistry of human large granular lymphocytes. *In* "NK Cells and Other Natural Effector Cells" (R. B. Herberman, ed.), p. 1. Academic Press, New York.
283. Manara, G. C. S. P., Ferrari, C., and De Panfilis, G. (1986). Natural killer cells expressing the Leu-11 antigen display phagocytic activity for 2-aminoethylisothiouronium bromide hydrobromide-treated sheep red blood cells. *Lab. Invest.* **55**, 412.
284. Kang, Y.-H., Carl, M., Watson, L., and Yaffe, L. (1986). Immunoultrastructural studies of human NK cells. II. Effector-target cell binding and phagocytosis. *Anat. Rec.* **217**, 290.
285. Huhn, D. (1968). Neue Organelle im Peripheren Lymphozyten? *Dtsch. Med. Wochenschr.* **3**, 2099.
286. Hovig, T., Jeremic, M., and Staven, P. (1968). A new type of inclusion body in lymphocytes. *Scand. J. Haematol.* **5**, 81.
287. Payne, C. M., and Tennican, P. M. (1982). A quantitative ultrastructural study of peripheral blood lymphocytes containing parallel tubular arrays in Epstein-Barr virus and cytomegalovirus mononucleosis. *Am. J. Pathol.* **106**, 71.
288. Payne, C. M., Jones, J. F., Sieber, O. F. J., and Fulginiti, V. A. (1977). Parallel tubular arrays in severe combined immunodeficiency disease: An ultrastructural study of peripheral blood lymphocytes. *Blood* **50**, 55.
289. Payne, C. M., Glasser, L., Fiederlein, R., and Lindberg, R. (1983). New ultrastructural observations: Parallel tubular arrays in human T-gamma lymphoid cells. *J. Immunol. Methods* **65**, 307.
290. Smit, J. W., Blom, N. R., Van Luyn, M., and Halie, M. R. (1983). Lymphocytes with parallel tubular structures: Morphologically as distinct subpopulation. *Blut* **46**, 311.
291. Smit, J. W., Blom, N. R., Van Luyn, M. J. A., and Halie, M. R. (1983). Susceptibility of the expression of parallel tubular structures in lymphocytes to the exposure to ammonium chloride buffer. *J. Immunol. Methods* **67**, 49.
292. Gruner, S. M., Cullis, P. R., Hope, M. J., and Tilcock, C. P. S. (1985). Lipid polymorphism: The molecular basis of nonbilayer phases. *Annu. Rev. Biophys. Chem.* **14**, 211.
293. Polli, N., Matutes, E., Robinson, D., and Catovsky, D. (1987). Morphological heterogeneity of Leu7, Leu11 and OKM$_1$ positive lymphocyte subsets: An ultrastructural study with the immunogold method. *Clin. Exp. Immunol.* **68**, 331.
294. Matutes, E., and Catovsky, D. (1982). The fine structure of normal lymphocyte subpopulations—A study with monoclonal antibodies and the immunogold technique. *Clin. Exp. Immunol.* **50**, 416.
295. Manara, G. C., De Panfilis, G., Ferrari, C., and Scandroglio, R. (1984). Immunoperoxidase-immunogold double labeling in immunoelectromicroscopy of large granular lymphocytes. *J. Immunol. Methods* **75**, 189.
296. Manara, G. C., De Panfilis, G., Ferrari, C., Bonati, A., and Scandroglio, R. (1984). The fine structure of HNK-1 (Leu 7) positive cells. A study using an immunoperoxidase technique. *Histochemistry* **81**, 153.
297. Manara, G. C., De Panfilis, G., and Ferrari, C. (1985). Ultrastructural characterization of human large granular lymphocyte subsets defined by the expression of HNK-1 (Leu-7), Leu-11, or both HNK-1 and Leu-11 antigens. *J. Histochem. Cytochem.* **33**, 1129.

298. Kang, Y.-H., Carl, M., Watson, L. P., and Yaffe, L. (1985). Immunoelectron microscopic identification of human NK cells by FITC-conjugated anti-Leu 11a and biotinylated anti-Leu-7 antibodies. *J. Immunol. Methods* **84**, 177.
299. Arancia, G., Fiorentini, C., Ferrari, C., De Panfilis, G., and Manara, G. C. (1986). Morphometric characterization of NK cell subset expressing the Leu-11 antigen in comparison to Leu-7 positive 11 negative cells. *Cell Biol. Int. Rep.* **10**, 845.
300. Zucker-Franklin, D., Grusky, G., and Yang, J.-S. (1983). Arylsulfatase in natural killer cells: Its possible role in cytotoxicity. *Proc. Natl Acad. Sci. U.S.A.* **80**, 6977.
301. Ferrarini, M., Cadoni, A., Franzi, A. T., Ghigliotti, C., Leprini, A., Zicca, A., and Grossi, C. E. (1980). Ultrastructure and cytochemistry of human peripheral blood lymphocytes. Similarities between the cells of the third population and T_G cells. *Eur. J. Immunol.* **10**, 562.
302. Landay, A., Clement, L. T., and Grossi, C. E. (1984). Phenotypically and functionally distinct subpopulations of human lymphocytes with T cell markers also exhibit different cytochemical patterns of staining for lysosomal enzymes. *Blood* **63**, 1067.
303. Monahan, R. A., Dvorak, H. F., and Dvorak, A. M. (1981). Ultrastructural localization of nonspecific esterase activity in guinea pig and human monocytes, macrophages, and lymphocytes. *Blood* **58**, 1089.
304. Prasthofer, F., Zarcone, D., and Grossi, C. E. (1988). Distinctive morphological features of human peripheral blood lymphocytes. *EOS—J. Immunol. Immunopharmacol.* **8**, 84.
305. Freundlich, B., Trinchieri, G., Perussia, B., and Zurier, R. B. (1984). The cytotoxic effector cells in preparations of adherent mononuclear cells from human peripheral blood. *J. Immunol.* **132** 1255.
306. Rolstad, B., Herberman, R. B., and Reynolds, C. W. (1986). Natural killer cell activity in the rat. V. The circulation patterns and tissue localization of peripheral blood large granular lymphocytes (LGL). *J. Immunol.* **136**, 2800.
307. Nieminen, P. (1986). The tissue distribution of NK-9 positive lymphoid cells including NK and AK cells and their precursors. *Acta Pathol. Microbiol. Immunol. Scand.* **94**, 119.
308. Fukui, H., Overton, W. R., Herberman, R. B., and Reynolds, C. W. (1987). Natural killer cell activity in the rat. VI. Characterization of rat large granular lymphocytes as effector cells in natural killer and antibody-dependent cellular cytotoxic activities. *J. Leuk. Biol.* **41**, 130.
309. Fresa, K. L., Korngold, R., and Murasko, D. M. (1985). Induction of natural killer cell activity of thoracic duct lymphocytes by polyinosinic–polycytidylic acid (polyI:C) or interferon. *Cell. Immunol.* **91**, 336.
310. Talpaz, M., and Spitzer, G. (1984). Low natural killer cell activity in the bone marrow of healthy donors with normal killer cell activity in the peripheral blood. *Exp. Hematol. (Copenhagen)* **12**, 629.
311. von Gaudecker, B., Pfingsten, U., and Müller-Hermelink, H. K. (1984). Localization and characterization of T-cell subpopulations and natural killer cells (HNK 1+ cells) in the human tonsilla palatina. An ultrastructural-immunocytochemical study. *Cell Tissue Res.* **238**, 135.
312. Christmas, S. E., Allan, G., and Moore, M. (1985). Naturally cytotoxic tonsillar leukocytes: Phenotypic characterization of the effector population. *Scand. J. Immunol.* **22**, 61.
313. Weissler, J. C., Nicod, L. P., Lipscomb, M. F.,and Toews, G. B. (1987). Natural

killer cell function in human lung is compartmentalized. *Am. Rev. Respir. Dis.* **135**, 941.
314. Prichard, M. G., Boerth, L. W., and Pennington, J. E. (1987). Compartmental analysis of resting and activated pulmonary natural killer cells. *Exp. Lung Res.* **12**, 239.
315. Mann, D. W., Sonnenfeld, G., and Stein-Streilein, J. (1985). Pulmonary compartmentalization of interferon and natural killer cell activity. *Proc. Soc. Exp. Biol. Med.* **180**, 224.
316. Luini, W., Boraschi, D., Alberti, S., Aleotti, A., and Tagliabue, A. (1981). Morphological characterization of a cell population responsible for natural killer activity. *Immunology* **43**, 663.
317. Ward, J. M., Argilan, F., and Reynolds, C. W. (1983). Immunoperoxidase localization of large granular lymphocytes in normal tissue and lesions of athymic nude rats. *J. Immunol.* **131**, 132.
318. Nauss, K. M., Pavlina, T. M., Kumar, V., and Newberne, P. M. (1984). Functional characteristics of lymphocytes isolated from the rat large intestine. Response to T-cell mitogens and natural killer cell activity. *Gastroenterology* **86**, 468.
319. Alberti, S., Colotta, F., Spreafico, F., Delia, D., Pasqualetto, E., and Luini, W. (1985). Large granular lymphocytes from murine blood and intestinal epithelium: Comparison of surface antigens, natural killer activity, and morphology. *Clin. Immunol. Immunopathol.* **36**, 227.
320. Carman, P. S., Ernst, P. B., Rosenthal, K. L., Clark, D. A., Befus, A. D., and Bienenstock, J. (1986). Intraepithelial leukocytes contain a unique subpopulation of NK-like cytotoxic cells active in the defense of gut epithelium to enteric murine coronavirus. *J. Immunol.* **136**, 1548.
321. Gibson, P. R., Dow, E. L., Selby, W. S., Strickland, R. G., and Jewell, D. P. (1984). Natural killer cells and spontaneous cell-mediated cytotoxicity in the human intestine. *Clin. Exp. Immunol.* **56**, 438.
322. Gibson, P. R., Verhaar, H. J., Selby, W. S., and Jewell, D. P. (1984). The mononuclear cells of human mesenteric blood, intestinal mucosa and mesenteric lymph nodes: Compartmentalization of NK cells. *Clin. Exp. Immunol.* **56**, 445.
323. Gibson, P. R., and Jewell, D. P. (1985). The nature of the natural killer (NK) cell of human intestinal mucosa and mesenteric lymph node. *Clin. Exp. Immunol.* **61**, 160.
324. Hogan, P. G., Hapel, A. J., and Doe, W. F. (1985). Lymphokine-activated and natural killer cell activity in human intestinal mucosa. *J. Immunol.* **135**, 1731.
325. Cerf-Bensussan, N., Guy-Grand, D., and Griscelli, C. (1985). Intraepithelial lymphocytes of human gut: Isolation, characterisation and study of natural killer activity. *Gut* **26**, 81.
326. Shanahan, F., Brogan, M., and Targan, S. (1987). Human mucosal cytotoxic effector cells. *Gastroenterology* **92**, 1951.
327. Wiltrout, R. H., Mathieson, B. J., Talmadge, J. E., Reynolds, C. W., Zhang, S. R., Herberman, R. B., and Ortaldo, J. R. (1984). Augmentation of organ-associated natural killer activity by biological response modifiers. Isolation and characterization of large granular lymphocytes from the liver. *J. Exp. Med.* **160**, 1431.
328. Cohen, S. A., Salazar, D., von Muenchhausen, W., Werner-Wasik, M., and Nolan, J. P. (1985). Natural antitumor defense system of the murine liver. *J. Leuk. Biol.* **37**, 559.

329. Zhang, S. R., Salup, R. R., Urias, P. E., Twilley, T. A., Talmadge, J. E., Herberman, R. B., and Wiltrout, R. H. (1986). Augmentation of NK activity and/or macrophage-mediated cytotoxicity in the liver by biological response modifiers including human recombinant interleukin 2. *Cancer Immunol. Immunother.* **21**, 19.
330. Malter, M., Friedrich, E., and Suss, R. (1986). Liver as a tumor cell killing organ: Kupffer cells and natural killers. *Cancer Res.* **46**, 3055.
331. Leung, K. H., Salazar, D., Ip, M. M., and Cohen, S. A. (1987). Characterization of natural cytotoxic effector cells isolated from rat liver. *Nat. Immun. Cell Growth Regul.* **6**, 150.
332. Malter, M., Suss, R., and Fischer, H. (1987). Natural cytotoxic cells from rat liver and spleen kill human glioma cells. *J. Cancer Res. Clin. Oncol.* **113**, 498.
333. Wisse, E., Van'T Noordende, J., Van Der Meulen, J., and Daems, W. T. (1976). Pit cell description of a new type of cell occurring in rat liver sinusoids and peripheral blood. *Cell Tissue Res.* **173**, 423.
334. Bouwens, L., Remels, L., Baekeland, M., Van Bossuyt, H., and Wisse, E. (1987). Large granular lymphocytes or "Pit cells" from rat liver: Isolation, ultrastructural characterization and natural killer activity. *Eur. J. Immunol.* **17**, 37.
335. Bouwens, L., and Wisse, E. (1987). Immuno-electron microscopic characterization of large granular lymphocytes (natural killer cells) from rat liver. *Eur. J. Immunol.* **17**, 1423.
336. Hornung, R. L., Salup, R. R., and Wiltrout, R. H. (1988). Tissue distribution and localization of IL2-activated killer cells after adoptive transfer in vivo. In "The Role of IL2 and IL2 Activated Killer Cells in Cancer" (E. Lotzova and R. B. Herberman, eds.), p. 5. CRC Press, Boca Raton, Florida.
337. Uksila, J., Lassila, O., Hirvonen, T., and Toivanen, P. (1985). Natural killer cell activity of human fetal liver cells after allogeneic stimulation. *Scand. J. Immunol.* **22**, 433.
338. Ueno, Y., Miyawaki, T., Seki, H., Matsuda, A., Taga, K., Sato, H., and Taniguchi, N. (1985). Differential effects of recombinant human interferon-gamma and interleukin 2 on natural killer cell activity of peripheral blood in early human development. *J. Immunol.* **135**, 180.
339. Uksila, J., Lassila, O., and Hirvonen, T. (1982). Natural killer cell function of human neonatal lymphocytes. *Clin. Exp. Immunol.* **48**, 649.
340. Lubens, R. G., Gard, S. F., Soderberg-Warner, M., and Stiehm, E. R. (1982). Lectin-dependent T-lymphocyte and natural killer cytotoxic deficiencies in human newborns. *Cell. Immunol.* **74**, 40.
341. Tarkkanen, J., and Säkselä, E. (1982). Umbilical-cord-blood-derived suppressor cells of the human natural killer cells activity are inhibited by interferon. *Scand. J. Immunol.* **15**, 149.
342. Abo, T., Miller, C. A., and Balch, C. M. (1984). Characterization of human granular lymphocyte subpopulations expressing HNK-1 (Leu-7) and Leu-11 antigens in the blood and lymphoid tissue from fetuses, neonates and adults. *Eur. J. Immunol.* **14**, 616.
343. Huh, N. D., Kim, Y. B., Koren, H. S., and Amos, D. B. (1981). Natural killing and antibody-dependent cellular cytotoxicity in specific-pathogen-free miniature swine and germ-free piglets. II. Ontogenic development of NK and ADCC. *Int. J. Cancer* **28**, 175.
344. Bender, B. S., Chrest, F. J., and Adler, W. H. (1986). Phenotypic expression of

natural killer cell associated membrane antigens and cytolytic function of peripheral blood cells from different aged humans. *J. Clin. Lab. Immunol.* **21**, 31.

345. Hu, C., Scorza-Smeraldi, R., Radelli, L., Fabio, G., and Vanoli, M. (1987). Age- and sex-dependent changes in natural killer cell activity. *Boll. Ist. Sieroter. Milan.* **66**, 289.

346. Tilden, A. B., Grossi, C. E., Itoh, K., Cloud, G. A., Dougherty, P. A., and Balch, C. M. (1986). Subpopulation analysis of human granular lymphocytes: Associations with age, gender and cytotoxic activity. *Nat. Immun. Cell Growth Regul.* **5**, 90.

347. Ligthart, G. J., Van Vlokhoven, P. C., Schuit, H. R., and Hijmans, W. (1986). The expanded null cell compartment in ageing: Increase in the number of natural killer cells and changes in T-cell and NK-cell subsets in human blood. *Immunology* **59**, 353.

348. Krishnaraj, R., and Blandford, G. (1987). Age-associated alterations in human natural killer cells. 1. Increased activity as per conventional and kinetic analysis. *Clin. Immunol. Immunopathol.* **45**, 268.

349. Krishnaraj, R., and Blandford, G. (1988). Age-associated alterations in human natural killer cells. 2. Increased frequency of selective NK subsets. *Cell. Immunol.* **114**, 137.

350. Facchini, A., Mariani, E., Mariani, A. R., Papa, S., Vitale, M., and Manzoli, F. A. (1987). Increased number of circulating Leu 11+ (CD 16) large granular lymphocytes and decreased NK activity during human ageing. *Clin. Exp. Immunol.* **68**, 340.

351. Pross, H. F., Rubin, P., and Baines, M. (1982). The assessment of natural killer cell activity in cancer patients. In "NK Cells and Other Natural Effector Cells" (R. B. Herberman, ed.), p. 1175. Academic Press, New York.

352. Gatti, G., Del Ponte, D., Cavallo, R., Sartori, M. L., Salvadori, A., Carignola, R., Carandente, F., and Angeli, A. (1987). Circadian changes in human natural killer (NK) activity. *Prog. Clin. Biol. Res.* **227**, 399.

353. Levi, F. A., Canon, C., Touitou, Y., Reinberg, A., and Mathé, G. (1988). Seasonal modulation of the circadian time structure of circulating T and natural killer lymphocyte subsets from healthy subjects. *J. Clin. Invest.* **81**, 407.

354. Hrushesky, W. J., Gruber, S. A., Sothern, R. B., Hoffman, R. A., and Lakatua, D. (1988). Natural killer cell activity: Age, estrous- and circadian-stage dependence and inverse correlation with metastatic potential. *J. Natl. Cancer Inst.* **80**, 1232.

355. Pati, A. K., Florentin, I., Chung, V., De Sousa, M., Levi, F., and Mathé, G. (1987). Circannual rhythm in natural killer activity and mitogen responsiveness of murine splenocytes. *Cell. Immunol.* **108**, 227.

356. Petranyi, G., Ivanyi, P., and Hollan, S. R. (1974). Relation of HL-A and Rh systems to immune reactivity. *Vox Sang.* **26**, 470.

357. Jakobisiak, M., Saidman, S., Schlaut, J., Pazderka, F., and Dossetor, J. B. (1986). Elevated natural killer cytotoxicity in HLA-B8 and HLA-DR3-positive individuals. *Immunol. Lett.* **12**, 61.

358. Warren, R. P., Lum, L. G., and Storb, R. (1985). Is the leukocyte group-5a antigen associated with reduced NK cell function? *Tissue Antigens* **25**, 107.

359. Kiessling, R., Klein, E., Pross, H., and Wigzell, H. (1975). "Natural" killer cells in the mouse. II. Cytotoxic cells with specificity for mouse Moloney leukemia cells. Characteristics of the killer cell. *Eur. J. Immunol.* **5**, 117.

360. Herberman, R. B., Nunn, M. F., and Lavrin, D. H. (1975). Natural cytotoxic

reactivity of mouse lymphoid cells against syngeneic and allogeneic tumors. II. Characterization of effector cells. *Int. J. Cancer* **16**, 230.
361. Cudkowicz, G., and Hochman, P. S. (1979). Do natural killer cells engage in regulated reaction against self to ensure homeostasis? *Immunol. Rev.* **44**, 13.
362. Clark, E. A., Engle, D., and Windsor, N. T. (1981). Immune responsiveness of SM/J mice; hyper NK cell activity mediated by NK1$^+$ Qa5$^-$ cells. *J. Immunol.* **127**, 2391.
363. Vaillier, D., Legrand, E., Labat, V., and Duplan, J. F. (1984). Thymic control in expression of natural killer activity in AKR and C57BL/6 mice. *Ann. Immunol. (Paris)* **135**, 1.
364. Lanza, E., and Djeu, J. Y. (1982). Persistence of natural killer activity in murine peripheral blood lymphocytes. *Fed. Proc., Fed. Am. Soc. Exp. Biol.* **41**, 601.
365. Kawakami, K., and Bloom, E. T. (1987). Lymphokine-activated killer cells and aging in mice: Significance for defining the precursor cell. *Mech. Ageing Dev.* **41**, 229.
366. Saxena, R. K., Saxena, Q. B., and Adler, W. H. (1984). Interleukin-2-induced activation of natural killer activity in spleen cells from old and young mice. *Immunology* **51**, 719.
367. Riccardi, C., Giampietri, A., Migliorati, G., Frati, L., and Herberman, R. B. (1986). Studies on the mechanism of low natural killer cell activity in infant and aged mice. *Nat. Immun. Cell Growth Regul.* **5**, 238.
368. Irimajiri, N., Bloom, E. T., and Makinodan, T. (1985). Suppression of murine natural killer cell activity by adherent cells from aging mice. *Mech. Ageing Dev.* **31**, 155.
369. Albright, J. W., and Albright, J. F. (1985). Age-associated decline in natural killer (NK) activity reflects primarily a defect in function of NK cells. *Mech. Ageing Dev.* **31**, 295.
370. Mysliwska, J., Mysliwski, A., and Witkowski, J. (1985). Age-dependent decline of natural killer and antibody-dependent cell mediated cytotoxicity activity of human lymphocytes is connected with decrease of their acid phosphatase activity. *Mech. Ageing Dev.* **31**, 1.
371. Bash, J. A., and Vogel, D. (1984). Cellular immunosenescence in F344 rats: Decreased natural killer (NK) cell activity involves changes in regulatory interactions between NK cells, interferon, prostaglandin and macrophages. *Mech. Ageing Dev.* **24**, 49.
372. Kiessling, R., and Wigzell, H. (1979). An analysis of the murine NK cell as to structure, function, and biological relevance. *Immunol. Rev.* **44**, 165.
373. Petranyi, G. G., Kiessling, R., Povey, S., Klein, G., Herzenberg, L., and Wigzell, H. (1976). The genetic control of natural killer cell activity and its association with in vivo resistance against a Moloney isograft. *Immunogenetics* **3**, 15.
374. Clark, E. A., and Harmon, R. C. (1980). Genetic control of natural cytotoxicity and hybrid resistance. *Adv. Cancer Res.* **31**, 227.
375. Fleisher, G., Koven, N., Kamiya, H., and Henle, W. (1982). A non-X-linked syndrome with susceptibility to severe Epstein-Barr virus infections. *J. Pediatr.* **100**, 727.
376. Kaminsky, S. G., Nakamura, I., and Cudkowicz, G. (1985). Genetic control of the natural killer cell activity in SJL and other strains of mice. *J. Immunol.* **135**, 665.
377. Biron, C. A., Byron, K. S., and Sullivan, J. L. (1988). Susceptibility to viral infections in an individual with a complete lack of natural killer cells. *Nat. Immun. Cell Growth Regul.* **7**, 47.

378. Ross, G. D., Thompson, R. A., Walport, M. J., Springer, T. A., Watson, J. V., Ward, R. H., Lida, J., Newman, S. L., Harrison, R. A., and Lachman, P. J. (1985). Characterization of patients with an increased susceptibility to bacterial infections and a genetic deficiency of leukocyte membrane complement receptor type 3 and the related membrane antigen LFA-1. *Blood* **66**, 882.
379. Seeley, J. K., Bechtold, T., Purtilo, D. T., and Lindsten, T. (1982). NK deficiency in X-linked lymphoproliferative syndrome. *In* "NK Cells and Other Effector Cells" (R. B. Herberman, ed.), p. 1211. Academic Press, New York.
380. Sullivan, J. L., Biron, K. S., Brewster, F. E., and Purtilo, D. T. (1980). Deficient natural killer cell activity in X-linked lymphoproliferative syndrome. *Science* **210**, 543.
381. White, J. G., and Clawson, C. C. (1980). The Chediak-Higashi syndrome; the nature of the giant neutrophil granules and their interactions with cytoplasm and foreign particulates. *Am. J. Pathol.* **98**, 151.
382. Dent, P. B., Fish, L. A., White, J. F., and Good, R. A. (1966). Chediak-Higashi syndrome. Observations on the nature of the associated malignancy. *Lab. Invest.* **15**, 1634.
383. Haliotis, T., Roder, J., Klein, M., Ortaldo, J., Fauci, A. S., and Herberman, R. B. (1980). Chediak-Higashi gene in humans. I. Impairment of natural-killer function. *J. Exp. Med.* **151**, 1039.
384. Klein, M., Roder, J., Haliotis, T., Korec, S., Jett, J. R., Herberman, R. B., Katz, P., and Fauci, A. S. (1980). Chediak-Higashi gene in humans. II. The selectivity of the defect in natural-killer and antibody-dependent cell-mediated cytotoxicity function. *J. Exp. Med.* **151**, 1049.
385. Roder, J. C., Haliotis, T., Klein, M., Korec, S., Jett, J. R., Ortaldo, J., Herberman, R. B., Katz, P., and Fauci, A. S. (1980). A new immunodeficiency disorder in humans involving NK cells. *Nature (London)* **284**, 553.
386. Roder, J. C., Haliotis, T., Laing, L., Kozbor, D., Rubin, P., Pross, H., Boxer, L. A., White, J. G., Fauci, A. S., Mostowski, H., and Matheson, D. S. (1982). Further studies of natural killer cell function in Chediak-Higashi patients. *Immunology* **46**, 555.
387. Brahmi, Z. (1983). Nature of natural killer cell hyporesponsiveness in the Chediak-Higashi syndrome. *Hum. Immunol.* **6**, 45.
388. Katz, P., Zaytoun, A. M., and Fauci, A. S. (1982). Deficiency of active natural killer cells in the Chediak-Higashi syndrome. Localization of the defect using a single cell cytotoxicity assay. *J. Clin. Invest.* **69**, 1231.
389. Targan, S., and Oseas, R. (1983). The "lazy" NK cells of Chediak-Higashi syndrome. *J. Immunol.* **130**, 2671.
390. Abo, T., Roder, J. C., Abo, W., Cooper, M. D., and Balch, C. M. (1982). Natural killer (HNK-1$^+$) cells in Chediak-Higashi patients are present in normal numbers but are abnormal in function and morphology. *J. Clin. Invest.* **70**, 193.
391. Grossi, C. E., Crist, W. M., Abo, T., Velardi, A., and Cooper, M. D. (1985). Expression of the Chediak-Higashi lysosomal abnormality in human peripheral blood lymphocyte subpopulations. *Blood* **65**, 837.
392. Windhorst, D. B., and Padgett, G. (1973). The Chediak-Higashi syndrome and the homologous trait in animals. *J. Invest. Dermatol.* **60**, 529.
393. Luevano, E., Kumar, V., and Bennett, M. (1981). Hybrid resistance to EL-4 lymphoma cells. II. Association between loss of hybrid resistance and detection of suppressor cells after treatment of mice with ^{89}Sr. *Scand. J. Immunol.* **13**, 563.
394. Roder, J. C., Lohmann-Matthes, M., Domzig, W., and Wigzell, H. (1979). The

beige mutation in the mouse. II. Selectivity of the natural killer (NK) cell defect. *J. Immunol.* **123**, 2174.
395. McGarry, R. C., Walker, R., and Roder, J. C. (1984). The cooperative effect of the satin and beige mutations in the suppression of NK and CTL activities in mice. *Immunogenetics* **20**, 527.
396. Koren, H. S., Amos, D. B., and Buckley, R. B. (1978). Natural killing in immunodeficient patients. *J. Immunol.* **120**, 796.
397. Lipinski, M., Dokhelar, M. C., and Tursz, T. (1982). NK cell activity in patients with high risk for tumors and in patients with cancer. *In* "NK Cells and Other Natural Effector Cells" (R. B. Herberman, ed.), p. 1183. Academic Press, New York.
398. Lipinski, M., Virelizier, J. L., Tursz, T., and Griscelli, C. (1980). Natural killer and killer cell activities in patients with primary immunodeficiencies or defects in immune interferon production. *Eur. J. Immunol.* **10**, 246.
399. Lopez, C., Kirkpatrick, D., Fitzgerald, P. A., Ching, C. Y., Pahwa, R. N., Good, R. A., and Smithwick, E. (1982). Studies of cell lineage of the effector cells that spontaneously lyse HSV-1-infected fibroblasts (NK(HSV-1)). *J. Immunol.* **129**, 824.
400. Peter. H. H., Friederich, W., Dopfer, R., Muller, W., Kortmann, C., Pichler, W., Heinz, F., and Rieger, C. H. L. (1983). NK cell function in severe combined immunodeficiency (SCID): Evidence of a common T cell defect in some but not all SCID patients. *J. Immunol.* **131**, 2332.
401. Peter, H. H., Rieger, C. R., Gendvilis, S., Eckert, G., Pichler, W. J., and Stangel, W. (1982). Spontaneous cell-mediated cytotoxicity (SCMC) in patients with myelodysplastic disorders and immunodeficiency syndromes. *Dev. Immunol.* **17**, 341.
402. Pross, H. F., Gupta, S., Good, R. A., and Baines, M. G. (1978). Spontaneous human lymphocyte-mediated cytotoxicity against tumor target cells. VII. The effect of immunodeficiency disease. *Cell. Immunol.* **43**, 160.
403. Tsuge, I., Matsuoka, H., Torii, S., Okada, J.-I., Mizuno, T., Matsuoka, M., Kodera, Y., and Takahashi, T. (1987). Preservation of natural killer and interleukin-2 activated killer cell activity in ataxiatelangectasia with T cell deficiency. *J. Clin. Lab. Immunol.* **23**, 7.
404. Sirianni, M. C., Businco, L., Seminara, R., and Aiuti, F. (1983). Severe combined immunodeficiencies, primary T-cell defects and DiGeorge syndrome in human: Characterization by monoclonal antibodies and natural killer cell activity. *Clin. Immunol. Immunopathol.* **28**, 361.
405. Messina, C., Kirkpatrick, D., Fitzgerald, P. A., O'Reilly, R. J., Siegal, F. P., Cunningham-Rundles, C., Blaese, M., Oleske, J., Pahwa, S., and Lopez, C. (1986). Natural killer cell function and interferon generation in patients with primary immunodeficiencies. *Clin. Immunol. Immunopathol.* **39**, 394.
406. Hiserodt, J., Britvan, L., and Targan, S. (1982). Differential effects of various pharmacologic agents on the cytolytic reaction mechanism of the human natural killer lymphocyte. *J. Immunol.* **129**, 2266.
407. Lotzova, E., Savary, C. A., Gray, K. N., Raulston, G. L., and Jardine, J. H. (1984). Natural killer cell profile of two random-bred strains of athymic rats. *Exp. Hematol. (Copenhagen)* **12**, 633.
408. Perussia, B., Santoli, D., and Trinchieri, G. (1980). Interferon modulation of natural killer cell activity. *Ann. N.Y. Acad. Sci.* **350**, 55.
409. Sindel, L. J., Buckley, R. H., Schiff, S. E., Ward, F. E., Mickey, G. H., Huang, A. T., Naspitz, C., and Koren, H. (1984). Severe combined immunodeficiency

with natural killer-cell predominance: Abrogation of graft-versus-host disease and immunologic reconstitution with HLA-identical bone marrow cells. *J. Allergy Clin. Immunol.* **73**, 829.

410. Buckley, R. H., Gard, S., Haynes, B. R., Sindel, L. J., Davis, K., Sampson, H. A., Ruff, M. E., and Koren, H. S. (1983). Severe combined immunodeficiency (SCID) with natural killer (NK) cell predominance. *Birth Defects, Orig. Artic. Ser.* **19**, 101.
411. Pierce, G. F., and Polmar, S. H. (1986). Natural cytotoxicity in immunodeficiency diseases: Preservation of natural killer activity and the in vivo appearance of radioresistant killing. *Hum. Immunol.* **15**, 85.
412. Hackett, J. J., Bosma, G. C., Bosma, M. J., Bennett, M., and Kumar, V. (1986). Transplantable progenitors of natural killer cells are distinct from those of T and B lymphocytes. *Proc. Natl. Acad. Sci. U.S.A.* **83**, 3427.
413. Dorshkind, K., Pollack, S. B., Bosma, M. J., and Phillips, R. A. (1985). Natural killer (NK) cells are present in mice with severe combined immunodeficiency (*scid*). *J. Immunol.* **134**, 3798.
414. Seaman, W. E., Gindhart, T. D., Greenspan, J. S., Blackman, M. A., and Talal, N. (1979). Natural killer cells, bone, and the bone marrow: Studies in estrogen-treated mice and in congenitally osteopetrotic (*mi/mi*) mice. *J. Immunol.* **122**, 2541.
415. Seaman, W. E., Merigan, T. C., and Talal, N. (1979). Natural killing in estrogen-treated mice responds poorly to poly I–C despite normal stimulation of circulating interferon. *J. Immunol.* **123**, 2903.
416. Komiyama, A., Kawai, H., Miyagawa, Y., and Akabane, T. (1982). Childhood lymphoblastic leukemia with natural killer activity; establishment of the leukemia cell lines retaining the activity. *Blood* **60**, 1429.
417. Komiyama, A., Yamada, S., Kawai, H., Miyagawa, Y., and Akabane, T. (1984). Childhood acute lymphoblastic leukemia with natural killer activity. Clinical and cellular features of three cases. *Cancer (Philadelphia)* **54**, 1547.
418. Kaplan, J., Ravindranath, Y., and Inoue, S. (1986). T-cell acute lymphoblastic leukemia with natural killer cell phenotype. *Am. J. Hematol.* **22**, 355.
419. McKenna, R. W., Parkin, J., Kersey, J. H., Gajl, K. J., Peterson, L., and Brunning, R. D. (1977). Chronic lymphoproliferative disorder with unusual clinical, morphologic, ultrastructural and membrane surface marker characteristics. *Am. J. Med.* **62**, 588.
420. Bom-van Noorloos, A. A., Pegels, H. G., Van Oers, R. H., Silberbusch, J., Feltkamp-Vroom, T. M., Goudsmit, R., Zeijlemaker, W. P., von dem Borne, A. E., and Melief, C. J. (1980). Proliferation of T gamma cells with killer-cell activity in two patients with neutropenia and recurrent infections. *N. Engl. J. Med.* **302**, 933.
421. Waldmann, T. A., Davis, M. M., Bongiovanni, K. F., and Korsmeyer, S. J. (1985). Rearrangements of genes for the antigen receptor on T cells as markers of lineage and clonality in human lymphoid neoplasms. *N. Engl. J. Med.* **313**, 776.
422. Loughran, T. P., Jr., Kadin, M. E., Starkebaum, G., Abkowitz, J. L., Clark, E. A., Disteche, C., Lum, L. G., and Slichter, S. J. (1985). Leukemia of large granular lymphocytes: Association with clonal chromosomal abnormalities and autoimmune neutropenia thrombocytopenia and hemolytic anemia. *Ann. Intern. Med.* **102**, 169.
423. Rambaldi, A., Pelicci, P., Allavena, P., Knowles, D. M., Rossini, S., Bassan, R., Barbui, T., Dalla-Favera, R., and Mantovani, A. (1985). T cell receptor β chain gene rearrangements in lymphoproliferative disorders of large granular lymphocytes/natural killer cells. *J. Exp. Med.* **162**, 2156.

424. Flug, F., Pelicci, P. G., Bonetti, F., Knowles, D. M., and Dalla-Favera, R. (1985). T-cell receptor gene rearrangements as markers of lineage and clonality in T-cell neoplasms. *Proc. Natl. Acad. Sci. U.S.A.* **82**, 3460.
425. Aisenberg, A. C., Krontiris, T. G., Mak, T. W., and Wilkes, B. M. (1985). Rearrangement of the gene for the beta chain of the T-cell receptor in T cell chronic lymphocytic leukemia and related disorders. *N. Engl. J. Med.* **313**, 529.
426. Minden, M. D., Toyonaga, B., Ha, K., Yanagi, Y., Chin, B., Gelfand, E., and Mak, T. (1985). Somatic rearrangement of T cell antigen receptor β gene in human T cell malignancies. *Proc. Natl. Acad. Sci. U.S.A.* **82**, 1224.
427. Foa, R., Pelicci, P-G., Migone, N., Lauria, F., Pizzolo, G., Flug, F., Knowles, D. M., and Dalla-Favera, R. (1986). Analysis of T cell receptor beta chain (Tβ) gene rearrangements demonstrates the monoclonal nature of T cell chronic lymphoproliferative disorders. *Blood* **67**, 247.
428. Berliner, N., Duby, A. D., Linch, D. C., Murre, C., Quertermous, T., Knott, L. J., Azin, T., Newland, A. C., Lewis, D. L., Galvin, M. C., and Seidman, J. D. (1986). T cell receptor β gene rearrangements define a monoclonal T cell proliferation in patients with T cell lymphocytosis and cytopenia. *Blood* **67**, 914.
429. Semenzato, G., Pizzolo, G., Ranucci, A., Agostini, C., Chilosi, M., Quinti, I., De Sanctis, G., Vercelli, B., and Pandolfi, F. (1984). Abnormal expansions of polyclonal large to small size granular lymphocytes: Reactive or neoplastic process? *Blood* **63**, 1271.
430. McKenna, R. W., Arthur, D. C., Gajl-Peczalska, K. J., Flynn, P., and Brunning, R. D. (1985). Granulated T cell lymphocytosis with neutropenia: Malignant or benign chronic lymphoproliferative disorder? *Blood* **66**, 259.
431. Van De Griend, R. J., and Bolhuis, R. L. H. (1985). In vitro expansion and analysis of cloned cytotoxic T cells derived from patients with chronic Tγ lymphoproliferative disorders. *Blood* **65**, 1002.
432. Pistoia, V., Prasthofer, E. F., Tilden, A. B., Barton, J. C., Ferrarini, M., Grossi, C. E., and Zuckerman, K. S. (1986). Large granular lymphocytes (LGL) from patients with expanded LGL populations acquire cytotoxic functions and release lymphokines upon *in vitro* activation. *Blood* **68**, 1095.
433. Rambaldi, A., Rossi, V., Allavena, P., Introna, M., Landolfo, S., Bassan, R., Barbui, T., and Mantovani, A. (1986). Lymphokine production in Tγ lymphoproliferative disorders. *Scand. J. Immunol.* **23**, 183.
434. Oshimi, K., Oshimi, Y., Akahoshi, M., Kobayashi, Y., Hirai, H., Takaku, F., Hattori, M., Asano, S., Kodo, H., Nishinarita, S., Iizuka, Y., and Mizoguchi, H. (1988). Role of T-cell antigens in the cytolytic activities of large granular lymphocytes (LGL) in patients with LGL lymphocytosis. *Blood* **71**, 473.
435. Pistoia, V., Carroll, A. J., Prasthofer, E. F., Tilden, A. B., Zuckerman, K. S., Ferrarini, M., and Grossi, C. E. (1986). Establishment of TAC-negative, IL-2 dependent cytotoxic cell lines from large granular lymphocytes (LGL) of patients with expanded LGL populations. *J. Clin. Immunol.* **6**, 457.
436. Landay, A., Gebel, H., Levin, S., Prasthofer, E., Pistoia, V., Downing, J., and Grossi, C. (1987). CD16$^+$ NK lymphoproliferative disorders: Cellular and molecular characterization. *Nat. Immun. Cell Growth Regul.* **6**, 141.
437. Chan, W. C., Link, S., Mawle, A., Check, I., Brynes, R. K., and Winton, E. G. (1986). Heterogeneity of large granular lymphocyte proliferations: Delineation of two major subtypes. *Blood* **68**, 1142.
438. Koizumi, S., Seki, H., Tachinami, T., Taniguchi, M., Matsuda, A., Taga, K., Nakarai, T., Kato, E., Taniguchi, N., and Nakamura, H. (1986). Malignant clonal

expansion of large granular lymphocytes with a Leu11+, Leu-7 surface phenotype: In vitro responsiveness of malignant cells to recombinant human interleukin 2. *Blood* **68**, 1065.
439. Kadin, M. E., Kamoun, M., and Lamberg, J. (1981). Erythrophagocytic Ty lymphoma: A clinicopathologic entity resembling malignant histiocytosis. *N. Engl. J. Med.* **304**, 648.
440. Pandolfi, F., Pezzutto, A., De Rossi, G., Pasqualetti, D., Semenzato, G., Quinti, I., Ranucci, A., Raimondi, R., Basso, G., Strong, D. M., Fontana, L., and Aiuti, F. (1984). Characterization of two patients with lymphomas of large granular lymphocytes. *Cancer (Philadelphia)* **53**, 445.
441. Sohn, C. C., Blayney, D. W., Misset, J. L., Mathé, G., Flandrin, G., Moran, E. M., Jensen, F. C., Winberg, C. D., and Rappaport, H. (1986). Leukopenic chronic T cell leukemia mimicking hairy cell leukemia: Association with human retroviruses. *Blood* **67**, 949.
442. Haller, O., and Wigzell, H. (1977). Suppression of natural killer cell activity with radioactive strontium: Effector cells are marrow dependent. *J. Immunol.* **118**, 1503.
443. Kumar, V., Ben-Ezra, J., Bennett, M., and Sonnenfeld, G. (1979). Natural killer cells in mice treated with 89 strontium: Normal target-binding cell numbers but inability to kill even after interferon administration. *J. Immunol.* **123**, 1832.
444. Levy, E. M., Kumar, V., and Bennett, M. (1981). Natural killer activity and suppressor cells in irradiated mice repopulated with a mixture of cells from normal and ^{89}Sr-treated mice. *J. Immunol.* **127**, 1428.
445. Haller, O., Kiessling, R., Orn, A., and Wigzell, H. (1977). Generation of natural killer cells: An autonomous function of the bone marrow. *J. Exp. Med.* **145**, 1411.
446. Roder, J. C. (1979). The beige mutation in the mouse. I. A stem cells predetermined impairment in natural killer cell function. *J. Immunol.* **123**, 2168.
447. Roder, J. C., and Duwe, A. (1979). The beige mutation in the mouse selectively impairs natural killer cell function. *Nature (London)* **278**, 451.
448. Johnson, G. R., and Metcalf, D. (1977). Pure and mixed erythroid colony formation *in vitro* stimulated by spleen conditioned medium with no detectable erythropoietin. *Proc. Natl. Acad. Sci. U.S.A.* **74**, 3879.
449. Stechschulte, D. J., Sharma, R., Dileepan, K. N., Simpson, K. M., Aggarwal, N., Clancy, J., Jr., and Jilka, R. L. (1987). Effect of the *mi* allele on mast cells, basophils, natural killer cells, and osteoclasts in C57BL/6J mice. *J. Cell. Physiol.* **132**, 565.
450. Blomgren, H., Baral, E., Edsmyr, F., Strender, L. E., Petrini, B., and Wasserman, J. (1980). Natural killer activity in peripheral lymphocyte population following local radiation therapy. *Acta Radiol.: Oncol., Radiat. Phys., Biol.* **19**, 139.
451. Brovall, C., and Schacter, B. (1981). Radiation sensitivity of human natural killer cell activity: Control by X-linked genes. *J. Immunol.* **126**, 2236.
452. Dean, D. M., Pross, H. F., and Kennedy, J. C. (1978). Spontaneous human lymphocyte-mediated cytotoxicity against tumor target cells. III. Stimulating and inhibitory effects of ionizing radiation. *Int. J. Radiat. Oncol., Biol., Phys.* **4**, 633.
453. Gorelik, E., and Herberman, R. B. (1982). Depression of natural antitumor resistance of C57BL/6 mice by leukemogenic doses of radiation and restoration of resistance by transfer of bone marrow or spleen cells from normal, but not beige, syngeneic jmice. *JNCI, J. Natl. Cancer Inst.* **69**, 89.
454. Hochman, P. S., Cudkowicz, G., and Dausset, J. (1978). Decline of natural killer cell activity in sublethally irradiated mice. *J. Natl. Cancer Inst.* **61**, 265.
455. Miller, S. C. (1982). Production and renweal of murine killer cells in the spleen and bone marrow. *J. Immunol.* **129**, 2282.

456. Onsrud, M., and Thorsby, E. (1981). Long term changes in natural killer activity after external pelvic radiotherapy. *Int. J. Radiat. Oncol., Biol., Phys.* **7**, 609.
457. Parkinson, D. R., Brightman, R. P., and Waksal, S. D. (1981). Altered natural killer cell biology in C57BL/6 mice after leukemogenic split-dose irradiation. *J. Immunol.* **126**, 1460.
458. Pollack, S. B., and Rosse, C. (1987). The primary role of murine bone marrow in the production of natural killer cells. A cytokinetic study. *J. Immunol.* **139**, 2149.
459. Nassiry, L., and Miller, S. C. (1987). Renewal of natural killer cells in mice having elevated natural killer cell activity. *Nat. Immun. Cell Growth Regul.* **6**, 250.
460. Rooney, C. M., Wimperis, J. Z., Brenner, M. K., Patterson, J., Hoffbrand, A. V., and Prentice, H. G. (1986). Natural killer cell activity following T-cell depleted allogeneic bone marrow transplantation. *Br. J. Haematol.* **62**, 413.
461. Lum, L. G. (1987). The kinetics of immune reconstitution after human marrow transplantation. *Blood* **69**, 369.
462. Keever, C. A., Welte, K., Small, T., Levick, J., Sullivan, M., Hauch, M., Evans, R. L., and O'Reilly, R. J. (1987). Interleukin 2-activated killer cells in patients following transplants of soybean lectin-separated and E rosette-depleted bone marrow. *Blood* **70**, 1893.
463. Hokland, M., Jacobsen, N., Ellegaard, J., and Hokland, P. (1988). Natural killer function following allogeneic bone marrow transplantation. Very early reemergence but strong dependence of cytomegalovirus infection. *Transplantation* **45**, 1080.
464. Sihvola, M., and Hurme, M. (1987). Simultaneous development of antibody-dependent cellular cytotoxicity (ADCC) and natural killer (NK) activity in irradiated mice reconstituted with bone marrow cells. *Cell. Immunol.* **109**, 115.
465. Ault, K. A., Antin, J. H., Ginsburg, D., Orkin, S. H., Rappeport, J. M., Keohan, M. L., Martin, P., and Smith, B. R. (1985). Phenotype of recovering lymphoid cell populations after marrow transplantation. *J. Exp. Med.* **161**, 1483.
466. Hercend, T., Takvorian, T., Nowill, A., Tantravahi, R., Moingeon, P., Anderson, K. C., Murray, C., Bohuon, C., Ythier, A., and Ritz, J. (1986). Characterization of natural killer cells with antileukemia activity following allogeneic bone marrow transplantation. *Blood* **67**, 722.
467. Dokhelar, M. C., Wiels, J., Lipinski, M., Tetaud, C., Devergie, A., Gluckman, E., and Tursz, T. (1981). Natural killer cell activity in human bone marrow recipients: Early reappearance of peripheral natural killer activity in graft-versus-host disease. *Transplantation* **31**, 61.
468. Bowden, R. A., Day, L. M., Amos, D. E., and Meyers, J. D. (1987). Natural cytotoxic activity against cytomegalovirus-infected target cells following marrow transplantation. *Transplantation* **44**, 504.
469. Hurme, M. (1984). Cell proliferation during the maturation of natural killer cells. *Scand. J. Immunol.* **19**, 379.
470. Hurme, M., and Sihvola, M. (1984). High expression of the Thy-1 antigen on natural killer cells recently derived from bone marrow. *Cell. Immunol.* **84**, 276.
471. Sihvola, M., and Hurme, M. (1984). The development of NK cell activity in thymectomized bone marrow chimaeras. *Immunology* **53**, 17.
472. Kaminsky, S. G., Milisauskas, V., Chen, P. B., and Nakamura, I. (1987). Defective differentiation of natural killer cells in SJL mice. Role of the thymus. *J. Immunol.* **138**, 1020.
473. Hackett, J. J., Bennett, M., and Kumar, V. (1985). Origin and differentiation of natural killer cells. I. Characteristics of a transplantable NK cell precursor. *J. Immunol.* **134**, 3731.

474. Miller, S. C. (1984). Fetal thymic pre-T cells neither demonstrate nor develop natural killer cell activity. *Cell. Immunol.* **84**, 194.
475. Riccardi, C., Rossi, R., Giampietri, A., Migliorati, G., and Biondi, R. (1984). Effects of interleukin-1 (IL-1) and interleukin-2 (IL-2) on the in vivo growth and differentiation of progenitors of natural killer (NK) cells. *Chemioterapia* **3**, 350.
476. Riccardi, C., Giampietri, A., Migliorati, G., Cannarile, L., D'Adamio, L., and Herberman, R. B. (1986). Generation of mouse natural killer (NK) cell activity: Effect of interleukin-2 (IL-2) and interferon (IFN) on the in vivo development of natural killer cells from bone marrow (BM) progenitor cells. *Int. J. Cancer* **38**, 553.
477. Kalland, T. (1987). Physiology of natural killer cells. In vivo regulation of progenitors by interleukin 3. *J. Immunol.* **139**, 3671.
478. Koo, G. C., Peppard, J. R., Hatzfeld, A., and Cayre, Y. (1981). Ontogeny of NK-1+ natural killer cells. *In* "NK Cells and Other Natural Effector Cells" (R. B. Herberman, ed.), p. 325. Academic Press, New York.
479. Koo, G. C., Peppard, J. R., and Mark, W. H. (1984). Natural killer cells generated from bone marrow culture. *J. Immunol.* **132**, 2300.
480. Klimpel, G. R., Sarzotti, M., Reyes, V. E., and Klimpel, K. D. (1985). Characterization of cytotoxic cells generated from in vitro cultures of murine bone marrow cells. *Cell. Immunol.* **92**, 1.
481. Kalland, T. (1986). Generation of natural killer cells from bone marrow precursors in vitro. *Immunology* **57**, 493.
482. Koo, G. C., Peppard, J. R., and Lattime, E. C. (1986). Characterization of cytotoxic cells generated from bone marrow culture. *Cell. Immunol.* **98**, 172.
483. Migliorati, G., Cannarile, L., Herberman, R. B., and Riccardi, C. (1987). Role of interleukin 2 (IL-2) and hemopoietin-1 (H-1) in the generation of mouse natural killer (NK) cells from primitive bone marrow precursors. *J. Immunol.* **138**, 3618.
484. Migliorati. G., Cannarile, L., D'Adamio, L., Herberman, R. B., and Riccardi, C. (1987). Interleukin-1 augments the interleukin-2-dependent generation of natural killer cells from the bone marrow precursors. *Nat. Immun. Cell Growth Regul.* **6**, 306.
485. Migliorati, G., Cannarile, L., Herberman, R. B.,and Riccardi, C. (1988). Role of interferons in natural killer cell generation from primitive bone marrow precursors. *Int. J. Immunopharmacol.* **10**, 665.
486. Migliorati, G., Carrarile, L., Herberman, R. B., and Riccardi, C. (1989). Effect of various cytokines and growth factors on the IL-2-dependent in vitro differentiation of NK cells from bone marrow. *Nat. Immun. Cell Growth Regul.* **8**, 48.
487. Kalland, T. (1986). Interleukin 3 is a major negative regulator of the generation of natural killer cells from bone marrow precursors. *J. Immunol.* **137**, 2268.
488. Yung, Y. P., Okumura, K., and Moore, M. A. (1985). Generation of natural killer cell lines from murine long-term bone marrow cultures. *J. Immunol.* **134**, 1462.
489. Lotzova, E., and Savary, C. A. (1987). Generation of NK cell activity from human bone marrow. *J. Immunol.* **139**, 279.
490. Yoda, Y., Kawakami, Z., Shibuya, A., and Abe, T. (1988). Characterization of natural killer cells cultured from human bone marrow cells. *Exp. Hematol. (Copenhagen)* **16**, 712.
491. Shau, H., and Golub, S. H. (1985). Depletion of NK cells with the lysosomotropic agent L-leucine methyl ester and the in vitro generation of NK activity from NK precursor cells. *J. Immunol.* **134**, 1136.
492. Warren, H. S. (1984). Differentiation of NK-like cells from OKT3−, OKT11+,

and OKM1 + small resting lymphocytes by culture with autologous T cell blasts and lymphokine. *J. Immunol.* **132**, 2888.
493. Warren, H. S., and Pembrey, R. G. (1986). Cyclosporin inhibits a two-signal mechanism for the generation of cytotoxic NK-like cells from small lymphocyte precursors. *Immunol. Lett.* **12**, 69.
494. Torten, M., Sidell, N., and Golub, S. H. (1982). Interleukin 2 and stimulator lymphoblastoid cells induce human thymocytes to bind and kill K562 targets. *J. Exp. Med.* **156**, 1545.
495. Toribio, M. L., De Landazuri, M. O., and Lopez-Botet, M. (1983). Induction of natural killer-like cytotoxicity in cultured human thymocytes. *Eur. J. Immunol.* **13**, 964.
496. Michon, J. M., Caligiuri, M. A., Hazanow, S. M., Levine, H., Schlossman, S. F., and Ritz, J. (1988). Induction of natural killer effectors from human thymus with recombinant IL-2. *J. Immunol.* **140**, 3660.
497. Blue, M. L., Levine, H., Daley, J. F., Craig, K. A., and Schlossman, S. F. (1987). Development of natural killer cells in human thymocyte culture: Regulation by accessory cells. *Eur. J. Immunol.* **17**, 669.
498. Ramsdell, F. J., Gray, J. D., and Golub, S. H. (1988). Similarities between LAK cells derived from human thymocytes and peripheral blood lymphocytes: Expression of the NKH-1 and CD3 antigens. *Cell. Immunol.* **114**, 209.
499. Laskay, T., and Kiessling, R. (1986). Interferon and butyrate treatment leads to a decreased sensitivity of NK target cells to lysis by homologous but not by heterologous effector cells. *Nat. Immun. Cell Growth Regul.* **5**, 211.
500. Henkart, P. A., Lewis, J. T., and Ortaldo, J. R. (1986). Preparation of target antigens specifically recognized by human natural killer cells. *Nat. Immun. Cell Growth Regul.* **5**, 113.
501. Roozemond, R. C., Van Der Geer, P., and Bonavida, B. (1986). Effect of altered membrane structure on NK cell-mediated cytotoxicity. II. Conversion of NK-resistant tumor cells into NK-sensitive targets upon fusion with liposomes containing NK-sensitive membranes. *J. Immunol.* **136**, 3921.
502. Timonen, T., Ortaldo, J. R., and Herberman, R. B. (1982). Analysis by a single cell cytotoxicity assay of natural killer (NK) cell frequencies among human large granular lymphocytes and of the effects of IFN on their activity. *J. Immunol.* **128**, 2514.
503. Trinchieri, G., Granato, D., and Perussia, B. (1981). Interferon-induced resistance of fibroblasts to cytolysis mediated by natural killer cells: Specificity and mechanism. *J. Immunol.* **126**, 335.
504. Wright, S. C., and Bonavida, B. (1982). Lysis of NK targets by natural killer cytotoxic factors (NKCF): Dual effects of interferon-treatment of effector or target cells. *Fed. Proc., Fed. Am. Soc. Exp. Biol.* **41**, 476 (abstr.).
505. Yefenof, E., Yron, I., and Klein, E. (1987). Complement-dependent cellular cytotoxicity due to alternative pathway C3 activation by the target cell membrane. *Cell. Immunol.* **87**, 698.
506. Kai, C., Sarmay, G., Ramos, O., Yefenof, E., and Klein, E. (1988). Elevated NK sensitivity of Raji cells carrying acceptor-bound C3 fragments. *Cell. Immunol.* **113**, 227.
507. Van De Griend, R. J., Bolhuis, R. L. H., Stoter, G., and Roozemond, R. C. (1987). Regulation of cytolytic activity in CD3$^-$ and CD3$^+$ killer cell clones by monoclonal antibodies (anti-CD16, anti-CD2, anti-CD3) depends on subclass specificity of target cell IgG-FcR. *J. Immunol.* **138**, 3137.
508. Titus, J. A., Perez, P., Kaubisch, A., Garrido, M. A., and Segal, D. M. (1987).

Human K/natural killer cells targeted with hetero-cross-linked antibodies specifically lyse tumor cells *in vitro* and prevent tumor growth *in vivo. J. Immunol.* **139**, 3153.
509. Segal, D. M., and Wunderlich, J. R. (1988). Targeting of cytotoxic cells heterocrosslinked antibodies. *Cancer Invest.* **6**, 83.
510. Bandyopadhyay, S., Perussia, B., Trinchieri, G., Miller, D. S., and Starr, S. E. (1986). Requirement for HLA-DR positive accessory cells in natural killing of cytomegalovirus-infected fibroblasts. *J. Exp. Med.* **164**, 180.
511. Bukowski, J. F., and Welsh, R. M. (1985). Inability of interferon to protect virus-infected cells against lysis by natural killer (NK) cells correlates with NK cell-mediated antiviral effects *in vivo. J. Immunol.* **135**, 3537.
512. Bishop, G. A., McCurry, L., Schwartz, S. A., and Glorioso, J. C. (1987). Activation of human natural killer cells by herpes simplex virus type 1-infected cells. *Intervirology* **28**, 78.
513. Borysiewicz, L. K., Rodgers, B., Morris, S., Graham, S., and Sissons, J. G. (1985). Lysis of human cytomegalovirus infected fibroblasts by natural killer cells: Demonstration of an interferon-independent component requiring expression of early viral proteins and characterization of effector cells. *J. Immunol.* **134**, 2695.
514. Uchida, A., and Yanagawa, E. (1984). Natural killer cell activity and autologous tumor killing activity in cancer patients: Overlapping involvement of effector cells as determined in two-target conjugate cytotoxicity assay. *J. Natl. Cancer Inst.* **73**, 1093.
515. Oshimi, K., Oshimi, Y., Yamada, O., and Mizoguchi, H. (1985). Lysis of lymphoma cells by autologous and allogeneic natural killer cells. *Blood* **65**, 638.
516. Ames, I. H., Gates, C. E., Garcia, A. M., John, P. A., Hennig, A. K., and Tomar, R. H. (1987). Lysis of fresh murine mammary tumor cells by syngeneic natural killer cells and lymphokine-activated killer cells. *Cancer Immunol. Immunother.* **25**, 161.
517. Lotzova, E., Savary, C. A., Freedman, R. S., Edwards, C. L., and Wharton, J. T. (1988). Recombinant IL-2-activated NK cells mediate LAK activity against ovarian cancer. *Int. J. Cancer* **42**, 225.
518. Moingeon, P., Ythier, A., Nowill, A., Delmon, L., Bayle, C., Pico, J. L., Bohuon, C., and Hercend, T. (1986). Short-term culture of acute myeloid leukemia blasts: Analysis of acquired susceptibility to activated natural killer cells. *Blood* **67**, 777.
519. Spitz, D. L., Zucker-Franklin, D., and Nabi, Z. F. (1988). Unmasking of cryptic natural killer (NK) cell recognition sites on chronic lymphocytic leukemia lymphocytes. *Am. J. Hematol.* **28**, 155.
520. Becker, S., Kiessling, R., Lee, N., and Klein, G. (1979). Modulation of sensitivity to natural killer (NK) cell lysis after *in vitro* explantation of a mouse lymphoma. *JNCI, J. Natl. Cancer Inst.* **61**, 1495.
521. Hansson, M., Kiessling, R., Andersson, B., and Welsh, R. M. (1980). Effect of interferon and interferon inducers on the NK sensitivity of normal mouse thymocytes. *J. Immunol.* **125**, 2225.
522. Timonen, T., Lehtovirta, P., and Säkselä, E. (1987). Interleukin-2-stimulated natural killer activity against malignant and benign endometrium. *Int. J. Cancer* **40**, 479.
523. Trimble, W. S., Johnson, P. W., Hozumi, N., and Roder, J. C. (1986). Inducible cellular transformation by a metallothionein-*ras* hybrid oncogene leads to natural killer cell susceptiblity. *Nature (London)* **321**, 782.
524. Lanza, L. A., Wilson, D. J., Ikejiri, B., Roth, J. A., and Grimm, E. A. (1986).

Human oncogene-transfected tumor cells display differential susceptibility to lysis by lymphokine-activated killer cells (LAK) and natural killer cells. *J. Immunol.* **137**, 2716.
525. Greenberg, A. H., Egan, S. E., Jarolim, L., and Wright, J. A. (1987). NK sensitivity of H-*ras* transfected fibroblasts is transformation-independent. *Cell. Immunol.* **109**, 444.
526. Nabi, Z. F., Zucker-Franklin, D., Lipkin, G., and Rosenberg, M. (1986). Susceptibility to NK cell lysis is abolished in tumor cells by a factor which restores their contact inhibited growth. *Cancer (Philadelphia)* **58**, 1461.
527. Lattime, E. C., Bykowsky, M. J., and Stutman, O. (1986). Susceptibility to lysis by natural killer and natural cytotoxic cells is independent of the mototic stage of the target cell cycle. *Cell. Immunol.* **100**, 79.
528. Landay, A. L., Zarcone, D., Grossi, C. E., and Bauer, K. (1987). Relationship between target cell cycle and susceptibility to natural killer lysis. *Cancer Res.* **47**, 2767.
529. Kiessling, R., and Wigzell, H. (1981). Surveillance of primitive cells by natural killer cells. *Curr. Top. Microbiol. Immunol.* **92**, 107.
530. Stern, P., Gidlund, M., Orn, A., and Wigzell, H. (1980). Natural killer cells mediate lysis of embryonal carcinoma cells lacking MHC. *Nature (London)* **285**, 341.
531. Hagner, G. (1984). Induction of erythroid differentiation in K562 cells and natural killer cell-mediated lysis: Distinct effects at the level of recognition and lysis in relation to target cell proliferation. *Immunobiology* **167**, 389.
532. Dokhelar, M. C., Garson, D., Wakasugi, H., Tabilio, A., Testa, U., Vainchecker, W., and Tursz, T. (1984). K562 cells induced to differentiate by phorbol ester tumor promoters resist NK lysis. *Cell. Immunol.* **87**, 389.
533. Dokhelar, M. C., Garson, D., Testa, U., and Tursz, T. (1984). Target structure for natural killer cells: Evidence against a unique role for transferrin receptor. *Eur. J. Immunol.* **14**, 340.
534. Zucker-Franklin, D., and Nabi, Z. F. (1987). Phorbol ester-induced loss of cell surface sialic acid enhances target cell sensitivity to cytolysis by natural killer (NK) cells. *Trans. Assoc. Am. Physicians* **100**, 339.
535. Kimber, I., Moore, M., and Harrison, C. J. (1984). Influence of 12-O-tetradecanoylphorbol-13-acetate (TPA) on the susceptibility of K562 to natural cytotoxicity: Evidence for clonal variation in differentiation-induced changes of lytic sensitivity. *Int. J. Cancer* **33**, 693.
536. Patarrayo, M., Biberfeld, P., Klein, E., and Klein, G. (1981). 12-O-tetradecanoylphorbol-13-acetate (TPA) treatment elevates the natural killer (NK) sensitivity of certain lymphoid cell lines. *Cell. Immunol.* **63**, 237.
537. Yogeeswaran, G., Gronberg, A., Hansson, M., Dalianis, T., Kiessling, R., and Welsh, R. M. (1981). Correlation of glycosphingolipids and sialic acid in YAC-1 lymphoma variants with their sensitivity to natural killer-cell-mediated lysis. *Int. J. Cancer* **28**, 517.
538. Einhorn, S., and Anderbring, E. (1985). Human peripheral blood monocytes are susceptible to interferon-activated natural killer cells. *J. Clin. Lab. Invest.* **16**, 197.
539. Djeu, J. Y., and Blanchard, D. K. (1988). Lysis of human monocytes by lymphokine-activated killer cells. *Cell. Immunol.* **111**, 55.
540. Hansson, M., Karre, K., Kiessling, R., Roder, J., Andersson, B., and Häyry, P. (1979). Natural NK-cell targets in the mouse thymus: Characteristics of the sensitive cell population. *J. Immunol.* **123**, 765.
541. Ljunggren, H. G., and Karre, K. (1986). Experimental strategies and interpretations

in the analysis of changes in MHC gene expression during tumour progression. Opposing influences of T cell and natural killer mediated resistance? *J. Immunogenet.* **13**, 141.
542. Karre, K., Ljunggren, H. G., Piontek, G., and Kiessling, R. (1986). Selective rejection of H-2-deficient lymphoma variants suggests alternative immune defence strategy. *Nature (London)* **319**, 675.
543. Piontek, G. E., Taniguchi, K., Ljunggren, H. G., Gronberg, A., Kiessling, R., Klein, G., and Karre, K. (1985). YAC-1 MHC class I variants reveal an association between decreased NK sensitivity and increased H-2 expression after interferon treatment or *in vivo* passage. *J. Immunol.* **135**, 4281.
544. Harel-Bellan, A., Quillet, A., Marchiol, C., DeMars, R., Tursz, T., and Fradelizi, D. (1986). Natural killer susceptibility of human cells may be regulated by genes in the HLA region on chromosome 6. *Proc. Natl. Acad. Sci. U.S.A.* **83**, 5688.
545. Storkus, W. J., Howell, D. N., Salter, R. D., Dawson, J. R., and Cresswell, P. (1987). NK susceptibility varies inversely with target cell class I HLA antigen expression. *J. Immunol.* **138**, 1657.
546. Yamasaki, T., Klein, G., Ljunggren, H. G., Hoglund, P., Ohlen, C., Petersson, M. G., and Karre, K. (1988). Effects of dimethyl sulfoxide treatment on H-2 expression and susceptibility to NK- or cytotoxic T-lymphocyte-mediated lysis of the YAC-1 lymphoma and its beta 2-microglobulin-deficient variant. *J. Natl. Cancer Inst.* **80**, 263.
547. Chervenak, R., and Wolcott, R. M. (1988). Target cell expression of MHC antigens is not (always) a turn-off signal to natural killer cells. *J. Immunol.* **140**, 3712.
548. Gorelik, E., Gunji, Y., and Herberman, R. B. (1988). H-2 antigen expression and sensitivity of BL6 melanoma cells to natural killer cell cytotoxicity. *J. Immunol.* **140**, 2096.
549. Gopas, J., Segal, S., Hammerling, G., Bar-Eli, M., and Rager-Zisman, B. (1988). Influence of H-2K transfection on susceptibility of fibrosarcoma tumor cells to natural killer (NK) cells. *Immunol. Lett.* **17**, 261.
550. Dennert, G., Landon, C., Lord, E. M., Bahler, D. W., and Frelinger, J. G. (1988). Lysis of a lung carcinoma by poly I:C-induced natural killer cells is independent of the expression of class I histocompatibility antigens. *J. Immunol.* **140**, 2472.
551. Sawada, Y., Fohring, B., Shenk, T. E., and Raska, K., Jr. (1985). Tumorigenicity of adenovirus-transformed cells: Region E1A of adenovirus 12 confers resistance to natural killer cells. *Virology* **147**, 413.
552. Lazarus, A. H., and Baines, M. G. (1985). Studies on the mechanism of specificity of human natural killer cells for tumor cells: Correlation between target cell transferrin receptor expression and competitive activity. *Cell. Immunol.* **96**, 255.
553. Alarcon, B., and Fresno, M. (1985). Specific effect of anti-transferrin antibodies on natural killer cells directed against tumor cells. Evidence for the transferrin receptor being one of the target structures recognized by NK cells. *J. Immunol.* **134**, 1286.
554. Zanyk, M. J., Banerjee, D., and McFarlane, D. L. (1988). Transferrin receptor and 4F2 expression by NK-sensitive and NK-resistant tumour cell lines. *Carcinogenesis (London)* **9**, 1377.
555. Bridges, K. R., and Smith, B. R. (1985). Discordance between transferrin receptor expression and susceptibility to lysis by natural killer cells. *J. Clin. Invest.* **76**, 913.
556. Rieber, E. P., Rank, G., and Riethmuller, G. (1986). Transferrin receptors on tumor and bone marrow cells: Lack of involvement as target structure for natural killer cells. *Klin. Wochenschr.* **64**, 1119.
557. Perl, A., Looney, R. J., Ryan, D. H., and Abraham, G. N. (1986). The low affinity

40,000 Fc gamma receptor and the transferrin receptor can be alternative or simultaneous target structures on cells sensitive for natural killing. *J. Immunol.* **136**, 4714.
558. Zarcone, D., Tilden, A. B., Friedman, H. M., and Crossi, C. E. (1987). Human leukemia-derived cell lines and clones as models for mechanistic analysis of natural killer cell-mediated cytotoxicity. *Cancer Res.* **47**, 2674.
559. Harris, J. F., Chin, J., Jewett, M. A., Kennedy, M., and Gorczynski, R. M. (1984). Monoclonal antibodies against SSEA-1 antigen: Binding properties and inhibition of human natural killer cell activity against target cells bearing SSEA-1 antigen. *J. Immunol.* **132**, 2502.
560. Chin, A. I., and Yen, T. S. (1987). Natural killer cell–target interactions: The role of 4F2 antigen in the human system. *Cell. Immunol.* **106**, 180.
561. Jaso-Friedmann, L., Evans, D. L., Grant, C. C., John, A. S., Harris, D. T., and Koren, H. S. (1988). Characterization by monoclonal antibodies of a target cell antigen complex recognized by nonspecific cytotoxic cells. *J. Immunol.* **141**, 2861.
562. Forbes, J. T., Beretthauser, R. K., and Oeltmann, T. N. (1981). Mannose 6-, fructose 1-, and fructose 6-phosphates inhibit human natural killer cell-mediated cytotoxicity. *Proc. Natl. Acad. Sci. U.S.A.* **78**, 5797.
563. Ortaldo, J. R., Timonen, T. T., and Herberman, R. B. (1984). Inhibition of activity of human NK and K cells by simple sugars: Discrimination between binding and postbinding events. *Clin. Immunol. Immunopathol.* **31**, 439.
564. Chambers, W. H., and Oeltmann, T. N. (1986). The effects of hexose 6-O-sulfate esters on human natural killer cell lytic function. *J. Immunol.* **137**, 1469.
565. Decker, J. M., Hinson, A., and Ades, E. W. (1984). Inhibition of human NK cell cytotoxicity against K562 cells with glycopeptides from K562 plasma membrane. *J. Clin. Lab. Immunol.* **15**, 137.
566. Werkmeister, J. A., and Pross, H. F. (1985). Studies on natural antibody-dependent, and interleukin-2-activated killer-cell activity of a patient with mucolipidosis III as a test of the mannose-6-phosphate lytic acceptor hypothesis. *J. Clin. Immunol.* **5**, 228.
567. Haubeck, H. D., Kolsch, E., Imort, M., Hasilik, A., and von Figura, K. (1985). Natural killer cell-mediated cytotoxicity does not depend on recognition of mannose 6-phosphate residues. *J. Immunol.* **134**, 65.
568. Pospisil, M., Kubrycht, J., Bezouska, T., Taborsky, O., Novak, M., and Kocourek, J. (1986). Lactosamine type asialooligosaccharide recognition in NK cytotoxicity. *Immunol. Lett.* **12**, 83.
569. Trinchieri, G., Santoli, D., Granato, D., and Perussia, B. (1981). Antagonistic effects of interferons on the cytotoxicity mediated by natural killer cells. *Fed. Proc., Fed. Am. Soc. Exp. Biol.* **40**, 2705.
570. Welsh, R. M., Karre, K., Hansson, M., Kunkel, L. A., and Kiessling, R. W. (1981). Interferon-mediated protection of normal and tumor target cells against lysis by mouse natural killer cells. *J. Immunol.* **126**, 219.
571. Wallach, D. (1983). Interferon-induced resistance to the killing by NK cells: A preferential effect of IFN-gamma. *Cell. Immunol.* **75**, 390.
572. Cunningham-Rundles, S. (1982). Control of natural cytotoxicity in the regional lymph node in breast cancer. In "NK Cells and Other Natural Effector Cells" (R. B. Herberman, ed.), p. 1133. Academic Press, New York.
573. Wright, S. C., and Bonavida, B. (1983). Studies on the mechanism of natural killer cell-mediated cytotoxicity. IV. Interferon-induced inhibition of NK target cell susceptibility to lysis is due to a defect in their ability to stimulate release of natural killer cytotoxic factors (NKCF). *J. Immunol.* **130**, 2965.

574. Uchida, A., Vanky, F., and Klein, E. (1985). Natural cytotoxicity of human blood lymphocytes and monocytes and their cytotoxic factors: Effect of interferon on target cell susceptibility. *J. Natl. Cancer Inst.* 75, 849.
575. Gronberg, A., Ferm, M. T., Ng, J., Reynolds, C. W., and Ortaldo, J. R. (1988). IFN-gamma treatment of K562 cells inhibits natural killer cell triggering and decreases the susceptibility to lysis by cytoplasmic granules from large granular lymphocytes. *J. Immunol.* 140, 4397.
576. De Fries, R. U., and Golub, S. H. (1988). Characteristics and mechanism of IFN-gamma-induced protection of human tumor cells from lysis by lymphokine-activated killer cells. *J. Immunol.* 140, 3686.
577. Djeu, J. Y., and Blanchard, D. K. (1988). Interferon-gamma-induced alterations of monocyte susceptibility to lysis by autologous lumphokine-activated killer (LAK) cells. *Int. J. Cancer* 42, 449.
578. Yogeeswaran, G., Fujinami, R., Kiessling, R., and Welsh, R. M. (1982). Interferon-induced alterations in sialic acid and glycoconjugates of L-929 cells. *Virology* 121, 363.
579. Reiter, Z., Fischer, D. G., and Rubinstein, M. (1988). The protective effect of interferon against natural killing activity is not mediated via the expression of class I MHC antigens. *Immunol. Lett.* 17, 323.
580. Zoller, M., Strubel, A., Hammerling, G., Andrighetto, G., Raz, A., and Ben-Zeev, A. (1988). Interferon-gamma treatment of B16 melanoma cells: Opposing effects for non-adaptive and adaptive immune defense and its reflection by metastatic spread. *Int. J. Cancer* 41, 256.
581. Tai, A., Safilian, B., and Warner, N. L. (1982). Identification of distinct target-specific subsets of NK cells in peripheral blood of normal donors. *Hum. Immunol.* 4, 123.
582. Takasugi, M., and Mickey, M. R. (1976). Interaction analysis of selective and nonselective cell-mediated cytotoxicity. *J. Natl. Cancer Inst. (U.S.)* 57, 255.
583. Bolhuis, R. L. H., Van De Griend, R. J., and Roteltap, C. P. H. (1983). Clonal expansion of human B73.1 positive NK cells or large granular lymphocytes exerting strong antibody dependent and independent cytotoxicity and occasionally lectin dependent cytotoxicity. *Nat. Immun. Cell Growth Regul.* 3, 61.
584. Krensky, A. M., Ault, K. A., Reiss, C. S., Strominger, J. L., and Burakoff, S. J. (1982). Generation of long-term human cytolytic cell lines with persistent natural killer activity. *J. Immunol.* 129, 1748.
585. Ciccone, E., Viale, O., Pende, D., Malnati, M., Biassoni, R., Melioli, G., Moretta, A., Long, E. O., and Moretta, L. (1988). Specific lysis of allogeneic cells after activation of CD3$^-$ lymphocytes in mixed lymphocyte culture. *J. Exp. Med.* 168, 2403.
586. Koide, Y., and Takasugi, M. (1977). Determination of specificity in natural cell-mediated cytotoxicity by natural antibodies. *J. Natl. Cancer Inst. (U.S.)* 59, 1099.
587. Takasugi, J., Koide, Y., and Takasugi, M. (1977). Reconstitution of natural cell-mediated cytotoxicity with specific antibodies. *Eur. J. Immunol.* 7, 887.
588. Dennert, G., Anderson, C. G., and Warner, J. (1986). Induction of bone marrow allograft rejection and hybrid resistance in non responder recipients by antibody: Is there avidence for a dual receptor interaction in acute marrow graft rejection? *J. Immunol.* 136, 3981.
589. Harfast, B., Torbjorn, A., Stejskal, V., and Perlmann, P. (1977). Interactions between human lymphocytes and paramyxovirus-infected cells: Adsorption and cytotoxicity. *J. Immunol.* 118, 1132.
590. Kay, H. D., Bonnard, G. D., and Herberman, R. B. (1979). Evaluation of the

role of IgG antibodies in human natural cell-mediated cytotoxicity against the myeloid cell line K562. *J. Immunol.* **122**, 675.

591. Trinchieri, G., Santoli, D., and Koprowski, H. (1978). Spontaneous cell-mediated cytotoxicity in humans. *J. Immunol.* **120**, 1849.
592. Cordier, G., Samarut, C., and Revillard, J. P. (1977). Changes of Fc receptor-related properties induced by interaction of human lymphocytes with insoluble immune complexes. *J. Immunol.* **119**, 1943.
593. Pape, G. R., Moretta, L., Troye, M., and Perlmann, P. (1979). Natural cytotoxicity of human Fc-receptor-positive T lymphocytes after surface modulation with immune complexes. *Scand. J. Immunol.* **9**, 291.
594. Ziegler, H. K., and Henney, C. S. (1977). Studies on the cytotoxic activity of human lymphocytes. II. Interactions between IgG and Fc receptors leading to inhibition of K cell function. *J. Immunol.* **119**, 1010.
595. Heiskala, M. (1987). Effect of interferons on the inhibition of human natural killers by primary monolayer cell cultures. *Immunology* **60**, 167.
596. Abrams, S. I., and Brahmi, Z. (1986). The functional loss of human natural killer cell activity induced by K562 is reversible via an interleukin-2-dependent mechanism. *Cell. Immunol.* **101**, 558.
597. Abrams, S. I., and Brahmi, Z. (1988). Target cell directed NK inactivation. Concomitant loss of NK and antibody-dependent cellular cytotoxicity activities. *J. Immunol.* **140**, 2090.
598. Brahmi, Z., Bray, R. A., and Abrams, S. I. (1985). Evidence for an early calcium-independent event in the activation of the human natural killer cell cytolytic mechanism. *J. Immunol.* **135**, 4108.
599. Seaman, W. E., Eriksson, E., Dobrow, R., and Imboden, J. B. (1987). Inositol trisphosphate is generated by a rat natural killer cell tumor in response to target cells or to crosslinked monoclonal antibody OX-34: Possible signaling role for the OX-34 determinant during activation by target cells. *Proc. Natl. Acad. Sci. U.S.A.* **84**, 4239.
600. Gerrard, J. M., Hildes, E., Atkinson, E. A., and Greenberg, A. H. (1987). Activation of inositol cycle in large granular lymphocyte leukemia RNK following contact with an NK-sensitive tumor. *Adv. Prostaglandin, Thromboxane Leukotriene Res.* **17A**, 573.
601. Steele, T. A., and Brahmi, Z. (1988). Phosphatidylinositol metabolism accompanies early activation events in tumor target cell-stimulated human natural killer cells. *Cell. Immunol.* **112**, 402.
602. Chow, S. C., Ng, J., Nordstedt, C., Fredholm, B. B., and Jondal, M. (1988). Phosphoinositide breakdown and evidence for protein kinase C involvement during human NK killing. *Cell. Immunol.* **114**, 96.
603. Jondal, M., Ng, J., Patarroyo, M., and Broliden, P. A. (1986). Phorbol ester regulation of Ca^{2+} flux during natural, lectin and antibody-dependent killing. *Immunology* **59**, 347.
604. Windebank, K. P., Abraham, R. T., Powis, G., Olsen, R. A., Barna, T. J., and Leibson, P. J. (1988). Signal transduction during human natural killer cell activation: Inositol phosphate generation and regulation by cyclic AMP. *J. Immunol.* **141**, 3951.
605. Pantaleo, G., Olive, D., Poggi, A., Pozzan, T., Moretta, L., and Moretta, A. (1987). Antibody-induced modulation of the CD3/T cell receptor complex causes T cell refractoriness by inhibiting the early metabolic steps involved in T cell activation. *J. Exp. Med.* **166**, 619.

606. Schrezenmeier, H., Ahnert-Hilger, G., and Fleischer, B. (1988). Inactivation of a T cell receptor-associated GTP-binding protein by antibody-induced modulation of the T cell receptor/CD3 complex. *J. Exp. Med.* **168**, 817.
607. Kohl, S., Springer, T. A., Schmalstieg, F. C., Loo, L. S., and Anderson, D. C. (1984). Defective natural killer cytotoxicity and polymorphonuclear leukocyte antibody-dependent cellular cytotoxicity in patients with LFA-1/OKM-1 deficiency. *J. Immunol.* **133**, 2972.
608. Mentzer, S. J., Krensky, A. M., and Burakoff, S. J. (1986). Mapping functional epitopes of the human LFA-1 glycoprotein: Monoclonal antibody inhibition of NK and CTL effectors. *Hum. Immunol.* **17**, 288.
609. Axberg, I., Ramstedt, U., Patarroyo, M., Beatty, P., and Wigzell, H. (1987). Inhibition of natural killer cell cytotoxicity by a monoclonal antibody directed against adhesion-mediating protein gp 90 (CD18). *Scand. J. Immunol.* **26**, 547.
610. Hart, M. K., Kornbluth, J., Main, E. K., Spear, B. T., Taylor, J., and Wilson, D. B. (1987). Lymphocyte function-associated antigen 1 (LFA-1) and natural killer (NK) cell activity: LFA-1 is not necessary for all killer:target cell interactions. *Cell. Immunol.* **109**, 306.
611. Schmidt, R. E., Bartley, G., Levine, H., Schlossman, S. F., and Ritz, J. (1985). Functional characterization of LFA-1 antigens in the interaction of human NK clones and target cells. *J. Immunol.* **135**, 1020.
612. Ramos, O. F., Kai, C., Yefenof, E., and Klein, E. (1988). The elevated natural killer sensitivity of targets carrying surface-attached C3 fragments require the availability of the iC3b receptor (CR3) on the effectors. *J. Immunol.* **140**, 1239.
613. Pawelec, G., Newman, W., Schwulera, U., and Wernet, P. (1985). Heterogeneity of human natural killer recognition demonstrated by cloned effector cells and differential blocking of cytotoxicity with monoclonal antibodies. *Cell. Immunol.* **92**, 31.
614. Starling, G. C., Davidson, S. E., McKenzie, J. L., and Hart, D. N. (1987). Inhibition of natural killer-cell mediated cytolysis with monoclonal antibodies to restricted and non-restricted epitopes of the leucocyte common antigen. *Immunology* **61**, 351.
615. Burns, G. F., Werkmeister, J. A., and Triglia, T. (1984). A novel antigenic cell surface protein associated with T200 is involved in the post-activation stage of human NK cell-mediated lysis. *J. Immunol.* **133**, 1391.
616. Werkmeister, J. A., Burns, G. F., and Triglia, T. (1984). Anti-idiotype antibodies to the 9.1C3 blocking antibody used to probe the lethal hit stage of NK cell-mediated cytolysis. *J. Immunol.* **133**, 1385.
617. Hiserodt, J. C., Laybourn, K. A., and Varani, J. (1985). Laminin inhibits the recognition of tumor target cells by murine natural killer (NK) and natural cytotoxic (NC) lymphocytes. *Am. J. Pathol.* **121**, 148.
618. Hiserodt, J. C., Laybourn, K. A., and Varani, J. (1985). Expression of a laminin-like substance on the surface of murine natural killer (NK) lymphocytes and its role in NK recognition of tumor target cells. *J. Immunol.* **135**, 1484.
619. Schwarz, R. E., Whiteside, T. L., and Hiserodt, J. C. (1989). A laminin B2-like surface receptor (human P48 protein equivalent) is involved in tumor cell recognition by lymphokine activated killer cells expressing a Leu19$^+$/CD3$^-$ or a Leu19$^+$/CD3$^+$ surface phenotype. *In* "Cellular Basis of Immune Modulation" (J. G. Kaplan and D. R. Green, eds.). Liss, New York (in press).
620. Schwarz, R. E., and Hiserodt, J. C. (1988). The expression and functional involvement of laminin-like molecules in non-MHC restricted cytotoxicity by human Leu-19$^+$/CD3$^-$ natural killer lymphocytes. *J. Immunol.* **141**, 3318.
621. Baum, L. L., James, K. K., Glaviano, R. R., and Gewurz, H. (1983). Possible

role for C-reactive protein in the human natural killer cell response. *J. Exp. Med.* **157**, 301.
622. Samberg, N. L., Bray, R. A., Gewurz, H., Landay, A. L., and Potempa, L. A. (1988). Preferential expression of neo-CRP epitopes on the surface of human peripheral blood lymphocytes. *Cell. Immunol.* **116**, 86.
623. Baum, L. L., Johnson, B., Berman, S., Graham, D., and Mold, C. (1987). C-reactive protein is involved in natural killer cell-mediated lysis but does not mediate effector–target cell recognition. *Immunology* **61**, 93.
624. Meuer, S. C., Hussey, R. E., Fabbi, M., Fox, D., Acuto, O., Fitzgerald, K. A., Hodgdon, J. C., Protentis, J. P., Schlossman, S. F., and Reinherz, E. L. (1984). An alternative pathway of T-cell activation: A functional role for the 50 Kd T11 sheep erythrocyte receptor protein. *Cell (Cambridge, Mass.)* **36**, 897.
625. Ythier, A., Delmon, L., Reinherz, E., Nowill, A., Mingeon, P., Mishal, Z., Bohuon, C., and Hercend, T. (1985). Proliferative responses of circulating human NK cells: Delineation of a unique pathway involving both direct and helper signals. *Eur. J. Immunol.* **15**, 1209.
626. Pantaleo, G., Zocchi, M. R., Ferrini, S., Poggi, A., Tambussi, G., Bottino, C., Moretta, L., and Moretta, A. (1988). Human cytolytic cell clones lacking surface expression of T cell receptor alpha/beta or gamma/delta. Evidence that surface structures other than CD3 or CD2 molecules are required for signal transduction. *J. Exp. Med.* **168**, 13.
627. Schmidt, R. E., Hercend, T., Fox, D. A., Bensussan, A., Bartley, G., Daley, J. F., Schlossman, S. F., Reinherz, E. L., and Ritz, J. (1985). The role of interleukin 2 and T11 E rosette antigen in activation and proliferation of human NK clones. *J. Immunol.* **135**, 672.
628. Schmidt, R. E., Michon, J. M., Woronicz, J., Schlossman, S. F., Reinherz, E. L., and Ritz, J. (1987). Enhancement of natural killer function through activation of the T11 E rosette receptor. *J. Clin. Invest.* **79**, 305.
629. Siliciano, R. F., Pratt, J. C., Schmidt, R. E., Ritz, J., and Reinherz, E. L. (1985). Activation of cytolytic T lymphocyte and natural killer cell function through the T11 sheep erythrocyte binding protein. *Nature (London)* **317**, 428.
630. Schmidt, R. E., Caulfield, J. P., Michon, J., Hein, A., Kamada, M. M., MacDermott, R. P., Stevens, R. L., and Ritz, J. (1988). T11/CD2 activation of cloned human natural killer cells results in increased conjugate formation and exocytosis of cytolytic granules. *J. Immunol.* **140**, 991.
631. Anasetti, C., Martin, P. J., June, C. H., Hellström, K. E., Ledbetter, J. A., Rabinovitch, P. S., Morishita, Y., Hellström, I., and Hansen, J. A. (1987). Induction of calcium flux and enhancement of cytolytic activity in natural killer cells by cross-linking of the sheep erythrocyte binding protein (CD2) and the Fc-receptor (CD16). *J. Immunol.* **139**, 1772.
632. Harris, D. T., Koren, H. S., Devlin, R. B., Jaso-Friedmann, L., and Evans, D. L. (1989). Analysis of a human natural killer cell antigen receptor. *In* "Natural Killer Cells and the Host Defense" (E. W. Ades and C. Lopez, eds.). Karger, Basel (in press).
633. Harris, D. T., Jaso-Friedman, L., Devlin, R. B., Koren, H. S., and Evans, D. L. (1989). Identification of a structure on human natural killer cells involved in antigen recognition. *J. Immunol.* (in press).
634. Ortaldo, J. R., Kantor, R. R. S., Segal, D., Giardina, S. L., and Bino, T. (1988). Definition of a proposed NK receptor. *Nat. Immun. Cell Growth Regul.* **7**, 62.
635. Timonen, T., Carpén, O., and Seppälä, I. (1988). Reactivity of anti-

immunoglobulin antibodies with functional determinants of natrual killer cells. *Nat. Immun. Cell Growth Regul.* **7**, 59.
636. Hiserodt, J. C. (1988). NK receptors and target antigens involved in cytotoxicity. *Nat. Immun. Cell Growth Regul.* **7**, 57.
637. Cassatella, M. A., Anegón, I., Cuturi, M. C., Griskey, P., Trinchieri, G., and Perussia, B. (1989). FcR (CD16) interaction with ligand induces Ca^{2+} mobilization and phosphoinositide turnover in human natural killer cells. Differential role of Ca^{2+} in FcR (CD16) and II-2-induced transcription and expression of lymphokine genes. *J. Exp. Med.* **169**, 549.
638. Young, J. D.-E., and Cohn, Z. A. (1987). Cellular and humoral mechanisms of cytotoxicity: Structural and functional analogies. *Adv. Immunol.* **41**, 269.
639. Carpén, O., and Säkselä, E. (1988). Directed exocytosis in the NK cell-mediated cytotoxicity. A review. *Nat. Immun. Cell. Growth Regul.* **7**, 1.
640. Roder, J. C., Argov, S., Klein, M., Petersson, C., Kiessling, R., Andersson, K. and Hansson, M. (1980). Target-effector cell interaction in the natural killer cell system. V. Energy requirements, membrane integrity, and the possible involvement of lysosomal enzymes. *Immunology* **40**, 107.
641. Roder, J. C., Kiessling, R., Biberfield, P., and Andersson, B. (1978). Target-effector interactions in the natural killer (NK) cell system. II. Isolation and characterization of the effector cells. *J. Immunol.* **121**, 2509.
642. Hiserodt, J., Britvan, L., and Targans, S. (1982). Characterization of the cytolytic reaction mechanism of the human natural killer lymphocyte. *J. Immunol.* **129**, 1782.
643. Quan, P. C., Ishizaka, T., and Bloom, B. R. (1982). Studies on the mechanism of NK cell lysis. *J. Immunol.* **128**, 1786.
644. Roder, J. C., and Haliotis, T. (1980). A comparative analysis of the NK cytolytic mechanism and regulatory genes. *In* "Natural Cell-Mediated Immunity against Tumors" (R. B. Herberman, ed.), p. 379. Academic Press, New York.
645. Hiserodt, J., Britvan, L., and Targans, S. (1982). Inhibition of human natural killer cytotoxicity by heterologous and monoclonal antibodies. *J. Immunol.* **129**, 2248.
646. Solovera, J. J., Alvarez-Mon, M., Casas, J., Carballido, J., and Durantez, A. (1987). Inhibition of human natural killer (NK) activity by calcium channel modulators and a calmodulin antagonist. *J. Immunol.* **139**, 876.
647. Ng, J., Fredholm, B. B., and Jondal, M. (1987). Studies on the calcium dependence of human NK cell killing. *Biochem. Pharmacol.* **36**, 3943.
648. Steele, T. A., and Brahmi, Z. (1988). Chlorpromazine inhibits human natural killer cell activity and antibody-dependent cell-mediated cytotoxicity. *Biochem. Biophys. Res. Commun.* **155**, 597.
649. Ullberg, M., Jondal, M., Lanefelt, F., and Fredholm, B. B. (1983). Inhibition of human NK cell cytotoxicity by induction of cyclic AMP depends on impaired target cell recognition. *Scand. J. Immunol.* **17**, 365.
650. Bancu, A. C., Gherman, M., Sulica, A., Goto, T., Farrar, W., and Herberman, R. B. (1988). Regulation of human natural cytotoxicity by IgG. II. Cyclic AMP as a mediator of monomeric IgG-induced inhibition of natural killer cell activity. *Cell. Immunol.* **114**, 246.
651. Frey, T., Petty, H. R., and McConnell, H. M. (1982). Electron microscopic study of natural killer cell-tumor cell conjugates. *Proc. Natl. Acad. Sci. U.S.A.* **79**, 5317.
652. Burns, E. R., Zucker-Franklin, D., and Valentine, F. (1982). Cytotoxicity of natural killer cells. Correlation with emperipolesis and surface enzymes. *Lab. Invest.* **47**, 99.

653. Hoffman, T., Hirata, F., Bougnoux, P., Fraser, B. A., Goldfarb, R. H., Herberman, R. B., and Axelrod, J. (1981). Phospholipid methylation and phospholipase A₂ activation in cytotoxicity by human natural killer cells. *Proc. Natl. Acad. Sci. U.S.A.* **78**, 3839.
654. Carine, K., and Hudig, D. (1984). Assessment of a role for phospholipase A2 and arachidonic acid metabolism in human lymphocyte natural cytotoxicity. *Cell. Immunol.* **87**, 270.
655. Leung, K. H., and Koren, H. S. (1984). Regulation of human natural killing. III. Mechanism for interferon induction of loss of susceptibility to suppression by cyclic AMP elevating agents. *J. Immunol.* **132**, 1445.
656. Ramstedt, U., Ng, J., Wigzell, H., Serhan, C. N., and Samuelsson, B. (1985). Action of novel eicosanoids lipoxin A and B on human natural killer cell cytotoxicity: Effects on intracellular cAMP and target cell binding. *J. Immunol.* **135**, 3434.
657. Imir, T., Sibbitt, W., and Bankhurst, A. (1987). The relative resistance of lymphokine activated killer cells to suppression by prostaglandins and glucocorticoids. *Prostaglandins, Leukotrienes Med.* **28**, 111.
658. Seaman, W. E. (1983). Human natural killer cell activity is reversibly inhibited by antagonists of lipoxygenation. *J. Immunol.* **131**, 2953.
659. Leung, K. H. (1988). Selective inhibition of leukotriene C4 synthesis and natural killer activity by ethacrynic acid. *Cell. Immunol.* **114**, 359.
660. Sevilla, C. L., Radcliff, G., Mahle, N. H., Swartz, S., Sevilla, M. D., Chores, J., and Callewaert, D. M. (1989). Multiple mechanisms of target cell disintegration are employed in cytotoxicity reaction mediated by human natural killer cells. *Nat. Immun. Cell Growth Regul.* **8**, 20.
661. Carpén, O., Virtanen, I., and Säkselä, E. (1981). The cytotxic activity of human natural killer cells requires an intact secretory apparatus. *Cell. Immunol.* **58**, 97.
662. Hiserodt, J., Britvan, L., and Targan, S. (1983). Studies on the mechanism of the human natural killer cell lethal hit. Analysis of the mechanism of protease inhibition of the lethal hit. *J. Immunol.* **131**, 2705.
663. Hiserodt, J., Britvan, L., and Targan, S. (1983). Studies on the mechanism of human natural killer cell lethal hit. Evidence for transfer of protease sensitive structures requisite for target cell lysis. *J. Immunol.* **131**, 2710.
664. Wright, S. C., and Bonavida, B. (1981). Selective lysis of NK-sensitive target cells by a soluble mediator released from murine spleen cells and human peripheral blood lymphocytes. *J. Immunol.* **126**, 1516.
665. Wright, S. C., and Bonavida, B. (1982). Studies on the mechanism of natural killer (NK) cell-mediated cytotoxicity (CMC). I. Release of cytotoxic factors specific for NK-sensitive target cells (NKCF) during coculture of NK effector cells with NK target cells. *J. Immunol.* **129**, 433.
666. Wright, S. C., and Bonavida, B. (1983). Studies on the mechanism of natural killer cytotoxicity. II. Coculture of human PBL with NK-sensitive or resistant cell lines stimulates release of natural killer cytotoxic factors (NKCF) selectively cytotoxic to NK-sensitive target cells. *J. Immunol.* **130**, 2479.
667. Farram, E., and Targan, S. R. (1983). Identification of human natural killer soluble cytotoxic factor(s) (NKCF) derived from NK-enriched lymphocyte populations: Specificity of generation and killing. *J. Immunol.* **130**, 1252.
668. Degliantoni, G., Murphy, M., Kobayashi, M., Francis, M.-K., Perussia, B., and Trinchieri, G. (1985). Natural killer (NK) cell-derived hematopoietic colony-inhibiting activity and NK cytotoxic factor. Relationship with tumor necrosis factor and synergism with immune interferon. *J. Exp. Med.* **162**, 1512.

669. Wright, S. C., and Bonavida, B. (1987). Studies on the mechanism of natural killer cell-mediated cytotoxicity. VII. Functional comparison of human natural killer cytotoxic factors with recombinant lymphotoxin and tumor necrosis factor. *J. Immunol.* **138**, 1791.
670. Ortaldo, J. R., Ransom, J. R., Sayers, T. J., and Herberman, R. B. (1986). Analysis of cytostatic/cytotoxic lymphokines: Relationship of natural killer cytotoxic factor to recombinant lymphotoxin, recombinant tumor necrosis factor, and leukoregulin. *J. Immunol.* **137**, 2857.
671. Bialas, T., Kolitz, J., Levi, E., Polivka, A., Oez, S., Miller, G., and Welte, K. (1988). Distinction of partially purified human natural killer cytotoxic factor from recombinant human tumor necrosis factor and recombinant human lymphotoxin. *Cancer Res.* **48**, 891.
672. Ortaldo, J. R., Winkler-Pickett, R., Morgan, A. C., Woodhouse, C., Kantor, R., and Reynolds, C. W. (1987). Analysis of rat natural killer cytotoxic factor (NKCF) produced by rat NK cell lines and the production of a murine monoclonal antibody that neutralizes NKCF. *J. Immunol.* **139**, 3159.
673. Liu, C.-C., Steffen, M., King, F., and Young, J. D. (1987). Identification, isolation, and characterization of a novel cytotoxin in murine cytolytic lymphocytes. *Cell (Cambridge, Mass.)* **51**, 393.
674. Lichtenheld, M. G., Olsen, K. J., Lu, P., Lowrey, D. M., Hameed, A., Hengartner, H., and Podack, E. R. (1988). Structure and function of human perforin. *Nature (London)* **335**, 448.
675. Liu, C.-C., Perussia, B., Cohn, Z. A., and Young, J. D. (1986). Identification and characterization of a pore-forming protein of human peripheral blood NK cells. *J. Exp. Med.* **164**, 2061.
676. Zalman, L. S., Brothers, M. A., and Müller-Eberhard, H. J. (1985). A C9 related channel forming protein in the cytoplasmic granules of human large granular lymphocytes. *Biosci. Rep.* **5**, 1093.
677. Shinkai, Y., Ishikawa, H., Hattori, M., and Okumura, K. (1988). Resistance of mouse cytolytic cells to pore-forming protein-mediated cytolysis. *Eur. J. Immunol.* **18**, 29.
678. Jiang, S., Pereschini, P., Zychlinsky, A., Liu, C.-C., Perussia, B., and Young, J. D. (1988). Resistance of cytolytic lymphocytes to perforin mediated killing: Lack of correlation with complement-associated homologous species restriction. *J. Exp. Med.* **168**, 2207.
679. Müller-Eberhard, H. J. (1988). The molecular basis of target cell killing by human lymphocytes and of killer cell self-protection. *Immunol. Rev.* **103**, 87.
680. Zalman, L. S., Brothers, M. A., and Müller-Eberhard, H. J. (1988). Self-protection of cytotoxic lymphocytes: A soluble form of homologous restriction factor in cytoplasmic granules. *Proc. Natl. Acad. Sci. U.S.A.* **85**, 4827.
681. Berke, G. (1988). Multiple mechanisms of lymphocyte-mediated killing. *Immunol. Today* **9**, 294.
682. Tirosh, R., and Berke, G. (1985). T-lymphocyte-mediated cytolysis as an excitatory process of the target. I. Evidence that the target cell may be the site of Ca^{2+} action. *Cell. Immunol.* **95**, 113.
683. Goldstein, P., and Smith, E. T. (1977). Mechanism of T-cell-mediated cytolysis: The lethal hit stage. *In* "Contemporary Topics in Immunology: T Cells" (O. Stutman, ed.), p. 273. Plenum, New York.
684. Trinchieri, G., and De Marchi, M. (1975). Antibody-dependent cell-mediated cytotoxicity in humans. II. Energy requirement. *J. Immunol.* **115**, 256.

685. Young, J. D., and Cohn, Z. A. (1987). Cellular and humoral mechanisms of cytotoxicity: Structural and functional analogies. *Adv. Immunol.* **41**, 269.
686. Russell, J. H. (1983). Internal disintegration model of cytotoxic lymphocyte-induced target damage. *Immunol. Rev.* **72**, 97.
687. Duke, R. C., Cohen, J. J., and Chervenak, R. (1986). Differences in target cell DNA fragmentation induced by mouse cytotoxic T lymphocytes and natural killer cells. *J. Immunol.* **137**, 1442.
688. Gromkowski, S. H., Brown, T. C., Cerutti, P. A., and Cerottini, J.-C. (1986). DNA of human Raji target cells is damaged upon lymphocyte-mediated lysis. *J. Immunol.* **136**, 752.
689. Christiaansen, J. E., and Sears, D. W. (1985). Lack of lymphocyte-induced DNA fragmentation in human targets during lysis represents a species-specific difference between human and murine cells. *Proc. Natl. Acad. Sci. U.S.A.* **82**, 4482.
690. Trinchieri, G., and De Marchi, M. (1976). Antibody-dependent cell-mediated cytotoxicity in humans. III. Effect of protease inhibitors and substrates. *J. Immunol.* **116**, 885.
691. Hudig, D., Haverty, T., Fulcher, C., Redelman, D., and Mendelsohn, J. (1981). Inhibition of human natural cytotoxicity by macromolecular antiproteases. *J. Immunol.* **126**, 1569.
692. Hudig, D., Redelman, D., and Minning, L. L. (1984). The requirement for proteinase activity for human lymphocyte-mediated natural cytotoxicity (NK): Evidence that the proteinase is serine dependent and has aromatic amino acid specficity of cleavage. *J. Immunol.* **133**, 2647.
693. Carpén, O., Säkselä, O., and Säkselä, E. (1986). Identification and localization of urokinase-type plasminogen activator in human NK-cells. *Int. J. Cancer* **38**, 355.
694. Young, J. D., Leong, L. G., Liu, C.-C., Damiano, A., Wall, D. A., and Cohn, Z. A. (1986). Isolation and characterization of a serine esterase from cytolytic T cell granules. *Cell (Cambridge, Mass.)* **47**, 183.
695. Gershenfeld, H. K., Hershberger, R. J., Shows, T. B., and Weissman, I. L. (1988). Cloning and chromosomal assignment of a human cDNA encoding a T cell- and natural killer cell-specific trypsin-like serine protease. *Proc. Natl. Acad. Sci. U.S.A.* **85**, 1184.
696. Trapani, J. A., Klein, J. L., White, P. C., and Dupont, B. (1988). Molecular cloning of an inducible serine esterase gene from human cytotoxic lymphocytes. *Proc. Natl. Acad. Sci. U.S.A.* **85**, 6924.
697. Krahenbuhl, O., Rey, C., Jenne, D., Lanzavecchia, A., Groscurth, P., Carrel, S., and Tschopp, J. (1988). Characterization of granzymes A and B isolated from granules of cloned human cytotoxic T lymphocytes. *J. Immunol.* **141**, 3471.
698. Zucker-Franklin, D., Yang, J., and Fuks, A. (1984). Different enzyme classes associated with human natural killer cells may mediate disparate functions. *J. Immunol.* **132**, 1451.
699. Hudig, D., Gregg, N. J., Kam, C.-M., and Powers, J. C. (1987). Lymphocyte granule-mediated cytolysis requires serine protease activity. *Biochem. Biophys. Res. Commun.* **149**, 882.
700. Zunino, S. J., Allison, N. J., Kam, C.-M., Powers, J. C., and Hudig, D. (1989). Localization, function and gene expression of chymotrypsin-like proteases of cytotoxic RNK-16 lymphocytes. *Biochim. Biophys. Acta* **967**, 331.
701. MacDermott, R. P., Schmidt, R. E., Caulfield, J. P., Hein, A., Bartley, G. T., Ritz, J., Schlossman, S. F., Austen, K. F., and Stevens, R. L. (1985). Proteoglycans in cell-mediated cytotoxicity. Identification, localization, and exocytosis of a

chondroitin sulfate proteoglycan from human cloned natural killer cells during target cell lysis. *J. Exp. Med.* **162**, 1771.

702. Schmidt, R. E., MacDermott, R. P., Bartley, G., Bertovich, M., Amato, D. A., Austen, K. F., Schlossman, S. F., Stevens, R. L., and Ritz, J. (1985). Specific release of proteoglycans from human natural killer cells during target lysis. *Nature (London)* **318**, 289.

703. Stevens, R. L., Otsu, K., Weis, J. H., Tantravahi, R. V., Austen, K. F., Henkart, P. A., Galli, M. C., and Reynolds, C. W. (1987). Co-sedimentation of chondroitin sulfate A glycosaminoglycans and proteoglycans with the cytolytic secretory granules of rat large granular lymphocyte (LGL) tumor cells, and identification of a mRNA in normal and transformed LGL that encodes proteoglycans. *J. Immunol.* **139**, 863.

704. Christmas, S. E., Steward, W. P., Lyon, M., Gallagher, J. T., and Moore, M. (1988). Chondroitin sulphate proteoglycan production by NK cells and T cells: Effects of xylosides on proliferation and cytotoxic function. *Immunology* **63**, 225.

705. Wolfe, S. A., Tracey, D. E., and Henney, C. S. (1976). Induction of "natural" killer cells by BCG. *Nature (London)* **262**, 584.

706. Trinchieri, G., Santoli, D., and Knowles, B. B. (1977). Tumor cell lines induce interferon in human lymphocytes. *Nature (London)* **270**, 611.

707. Weigent, D. A., Langford, M. P., Fleishmann, W. R., and Stanton, G. J. (1982). Enhancement of natural killing activity by different types of interferon. In "Human Lymphokines" (A. Khan and N. O. Hill, eds.), p. 539. Academic Press, New York.

708. Trinchieri, G., Matsumoto-Kobayashi, M., Clark, S. C., Sheehra, J., London, L., and Perussia, B. (1984). Response of resting human peripheral blood natural killer cells to interleukin-2. *J. Exp. Med.* **160**, 1147.

709. Platsoucas, C. D. (1986). Regulation of natural killer cytotoxicity by *Escherichia coli*-derived human interferon gamma. *Scand. J. Immunol.* **24**, 93.

710. Brunda, M. J., Tarnowski, D., and Davatelis, V. (1986). Interaction of recombinant interferons with recombinant interleukin-2: Differential effects on natural killer cell activity and interleukin-2-activated killer cells. *Int. J. Cancer* **37**, 787.

711. Weigent, D. A., Stanton, G. J., and Johnson, H. M. (1983). Recombinant gamma interferon enhances natural killer cell activity similar to natural gamma interferon. *Biochem. Biophys. Res. Commun.* **111**, 525.

712. Faltynek, C. R., Princler, G. L., and Ortaldo, J. R. (1986). Expression of IFN-alpha and IFN-gamma receptors on normal human small resting T lymphocytes and large granular lymphocytes. *J. Immunol.* **136**, 4134.

713. Black, P. L., Henderson, E. E., Pfleiderer, W., Charubala, R., and Suhadolnik, R. J. (1984). 2′, 5′-Oligoadenylate trimer core and the cordycepin analog augment the tumoricidal activity of human natural killer cells. *J. Immunol.* **133**, 2773.

714. Schmidt, A., Crisp, B., Krause, D., Silverman, R. H., Herberman, R. B., and Ortaldo, J. R. (1987). Involvement of the 2′-5′ A pathway in the augmentation of natural killer activity. *Nat. Immun. Cell Growth Regul.* **6**, 19.

715. Ortaldo, J. R., Herberman, R. B., Harvey, C., Osheroff, P., Pan, Y. C., Kelder, B., and Pestka, S. (1984). A species of human alpha interferon that lacks the ability to boost human natural killer activity. *Proc. Natl. Acad. Sci. U.S.A.* **81**, 4926.

716. Langer, J. A., Ortaldo, J. R., and Pestka, S. (1986). Binding of human alpha-interferons to natural killer cells. *J. Interferon Res.* **6**, 97.

717. Vanky, F., Argov, S., Einhorn, S., and Klein, E. (1980). The role of alloantigens in natural killing. Allogeneic but not autologous tumor biopsy cells are sensitive for interferon induced cytotoxicity of human blood lymphocytes. *J. Exp. Med.* **151**, 1151.

718. Säkselä, E., Timonen, T., and Cantell, K. (1979). Human natural killer cell activity is augmented by interferon via recruitment of "pre-NK" cells. *Scand. J. Immunol.* **10**, 257.
719. Silva, A., Bonavida, B., and Targan, S. (1980). Mode of action of interferon-mediated modulation of natural killer cytotoxic activity: Recruitment of pre-NK cells and enhanced kinetics of lysis. *J. Immunol.* **125**, 479.
720. Targan, S., and Dorey, F. (1980). Interferon activation of "pre-spontaneous killer" (pre-SK) cells and alteration in kinetics of lysis of both 'pre-SK' and active SK cells. *J. Immunol.* **124**, 2157.
721. Targan, S., and Dorey, F. (1980). Dual mechanism of interferon augmentation of natural killer cytotoxicity (NKCC). *Ann. N.Y. Acad. Sci.* **350**, 121.
722. Droller, M. J., Borg, H., and Perlmann, P. (1979). In vitro enhancement of natural and antibody-dependent lymphocyte-mediated cytotoxicity against tumor target cells by interferon. *Cell. Immunol.* **47**, 248.
723. Herberman, R. B., Ortaldo, J. R., and Bonnard, G. D. (1979). Augmentation by interferon of human natural and antibody-dependent cell-mediated cytotoxicity. *Nature (London)* **277**, 221.
724. Ortaldo, J. R., Pestka, S., Slease, R. B., Rubinstein, N., and Herberman, R. B. (1980). Augmentation of human K-cell activity with interferon. *Scand. J. Immunol.* **12**, 365.
725. Rumpold, H., Kraft, D., Scheiner, O., Meindl, P., and Bodo, G. (1980). Enhancement of NK, but not K cell activity by different interferons. *Int. Arch. Allergy Appl. Immunol.* **62**, 152.
726. Warren, R., Kalamasz, D., and Storb, R. (1982). Enhancement of human ADCC with interferon. *Clin. Exp. Immunol.* **50**, 183.
727. Basham, T. Y., Smith, W. K., and Merigan, T. C. (1984). Interferon enhances antibody-dependent cellular cytotoxicity when suboptimal concentrations of antibody are used. *Cell. Immunol.* **88**, 393.
728. Einhorn, S., Blomgren, H., and Strander, H. (1978). Interferon and spontaneous cytotoxicity in man. II. Studies in patients receiving exogenous leukocyte interferon. *Acta Med. Scand.* **204**, 477.
729. Huddlestone, J. F., Merigan, T. C., and Oldstone, M. B. (1979). Induction and kinetics of natural killer cells in humans following interferon therapy. *Nature (London)* **282**, 417.
730. Kariniemi, A. L., Timonen, T., and Kousa, M. (1980). Effect of leukocyte interferon on natrual killer cells in healthy volunteers. *Scand. J. Immunol.* **12**, 371.
731. Lotzova, E., Savary, C. A., Gutterman, J. U., and Hersh, E. M. (1982). Modulation of natural killer cell-mediated cytotoxicity by partially purified and cloned interferon. *Cancer Res.* **42**, 2480.
732. Pape, G. R., Hadam, M. R., Eisenburg, J., and Riethmuller, G. (1981). Kinetics of natural cytotoxicity in patients treated with human fibroblast interferon. *Cancer Immunol. Immunother.* **11**, 1.
733. Maluish, A. E., Ortaldo, J. R., Conlon, J. C., Sherwin, S. A., Leavitt, R., Strong, D. M., Wirnik, P., Oldham, R., and Herberman, R. B. (1983). Depression of natural killer cytotoxicity after in vivo administration of recombinant leukocyte interferon. *J. Immunol.* **131**, 503.
734. Biron, C. A., Sonnenfeld, G., and Welsh, R. M. (1984). Interferon induces natural killer cell blastogenesis *in vivo*. *J. Leuk. Biol.* **35**, 31.
735. Brunda, M. J., Taramelli, D., Holden, H. T., and Varesio, L. (1982). Suppression of murine natural killer cell activity by normal peritoneal macrophages. *In* "NK

Cells and Other Natural Effector Cells" (R. B. Herberman, ed.), p. 535. Academic Press, New York.

736. Hochman, P. S., Cudkowicz, G., and Evans, P. D. (1981). Carrageenan-induced decline of natural killer activity. II. Inhibition of cytolysis by adherent non-T Ia-negative suppressor cells activated in vivo. *Cell. Immunol.* **61**, 200.

737. Brunda, M. J., Taramelli, D., Holden, H. T., and Varesio, L. (1983). Suppression of *in vitro* maintenance and interferon-mediated augmentation of natural killer cell activity by adherent peritoneal cells from normal mice. *J. Immunol.* **130**, 1974.

738. Nair, M. P., Schwartz, S. A., Fernandes, G., Pahwa, R., Ikehara, S., and Good, R. A. (1981). Suppression of natural killer (NK) cell activity of spleen cells by thymocytes. *Cell. Immunol.* **58**, 9.

739. Riccardi, C., Santoni, A., Barlozzari, T., and Herberman, R. B. (1981). Suppression of natural killer (NK) activity by splenic adherent cells of low NK-reactive mice. *Int. J. Cancer* **28**, 811.

740. Santoni, A., Riccardi, C., Barlozzari, T., and Herberman, R. B. (1980). Suppression of activity of mouse natural killer (NK) cells by activated macrophages from mice treated with pyran copolymer. *Int. J. Cancer* **26**, 837.

741. Zoller, M., and Wigzell, H. (1982). Normally occurring inhibitory cells for natural killer cell activity. I. Organ distribution. *Cell. Immunol.* **74**, 14.

742. Zoller, M., and Wigzell, H. (1982). Normally occurring inhibitory cells for natural killer cell activity. II. Characterization of the inhibitory cell. *Cell. Immunol.* **74**, 27.

743. Brunda, M. J., Herberman, R. B., and Holden, H. T. (1980). Inhibition of murine natural killer cell activity by prostaglandins. *J. Immunol.* **124**, 2682.

744. Tanaka, Y. (1981). Natural killer (NK) activity of normal human peripheral blood lymphocytes against erythroleukemic cell lines K562. *Hiroshima J. Med. Sci.* **30**, 115.

745. Yang, J., and Zucker-Franklin, D. (1984). Modulation of natural killer (NK) cells by autologous neutrophils and monocytes. *Cell. Immunol.* **86**, 171.

746. Allavena, P., Introna, M., Mangioni, C., and Mantovani, A. (1981). Inhibition of natural killer activity by tumor-associated lymphoid cells from ascites ovarian carcinomas. *JNCI, J. Natl. Cancer Inst.* **67**, 319.

747. Eremin, O., Coombs, R. R.,and Ashby, J. (1981). Lymphocytes infiltrating human breast cancers lack K cell activity and show low levels of NK cell activity. *Br. J. Cancer* **44**, 166.

748. Herberman, R. B., Holden, H. T., Djeu, J. Y., Jerrells, T. R., Varesio, L., Tagliabue, A., White, S. L., Oehler, J. R., and Dean, J. H. (1979). Macrophages as regulators of immune responses against tumors. *Adv. Exp. Med. Biol.* **121B**, 361.

749. Uchida, A., and Micksche, M. (1981). Suppressor cells for natural killer activity in carcinoma pleural effusions of cancer patients. *Cancer Immunol. Immunother.* **11**, 255.

750. Young, M. R., Wheeler, E., and Newby, M. (1986). Macrophage-mediated suppression of natural killer cell activity in mice bearing Lewis lung carcinoma. *J. Natl. Cancer Inst.* **76**, 745.

751. Koren, H. S., and Leung, K. H. (1982). Modulation of human NK cells by interferon and prostaglandin E_2. *Mol. Immunol.* **19**, 1341.

752. Droller, M. J., Schneider, M. U., and Perlmann, P. (1978). A possible role of prostaglandins in the inhibition of natural and antibody-dependent cell-mediated cytotoxicity against tumor cells. *Cell. Immunol.* **39**, 165.

753. Kendall, R. A., and Targan, S. (1980). The dual effect of prostaglandin (PGE_2) and ethanol on the natural killer cytolytic process: Effector activation and NK-cell–target cell conjugate lytic inhibition. *J. Immunol.* **125**, 2770.

754. Lang, N. P., Ortaldo, J. R., Bonnard, G. D., and Herberman, R. B. (1982). Interferon and prostaglandin: Effects of human natural and lectin-induced cytotoxicity. *JNCI, J. Natl. Cancer Inst.* **69**, 339.
755. Leung, K. H., and Koren, H. S. (1982). Regulation of cytotoxic reactivity of NK cells by interferon and PGE2. *In* "NK Cells and Other Natural Effector Cells" (R. B. Herberman, ed.), p. 615. Academic Press, New York.
756. D'Amore, P. J., and Golub, S. H. (1985). Suppression of human NK cytotoxicity by an MLC-generated cell population. *J. Immunol.* **134**, 272.
757. Nair, M. P., and Schwartz, S. A. (1981). Suppression of natural killer activity and antibody-dependent cellular cytotoxicity by cultured human lymphocytes. *J. Immunol.* **126**, 2221.
758. Rook, A. H., Kehrl, J. H., Wakefield, L. M., Roberts, A. B., Sporn, M. B., Burlington, D. B., Lane, H. C., and Fauci, A. S. (1986). Effects of transforming growth factor beta on the functions of natural killer cells: Depressed cytolytic activity and blunting of interferon responsiveness. *J. Immunol.* **136**, 3916.
759. Gersuk, G. M., Holloway, J. M., Chang, W. C., and Pattengale, P. K. (1986). Inhibition of human natural killer cell activity by platelet-derived growth factor. *Nat. Immun. Cell Growth Regul.* **5**, 283.
760. Henney, C. S., Kuribayashi, K., Kern, D. E., and Gillis, S. (1981). Interleukin 2 augments natural killer cell activity. *Nature (London)* **291**, 335.
761. Weigent, D. A., Stanton, G. J., and Johnson, H. M. (1983). Interleukin 2 enhances natural killer cell activity through induction of gamma interferon. *Infect. Immun.* **41**, 992.
762. Hefeneider, S. H., Henney, C. S., and Gillis, S. (1982). In vivo interleukin-2 induced augmentation of natural killer cell activity. *In* "NK Cells and Other Natural Effector Cells" (R. B. Herberman, ed.), p. 421. Academic Press, New York.
763. Ortaldo, J. R., Mason, A. T., Gerard, J. P., Henderson, L. E., Farrar, W., and Hopkins, R. F. (1984). Effects of natural and recombinant IL 2 on regulation of IFN gamma production and natural killer activity: Lack of involvement of the Tac antigen for these immunoregulatory effects. *J. Immunol.* **133**, 779.
764. Phillips, J. H., Gemlo, B. T., Myers, W. W., Rayner, A. A., and Lanier, L. L. (1987). In vivo and in vitro activation of natural killer cells in advanced cancer patients undergoing combined recombinant interleukin-2 and LAK cell therapy. *J. Clin. Oncol.* **5**, 1933.
765. Sharon, M., Klausner, R. D., Cullen, B. R., Chizzonite, R., and Leonard, W. J. (1986). Novel interleukin 2 receptor subunit detected by crosslinking under high affinity conditions. *Science* **234**, 859.
766. Kehrl, J. H., Dukovich, M., Whalen, G., Katz, P., Fauci, A. S., and Greene, W. C. (1988). Novel interleukin 2 (IL-2) receptor appears to mediate IL-2-induced activation of natural killer cells. *J. Clin. Invest.* **81**, 200.
767. Siegel, J. P., Sharon, M., Smith, P. L., and Leonard, W. J. (1987). The IL-2 receptor beta chain (p70): Role in mediating signals for LAK, NK, and proliferative activities. *Science* **238**, 75.
768. Sayers, T. J., Mason, A. T., and Ortaldo, J. R. (1986). Regulation of human natural killer cell activity by interferon-gamma: Lack of a role in interleukin 2-mediated augmentation. *J. Immunol.* **136**, 2176.
769. Kabelitz, D., Kirchner, H., Armerding, D., and Wagner, H. (1985). Recombinant interleukin 2 rapidly augments human natural killer cell activity. *Cell. Immunol.* **93**, 38.

770. Svedersky, L. P., Shepard, H. M., Spencer, S. A., and Shalaby, M. R. (1984). Augmentation of human natural cell-mediated cytotoxicity by recombinant human interleukin 2. *J. Immunol.* **133**, 714.
771. Brunda, M. J., Tarnowski, D., and Davatelis, V. (1986). Interaction of recombinant interferons with recombinant interleukin-2: Differential effects on natural killer cell activity and interleukin-2-activated killer cells. *Int. J. Cancer* **37**, 787.
772. Vose, B. M., Riccardi, C., Bonnard, G. B., and Herberman, R. B. (1983). Limiting dilution analysis of the frequency of human T cells and large granular lymphocytes proliferating in response to interleukin 2. II. Regulatory role of interferon on proliferative and cytotoxic precursors. *J. Immunol.* **130**, 768.
773. Itoh, K., Shiiba, K., Shimizu, Y., Suzuki, R., and Kumagai, K. (1985). Generation of activated killer (AK) cells by recombinant interleukin 2 (rIL 2) in collaboration with interferon-γ (IFN-γ). *J. Immunol.* **134**, 3124.
774. Landolfo, S., Cofano, F., Giovarelli, M., Prat, M., Cavallo, G., and Forni, G. (1985). Inhibition of interferon-gamma may suppress allograft reactivity by T lymphocytes in vitro and in vivo. *Science* **229**, 176.
775. Lanier, L. L., Buck, D. W., Rhodes, L., Ding, A., Evans, E., Barney, C., and Phillips, J. H. (1988). Interleukin 2 activation of natural killer cells rapidly induces the expression and phosphorylation of the Leu-23 activation antigen. *J. Exp. Med.* **167**, 1572.
776. Grimm, E. A., Mazumder, A., Zhang, H. Z., and Rosenberg, S. A. (1982). Lymphokine-activated killer cells phenomenon. Lysis of natural killer-resistant fresh solid tumor cells by interleukin 2-activated autologous human peripheral blood lymphocytes. *J. Exp. Med.* **155**, 1823.
777. Grimm, E. A., Ramsey, K. M., Mazumder, A., Wilson, D. J., Djeu, J. Y., and Rosenberg, S. A. (1983). Lymphokine activated killer cell phenomenon. II. Precursor phenotype is serologically distinct from peripheral T lymphocytes, memory cytotoxic thymus-derived lymphocytes and natural killer cells. *J. Exp. Med.* **157**, 884.
778. Grimm, E. A., Robb, R. J., Roth, J. A., Neckers, L. M., Lachman, L. B., Wilson, D. J., and Rosenberg, S. A. (1983). Lymphokine activated killer cell phenomenon. III. Evidence that IL-2 alone is sufficient for direct activation of PBL to LAK. *J. Exp. Med.* **158**, 1356.
779. Itoh, K., Tilden, A. B., Kumagai, K., and Balch, C. M. (1985). Leu-11+ lymphocytes with natural killer (NK) activity are precursors of recombinant interleukin 2 (rIL 2)-induced activated killer (AK) cells. *J. Immunol.* **134**, 802.
780. Shau, H., Gray, D., and Mitchell, M. S. (1988). Studies on the relationship of human natural killer and lymphokine-activated killer cells with lysosomal staining and analysis of surface marker phenotypes. *Cell. Immunol.* **115**, 13.
781. Atzpodien, J., Wisniewski, D., Gulati, S., Welte, K., Knowles, R., and Clarkson, B. (1987). Interleukin-2- and mitogen-activated NK-like killer cells from highly purified human peripheral blood T cell ($CD3^+$ $N901^-$) cultures. *Nat. Immun. Cell Growth Regul.* **6**, 129.
782. Bolhuis, R. L. H., and Schellekens, H. (1981). Induction of natural killer cell activity and allocytotoxicity in human peripheral blood lymphocytes after mixed lymphocyte culture. *Scand. J. Immunol.* **13**, 401.
783. Rimm, I. J., Schlossman, S. F., and Reinherz, E. L. (1981). Antibody-dependent cellular cytotoxicity and natural killer-like activity are mediated by subsets of activated T cells. *Clin. Immunol. Immunopathol.* **21**, 134.
784. Seeley, J. K., Masucci, G., Poros, A., Klein, E., and Golub, S. H. (1979). Studies

on cytotoxicity generated in human mixed lymphocyte cultures. II. Anti K562 effectors are distinct from allospecific CTL and can be generated from NK-depleted T cells. *J. Immunol.* **123**, 1303.
785. Strassman, G., Back, F. H., and Zarling, J. M. (1983). Depletion of human NK cells with monoclonal antibodies allows the generation of cytotoxic T lymphocytes without NK-like cells in mixed cultures. *J. Immunol.* **130**, 1556.
786. Zarling, J. M., Bach, F. H., and Kung, P. C. (1981). Sensitization of lymphocytes against pooled allogeneic cells. II. Characterization of effector cells cytotoxic for autologous effector cell lines. *J. Immunol.* **126**, 375.
787. Bottazzi, B., Introna, M., Allavena, P., Villa, A., and Mantovani, A. (1985). In vitro migration of human large granular lymphocytes. *J. Immunol.* **134**, 2316.
788. Pohajdak, B., Gomez, J., Orr, F. W., Khalil, N., Talgoy, M., and Greenberg, A. H. (1986). Chemotaxis of large granular lymphocytes. *J. Immunol.* **136**, 278.
789. Polentarutti, N., Bottazzi, B., Balotta, C., Erroi, A., and Mantovani, A. (1986). Modulation of the locomotory capacity of human large granular lymphocytes. *Cell. Immunol.* **101**, 204.
790. Pirelli, A., Allavena, P., and Mantovani, A. (1988). Activated adherent large granular lymphocytes/Natural Killer (LGL/NK) cells change their migratory behavior. *Immunology* **65**, 651.
791. Ramos, O. F., Masucci, M. G., Bejarano, M. T., and Klein, E. (1983). The tumor promoter phorbol-12,13-dibutyrate P(Bu)^2 stimulates cytotoxic activity of human blood lymphocytes. *Immunobiology* **165**, 403.
792. Argov, S., Hebdon, M., Cuatrecasas, P., and Koren, H. S. (1985). Phorbol ester-induced lymphocyte adherence: Selective action of NK cells. *J. Immunol.* **134**, 2215.
793. Bender, J. R., Pardi, R., Karasek, M. A., and Engleman, E. G. (1987). Phenotypic and functional characterization of lymphocytes that bind human microvascular endothelial cells in vitro Evidence for preferential binding of natural killer cells. *Clin. Invest.* **79**, 1679.
794. Aronson, F. R., Libby, P., Brandon, E. P., Janicka, M. W., and Mier, J. W. (1988). IL-2 rapidly induces natural killer cell adhesion to human endothelial cells. A potential mechanism for endothelial injury. *J. Immunol.* **141**, 158.
795. Vujanovic, N. L., Herberman, R. B., Maghazachi, A. A., and Hiserodt, J. C. (1988). Lymphokine-activated killer cells in rats. III. A simple method for the purification of large granular lymphocytes and their rapid expansion and conversion into lymphokine-activated killer cells. *J. Exp. Med.* **167**, 15.
796. Melder, R. J., Whiteside, T. L., Vujanovic, N. L., Hiserodt, J. C., and Herberman, R. B. (1988). A new approach to generating antitumor effectors for adoptive immunotherapy using human adherent lymphokine-activated killer cells. *Cancer Res.* **48**, 3461.
797. Hercend, T., Meuer, S. C., Reinherz, E. L., Schlossman, S. F., and Ritz, J. (1982). Generation of a cloned NK cell line derived from the "null cell" fraction of human peripheral blood. *J. Immunol.* **129**, 1299.
798. Phillips, J. H., and Lanier, L. L. (1985). A model for the differentiation of human natural killer cells. Studies on the *in vitro* activation of Leu 11$^+$ granular lymphocytes with a natural killer-sensitive tumor cell, K562. *J. Exp. Med.* **161**, 1464.
799. Cuturi, M. C., Anegón, I., Sherman, F., Loudon, R., Clark, S. C., Perussia, B., and Trinchieri, G. (1989). Production of hematopoietic colony-stimulating factors by human natural killer cells. *J. Exp. Med.* **169**, 569.
800. Procopio, A., Gismondi, A., Paolini, R., Morrone, S., Testi, R., Piccoli, M.,

rati, L., Herberman, R. B., and Santoni, A. (1988). Proliferative effects of 12-O-tetradecanoylphorbol-13-acetate (TPA) and calcium ionophores on human large granular lymphocytes (LGL). *Cell. Immunol.* **113**, 70.
801. Spits, H., Yssel, H., Paliard, X., Kastelein, R., Figdor, C., and De Vries, J. E. (1988). IL-4 inhibits IL-2-mediated induction of human lymphokine-activated killer cells, but not the generation of antigen-specific cytotoxic T lymphocytes in mixed leukocyte cultures. *J. Immunol.* **141**, 29.
802. Nagler, A., Lanier, L. L., and Phillips, J. H. (1988). The effects of IL-4 on human natural killer cells. A potent regulator of IL-2 activation and proliferation. *J. Immunol.* **141**, 2349.
803. Mule, J. J., Smith, C. A., and Rosenberg, S. A. (1987). Interleukin 4 (B cell stimulatory factor 1) can mediate the induction of lymphokine-activated killer cell activity directed against fresh tumor cells. *J. Exp. Med.* **166**, 792.
804. Peace, D. J., Kern, D. E., Schultz, K. R., Greenberg, P. D., and Cheever, M. A. (1988). IL-4-induced lymphokine-activated killer cells. Lytic activity is mediated by phenotypically distinct natural killer-like and T cell-like large granular lymphocytes. *J. Immunol.* **140**, 3679.
805. Dinarello, C. A., Conti, P., and Mier, J. W. (1986). Effects of human interleukin-1 on natural killer cell activity: Is fever a host defense mechanism for tumor killing? *Yale J. Biol. Med.* **59**, 97.
806. Shirakawa, F., Tanaka, Y., Eto, S., Suzuki, H., Yodoi, J., and Yamashita, U. (1986). Effect of interleukin 1 on the expression of interleukin 2 receptor (Tac antigen) on human natural killer cells and natural killer-like cell line (YT cells). *J. Immunol.* **137**, 551.
807. Ostensen, M. E., Thiele, D. L., and Lipsky, P. E. (1987). Tumor necrosis factor-alpha enhances cytolytic activity of human natural killer cells. *J. Immunol.* **138**, 4185.
808. Chouaib, S., Bertoglio, J., Blay, J. Y., Marchiol, F. C., and Fradelizi, D. (1988). Generation of lymphokine-activated killer cells: Synergy between tumor necrosis factor and interleukin 2. *Proc. Natl. Acad. Sci. U.S.A.* **85**, 6875.
809. Gomez, J., Pohajdak, B., O'Neill, S., Wilkins, J., and Greenberg, A. H. (1985). Activation of rat and human alveolar macrophage intracellular microbial activity by a preformed LGL cytokine. *J. Immunol.* **135**, 1194.
810. Greenberg, A. H., Khalil, N., Pohajdak, B., Talgoy, M., Henkart, P., and Orr, F. W. (1986). NK-leukocyte chemotactic factor (NK-LCF): A large granular lymphocyte (LGL) granule-associated chemotactic factor. *J. Immunol.* **137**, 3224.
811. Roussel, E., and Greenberg, A. H. (1989). Identification of a macrophage activating factor (MAF) in granules of the RNK large granular leukemia. *J. Immunol.* **142**, 543.
812. Pohajdak, B., Gomez, J. L., Wilkins, J. A., and Greenberg, A. H. (1984). Tumor-activated NK cells trigger monocyte oxidative metabolism. *J. Immunol.* **133**, 2430.
813. Helfand, S. L., Werkmeister, J., and Roder, J. C. (1982). Chemiluminescence response of human natural killer cells. *J. Exp. Med.* **156**, 492.
814. Werkmeister, J., Helfand, S., Roder, J., and Pross, H. (1983). The chemiluminescence response of human natural killer cells. II. Assocation of a decreased response with low natural killer activity. *Eur. J. Immunol.* **13**, 514.
815. Duwe, A. K., and Roder, J. C. (1984). Involvement of hydroxyl free radical, but not superoxide, in the cytolytic pathway of natural killer cells. Revision of an earlier hypothesis. *Med. Biol.* **62**, 95.

816. Ramstedt, U., Rossi, P., Kullman, C., Warren, E., Palmblad, J., and Jondal, M. (1984). Free oxygen radicals are not detectable by chemiluminescence during human natural killer cell cytotoxicity. *Scand. J. Immunol.* **19**, 457.
817. Storkus, W. J., and Dawson, J. R. (1986). Oxygen-reactive metabolites are not detected at the effector-target interface during natural killing. *J. Leuk. Biol.* **39**, 547.
818. El Hag, A., and Clark, R. A. (1984). Intact natural killer activity in chronic granulomatous disease: Evidence against an oxygen-dependent cytotoxic mechanism. *J. Immunol.* **132**, 569.
819. Suthanthiran, M., Solomon, S. D., Williams, P. S., and Rubin, A. L. (1984). Hydroxyl radical scavengers inhibit human natural killer cell activity. *Nature (London)* **307**, 276.
820. Gibboney, J. J., Haak, R. A., Kleinhaus, F. W., and Brahmi, Z. (1988). Electron spin spectroscopy does not reveal hydroxyl radical production in activated natural killer lymphocytes. *J. Leuk. Biol.* **44**, 545.
821. Djeu, J. Y., Stocks, N., Zoon, K., Stanton, G. J., Timonen, T., and Herberman, R. B. (1982). Positive self regulation of cytotoxicity in human natural killer cells by production of interferon upon exposure to influenza and herpes virus. *J. Exp. Med.* **156**, 1222.
822. Trinchieri, G., Perussia, B., and Santoli, D. (1980). Interferon production in lymphocytes cultured with tumor-derived cells. In "Natural Cell-Mediated Cytotoxicity Against Tumors" (R. B. Herberman, ed.), p. 1199. Academic Press, New York.
823. Djeu, J. Y., Timonen, T., and Herberman, R. B. (1982). Production of interferon by human natural killer cells in response to mitogens, viruses and bacteria. In "NK Cells and Other Natural Effector Cells" (R. B. Herberman, ed.), p. 669. Academic Press, New York.
824. Kasahara, T., Djeu, J. Y., Dougherty, S. F., and Oppenheim, J. S. (1983). Capacity of human large granular lymphocytes (LGL) to produce mutiple lymphokines: Interleukin 2, interferon and colony stimulating factor. *J. Immunol.* **131**, 2379.
825. Saksela, E. (1982). Interferon and natural killer cells. In "Interferon 3" (I. Gresser, ed.), p. 46. Academic Press, London.
826. Timonen, T., Säksela, E., Virtanen, I., and Cantell, K. (1980). Natural killer cells are responsible for the interferon production induced in human lymphocytes by tumor cell contact. *Eur. J. Immunol.* **10**, 422.
827. Abb, J., Abb, H., and Deinhardt, F. (1983). Phenotype of human α-interferon producing leukocytes identified by monoclonal antibodies. *Clin. Exp. Immunol.* **52**, 179.
828. Perussia, B., Fanning, V., and Trinchieri, G. (1984). Characterization of human peripheral blood IFNα-producing cells. In "'Natural Killer Activity and Its Regulation" (T. Hoshino, ed.), p. 107. Excerpta Medica, Tokyo.
829. Ronnblom, L., Ramstedt, U., and Alm, G. V. (1983). Properties of human natural interferon-producing cells stimulated by tumor cell lines. *Eur. J. Immunol.* **13**, 471.
830. Young, H. A., and Ortaldo, J. R. (1987). One-signal requirement for interferon-production by human large granular lymphocytes. *J. Immunol.* **139**, 724.
831. Wilson, A. B., Harris, J. M., and Coombs, R. R. (1988). Interleukin-2-induced production of interferon-gamma by resting human T cells and large granular lymphocytes: Requirement for accessory cell factors, including interleukin-1. *Cell. Immunol.* **113**, 130.
832. Domzig, W., and Stadler, B. M. (1982). The relation between human natural killer

cells and interleukin 2. *In* "NK Cells and Other Natural Effector Cells" (R. B. Herberman, ed.), p. 409. Academic Press, New York.
833. Mingari, M. C., Ferrini, S., Pende, D., Bottino, C., Prigione, I., Moretta, A., and Moretta, L. (1987). Phenotypic and functional analysis of human CD3+ and CD3− clones with "lymphokine-activated killer" (LAK) activity. Frequent occurrence of CD3+ LAK clones which produce interleukin-2. *Int. J. Cancer* **40**, 495.
834. Pistoia, V., Cozzolino, F., Torcia, M., Castigli, E., and Ferrarini, M. (1985). Production of B cell growth factor by a Leu7+, OKM1+ non-T cell with the features of large granular lymphocytes (LGL). *J. Immunol.* **134**, 3179.
835. Procopio, A. D., Allavena, P., and Ortaldo, J. R. (1985). Noncytotoxic functions of natural killer (NK) cells: Large granular lymphocytes (LGL) produce a B cell growth factor (BCGF). *J. Immunol.* **135**, 3264.
836. Yamamoto, R. S., Ware, C. F., and Granger, G. A. (1986). The human LT system. XI. Identification of LT and "TNF-like" forms from stimulated natural killers, specific and nonspecific cytotoxic human T cells in vitro. *J. Immunol.* **137**, 1878.
837. Peters, P. M., Ortaldo, J. R., Shalaby, M. R., Svedersky, L. P., Nedwin, G. E., Bringman, T. S., Hass, P. E., Aggarwal, B. B., Herberman, R. B., Goeddel, D. V., and Palladino, M. A., Jr. (1986). Natural killer-sensitive targets stimulate production of TNF-alpha not TNF-beta (lymphotoxin) by highly purified human peripheral blood large granular lymphocytes. *J. Immunol.* **137**, 2592.
838. Rambaldi, A., Alessio, G., Rossi, V., Donati, M. B., Semeraro, N., and Mantovani, A. (1985). Production of interleukin 1 but not of procoagulant activity by large granular lymphocytes. *Scand. J. Immunol.* **22**, 363.
839. Scala, G., Allavena, P., Djeu, J. Y., Kasahara, T., Ortaldo, J. R., Herberman, R. B., and Oppenheim, J. J. (1984). Human large granular lymphocytes are potent producers of interleukin-1. *Nature (London)* **309**, 56.
840. Payan, D. G., and McGillis, J. P. (1986). Neuroimmunology. *Adv. Immunol.* **39**, 244.
841. Cross, R. J., Markesbery, W. R., Brooks, W. H., and Roszman, T. L. (1984). Hypothalamic–immune interactions: Neuromodulation of natural killer activity by lesioning of the anterior hypothalamus. *Immunology* **51**, 399.
842. Belluardo, N., Mudo, G., Cella, S., Santoni, A., Forni, G., and Bindoni, M. (1987). Hypothalamic control of certain aspects of natural immunity in the mouse. *Immunology* **62**, 321.
843. Aoki, T., Usuda, Y., Miyakoshi, H., Tamura, K., and Herberman, R. B. (1987). Low natural killer syndrome: Clinical and immunologic features. *Nat. Immun. Cell Growth Regul.* **6**, 116.
844. Caligiuri, M., Murray, C., Buchwald, D., Levine, H., Cheney, P., Peterson, D., Komaroff, A. L., and Ritz, J. (1987). Phenotypic and functional deficiency of natural killer cells in patients with chronic fatigue syndrome. *J. Immunol.* **139**, 3306.
845. Irwin, M., Smith, T. L., and Gillin, J. C. (1987). Low natural killer cytotoxicity in major depression. *Life Sci.* **41**, 2127.
846. Levy, S., Herberman, R. B., Lippman, M., and D'Angelo, T. (1987). Correlation of stress factors with sustained depression of natural killer cell activity and predicted prognosis in patients with breast cancer. *J. Clin. Oncol.* **5**, 348.
847. Irwin, M., Daniels, M., Smith, T. L., Bloom, E., and Weiner, H. (1987). Impaired natural killer cell activity during bereavement. *Brain Behav. Immunol.* **1**, 98.
848. Irwin, M., Daniels, M., Risch, S. C., Bloom, E., and Weiner, H. (1988). Plasma

cortisol and natural killer cell activity during bereavement. *Biol. Psychiatry* **24**, 173.
849. Glaser, R., Rice, J., Speicher, C. E., Stout, J. C., and Kiecolt-Glaser, J. K. (1986). Stress depresses interferon production by leukocytes concomitant with a decrease in natural killer cell activity. *Behav. Neurosci.* **100**, 675.
850. Locke, S. E., Kraus, L., Leserman, J., Hurst, M. W., Heisel, J. S., and Williams, R. M. (1984). Life change stress, psychiatric symptoms, and natural killer cell activity. *Psychosom. Med.* **46**, 441.
851. Yoshihara, H., Tanaka, N., and Orita, K. (1986). Suppression of natural killer cell activity by surgical stress in cancer patients and the underlying mechanisms. *Acta Med. Okayama* **40**, 113.
852. Tønnesen, E., Brinklv, M. M., Christensen, N. J., Olesen, A. S., and Madsen, T. (1987). Natural killer cell activity and lymphocyte function during and after coronary artery bypass grafting in relation to the endocrine stress response. *Anesthesiology* **67**, 526.
853. Pollock, R. E., and Lotzova, E. (1987). Surgical-stress-related suppression of natural killer cell activity: A possible role in tumor metastasis. *Nat. Immun. Cell Growth Regul.* **6**, 269.
854. Ghoneum, M., Gill, G., Assanah, P., and Stevens, W. (1987). Susceptibility of natural killer cell activity of old rats to stress. *Immunology* **60**, 461.
855. Okimura, T., Ogawa, M., and Yamauchi, T. (1986). Stress and immune responses. III. Effect of restraint stress on delayed type hypersensitivity (DTH) response, natural killer (NK) activity and phagocytosis in mice. *Jpn. J. Pharmacol.* **41**, 229.
856. Kandil, O., and Borysenko, M. (1987). Decline of natural killer cell target binding and lytic activity in mice exposed to rotation stress. *Health Psychol.* **6**, 89.
857. Aguila, H. N., Pakes, S. P., Lai, W. C., and Lu, Y. S. (1988). The effect of transportation stress on splenic natural killer cell activity in C57BL/6J mice. *Lab. Anim. Sci.* **38**, 148.
858. Shavit, Y., Lewis, J. W., Terman, G. W., Gale, R. P., and Liebeskind, J. C. (1984). Opioid peptides mediate the suppressive effect of stress on natural killer cell cytotoxicity. *Science* **223**, 188.
859. Shavit, Y., Terman, G. W., Lewis, J. W., Zane, C. J., and Gale, R. P. (1986). Effects of footshock stress and morphine on natural killer lymphocytes in rats: Studies of tolerance and cross-tolerance. *Brain Res.* **372**, 382.
860. Shavit, Y., Martin, F. C., Yirmiya, R., Ben-Eliyahu, S., Terman, G. W., Weiner, H., Gale, R. P., and Liebeskind, J. C. (1987). Effects of a single administration of morphine or footshock stress on natural killer cell cytotoxicity. *Brain Behav. Immunol.* **1**, 318.
861. Shavit, Y., Depaulis, A., Martin, F. C., Terman, G. W., Pechnick, R. N., Zane, C. J., Gale, R. P., and Liebeskind, J. C. (1986). Involvement of the brain opiate receptors in the immune suppressive effects of morphine. *Proc. Natl. Acad. Sci. U.S.A.* **83**, 7114.
862. Irwin, M. R., Vale, W., and Britton, K. T. (1987). Central corticotropin-releasing factor suppresses natural killer cytotoxicity. *Brain Behav. Immunol.* **1**, 81.
863. Hellstrand, K., Hermodsson, S., and Strannegard, O. (1985). Evidence for a β-adrenoreceptor-mediated regulation of human natural killer cells. *J. Immunol.* **134**, 4095.
864. Kraut, R. P., and Greenberg, A. H. (1986). Effects of endogenous and exogenous opioids on splenic natural killer cell activity. *Nat. Immun. Cell Growth Regul.* **5**, 28.

865. Faith, R. E., Liang, H. J., Murgo, A. J., and Plotnikoff, N. P. (1984). Neuroimmunomodulation with enkephalins: Enhancement of human natural killer (NK) cell activity *in vitro. Clin. Immunol. Immunopathol.* **31**, 412.
866. Faith, R. E., Liang, H. J., Plotnikoff, N. P., Murgo, A. J., and Nimeh, N. F. (1987). Neuroimmunomodulation with enkephalins: *In vitro* enhancement of natural killer cell activity in peripheral blood lymphocytes from cancer patients. *Nat. Immun. Cell Growth Regul.* **6**, 88.
867. Froelich, C. J., and Bankhurst, A. D. (1984). The effect of β-endorphin on natural cytotoxicity and antibody dependent cellular cytotoxicity. *Life Sci.* **35**, 261.
868. Mandler, R. N., Biddison, W. E., Mandler, R., and Serrate, S. A. (1986). β-Endorphin augments the cytolytic activity and interferon production of natural killer cells. *J. Immunol.* **136**, 934.
869. Wybran, J. (1985). Enkephalins and endorphins: Activation molecules for the immune system and natural killer activity? *Neuropeptides (Edinburgh)* **5**, 371.
870. Williamson, S. A., Knight, R. A., Lightman, S. L., and Hobbs, J. R. (1987). Differential effects of β-endorphin fragments on human natural killing. *Brain Behav. Immunol.* **1**, 329.
871. Kay, N., Morley, J. E., and Van Ree, J. M. (1987). Enhancement of human lymphocyte natural killing function by non-opioid fragments of β-endorphin. *Life Sci.* **40**, 1083.
872. Mathews, P. M., Froelich, C. J., Sibbitt, W. L., and Bankhurst, A. D. (1983). Enhancement of natural cytotoxicity by β-endorphin. *J. Immunol.* **130**, 1658.
873. Pross, H, Mitchell, H., and Werkmeister, J. (1985). The sensitivity of placental trophoblast cells to intraplacental and allogeneic cytotoxic lymphocytes. *Am. J. Reprod. Immunol. Microbiol.* **8**, 1.
874. Gruber, S. A., Hoffman, R. A., Sothern, R. B., Lakatua, D., Carlson, A., Simmons, R. L., and Hrushesky, W. J. (1988). Splenocyte natural killer cell activity and metastatic potential are inversely dependent on estrous stage. *Surgery (St. Louis)* **104**, 398.
875. Okamura, K., Furukawa, K., Nakakuki, M., Yamada, K., and Suzuki, M. (1984). Natural killer cell activity during pregnancy. *Am. J. Obstet. Gynecol.* **149**, 396.
876. Russell, A. S., and Miller, C. L. (1986). Sequential studies of NK cell activity in human pregnancy. *J. Clin. Lab. Immunol.* **19**, 5.
877. Gregory, C. D., Lee, H., Rees, G. B., Scott, I. V., Shah, L. P., and Golding, P. R. (1985). Natural killer cells in normal pregnancy: Analysis using monoclonal antibodies and single-cell cytotoxicity assays. *Clin. Exp. Immunol.* **62**, 121.
878. Lee, H., Gregory, C. D., Rees, G. B., Scott, I. V., and Golding, P. R. (1987). Cytotoxic activity and phenotypic analysis of natural killer cells in early normal human pregnancy. *J. Reprod. Immunol.* **12**, 35.
879. Vaquer, S., De La Hera, A., Jorda, J., Martinez, C., Escudero, M., and Alvarez-Mon, M. (1987). Diminished natural killer activity in pregnancy: Modulation by interleukin 2 and interferon gamma. *Scand. J. Immunol.* **26**, 691.
880. Gregory, C. D., Lee, H., Scott, I. V., and Golding, P. R. (1987). Phenotypic heterogeneity and recycling capacity of natural killer cells in normal human pregnancy. *J. Reprod. Immunol.* **11**, 135.
881. Gabrilovac, J., Zadjelovic, J., Osmak, M., Suchanek, E., Zupanovic, Z., and Boranic, M. (1988). NK cell activity and estrogen hormone levels during normal human pregnancy. *Gynecol. Obstet. Invest.* **25**, 165.

882. Kalland, T. (1984). Exposure of neonatal female mice to diethylstilbestrol persistently impairs NK activity through reduction of effector cells at the bone marrow level. *Immunopharmacology* **7**, 127.
883. Pfeifer, R. W., and Patterson, R. M. (1985). Modulation of nonpsecific cell-mediated growth inhibition by estrogen metabolites. *Immunopharmacology* **10**, 127.
884. Screpanti, I., Santoni, A., Gulino, A., Herberman, R. B., and Frati, L. (1987). Estrogen and antiestrogen modulation of the levels of mouse natural killer activity and large granular lymphocytes. *Cell. Immunol.* **106**, 191.
885. Kalland, T., and Campbell, T. (1984). Effects of diethylstilbestrol on human natural killer cells *in vitro*. *Immunopharmacology* **8**, 19.
886. Ferguson, M. M., and McDonald, F. G. (1985). Oestrogen as an inhibitor of human NK cell cytolysis. *FEBS Lett.* **191**, 145.
887. Ablin, R. J., Bartkus, J. M., and Gonder, M. J. (1988). *In vitro* effects of diethylstilbestrol and the LHRH analogue leuprolide on natural killer cell activity. *Immunopharmacology* **15**, 95.
888. Sulke, A. N., Jones, D. B., and Wood, P. J. (1985). Hormonal modulation of human natural killer cell activity *in vitro*. *J. Reprod. Immunol.* **7**, 105.
889. Uksila, J. (1985). Human NK activity is not inhibited by pregnancy and cord serum factors and female steroid hormones *in vitro*. *J. Reprod. Immunol.* **7**, 111.
890. Ritson, A., and Bulmer, J. N. (1987). Endometrial granulocytes in human decidua react with a natural-killer (NK) cell marker, NKH1. *Immunology* **62**, 329.
891. Croy, B. A., Waterfield, A., Wood, W., and King, G. J. (1988). Normal murine and porcine embryos recruit NK cells to the uterus. *Cell. Immunol.* **115**, 471.
892. Croy, B. A., Gambel, P., Rossant, J., and Wegmann, T. G. (1985). Characterization of murine decidual natural killer (NK) cells and their relevance to the success of pregnancy. *Cell. Immunol.* **93**, 315.
893. Starkey, P. M., Sargent, I. L., and Redman, C. W. G. (1988). Cell populations in human early pregancy decidua: Characterization and isolation of large granular lymphocytes by flow cytometry. *Immunology* **65**, 129.
894. Bulmer, J. N., and Sunderland, C. A. (1984). Immunohistological characterization of lymphoid cell populations in the early human placental bed. *Immunology* **52**, 349.
895. Bulmer, J. N., and Sunderland, C. A. (1983). Bone-marrow origin of endometrial granulocytes in the early human placental bed. *J. Reprod. Immunol.* **5**, 383.
896. Kearns, M., and Lala, P. K. (1985). Characterization of hematogenous cellular constituents of the murine decidua: A surface marker study. *J. Reprod. Immunol.* **8**, 213.
897. Zuckerman, F. A., and Head, J. R. (1988). Murine trophoblast resists cell-mediate lysis. II. Resistance to natural cell-mediated cytotoxicity. *Cell. Immunol.* **116**, 274.
898. Athanassakis, I., Bleackley, R. C., Paetkau, V., Guilbert, L., Barr, P. J., and Wegmann, T. G. (1987). The immunostimulatory effect of T cells and T cell lymphokines on murine fetally derived placental cells. *J. Immunol.* **138**, 37.
899. McIntyre, K. W., and Welsh, R. M. (1986). Accumulation of natural killer and cytotoxic T large granular lymphocytes in the liver during virus infection. *J. Exp. Med.* **164**, 1667.
900. Kolb, J. P., Chaouat, G., and Chassoux, D. (1984). Immunoactive products of placenta. III. Suppression of natural killing activity. *J. Immunol.* **132**, 2305.
901. Clark, D. A., and Chaouat, G. (1986). Characterization of the cellular basis for the inhibition of cytolytic effector cells by murine placenta. *Cell. Immunol.* **102**, 43.

902. Slapsys, R. M., Richards, C. D., and Clark, D. A. (1986). Active suppression of host-versus-graft reaction in pregnant mice. VIII. The uterine decidua-associated suppressor cell is distinct from decidual NK cells. *Cell. Immunol.* **99**, 140.
903. Szekeres-Bartho, J., Hadnagy, J., Csernus, V., Balazs, L., Magyarlaki, T., and Pacsa, A. S. (1985). Increased NK activity is responsible for higher cytotoxicity to HEF cells by lymphocytes of women with threatened preterm delivery. *AJRI, Am. J. Reprod. Immunol., Microbiol.* **7**, 22.
904. Gendron, R. L., and Baines, M. G. (1988). Infiltrating decidual natural killer cells are associated with spontaneous abortion in mice. *Cell. Immunol.* **113**, 261.
905. De Fougerolles, A. R., and Baines, M. G. (1987). Modulation of the natural killer cell activity in pregnant mice alters the spontaneous abortion rate. *J. Reprod. Immunol.* **11**, 147.
906. Bagby, G. C., Lawrence, H. J., and Neerhout, R. C. (1983). T-lymphocyte-mediated granulopoietic failure. In vitro identification of prednisone-responsive patients. *N. Engl. J. Med.* **309**, 1073.
907. Cudkowicz, G., and Stimpfling, J. H. (1964). Deficient growth of C57BL mouse marrow cells transplanted in F1 hybrid mice. Association with the histocompatibility-2 locus. *Immunology* **7**, 291.
908. Kiessling, R., Hochman, P. S., Haller, O., Shearer, G. M., Wigzell, H., and Cudkowicz, G. (1977). Evidence for a similar or common mechanism for natural killer cell activity and resistance to hemopoietic grafts. *Eur. J. Immunol.* **7**, 655.
909. Cudkowicz, G., and Bennett, M. (1971). Peculiar immunobiology of bone marrow allografts. I. Graft rejection by heavily "responder" mice. *J. Exp. Med.* **134**, 83.
910. Okumura, K., Habu, S. and Shimamura, K. (1982). The role of asialo GM1+ (GA1+) cells in the resistance to transplants of bone marrow or other tissues. In "NK Cells and Other Natural Effector Cells" (R. B. Herberman, ed.), p. 1527. Academic Press, New York.
911. Lotzova, E., Pollack, S. B., and Savary, C. A. (1982). Direct evidence for the involvement of natural killer cells in bone marrow transplantation. In "NK Cells and Other Natural Effector Cells" (R. B. Herberman, ed.), p. 1535. Academic Press, New York.
912. Harrison, D. E., and Carlson, G. A. (1983). Effect of the beige mutation on natural resistance to marrow grafts. *J. Immunol.* **130**, 484.
913. Warner, J. F., and Dennert, G. (1982). Effects of a cloned cell line with NK activity on bone marrow transplants, tumor development and metastasis in vivo. *Nature (London)* **300**, 31.
914. Bodignon, C., Daley, J. P., and Nakamura, I. (1985). Hematopoietic histoincompatibility reactions by NK cells *in vitro*: Model for genetic resistance to marrow grafts. *Science* **230**, 1398.
915. Holmberg, L. A., Miller, B. A., and Ault, K. (1984). The effect of natural killer cells on the development of syngeneic hematopoietic progenitors. *J. Immunol.* **133**, 2933.
916. Daley, J. P., and Nakamura, I. (1984). Natural resistance of lethally irradiated F1 hybrid mice to parental marrow grafts is a function of H-2/Hh restricted effectors. *J. Exp. Med.* **159**, 1132.
917. Warner, J. F., and Dennert, G. (1985). Bone marrow graft rejection as a function of antibody-directed natural killer cells. *J. Exp. Med.* **161**, 563.
918. Randrup-Thomsen, A., Pisa, P., Bro-Jorgensen, K., and Kiessling, R. (1986).

Mechanisms of lymphocytic choriomeningitis virus-induced hemopoietic dysfunction. *J. Virol.* **59**, 428.
919. Bro-Jorgensen, K. (1978). The interplay between lymphocytic choriomeningitis virus, immune function, and hemopoiesis in mice. *Adv. Virus Res.* **22**, 327.
920. Bro-Jorgensen, K., and Knudtzon, S. (1977). Changes in hemopoiesis during the course of the acute LCM virus infection in mice. *Blood* **49**, 47.
921. Welsh, R. M. (1978). Cytotoxic cells induced during lymphocytic choriomeningitis virus infection of mice. I. Characterization of natural killer cell induction. *J. Exp. Med.* **148**, 163.
922. Biron, C. A., and Welsh, R. M. (1982). Blastogenesis of natural killer cells during viral infection *in vivo*. *J. Immunol.* **129**, 2788.
923. Hansson, M., Petersson, M., Koo, G. C., Wigzell, H.,and Kiessling, R. (1988). In vivo function of natural killer cells as regulators of myeloid precursor cells in the spleen. *Eur. J. Immunol.* **18**, 485.
924. Bagby, G. C. (1981). T lymphocytes involved in inhibition of granulopoiesis in two neutropenic patients are of the cytotoxic/suppressor (T3$^+$ T8$^+$) subset. *J. Clin. Invest.* **68**, 1597.
925. Zoumbos, N. C., Gascon, P., Djeu, J., Trost, S. R., and Young, N. S. (1985). Circulating activated suppressor T lymphocytes in aplastic anemia. *N. Engl. J. Med.* **312**, 275.
926. Tagawa, S., Tokumine, Y., Ueda, E., Waki, K., Kanayama, Y., Taniguchi, N., Nakanishi, T., Inoue, R., and Kitani, T. (1986). Leu11+ T cell chronic lymphocytic leukemia with partially activated natural killer function and its further activation by recombinant IL-2 in vitro. *Blood* **68**, 846.
927. Grillot-Courvalin, C., Vinci, G., Tsapis, A., Dokhelar, M. C., Vainchenker, W., and Brouet, J. C. (1987). The syndrome of T8 hyperlymphocytosis: Variation in phenotype and cytotoxic activities of granular cells and evaluation of their role in associated neutropenia. *Blood* **69**, 1204.
928. Freimark, B., Lanier, L., Phillips, J., Quertermous, T., and Fox, R. (1987). Comparison of T cell receptor gene rearrangements in patients with large granular T cell leukemia and Felty's syndrome. *J. Immunol.* **138**, 1724.
929. Loughran, T. P. J., Clark, E. A., Price, T. H., and Hammond, W. P. (1986). Adult-onset cyclic neutropenia is associated with increased large granular lymphocytes. *Blood* **68**, 1082.
930. Linch, D. C., Newland, A. C., Turnbull, A. L., Knott, L. J., MacWhannel, A., and Beverley, P. (1984). Unusual T cell proliferations and neutropenia in rheumatoid arthritis.: Comparison with classical Felty's syndrome. *Scand. J. Haematol.* **33**, 342.
931. Hansson, M., Kiessling, R., Andersson, B., Karre, K., and Roder, J. (1979). Natural killer (NK) sensitive T-cell subpopulation in the thymus: Inverse correlation to NK activity of the host. *Nature (London)* **278**, 174.
932. Riccardi, C., Santoni, A., Barlozzari, T., and Herberman, R. B. (1981). In vivo reactivity of mouse natural killer (NK) cells against normal bone marrow cells. *Cell. Immunol.* **60**, 136.
933. Gidlund, M., Nose, M., Axberg, I., Wigzell, H., Totterman, T., and Nilsson, K. (1982). Analysis of differentiation events causing changes in NK cell tumor-target sensitivity. *In* "NK Cells and Other Natural Effector Cells" (R. B. Herberman, ed.), p. 733. Academic Press, New York.
934. Morris, T. C. M., Vincent, P. C., Sutherland, R., and Hersey, P. (1980). Inhibi-

tion of normal granulopoiesis *in vitro* by non-B non-T lymphocytes. *Br. J. Haematol.* **45**, 541.
935. Barr, R. D., and Stevens, C. A. (1982). The role of autologous helper and suppressor T cells in the regulation of human granulopoiesis. *Am. J. Hematol.* **12**, 323.
936. Hansson, M., Beran, M., Andersson, B., and Kiessling, R. (1982). Inhibition of *in vitro* granulopoiesis by autologous and allogeneic human NK cells. *J. Immunol.* **129**, 126.
937. Spitzer, G., and Verma, D. S. (1982). Cells with Fc receptors form normal donors suppress granulocyte-macrophage colony formation. *Blood* **60**, 758.
938. Degliantoni, G., Perussia, B., Mangoni, L., and Trinchieri, G. (1985). Inhibition of bone marrow colony formation by human natural killer cells and by natural killer cell-derived colony-inhibiting activity. *J. Exp. Med.* **161**, 1152.
939. Mangan, K. F., Chikkappa, G., Bieler, L. F., Scharfman, W. B., and Parkinson, D. R. (1982). Regulation of human blood erythroid burst-forming unit (BFU-E) proliferation by T-lymphocyte subpopulations defined by Fc receptors and monoclonal antibodies. *Blood* **59**, 990.
940. Nagler, A., Greenberg, P. L., Lanier, L. L., and Phillips, J. H. (1988). The effects of recombinant interleukin 2-activated natural killer cells on autologous peripheral blood hematopoietic progenitors. *J. Exp. Med.* **168**, 47.
941. Beran, M., Hansson, M., and Kiessling, R. (1983). Human natural killer cells can inhibit clonogenic growth of fresh leukemic cells. *Blood* **61**, 596.
942. Herrmann, F., Schmidt, R. E., Ritz, J., and Griffin, J. D. (1987). *In vitro* regulation of human hematopoiesis by natural killer cells: Analysis at a clonal level. *Blood* **69**, 246.
943. Dickinson, A. M., Jacobs, E. A., Williamson, I. K., Reid, M. M., and Proctor, S. J. (1988). Suppression of human granulocyte-macrophage colony formation *in vitro* by natural killer cells. *Clin. Immunol. Immunopathol.* **49**, 83.
944. Goss, G. D., Wittwer, M. A., Bezwoda, W. R., Herman, J., Rabson, A., Seymour, L., Derman, D. P., and Mendelow. B. (1985). Effect of natural killer cells on syngeneic bone marrow: *In vitro* and *in vivo* studies demonstrating graft failure due to NK cells in an identical twin treated by bone marrow transplantation. *Blood* **66**, 1043.
945. Pistoia, V., Ghio, R., Nocera, A., Leprini, A., Perata, A., and Ferrarini, M. (1985). Large granular lymphocytes have a promoting activity on human peripheral blood erythroid burst-forming units. *Blood* **65**, 464.
946. Gewirtz, A. M., Xu, W. Y., and Mangan, K. F. (1987). Role of natural killer cells, in comparison with T lymphocytes and monocytes, in the regulation of normal human megakaryocytopoiesis *in vitro*. *J. Immunol.* **139**, 2915.
947. Zoumbos, N., Raefsky, E., and Young, N. (1986). Lymphokines and hematopoiesis. *Prog. Hematol.* **14**, 201.
948. Zoumbos, N. C., Gascon, P., Djeu, J. Y., and Young, N. S. (1985). Interferon is a mediator of hematopoietic suppression in aplastic anemia *in vitro* and possibly *in vivo*. *Proc. Natl. Acad. Sci. U.S.A.* **82**, 188.
949. Murphy, M., Loudon, R., Kobayashi, M., and Trinchieri, G. (1986). Gamma interferon and lymphotoxin, released by activated T cells, synergize to inhibit granulocyte-monocyte colony formation. *J. Exp. Med.* **164**, 263.
950. Broxmeyer, H. E., Williams, D. E., Lu, L., Cooper, S., Anderson, S. L., Beyer, G. S., Hoffman, R., and Rubin, B. Y. (1986). The suppressive influences of human tumor necrosis factors on bone marrow hematopoietic progenitor cells from normal

donors and patients with leukemia: Synergism of tumor necrosis factor and interferon-γ. *J. Immunol.* **136**, 4487.
951. Murphy, M., Perussia, B., and Trinchieri, G. (1988). Effects of recombinant tumor necrosis factor, lymphotoxin and immune interferon on proliferation and differentiation of enriched hematopoietic precursor cells. *Exp. Hematol.* **16**, 131.
952. Kannourakis, G., Begley, C. G., Johnson, G. R., Werkmeister, J. A., and Burns, G. F. (1988). Evidence for interactions between monocytes and natural killer cells in the regulation of *in vitro* hemopoiesis. *J. Immunol.* **140**, 2489.
953. Lopez, C., Fitzgerald, P., and Kirkpatrick, D. (1982). *In vivo* role of NK (HSV-1) in the induction of graft versus host disease in bone marrow transplant recipients. *In* "NK Cells and Other Natural Effector Cells" (R. B. Herberman, ed.), p. 1561. Academic Press, New York.
954. Lopez, C., Kirkpatrick, D., Livnat, S., and Storb, R. (1980). Natural killer cells in bone marrow transplantation. *Lancet* **2**, 1025 (abstr.).
955. Lopez, C., Sorell, M., Kirkpatrick, D., O'Reilly, R. J., Ching, C., and Bone Marrow Transplantation Unit (1979). Association between pre-treatment natural kill and graft-versus-host disease after stem-cell transplantation. *Lancet* **2**, 1103.
956. Livnat, S., Seigneuret, M., Storb, R., and Prentice, R. L. (1980). Analysis of cytotoxic effector cell function in patients with leukemia or aplastic anemia before and after marrow transplantation. *J. Immunol.* **124**, 481.
957. Gratama, J. W., Lipovich-Oosterveer, M. A., Ronteltap, C., Sinnige, L. G., Jansen, J., Van Der Griend, R. J., and Bolhuis, R. L. (1985). Natural immunity and graft-vs-host disease. *Transplantation* **40**, 256.
958. Weisdorf, S. A., Platt, J. L., and Snover, D. C. (1983). In situ analysis of T and killer lymphocyte subpopulations in rectal biopsies from bone marrow transplant patients. *Gastroenterology* **84**, 1348.
959. Murphy, G. F., Merot, Y., Tong, A. K. F., and Smith, B. (1985). Identification of distinctive lymphocyte subpopulation in cutaneous graft-versus-host disease (GVHD). *Lab. Invest.* **52**, 46A.
960. Guillen, F. J., Ferrara, J., Hancock, W. W., Messadi, D., Fonferko, E., Burakoff, S. J., and Murphy, G. F. (1986). Acute cutaneous graft-versus-host disease to minor histocompatibility antigens in a murine model. Evidence that large granular lymphocytes are effector cells in the immune response. *Lab. Invest.* **55**, 35.
961. Piguiet, P.-F., Grau, G. E., Allet, B., and Vassalli, P. (1987). Tumor necrosis factor/cachectin is an effector of skin and gut lesions of the acute phase of graft-versus-host disease. *J. Exp. Med.* **166**, 1280.
962. Korngold, R., and Sprent, J. (1978). Lethal graft-versus-host disease after bone marrow transplantation across minor histocompatibility barriers in mice. Prevention by removing mature T cells from mice. *J. Exp. Med.* **148**, 1678.
963. Reisner, Y., Kapoor, N., Kirkpatrick, D., Pollack, M. S., Cunninghma-Rundles, S., Dupont, B., Hodes, M. Z., Good, R. A., and O'Reilly, R. J. (1983). Transplantation for severe combined immunodeficiency with HLA-A,B,D,DR incompatible parental marrow cells fractionated by soybean agglutinin and sheep red blood cells. *Blood* **61**, 341.
964. Ghayur, T., Seemayer, T. A., Kongshavn, P. A., Gartner, J. G., and Lapp, W. S. (1987). Graft-versus-host reactions in the beige mouse. An investigation of the role of host and donor natural killer cells in the pathogenesis of graft-versus-host disease. *Transplantation* **44**, 261.
965. Ghayur, T., Seemayer, T. A., and Lapp, W. S. (1988). Prevention of murine graft-

versus-host disease by inducing and eliminating ASGM1+ cells of donor origin. *Transplantation* **45**, 586.

966. Blazar, B. R., Soderling, C. C., Koo, G. C., and Vallera, D. A. (1988). Absence of a facilitory role for NK 1.1-positive donor cells in engraftment across a major histocompatibility barrier in mice. *Transplantation* **45**, 876.
967. Varkila, K. (1987). Depletion of asialo-GM_1^+ cells from the F1 recipient mice prior to irradiation and transfusion of parental spleen cells prevents mortality to acute graft-versus-host disease and induction of anti-host specific cytotoxic T cells. *Clin. Exp. Immunol.* **69**, 652.
968. Mowat, A. M., and Felstein, M. V. (1987). Experimental studies of immunologically mediated enteropathy. II. Role of natural killer cells in the intestinal phase of murine graft-versus-host reaction. *Immunology* **61**, 179.
969. Mowat, A. M., Felstein, M. V., Borland, A., and Parrott, D. M. (1988). Experimental studies of immunologically mediated enteropathy. Development of cell mediated immunity and intestinal pathology during a graft-versus-host reaction in irradiated mice. *Gut* **29**, 949.
970. Biron, C. A., Habu, S., Okumura K., and Welsh, R. M. (1984). Lysis of uninfected and virus-infected cells *in vivo*: A rejection mechanism in addition to that mediated by natural killer cells. *J. Virol.* **50**, 698.
971. Stitz, L., Althage, A., Hengartner, H., and Zinkernagel, R. (1985). Natural killer cells vs. cytotoxic T cells in the peripheral blood of virus-infected mice. *J. Immunol.* **134**, 598.
972. Biron, C. A., Turgiss, L. R., and Welsh, R. M. (1983). Increase in NK cell number and turnover rate during acute viral infection. *J. Immunol.* **131**, 1539.
973. Natuk, R. J., and Welsh, R. M. (1987). Accumulation and chemotaxis of large granular lymphocytes at sites of virus replication. *J. Immunol.* **138**, 877.
974. Welsh, R. M., and Kiessling, R. W. (1980). Natural killer cell response to lymphocytic choriomeningitis virus in beige mice. *Scand. J. Immunol.* **11**, 363.
975. Welsh, R. M., Biron, C. A., Bukowski, J. F., McIntyre, K., and Yang, H. (1984). Role of natural killer cells in virus infections of mice. *Surv. Synth. Pathol. Res.* **3**, 409.
976. Bukowski, J. F., Woda, B. A., Habu, S., Okumura, K., and Welsh, R. M. (1983). Natural killer cell depletion enhances virus synthesis and virus-induced hepatitis *in vivo. J. Immunol.* **131**, 1531.
977. Allan, J. E., and Doherty, P. C. (1986). Natural killer cells contribute to inflammation but do not appear to be essential for the induction of clinical lymphocytic choriomeningitis. *Scand. J. Immunol.* **24**, 153.
978. Wabuke-Bunoti, M. A., Bennink, J. R., and Plotkin, S. A. (1986). Influenza virus-induced encephalopathy in mice: Interferon production and natural killer cell activity during acute infection. *J. Virol.* **60**, 1062.
979. Bukowski, J. F., Warner, J. F., Dennert, G., and Welsh, R. M. (1985). Adoptive transfer studies demonstrate the antiviral effect of NK cells *in vivo. J. Exp. Med.* **161**, 40.
980. Bukowski, J. F., Woda, B. A., and Welsh, R. M. (1984). Pathogenesis of murine cytomegalovirus infection in natural killer cell-depleted mice. *J. Virol.* **52**, 119.
981. Stein-Streilein, J., and Guffee, J. (1986). *In vivo* treatment of mice and hamsters with antibodies to asialo GM_1 increases morbidity and mortality to pulmonary influenza infection. *J. Immunol.* **136**, 1435.
982. Welsh, R. M. (1986). Regulation of virus infections by natural killer cells. A review. *Nat. Immun. Cell Growth Regul.* **5**, 169.

983. Habu, S., Akamatsu, K., Tamaoki, N., and Okumura, K. (1984). In vivo significance of NK cells on resistance against virus (HSV-1) infections in mice. *J. Immunol.* **133**, 2743.
984. Bukowski, J. F., and Welsh, R. M. (1986). The role of natural killer cells and interferon in resistance to acute infection of mice with herpes simplex virus type 1. *J. Immunol.* **137**, 3481.
985. Rager-Zisman, B., Quan, P. C., Rosner, M., Moller, J. R., and Bloom, B. R. (1987). Role of NK cells in protection of mice against herpes simplex virus-1 infection. *J. Immunol.* **138**, 884.
986. Ausiello, C., Valeri, M., Piazza, A., Antonelli, G., Adorno, D., and Casciani, C. U. (1983). Augmentation of natural killer activity during cytomegalovirus infection in one renal transplant recipient and one uremic patient. *Transplant Proc.* **15**, 1793.
987. Ennis, F. A., Beare, A. S., Riley, D., Schild, G. C., Meager, A., Qi, Y.-H., Schwarz, G., and Rook, A. H. (1981). Interferon induction and increased natural killer cell activity in influenza infections in man. *Lancet* **1**, 891.
988. Meguro, H., Kervina, M., and Wright, P. F. (1979). Antibody-dependent cell-mediated cytotoxicity against cells infected with respiratory syncitial virus: Characterization of *in vitro* and *in vivo* properties. *J. Immunol.* **122**, 2521.
989. Perrin, L., Tishon, A., and Oldstone, M. (1977). Immunological injury in measles virus infection. III. Presence and characterization of human cytotoxic lymphocytes. *J. Immunol.* **118**, 282.
990. Quinnan, G. V. J., Kirmani, N., Esber, E., Saral, R., Manischewitz, J. R., Rogers, J. L., Rook, A. H., Santos, G. W., and Burns, W. H. (1981). HLA-restricted cytotoxic T lymphocyte and nonthymic cytotoxic lymphocyte responses to cytomegalovirus infection of bone marrow transplant recipients. *J. Immunol.* **126**, 2036.
991. Lewis, D. E., Gilbert, B. E., and Knight, V. (1986). Influenza virus infection induces functional alterations in peripheral blood lymphocytes. *J. Immunol.* **137**, 3777.
992. Cauda, R., Prasthofer, E. F., Grossi, C. E., Whitley, R. J., and Pass, R. F. (1987). Congenital cytomegalovirus: Immunological alterations. *J. Med. Virol.* **23**, 41.
993. Quinnan, G. V. J., Kirmani, N., Rook, A. H., Manischewitz, J. F., Jackson, L., Moreschi, G., Santos, G. W., Saral, R., and Burns, W. H. (1982). Cytotoxic T cells in cytomegalovirus infection: HLA-restricted T-lymphocyte and non-T-lymphocyte cytotoxic responses correlate with recovery from cytomegalovirus infection in bone-marrow-transplant recipients. *N. Engl. J. Med.* **307**, 7.
994. Lopez, C., Kirkpatrick, D., and Fitzgerald, P. (1982). The role of NK (HSV-1) effector cells in the resistance to herpes virus infections in man. *In* "NK Cells and Other Natural Effector Cells" (R. B. Herberman, ed.), p. 1445. Academic Press, New York.
995. Moller-Larsen, A., Heron, I., and Haahr, S. (1977). Cell-mediated cytotoxicity to herpes-infected cells in humans: Dependence on antibodies. *Infect. Immun.* **16**, 43.
996. Rager-Zisman, B., Grose, C., and Bloom, B. R. (1976). Mechanism of selective nonspecific cell-mediated cytotoxicity of virus-infected cells. *Nature (London)* **260**, 369.
997. Harfast, B., Andersson, T., and Perlmann, P. (1975). Human lymphocyte cytotoxicity against mumps virus-infected target cells. Requirement for non-T cells. *J. Immunol.* **114**, 1820.
998. Santoli, D., Trinchieri, G., and Lief, F. S. (1978). Cell-mediated cytotoxicity against

virus-infected cells in humans. I. Characterization of the effector lymphocyte. *J. Immunol.* **121**, 526.

999. Kurane, I., Hebblewaite, D., and Ennis, F. A. (1986). Characterization with monoclonal antibodies of human lymphcoytes active in natural killing and antibody-dependent cell-mediated cytotoxicity of dengue virus-infected cells. *Immunology* **58**, 429.

1000. Bishop, G. A., Marlin, S. D., Schwartz, S. A., and Glorioso, J. C. (1984). Human natural killer cell recognition of herpes simplex virus type 1. Glycoproteins: Specificity analysis with the use of monoclonal antibodies and antigenic variants. *J. Immunol.* **133**, 2206.

1001. Casali, P., Sissons, J. G. P., Buchmeier, M. J., and Oldstone, M. B. A. (1981). Generation of human cytotoxic lymphocytes by virus. Viral glycoproteins induce nonspecific cell-mediated cytotoxicity without release of interferon *in vitro. J. Exp. Med.* **154**, 840.

1002. Harfast, B., Orvell, C., Alsheikhly, A., Andersson, T., Perlmann, P., and Norrby, E. (1980). The role of viral glycoproteins in mumps-virus dependent lymphocyte-mediated cytotoxicity *in vitro. Scand. J. Immunol.* **11**, 391.

1003. Alsheikhly, A.-R., Orvell, C., Andersson, T., and Perlmann, P. (1985). The role of serologically defined epitopes on mumps virus HN-glycoproteins in the induction of virus dependent cell-mediated cytotoxicity (VDCC) *in vitro*. Analysis with monoclonal antibodies. *Scand. J. Immunol.* **22**, 529.

1004. Harfast, B., Andersson, T., and Perlmann, P. (1980). Immunoglobulin-independent natural cytotoxicity of Fc receptor-bearing human blood lymphocytes to mumps virus-infected Farget cells. *J. Immunol.* **121**, 755.

1005. Alsheikhly, A.-R., Andersson, T., and Perlmann, P. (1985). Virus-dependent cellular cytotoxicity *in vitro*: Mechanisms of induction and effector cell characterization. *Scand. J. Immunol.* **21**, 329.

1006. Alsheikhly, A.-R., Andersson, T., and Perlmann, P. (1984). Virus-mediated induction in human lymphocytes of antibody-independent cytotoxicity (VDCC) and enhancement of antibody-dependent cytotoxicity (ADCC) against natural killer-resistant tumor target cells. *Cell. Immunol.* **88**, 511.

1007. Tang, J., DeLong, D. C., Butler, L. D., Marder, P., and Ades, E. W. (1986). Murine thymocytes mediate a natural killer-like activity against herpes virus-infected target cells but not YAC-1 target cells. *Scand. J. Immunol.* **24**, 115.

1008. Hendricks, R. L., and Sugar, J. (1984). Lysis of herpes simplex virus-infected targets. II. Nature of the effector cells. *Cell. Immunol.* **83**, 262.

1009. Yasukawa, M., and Zarling, J. M. (1983). Autologous herpes simplex virus-infected cells are lysed by human natural killer cells. *J. Immunol.* **131**, 2011.

1010. Tilden, A. B., Cauda, R., Grossi, C. E., Balch, C. M., Lakeman, A. D., and Whitley, R. J. (1986). Demonstration of NK cell-mediated lysis of varicella-zoster virus (VZV)-infected cells: Characterization of the effector cells. *J. Immunol.* **136**, 4243.

1011. Colmenares, C., and Lopez, C. (1986). Enhanced lysis of herpes simplex virus type 1-infected mouse cell lines by NC and NK effectors. *J. Immunol.* **136**, 3473.

1012. Paya, C. V., Kenmotsu, N., Schoon, R. A., and Leibson, P. J. (1988). Tumor necrosis factor and lymphotoxin secretion by human natural killer cells leads to antiviral cytotoxicity. *J. Immunol.* **141**, 1989.

1013. Casali, P., and Oldstone, M. B. A. (1982). Mechanisms of killing of measles virus

infected cells by human lymphocytes: Interferon associated and unassociated cell-mediated cytotoxicity. *Cell. Immunol.* **70**, 330.
1014. Arora, D. J., and Justewicz, D. M. (1986). Influenza viral glycoproteins induced cell-mediated cytotoxicity by an interferon-independent mechanism. *Cell. Immunol.* **97**, 102.
1015. Rees, R. C., Dalton, B. J., Young, J. F., Hanna, N., and Poste, G. (1987). Augmentation of human natural killer cell activity by influenza virus antigens produced in *Escherichia coli*. *J. Biol. Response Modif.* **6**, 69.
1016. Fitzgerald, P. A., von Wussow, P., and Lopez, C. (1982). Role of interferon in natural kill of HSV-1 infected fibroblasts. *J. Immunol.* **129**, 819.
1017. Fitzgerald, P. A., Mendelsohn, M., and Lopez, C. (1985). Human natural killer cells limit replication of herpes simplex virus type I *in vitro*. *J. Immunol.* **134**, 2666.
1018. Bishop, G. A., Glorioso, J. C., and Schwartz, S. A. (1983). Role of interferon in human natural killer activity against target cells infected with HSV-1. *J. Immunol.* **131**, 1849.
1019. Fitzgerald, P. A., Schindler, T. E., Siegal, F. P., and Lopez, C. (1984). Independence of interferon production and natural killer function and association with opportunistic infection in acquired immune deficiency syndrome. *In* "Natural Killer Activity and Its Regulation" (T. Hoshino, H. S. Koren, and A. Uchida, eds.), p. 414. Excerpta Medica, Amsterdam.
1020. Blalock, J. E., and Stanton, G. J. (1978). Efficient transfer of interferon-induced virus resistance between human cells. *J. Gen. Virol.* **41**, 325.
1021. Weigent, D. A., Blalock, J. E., and Stanton, G. J. (1985). Interferon-induced transfer of natural cytotoxic activity between human leukocytes. *J. Biol. Response Modif.* **4**, 60.
1022. Abb, J., Abb, H., and Deinhardt, F. (1984). Relationship between natural killer (NK) cells and interferon (IFN) alpha-producing cells in human peripheral blood. Studies with a monoclonal antibody with specificity for human natural killer cells. *Immunobiology* **167**, 359.
1023. Oh, S. H., Bandyopadhyay, S., Miller, D. S., and Starr, S. E. (1987). Cooperation between CD16 (Leu-11b)$^+$ NK cells and HLA-DR$^+$ cells in natural killing of herpesvirus-infected fibroblasts. *J. Immunol.* **139**, 2799.
1024. Bartizal, K. F., Salkowski, C., Pleasants, J. R., and Balish, E. (1984). The effect of microbial flora, diet, and age on the tumoricidal activity of natural killer cells. *J. Leuk. Biol.* **36**, 739.
1025. Kearns, R. J., and Leu, R. W. (1984). Modulation of natural killer activity in mice following infection with *Listeria monocytogenes*. *Cell Immunol.* **84**, 361.
1026. Williams, D. M., Schachter, J., and Grubbs, B. (1987). Role of natural killer cells in infection with the mouse pneumonitis agent (murine *Chlamydia trachomatis*). *Infect. Immun.* **55**, 223.
1027. Wood, P., and Cheers, C. (1985). Activation of non-specific cytotoxic cells in *Listeria*-susceptible and -resistant mouse strains. *Immunology* **54**, 113.
1028. Morahan, P. S., Dempsey, W. L., Volkman, A., and Connor, J. (1986). Antimicrobial activity of various immunomodulators: Independence from normal levels of circulating monocytes and natural killer cells. *Infect. Immun.* **51**, 87.
1029. Nencioni, L., Villa, L., Boraschi, D., Berti, B., and Tagliabue, A. (1983). Natural and antibody-dependent cell-mediated activity against *Salmonella typhimurium* by peripheral and intestinal lymphoid cells in mice. *J. Immunol.* **130**, 903.

1030. Morgan, D. R., Dupont, H. L., Gonik, B., and Kohl, S. (1984). Cytotoxicity of human peripheral blood and colostral leukocytes against *Shigella* species. *Infect. Immun.* **46**, 25.
1031. Klimpel, G. R., Niesel, D. W., and Klimpel, K. D. (1986). Natural cytotoxic effector cell activity against *Shigella flexneri*-infected HeLa cells. *J. Immunol.* **136**, 1081.
1032. Blanchard, D. K., Stewart, W. E., II, Klein, T. W., Friedman, H., and Djeu, J. Y. (1987). Cytolytic activity of human peripheral blood leukocytes against *Legionella pneumophila*-infected monocytes: Characterization of the effector cell and augmentation by interleukin 2. *J. Immunol.* **139**, 551.
1033. Blanchard, D. K., Bia Michelini-Norris, M., Friedman, H., and Djeu, J. Y. (1989). Lysis of mycobacteria-infected monocytes by IL-2-activated killer cells: Role of LFA-1. *Cell. Immunol.* (in press).
1034. Garcia-Penarrubia, P. Koster, F. T., Kelley, R. O., McDowell, T. D., and Bankhurst, A. D. (1989). Antibacterial activity of human natural killer cells. *J. Exp. Med.* **169**, 99.
1035. Tarkkanen, J., Saxén, H., Nurminen, M., Mäkelä, P. H., and Säkselä, E. (1986). Bacterial induction of human activated lymphocyte killing and its inhibition by lipopolysaccharide (LPS). *J. Immunol.* **136**, 2662.
1036. Tarkkanen, J., Säkselä, E., and Lanier, L. L. (1986). Bacterial activation of human natural killer cells. Characteristics of the activation process and identification of the effector cells. *J. Immunol.* **137**, 2428.
1037. Klimpel, G. R., Niesel, D. W., Asuncion, M., and Klimpel, K. D. (1988). Natural killer cell activation and interferon produced by peripheral blood lymphocytes after exposure to bacteria. *Infect. Immun.* **56**, 1436.
1038. Blanchard, D. K., Friedman, H., Stewart, W. E., II, Klein, T. W., and Djeu, J. Y. (1988). Role of gamma interferon in induction of natural killer activity by *Legionella pneumophila in vitro* and in an experimental murine infection model. *Infect. Immun.* **56**, 1187.
1039. Lindemann, R. A. (1988). Bacterial activation of human natural killer cells: Role of cell surface lipopolysaccharide. *Infect. Immun.* **56**, 1301.
1040. Kang, Y. H., Carl, M., Maheshwari, R. K., Watson, L. P., Yaffe, L., and Grimley, P. M. (1988). Incorporation of bacterial lipopolysaccharide by human Leu-11a[+] natural killer cells. Ultrastructural and functional correlations. *Lab. Invest.* **58**, 196.
1041. Lapham, C., John, P. A., and Tomar, R. H. (1986). The mechanism of enhancement of natural killer cell activity by soluble streptococcal products. *Clin. Immunol. Immunopathol.* **40**, 335.
1042. Uchida, A., and Klein, E. (1985) Activation of human blood lymphocytes and monocytes by the streptococcal preparation OK432: Enhanced generation of soluble cytotoxic factors. *Immunol. Lett.* **10**, 177.
1043. Pollack, S. B. (1987). OK-432 stimulates primary production and activity of murine natural killer cells. *Nat. Immun. Cell Growth Regul.* **6**, 224.
1044. Nabavi, N., and Murphy, J. W. (1985). *In vitro* binding of natural killer cells to *Cryptococcus neoformans* targets. *Infect. Immun.* **50**, 50.
1045. Jimenez, B. E., and Murphy, J. W. (1984). *In vitro* effects of natural killer cells against *Paracoccidioides brasiliensis* yeast phase. *Infect. Immun.* **46**, 552.
1046. Petkus, A. F., and Baum, L. L. (1987). Natural killer cell inhibition of young spherules and endospores of *Coccidioides immitis*. *J. Immunol.* **139**, 3107.

1047. Hidore, M. R., and Murphy, J. W. (1986). Natural cellular resistance of beige mice against *Cryptococcus neoformans. J. Immunol.* **137**, 3624.
1048. Hidore, M. R., and Murphy, J. W. (1986). Correlation of natural killer cell activity and clearance of *Cryptococcus neoformans* from mice after adoptive transfer of splenic nylon wool-nonadherent cells. *Infect. Immun.* **51**, 547.
1049. Lipscomb, M. F., Alvarellos, T., Toews, G. B., Tompkins, R., Evans, Z., Koo, G., and Kumar, V. (1987). Role of natural killer cells to resistance to *Cryptococcus neoformans* infections in mice. *Am. J. Pathol.* **128**, 354.
1050. Marconi, P., Scaringi, L., Tissi, L., Boccanera, M., Bistoni, F., Bonmassar, E., and Cassone, A. (1985). Induction of natural killer cell activity by inactivated *Candida albicans* in mice. *Infect. Immun.* **50**, 297.
1051. Djeu, J. Y., Blanchard, D. K., Richards, A. L., and Friedman, H. (1988). Tumor necrosis factor induction by *Candida albicans* from human natural killer cells and monocytes. *J. Immunol.* **141**, 4047.
1052. Zunino, S. J., and Hudig, D. (1988). Interactions between human natural killer (NK) lymphocytes and yeast cells: Human NK cells do not kill *Candida albicans*, although *C. albicans* blocks NK lysis of K562 cells. *Infect. Immun.* **56**, 564.
1053. Djeu, J. Y., and Blanchard, D. K. (1987). Regulation of human polymorphonuclear neutrophil (PMN) activity against *Candida albicans* by large granular lymphocytes via release of a PMN-activating factor. *J. Immunol.* **139**, 2761.
1054. Kamiyama, T. (1984). Toxoplasma-induced activities of peritoneal and spleen natural killer cells from beige mice against thymocytes and YAC-1 lymphoma targets. *Infect. Immun.* **43**, 973.
1055. Ojo-Amaize, E. A., Vilcek, J., Cochrane, A. H., and Nussenzweig, R. S. (1984). *Plasmodium berghei* sporozoites are mitogenic for murine T cells, induce interferon, and activate natural killer cells. *J. Immunol.* **133**, 1005.
1056. Solomon, J. B., Forbes, M. G., and Solomon, G. R. (1985). A possible role for natural killer cells in providing protection against *Plasmodium berghei* in early stages of infection. *Immunol. Lett.* **9**, 349.
1057. Hauseer, W. E., Jr., and Tsai, V. (1986) Acute toxoplasma infection of mice induces spleen NK cells that are cytotoxic for *T. gondii in vitro. J. Immunol.* **136**, 313.
1058. Kirkpatrick, C. E., and Farrell, J. P. (1984). Splenic natural killer-cell activity in mice infected with *Leishmania donovani. Cell Immunol.* **85**, 201.
1059. Kirkpatrick, C. E., Farrell, J. P., Warner, J. F., and Dennert, G. (1985). Participation of natural killer cells in the recovery of mice from visceral leishmaniasis. *Cell. Immunol.* **92**, 163.
1060. Albright, J. W., Munger, W. E., Henkart, P. A., and Albright, J. F. (1988). The toxicity of rat large granular lymphocyte tumor cells and their cytoplasmic granules for rodent and African trypanosomes. *J. Immunol.* **140**, 2774.
1061. Moretta, L., Webb, S. R., Grossi, C. E., Lydyard, P. M., and Cooper, M. D. (1977). Functional analysis of two human T-cell subpopulations: Help and suppression of B-cell responses by T-cells bearing receptors for IgM or IgG. *J. Exp. Med.* **146**, 184.
1062. Lobo, P. I. (1981). Characterization of a non-T, non-B human lymphocyte (L cell) with use of monoclonal antibodies. Its regulatory role in B lymphocyte function. *J. Clin. Invest.* **68**, 431.
1063. Arai, S., Yamamoto, H. Itoh, K., and Kumagai, K. (1983). Suppressive effect of human natural killer cells on pokeweed mitogen-induced B cell differentiation. *J. Immunol.* **131**, 651.
1064. Nabel, G., Allard, W. J., and Cantor, H. (1982). A cloned cell line mediating

natural killer cell function inhibits immunoglobulin secretion. *J. Exp. Med.* **156**, 658.
1065. Storkus, W. J., and Dawson, J. R. (1986). B cell sensitivity to natural killing: Correlation with target cell stage of differentiation and state of activation. *J. Immunol.* **136**, 1542.
1066. Robles, C. P., Pereira, P., Wortley, P., and Pollack, S. B. (1985). Regulation of the B cell response by NK cells. *In* "Mechanisms of Cytotoxicity by NK Cells" (R. B. Herberman and D. M. Callewaert, eds.), p. 499. Academic Press, Orlando, Florida.
1067. Froelich, C. J., and Guiffaut, S. (1987). Natural killer cells do not lyse resting or mitogen-stimulated B cells. *Nat. Immun. Cell Growth Regul.* **6**, 12.
1068. Tilden, A. B., Abo, T., and Balch, C. M. (1983). Suppressor cell function of human granular lymphocytes identified by the HNK-1 (Leu 7) monoclonal antibody. *J. Immunol.* **130**, 1171.
1069. Brieva, J. A., Targan, S., and Stevens, R. H. (1984). NK and T cell subsets regulate antibody production by human *in vivo* antigen-induced lymphoblastoid B cells. *J. Immunol.* **132**, 611.
1070. Kuwano, K., Arai, S., Munakata, T., Tomita, Y., Yoshitake, Y., and Kumagai, K. (1986). Suppressive effect of human natural killer cells on Epstein-Barr virus-induced immunoglobulin synthesis. *J. Immunol.* **137**, 1462.
1071. Takeuchi, T., DiMaggio, M., Levine, H., Schlossman, S. F. and Morimoto, C. (1988). CD11 molecule defines two types of suppressor cells within the T8$^+$ population. *Cell. Immunol.* **111**, 398.
1072. Kimata, H., Shanahan, F., Brogan, M., Targan, S., and Saxon, A. (1987). Modulation of ongoing human immunoglobulin synthesis by natural killer cells. *Cell. Immunol.* **107**, 74.
1073. Targan, S., Brieva, J., Newman, W., and Stevens, R. (1985). Is the NK lytic process involved in the mechanism of NK suppression of antibody-producing cells? *J. Immunol.* **134**, 666.
1074. Brieva, J. A.,and Stevens, R. H. (1984). Involvement of the transferrin receptor in the production and NK-induced suppression of human antibody synthesis. *J. Immunol.* **133**, 1288.
1075. Mortari, F., and Singhal, S. K. (1988). Production of human bone marrow-derived suppressor factor. Effect on antibody synthesis and lectin-activated cell proliferation. *J. Immunol.* **141**, 3037.
1076. Azuma, E., and Kaplan, J. (1988). Role of lymphokine-activated killer cells as mediators of veto and natural suppression. *J. Immunol.* **141**, 2601.
1077. Poppema, S., Visser, L., and De Leij, L. (1983). Reactivity of presumed anti-natural killer cell antibody Leu 7 with intrafollicular T lymphocytes. *Clin. Exp. Immunol.* **54**, 834.
1078. Robles, C. P., and Pollack, S. B. (1986). Regulation of the secondary *in vitro* antibody response by endogenous natural killer cells: Kinetics, isotype preference, and non-identity with T suppressor cells. *J. Immunol.* **137**, 2418.
1079. Khater, M., Macai, J., Genyea, C., and Kaplan, J. (1986). Natural killer cell regulation of age-related and type-specific variations in antibody responses to pneumococcal polysaccharides. *J. Exp. Med.* **164**, 1505.
1080. Abruzzo, L. U., and Rowley, D. A. (1983). Homeostasis of the antibody response: Immunoregulation by NK cells. *Science* **222**, 581.
1081. Abruzzo, L. V., Mullen, C. A., and Rowley, D. A. (1986). Immunoregulation by natural killer cells. *Cell. Immunol.* **98**, 266.

1082. Shah, P. D., Keij, J., Gilbertson, S. M., and Rowley, D. A. (1986). Thy-1$^+$ and Thy-1$^-$ natural killer cells. Only Thy-1$^-$ natural killer cells suppress dendritic cells. *J. Exp. Med.* **163**, 1012.
1083. Brunswick, M., and Lake, P. (1985). Obligatory role of gamma interferon in T cell-replacing factor-dependent, antigen-specific murine B cell responses. *J. Exp. Med.* **161**, 953.
1084. Mond, J. J., and Brunswick, M. (1987). A role for IFN-gamma and NK cells in immune response to T cell-regulated antigens types 1 and 2. *Immunol. Rev.* **99**, 105.
1085. Kimata, H., Sherr, E. H., and Saxon, A. (1988). Human natural killer (NK) cells produce a late-acting B-cell differentiation activity. *J. Clin. Immunol.* **8**, 381.
1086. Brenner, M. K., Vyakarnam, A., Reittie, J. E., Wimperis, J. Z., Grob, J. P., Hoffbrand, A. V., and Prentice, H. G. (1987). Human large granular lymphocytes induce immunoglobulin synthesis after bone marrow transplantation. *Eur. J. Immunol.* **17**, 43.
1087. Brenner, M. K., Reittie, J. E., Grob, J. P., Wimperis, J. Z., Stephens, S., Patterson, J., Hoffbrand, A. V., and Prentice, H. G. (1986). The contribution of large granular lymphocytes to B cell activation and differentiation after T-cell-depleted allogeneic bone marrow transplantation. *Transplantation* **42**, 257.
1088. Kimata, H., and Saxon, A. (1988). Subset of natural killer cells is induced by immune complexes to display Fc receptors for IgE and IgA and demonstrates isotype regulatory function. *J. Clin. Invest.* **82**, 160.
1089. Swendeman, S., and Thorley-Dawson, D. A. (1987). The activation antigen BLAST-2, when shed, is an autocrine BCGF for normal and transformed B cells. *EMBO J.* **6**, 1637.
1090. Vyakarnam, A., Brenner, M. K., Reittie, J. E., Houlker, C. H., and Lachmann, P. J. (1985). Human clones with natural killer function can activate B cells and secrete B cell differentiation factors. *Eur. J. Immunol.* **15**, 606.
1091. Varkila, K., Silvennoinen, O., and Hurme, M. (1987). Asialo GM$_1^+$ NK cells have opposite role in the activation of alloreactive cytotoxic T lymphocyte (CTL) response *in vitro* and *in vivo*. *Acta Pathol. Microbiol. Immunol. Scand.* **95**, 141.
1092. Suzuki, R., Suzuki, S., Ebina, N., and Kumagai, K. (1985). Suppression of alloimmune cytotoxic T lymphocyte (CTL) generation by depletion of NK cells and restoration by interferon and/or interleukin 2. *J. Immunol.* **134**, 2139.
1093. Schaaf-Lafontaine, N., Boniver, J., Huygen, K., and Degiovanni, G. (1984). Suppression of CTL responses *in vitro* by large granular T cells. *Immunol. Lett.* **8**, 201.
1094. Gilbertson, S. M., Shah, P. D., and Rowley, D. A. (1986). NK cells suppress the generation of Lyt-2$^+$ cytolytic T cells by suppressing or eliminating dendritic cells. *J. Immunol.* **136**, 3567.
1095. Pope, R. M., McChesney, L., Stebbing, N., Goldstein, L., and Talal, N. (1985). Regulation of T cell proliferation by cloned interferon-alpha mediated by Leu-11b-positive cells. *J. Immunol.* **135**, 4048.
1096. Shah, P. D., Gilbertson, S. M., and Rowley, D. A. (1985). Dendritic cells that have interacted with antigen are targets for natural killer cells. *J. Exp. Med.* **162**, 625.
1097. Shah, P. D. (1987). Dendritic cells but not macrophages are targets for immune regulation by natural killer cells. *Cell. Immunol.* **104**, 440.
1098. Scala, G., Allavena, P., Ortaldo, J. R., Herberman, R. B., and Oppenheim, J. J. (1985). Subsets of human large granular lymphocytes (LGL) exhibit accessory cell functions. *J. Immunol.* **134**, 3049.

1099. Burlington, D. B., Djeu, J. Y., Wells, M. A., Kiley, S. C., and Quinnan, G. V., Jr. (1984). Large granular lymphocytes provide an accessory function in the *in vitro* development of influenza A virus-specific cytotoxic T cells. *J. Immunol.* **132**, 3154.
1100. Silvennoinen, O. (1988). Purified human NK cells do not function as accessory cells in T-cell proliferative responses. *Immunology* **64**, 495.
1101. Weissler, J. C., Yarbrough, W. C., Jr., Toews, G. B., and Nicod, L. P. (1988). Human natural killer cells enhance a mixed leukocyte reaction. *J. Leuk. Biol.* **43**, 291.
1102. Kiessling, R., Petranyi, G., Klein, G., and Wigzell, H. (1976). Non-T-cell resistance against a mouse Maloney sarcoma. *Int. J. Cancer* **17**, 275.
1103. Hanna, N., and Burton, R. C. (1981). Definitive evidence that natural killer (NK) cells inhibit experimental tumor metastasis in vivo. *J. Immunol.* **127**, 1754.
1104. Gorelik, E., Fogel, M., Feldman, M., and Segal, S. (1979). Differences in resistance of metastatic tumor cells and cells from local tumor growth to cytotoxicity of natural killer cells. *JNCI, J. Natl. Cancer Inst.* **63**, 1397.
1105. Riccardi, C., Santoni, A., Barlozzari, T., Puccetti, P., and Herberman, R. B. (1980). In vivo natural reactivity of mice against tumor cells. *Int. J. Cancer* **25**, 475.
1106. Haller, O., Hansson, M., Kiessling, R., and Wigzell, H. (1977). Role of nonconventional natural killer cells in resistance against syngeneic tumor cells in vivo. *Nature (London)* **270**, 609.
1107. Karre, K., Klein, G. O., Kiessling, R., Klein, G., and Roder, J. C. (1980). In vitro NK-activity and in vivo resistance to leukemia: Studies of beige, beige/nude and wild type hosts in C57BL background. *Int. J. Cancer* **26**, 789.
1108. Talmadge, J. E., Meyers, K. M., Prieur, D. J., and Starkey, J. R. (1980). Role of NK cells in tumor growth and metastasis in beige mice. *Nature (London)* **284**, 622.
1109. Bukowski, J. F., Biron, C. A., and Welsh, R. M. (1983). Elevated natural killer cell-mediated cytotoxicity, plasma interferon, and tumor cell rejection in mice persistently infected with lymphocytic choriomeningitis virus. *J. Immunol.* **131**, 991.
1110. Minato, N., Bloom, B. R., Jones, C., Holland, J., and Reid, L. M. (1979). Mechanism of rejection of virus persistently infected tumor cells by athymic nude mice. *J. Exp. Med.* **149**, 1117.
1111. Ojo, E. (1979). Positive correlation between the levels of natural killer cells and the *in vivo* resistance to syngeneic tumor transplant as influenced by various routes of administration of *corynebacterium parvum* bacteria. *Cell. Immunol.* **45**, 182.
1112. Habu, S., Fukui, H., Shimamura, K., Kasai, M., Nagai, Y., and Okomura, K. (1981). In vivo effects of anti-asialo GM1. I. Reduction of NK activity and enhancement of transplanted tumor growth in nude mice. *J. Immunol.* **127**, 34.
1113. Pollack, S. B., and Hallenbeck, L. A. (1982). *In vivo* reduction of NK activity with anti-NK1 serum: Direct evaluation of NK cells in tumor clearance. *Int. J. Cancer* **29**, 203.
1114. Pollack, S. B. (1982). Direct evidence for anti-tumor activity by NK cells in vivo: Growth of B16 melanoma in anti-NK1.1 treated mice. *In* "NK Cells and Other Natural Effector Cells" (R. B. Herberman, ed.), p. 1347. Academic Press, New York.
1115. Seaman, W. E., Sleisenger, M., Eriksson, E., and Koo, G. C. (1987). Depletion of natural killer cells in mice by monoclonal antibody to NK-1.1. Reduction in host defense against malignancy without loss of cellular or humoral immunity. *J. Immunol.* **138** 4539.

1116. Reid, L. M., Minato, N., Gresser, I., Holland, J., Kadish, A., and Bloom, B. R. (1981). Influence of anti-mouse interferon serum on the growth and metastasis of tumor cells persistently infected with virus and of human prostatic tumors in athymic nude mice. *Proc. Natl. Acad. Sci. U.S.A.* **78**, 1171.
1117. Barlozzari, T., Leonhardt, J., Wiltrout, R. H., and Herberman, R. B. (1985). Direct evidence for the role of LGL in the inhibition of experimental tumor metastases. *J. Immunol.* **134**, 2783.
1118. Strong, D. M., Pandolfi, F., Slease, R. B., Budd, J. E., and Woody, J. N. (1981) Antigenic characterization of a T-CLL with heteroantisera and monoclonal antibodies: Evidence for the T cell lineage of an Ia-positive, Fc-IgG positive, suppressor-cell subpopulation. *J. Immunol.* **126**, 2205.
1119. Loutit, J. F., Townsend, K. M. S., and Knowles, J. F. (1980). Tumor surveillance in beige mice. *Nature (London)* **285**, 66.
1120. Fidler, I. J., Gersten, D. M., and Hart, I. R. (1978). The biology of cancer invasion and metastasis. *Adv. Cancer Res.* **28**, 149.
1121. Wiltrout, R. H., Herberman, R. B., Zhang, S. R. and Chirigos, M. A. (1985). Role of organ-associated NK cells in decreased formation of experimental metastases in lung and liver. *J. Immunol.* **134**, 4267.
1122. Schwarz, R. E., Vujanovic, N. L., and Hiserodt, J. C. (1989). Lymphokine-activated killer cells in rats: Enhanced anti-metastatic activity of LAK cells purified and expanded by their adherence to plastic. *Cancer Res.* **49**, 1441.
1123. Pross, H. F., and Baines, M. G. (1986). Alterations in natural killer cell activity in tumor-bearing hosts. In "Immunobiology of Natural Killer Cells" (E. Lotzova and R. B. Herberman, eds.), Vol. 1, p. 57. CRC Press, Boca Raton, Florida.
1124. Cunningham-Rundles, S., Filippa, D. A., Braun, D. W., Antonelli, P., and Ashikari, H. (1981). Natural cytotoxicity of peripheral blood lymphocytes and regional lymph node cells in breast cancer in women. *JNCI, J. Natl. Cancer Inst.* **67**, 585.
1125. Kadish, A. S., Doyle, A. T., Steinhauer, E. H., and Ghossein, N. A. (1981). Natural cytotoxicity and interferon production in human cancer: Deficient natural killer activity and normal interferon production in patients with advanced disease. *J. Immunol.* **127**, 1817.
1126. Pandolfi, F., Semenzato, G., De Rossi, G., Strong, D. M., Quinti, I., Pezzutto, A., Mandelli, F., and Aiuti, F. (1982). Heterogeneity of T-CLL defined by monoclonal antibodies in nine patients. *Clin. Immunol. Immunopathol.* **24**, 330.
1127. Pross, H. F., and Baines, M. G. (1976). Spontaneous human lymphocyte-mediated cytotoxicity against tumor target cells. I. The effect of malignant disease. *Int. J. Cancer* **18**, 593.
1128. Takasugi, M., Ramseyer, A., and Takasugi, J. (1977). Decline of natural nonselective cell-mediated cytotoxicity in patients with tumor progression. *Cancer Res.* **37**, 413.
1129. Golub, S. H., Niitsuma, M., Kawate, N., Cochran, A. J., and Holmes, E. C. (1982). NK activity of tumor infiltrating and lymph node lymphocytes in human pulmonary tumors. In "NK Cells and Other Natural Effector Cells" (R. B. Herberman, ed.), p. 1113. Academic Press, New York.
1130. Mantovani, A., Allavena, P., Sessa, C., Bolis, G., and Mangioni, C. (1980). Natural killer activity of lymphoid cells isolated from human ascitic ovarian tumors. *Int. J. Cancer* **25**, 573.
1131. Vose, B. M., Vanky, F., Argov, S., and Klein, E. (1977). Natural cytotoxicity in man: Activity of lymph node and tumor-infiltrating lymphocytes. *Eur. J. Immunol.* **7**, 753.

1132. Introna, M., Allavena, P., Biondi, A., Colombo, N., Villa, A., and Mantovani, A. (1983). Defective natural killer activity within human ovarian tumors: Low numbers of morphologically defined effectors present in situ. *J. Natl. Cancer Inst.* **70**, 21.

1133. Uchida, A., and Micksche, M. (1981). Natural killer cells in carcinomatous pleural effusions. *Cancer Immunol. Immunother.* **11**, 131.

1134. Moy, P., Holmes, E., and Golub, S. (1985). Depression of natural killer cytotoxic activity in lymphocytes infiltrating human pulmonary tumors. *Cancer Res.* **45**, 57.

1135. Uchida, A. and Micksche, M. (1983). Lysis of fresh human tumor cells by autologous large granular lymphocytes from peripheral blood and pleural effusions. *Int. J. Cancer* **32**, 37.

1136. Blanchard, D. K., Kavanagh, J. J., Sinkovics, J. G., Cavanagh, D., Hewitt, S. M., and Djeu, J. Y. (1988). Infiltration of interleukin-2-inducible killer cells in ascitic fluid and pleural effusions of advanced cancer patients. *Cancer Res.* **48**, 6321.

1137. Kerndrup, G., Meyer, K., Ellegaard, J., and Hokland, P. (1984). Natural killer (NK)-cell activity and antibody-dependent cellular cytotoxicity (ADCC) in primary preleukemic syndrome. *Leuk. Res.* **8**, 239.

1138. Takagi, S., Kitagawa, S., Takeda, A., Minato, N., Takaku, F., and Miura, Y. (1984). Natural killer–interferon system in patients with preleukaemic states. *Br. J. Haematol.* **58**, 71.

1139. Srskaar, D., Frre, O., Albrechtsen, D., and Stavem, P. (1986). Decreased natural killer cell activity versus normal natural killer cell markers in mononuclear cells from patients with smouldering leukemia. *Scand. J. Haematol.* **37**, 154.

1140. Okabe, M., Minagawa, T., Nakane, A., Sakurada, K., and Miyazaki, T. (1986). Impaired alpha-interferon production and natural killer activity in blood mononuclear cells in myelodysplastic syndrome. *Scand. J. Haematol.* **37**, 111.

1141. Galvani, D. W., Nethersell, A. B., and Cawley, J. C. (1988). Alpha-interferon in myelodysplasia; clinical observations and effects on NK cells. *Leuk. Res.* **12**, 257.

1142. Mangan, K. F., Chikkappa, G., and Farley, P. C. (1982). T gamma (Tγ) cells suppress growth of erythroid colony-forming units in vitro in the pure red aplasia of B-cell chronic lymphocytic leukemia. *J. Clin. Invest.* **70**, 1148.

1143. Fujimiya, Y., Chang, W. C., Bakke, A., Horwitz, D., and Pattengale, P. K. (1987). Natural killer (NK) cell immunodeficiency in patients with chronic myelogenous leukemia. II. Successful cloning and amplification of natural killer cells. *Cancer Immunol. Immunother.* **24**, 213.

1144. Mangan, K. F., and D'Allesandro, L. (1985). Hypoplastic anemia in B cell chronic lymphocytic leukemia: Evolution of T cell-mediated suppression of erythropoiesis in early stage and late stage disease. *Blood* **66**, 533.

1145. Trinchieri, G., Murphy, M., and Perussia, B. (1987). Regulation of hematopoiesis by T lymphocytes and natural killer cells. *CRC Crit. Rev. Oncol./Hematol.* **7**, 219.

1146. Pross, H. F., and Herberman, R. B. (1989). Clinical application of natural killer cells. *In* "Proceedings of the Fifth NK Workshop" (E. W. Ades and C. Lopez, eds.). Karger, Basel (in press).

1147. Hersey, P., Honeyman, E. M., and McCarthy, W. H. (1979). Low natural-killer-cell activity in familial melanoma patients and their relatives. *Br. J. Cancer* **40**, 113.

1148. Hersey, P., Edwards, A., McCarthy, W., and Milton, G. (1982). Tumor related changes and prognostic significance of natural killer cell activity in melanoma patients. *In* "NK Cells and Other Natural Effector Cells" (R. B. Herberman, ed.), p. 1167. Academic Press, New York.

1149. Strayer, D. R., Carter, W. A., Mayberry, S. D., Pequignot, E., and Brodsky, I.

(1984). Low natural cytotoxicity of peripheral blood mononuclear cells in individuals with high familial incidence of cancer. *Cancer Res.* **44**, 370.

1150. Pross, H. F., Sterns, E., and MacGillis, D. R. R. (1984). Natural killer activity in women at "high risk" for breast cancer, with and without benign breast syndrome. *Int. J. Cancer* **34**, 303.

1151. Pross, H. F. (1986). The involvement of natural killer cells in human malignant disease. *In* "Immunobiology of Natural Killer Cells" (E. Lotzova and R. B. Herberman, eds.), Vol. 2, p. 11. CRC Press, Boca Raton, Florida.

1152. Schantz, S. P., Brown, B. W., Lira, E., Taylor, D. L., and Beddingfield, N. (1987). Evidence for the role of natural immunity in the control of metastatic spread of head and neck cancer. *Cancer Immunol. Immunother.* **25**, 141.

1153. Pross, H. F. (1986). Natural killer cell activity in human malignant disease. *In* "Natural Immunity, Cancer and Biological Response Modification" (E. Lotzova and R. B. Herberman, eds.), p. 196. Karger, Basel.

1154. Sibbitt, W. L., Jr., and Bankhurst, A. D. (1985). Natural killer cells in connective tissue disorders. *Clin. Rheum. Dis.* **11**, 507.

1155. Sibbitt, W. L., Jr., Gibbs, D. L., Kenny, C., Bankhurst, A. D., Searles, R. P., and Ley, K. D. (1985). Realtionship between circulating interferon and antiinterferon antibodies and impaired natural killer cell activity in systemic lupus erythematosus. *Arthritis Rheum.* **28**, 624.

1156. Pan, L. Z., Dauphinee, M. J., Ansar-Ahmed, S., and Talal, N. (1986). Altered natural killer and natural cytotoxic cellular activities in *lpr* mice. *Scand. J. Immunol.* **23**, 415.

1157. Magilavy, D. B., Steinberg, A. D., and Latta, S. L. (1987). High hepatic natural killer cell activity in murine lupus. *J. Exp. Med.* **166**, 271.

1158. Karashima, A., Taniguchi, K., Himeno, K., Kawano, Y., Toshitani, A., and Nomoto, K. (1988). Does depression of NK activity cause lymphadenopathy in *lpr* mice? *Cell. Immunol.* **115**, 484.

1159. Seaman, W. E., Blackman, M. A., Greenspan, J. S., and Talal, N. (1980). Effect of ^{89}Sr on immunity and autoimmunity in NZB/NZW F_1 mice. *J. Immunol.* **124**, 812.

1160. MacKay, P., Jacobson, J., and Rabinovitch, A. (1986). Spontaenous diabetes mellitus in the Bio-Breeding/Worcester rat. Evidence in vitro for natural killer cell lysis of islet cells. *J. Clin. Invest.* **77**, 916.

1161. Woda, B. A., and Biron, C. A. (1986). Natural killer cell number and function in the spontaneously diabetic BB/W rat. *J. Immunol.* **137**, 1860.

1162. Like, A. A., Biron, C. A., Weringer, E. J., Byman, K., Sroczynski, E., and Guberski, D. L. (1986). Prevention of diabetes in BioBreeding/Worcester rats with monoclonal antibodies that recognize T lymphocytes or natural killer cells. *J. Exp. Med.* **164**, 1145.

1163. Negishi, K., Gupta, S., Chandy, K. G., Waldeck, N., Kershnar, A., Buckingham, B., and Charles, M. A. (1988). Interferon responsiveness of natural killer cells in type I human diabetes. *Diabetes Res.* **7**, 49.

1164. Neishi, K., Waldeck, N., Chandy, G., Buckingham, B., Kershnar, A., Fisher, L., Gupta, S., and Charles, A. M. (1987). Natural killer cell and islet killer cell activities in human type 1 diabetes. *Exp. Clin. Endocrinol.* **89**, 345.

1165. Hussain, M. J., Alviggi, L., Millward, B. A., Leslie, R. D., Pyke, D. A., and Vergani, D. (1987). Evidence that the reduced number of natural killer cells in type 1 (insulin-dependent) diabetes may be genetically determined. *Diabetologia* **30**, 907.

1166. Neighbour, P. A. (1984). Studies of interferon production and natural killing by lymphocytes from multiple sclerosis patients. *Ann. N.Y. Acad. Sci.* **436**, 181.
1167. Santoli, D., Hall, W., Kastrukoff, L., Lissak, R. P., Perussia, B., Trinchieri, G., and Koprowski, H. (1981). Cytotoxic activity and interferon production by lymphocytes from patients with multiple sclerosis. *J. Immunol.* **126**, 1274.
1168. Legendre, C. M., Guttmann, R. D., and Yip, G. H. (1986). Natural killer cell subsets in long-term renal allograft recipients. A phenotypic and functional study. *Transplantation* **42**, 347.
1169. Lefkowitz, M., Jorkasky, D., and Kornbluth, J. (1987). Increase in natural killer activity in cyclosporine-treated renal allograft recipients during rejection. *Hum. Immunol.* **19**, 139.
1170. Hoffman, R. A., Ascher, N. L., Jordan, M. L., Migliori, R. J., and Simmons, R. L. (1988). Characterization of natural killer activity in sponge matrix allografts. *J. Immunol.* **140**, 1702.
1171. Nemlander, A, Soots, A., and Häyry, P. (1984). In situ effector pathways of allograft destruction. 1. Generation of the "cellular" effector response in the graft and the graft recipient. *Cell. Immunol.* **89**, 409.
1172. Lefkowitz, M., Kornbluth, J., Tomaszewski, J. E., and Jorkasky, D. K. (1988). Natural killer-cell activity in cyclosporine-treated renal allograft recipients. *J. Clin. Immunol.* **8**, 121.
1173. Fontana, L., Sirianni, M. C., De Sanctis, G., Carbonari, M., Ensoli, B., and Aiuti, F. (1986). Deficiency of natural killer activity, but not of natural killer binding, in patients with lymphoadenopathy syndrome positive for antibodies to HTLV-III. *Immunobiology* **171**, 425.
1174. Bonavida, B., Katz J., and Gottlieb, M. (1986). Mechanism of defective NK cell activity in patients with acquired immunodeficiency syndrome (AIDS) and AIDS-related complex. I. Defective trigger on NK cells for NKCF production by target cells, and partial restoration by IL 2. *J. Immunol.* **137**, 1157.
1175. Katzman, M., and Lederman, M. M. (1986). Defective postbinding lysis underlies the impaired natural killer activity in factor VIII-treated, human T lymphotropic virus type III seropositive hemophiliacs. *J. Clin. Invest.* **77**, 1057.
1176. Sirianni, M. C., Soddus, S., Malorni, W., Arancia, G., and Aiuti, F. (1988). Mechanism of defective natural killer cell activity in patients with AIDS is associated with defective distribution of tubulin. *J. Immunol.* **140**, 2565.
1177. Vuillier, F., Bianco, N. E., Montagnier, L., and Dighiero, G. (1988). Selective depletion of low-density CD8+, CD16+ lymphocytes during HIV infection. *AIDS Res. Hum. Retroviruses* **4**, 121.
1178. Robinson, W. E., Jr., Mitchell, W. M., Chambers, W. H., Schuffman, S. S., Montefiori, D. C., and Oeltmann, T. N. (1988). Natural killer cell infection and inactivation in vitro by the human immunodeficiency virus. *Hum. Pathol.* **19**, 535.
1179. Lau, A. S., Read, S. E., and Williams, B. R. G. (1988). Downregulation of interferon α but not γ receptor expression in vivo in the acquired immunodeficiency syndrome. *J. Clin. Invest.* **82**, 1415.
1180. Lopez, C., Fitzgerald, P. A., Siegal, F. P., Landesman, S., Gold, J., and Krown, S. E. (1984). Deficiency of interferon-alpha generating capacity is associated with susceptibility to opportunistic infections in patients with AIDS. *Ann. N.Y. Acad. Sci.* **437**, 39.
1181. Cauda, R., Tumbarelo, M., Ortona, L., Kanda, P., Kennedy, R. C., and Chanh, T. C. (1988). Inhibition of normal human natural killer cell activity by human immunodeficiency virus synthetic transmembrane peptides. *Cell. Immunol.* **115**, 57.

1182. Harris, D. T., Cianciolo, G. J., Snyderman, R., Argov, S., and Koren, H. S. (1987). Inhibition of human natural killer cell activity by a synthetic peptide homologous to a conserved region in the retroviral protein, p15E. *J. Immunol.* **138**, 889.

This article was accepted for publication on 23 January 1989.

The Immunopathogenesis of HIV Infection

ZEDA F. ROSENBERG AND ANTHONY S. FAUCI

National Institute of Allergy and Infectious Diseases,
National Institutes of Health,
Bethesda, Maryland 20892

I. Introduction

The human immunodeficiency virus (HIV) has already infected an estimated 1-1.5 million individuals (A. R. Lifson et al., 1988) and is expected to infect at least 5 million people worldwide by 1993 (J. M. Mann et al., 1988). Although the vast majority of HIV-infected individuals are at present without symptoms, HIV has the ability to cause an insidious and progressive deterioration of the host's immune function, leading to profound immunosuppression (Bowen et al., 1985). HIV-induced immunosuppression results in the emergence of opportunistic infections and neoplasms that are pathognomonic for the acquired immunodeficiency syndrome (AIDS). Infection with HIV also results in a syndrome of neurological abnormalities, which has been termed the AIDS-dementia complex (Price et al., 1988).

In the United States alone, as of January 1989, more than 84,000 cases of AIDS have been diagnosed. More than 47,000 of these individuals have died (Centers for Disease Control, 1989). It is currently estimated that between 26 and 36% of HIV-infected individuals will develop AIDS within 7 years of infection, while an additional 40% will develop other signs of immune dysfunction (Curran et al., 1988). Thus, even if the transmission of HIV were completely halted, an estimated 365,000 cases will have occurred by 1992 if no effective treatment is found which will prevent the onset of AIDS in HIV-infected individuals (U.S. Public Health Service, 1988).

Efforts to control AIDS require a fundamental knowledge of the etiological agent itself, the mechanisms by which HIV destroys the immune system, and the nature of the immune response against HIV. Fortunately, longstanding basic research both on retroviruses and on the immune system laid the groundwork for rapid advances in the accrual of knowledge of HIV and the immunopathogenic mechanisms of HIV infection. This chapter will present a review of our state of knowledge concerning the structure and function of the HIV genome, virus cell tropism, cytotoxic and noncytotoxic effects of HIV on both the immune system and the central nervous system (CNS), latent HIV infection and virus activation, and the immune response to HIV.

II. The Etiological Agent

A. HIV

The discovery and isolation of the first recognized human retrovirus, human T cell leukemia–lymphoma virus (HTLV)-I, from mature T cells of individuals with adult T cell malignancies (Poiesz *et al.*, 1980, 1981) only a few years before the first cases of AIDS were described were crucial steps in the identification of another human retrovirus of the lentivirus subfamily, HIV, as the cause of AIDS. HIV, originally termed human T lymphotropic virus (HTLV)-III, lymphadenopathy-associated virus (LAV), or AIDS-associated retrovirus, was shown to be a distinct member of the HTLV group of viruses (Barré-Sinoussi *et al.*, 1983; Gallo *et al.*, 1984; Levy *et al.*, 1984). Unlike HTLV-I, however, HIV is cytopathic for its target cells and causes syncytia formation between infected and uninfected cells (Popovic *et al.*, 1984).

HIV shares many morphological, biological, and molecular properties with the nononcogenic, cytopathic lentiviruses of sheep, horses, and goats (Gonda *et al.*, 1985, 1986) as well as the more recently described bovine immunodeficiency-like virus (Gonda *et al.*, 1987) and feline immunodeficiency virus (Pedersen *et al.*, 1987). In addition, a cytopathic, T cell tropic virus, simian immunodeficiency virus (SIV), related to HIV has been isolated from macaques (Daniel *et al.*, 1985) and has been shown to induce an AIDS-like disease in inoculated rhesus monkeys (Letvin *et al.*, 1985). Like HIV, these animal lentiviruses can cause persistent and slowly progressive, fatal infections in their hosts after a prolonged incubation period. The persistent viremic phase is associated with a weak neutralizing antibody response, genetic variation of the virus, CNS involvement, and cytolytic effects on the target cells (Desrosiers and Letvin, 1987).

The overall structure of HIV resembles that of other retroviruses. The virus particle consists of two identical single-stranded RNA molecules and viral enzymes within a viral protein core that is surrounded by an envelope derived from a combination of the host cell membrane and virus-specific glycoproteins (Varmus, 1988). The dense viral core of HIV is bar shaped, most closely resembling viruses within the lentivirus family (Rabson and Martin, 1985). In addition, nucleotide sequence analysis of the polymerase genes of several lentiviruses and oncogenic retroviruses revealed that HIV is more closely related to ungulate lentiviruses than to other retroviruses (Chiu *et al.*, 1985).

B. THE LIFE CYCLE OF HIV

During initial attempts to isolate and culture HIV from AIDS patients, it was noted that HIV displayed a tropism for T4 lymphocytes (Gallo *et al.*, 1984; Popovic *et al.*, 1984; Klatzmann *et al.*, 1984b). It was subsequently shown that the CD4 molecule, a 55- to 58-kDa glycoprotein originally described as a T cell differentiation antigen (Reinherz *et al.*, 1979; Reinherz and Schlossman, 1980; Ledbetter *et al.*, 1981), is a high-affinity receptor for HIV (Dalgleish *et al.*, 1984; Klatzmann *et al.*, 1984a). The binding of the viral external glycoprotein, gp120, to the CD4 receptor that is present on the surface of T4 lymphocytes (McDougal *et al.*, 1986) is the first step in the HIV life cycle (Fig. 1). Although early work suggested that HIV entered the cell via receptor-mediated endocytosis (Maddon *et al.*, 1986), it was subsequently shown that HIV could enter T4 lymphocytes even when receptor-mediated endocytosis is inhibited by treatment with lysomotropic agents (Stein *et al.*, 1987; McClure *et al.*, 1988). Later studies utilizing CD4$^+$ cells whose CD4 molecules were unable to undergo endocytosis confirmed that HIV infection of cells can occur by direct fusion of the HIV envelope with the host cell membrane (Hoxie *et al.*, 1988; Bedinger *et al.*, 1988; Maddon *et al.*, 1988). The prospect that other human proteins may be required for HIV infection is suggested by the observation that murine cells that express human CD4 and can bind HIV are nevertheless resistant to HIV infection (Maddon *et al.*, 1986). It has been hypothesized that human leukocyte

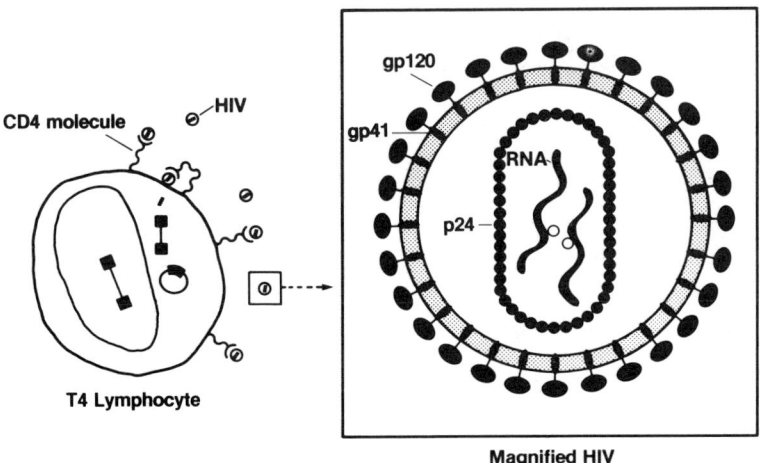

FIG. 1. The binding of HIV via its gp120 env protein to the CD4 molecule on T4 lymphocytes.

antigen (HLA)-DR may be involved in the binding site for HIV on cells expressing major histocompatibility complex (MHC) class II antigens (D. L. Mann et al., 1988).

Like other retroviruses, upon entry of the virion into the cell, the enveloped particle is converted into an enzymatically active nucleoprotein complex (Varmus, 1988). After the virion-associated reverse transcriptase transcribes the RNA genome into unintegrated double-stranded DNA, the virally encoded endonuclease (integrase) enables the viral DNA to integrate into the host cell's chromosomal DNA (Rabson, 1988). In most retroviral systems the unintegrated viral DNA is a short-lived intermediate stage between the virion RNA and the integrated viral DNA. In other retroviral systems persistence of unintegrated retroviral DNA has been associated with a cytopathic effect (Keshet and Temin, 1979; Weller et al., 1980). In HIV infection, a substantial amount of HIV DNA exists in an unintegrated form, potentially contributing to the cytopathicity observed in HIV infection (Shaw et al., 1984).

Once the HIV proviral DNA is integrated into the host cell's chromosomal DNA, viral replication may enter a restricted, latent phase, depending on the state of activation of the infected cell (Ho et al., 1987a). In an activated cell, host cell signals initiate the transcription of viral DNA into genomic RNA and mRNA. The mRNAs are spliced and translated into viral proteins that subsequently undergo posttranslational modifications, including cleavage and glycosylation. The virion RNA and core proteins associate with viral envelope proteins that are located at the cell membrane, and the mature virion forms by budding from the cell surface. Viral regulatory proteins (see Section II,C,1) influence the levels of viral RNA transcription, splicing of mRNAs, and packaging of mature virions (Ho et al., 1987a; Varmus, 1988).

C. The HIV Genome

1. Structure and Function of the Genome

Rapid molecular cloning (Hahn et al., 1984; Alizon et al., 1984; Luciw et al., 1984) and the complete sequencing (Ratner et al., 1985; Wain-Hobson et al., 1985; Sanchez-Pescador et al., 1985; Muesing et al., 1985) of HIV have resulted in a detailed depiction of the viral genome. Depending on the particular HIV isolate, the length of the genome is approximately 9.2–9.7 kb. Analogous to other retroviruses, the coding sequences for the core proteins (gag), retroviral enzymes (pol), and envelope proteins (env) are located within the flanking long terminal repeats (LTRs). The LTR contains characteristic regulatory elements, such as the polyadenylation signal sequence and the TATAA promoter sequence, in addition to *cis*-acting regions which are involved in the regulation of HIV expression. These regions include a negative regulatory element (NRE), an enhancer region (NFkB), Sp1 binding sites, and *trans*-acting responsive (TAR) sequences (Starcich *et al.*, 1985; Rosen *et al.*, 1985; Wright *et al.*, 1986).

The gag gene product is a p55 polyprotein precursor that is processed into the viral core proteins, p17, p24, and p15. The *pol* gene encodes three enzymes: reverse transcriptase, integrase, and protease. The functions of the reverse transcriptase and integrase were discussed in Section II,B. The HIV protease gene product has been shown to cleave the gag p55 translation product into p24 and p17, a function that is required for viral infectivity (Kohl *et al.*, 1988). The primary env gene product is a polyprotein, gp160, that is processed intracellularly into an env protein, gp120, and a transmembrane protein, gp41 (diMarzo Veronese *et al.*, 1985). It has been shown that the endoproteolytic cleavage of gp160 into gp120 and gp41 is required for viral infectivity (McCune *et al.*, 1988b).

In addition to the *gag*, *pol*, and *env* genes, HIV contains at least six other regulatory genes which may play an important role in the pathogenesis of HIV infection. The *tat* gene, located immediately 5' to the *env* gene (Arya *et al.*, 1985; Sodroski *et al.*, 1985) encodes a 14- to 15-kDa protein (Arya and Gallo, 1986) that is essential for HIV replication (Dayton *et al.*, 1986; Fisher *et al.*, 1986a). The target for *tat*-mediated up-regulation of HIV expression is the TAR region of the LTR (Rosen *et al.*, 1985). Although it was originally thought that *tat* functioned primarily at a posttranscriptional level (Rosen *et al.*, 1986; Feinberg *et al.*, 1986), later studies suggested that *tat* directs an increase in the accumulation of HIV mRNA (Peterlin *et al.*, 1986; Muesing *et al.*, 1987) either by removing a block to the elongation of mRNA transcripts (Kao *et al.*, 1987) or by increasing the transcription rate of the HIV LTR (Rice and Mathews, 1988).

The *rev* gene (previously designated *trs* or *art*) encodes a protein of approximately 20 kDa that acts posttranslationally to secure expression of gag and env proteins (Feinberg *et al.*, 1986; Sodroski *et al.*, 1986a; Knight *et al.*, 1987) and is required for HIV replication (Terwilliger *et al.*, 1988). In the absence of *rev*, gag and env mRNA transcripts are multiply spliced, resulting in the absence of gag and env proteins (Feinberg *et al.*, 1986; Knight *et al.*, 1987). In addition, *rev* may also function as a down-regulator of viral mRNA transcription (Sadaie *et al.*, 1988).

The function of the *nef* gene (previously designated 3' open reading frame, B, E', or F) was initially observed by Fisher *et al.* (1986b), who showed that *nef* deletion mutants displayed enhanced cytopathicity. Additional experiments demonstrated that the highly cytopathic *nef* mutants replicated to higher levels than wild-type virus and produced more viral DNA (Luciw et al., 1987). The 27-kDa nef protein (Arya and Gallo, 1986) has been shown to suppress HIV replication when added in *trans* and to down-regulate transcription from the HIV LTR by interacting with the NRE domain (Ahmad and Venkatesan, 1988). In addition, the nef protein shares structural homology with the ATP-binding site of protein kinases (Samuel et al., 1987); is phosphorylated by protein kinase C; displays GTPase, autophosphorylation, and GTP-binding activities; and can down-regulate CD4 expression (Guy et al., 1987). Thus, *nef* may be important in the maintenance of low-level or latent HIV infection.

Like *nef*, the product of the *vif* gene (previously designated *sor*, A, P', or Q), a protein of approximately 24 kDa (Lee et al., 1986; Arya and Gallo, 1986), is not necessary for HIV replication or cytopathicity in $CD4^+$ lymphoid cell lines (Sodroski et al., 1986b). However, viruses that have deletions in the *vif* gene are approximately 100- to 1000-fold less infectious than wild-type virus, apparently spreading in cultures through cell-to-cell contact rather than by free virus infection (Strebel et al., 1987; Fisher et al., 1987).

The function of the eighth gene of HIV, *vpr*, which codes for a protein that reacts with the sera of some HIV-infected individuals, is presently unknown (Wong-Staal et al., 1987). The ninth HIV gene, *vpu*, has recently been identified and shown to code for a 16-kDa protein that is recognized by the sera of HIV-infected individuals (Cohen et al., 1988; Strebel et al., 1988; Matsuda et al., 1988). While expression of the major viral proteins was not altered by a defective *vpu* gene, a five- to tenfold decrease in progeny virions was observed in T cells after infection with a *vpu* mutant HIV, suggesting an effect of *vpu* on assembly or maturation of a new virus (Strebel et al., 1988). Although there is, at present, no identified tenth gene or gene product, Miller (1988) has identified a region on the DNA plus strand of the HIV-replicative intermediate that may represent another functional domain.

It is clear that HIV is an extremely complex virus with genes that may facilitate high levels of virus production and cell death, restricted chronic virus replication, or latent infection (Fig. 2). The HIV-regulatory genes can interact with each other in a regulatory network that may switch from one pathway to another, depending on cellular factors (Haseltine, 1988). The interaction of cellular factors and the HIV genome is thought to play a major role in the maintenance of the long and variable asymptomatic phase in the infected individual and the subsequent progressive immunological deterioration This work will be discussed in detail in Section III,G.

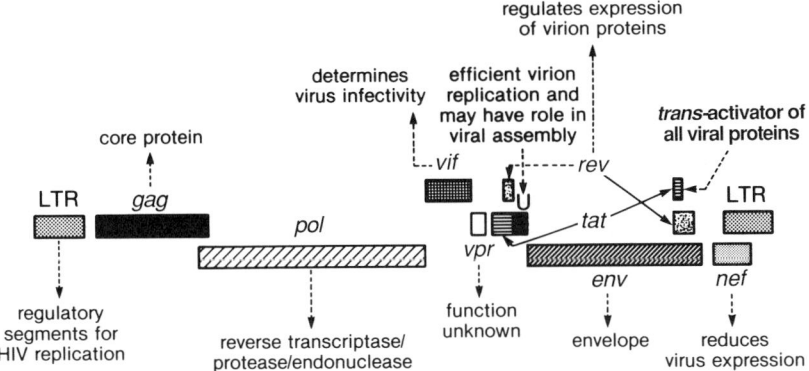

FIG. 2. HIV genes and their functions. [Adapted with permission from Fauci, A. S. (1988). *Science* **239**, 618. Copyright 1988 by the AAAS.]

2. Heterogeneity of HIV Isolates

The ability of HIV to evade the host's immune response and persist in the infected individual for long periods may be the result of the generation of antigenic variants. Variation of HIV isolates from one patient to another has been shown by restriction endonuclease analyses (Luciw *et al.*, 1984; Shaw *et al.*, 1984; Wong-Staal *et al.*, 1985; Benn *et al.*, 1985; Laure *et al.*, 1987). Comparison of the nucleotide sequences of different HIV isolates demonstrated that variation exists throughout the HIV genome, with the region of greatest variability occurring in the *env* gene (Starcich *et al.*, 1986; Alizon *et al.*, 1986). Within the *env* gene, both conserved and hypervariable regions have been identified (Starcich *et al.*, 1986; Willey *et al.*, 1986; Gurgo *et al.*, 1988).

Hahn *et al.* (1986) have shown that HIV isolates obtained sequentially from individual patients over time also display heterogeneity throughout the viral genome, with a tenfold higher rate of divergence for *env* sequences than for *gag* sequences (10^{-3} and 10^{-4} nucleotide substitutions per site per year, respectively). While mutation rates for retroviruses as a group are notably high (Dougherty and Temin, 1988; Leider *et al.*, 1988), the low fidelity of the HIV reverse transcriptase may be the cause of the exceptionally high variability seen in the HIV genome. Takeuchi *et al.* (1988) have shown that the fidelity of the reverse transcriptase of HIV was approximately one third that of other retroviruses. Using different assays, other researchers have demonstrated that the HIV-1 reverse transcriptase has an error rate ranging from one in 1700 to one in 4000 errors per detectable nucleotide incorporated, approximately ten times higher than polymerases from other retroviruses (Preston *et al.*, 1988; Roberts *et al.*, 1988).

It has been well established that independent HIV isolates exhibit differences in cell tropism, replicative capacity, and cytopathic characteristics (Evans *et al.*, 1987; Dahl *et al.*, 1987; Fenyo *et al.*, 1988). Investigators have determined that, *in vivo*, independent isolates of HIV are comprised of multiple variants with different target cell susceptibilities (Bolton *et al.*, 1987; von Briesen *et al.*, 1987; Saag *et al.*, 1988; Fisher *et al.*, 1988b; Sakai *et al.*, 1988). Sakai *et al.* (1988) have also shown that HIV variants isolated simultaneously from the same patient display differences in replicative capacity and cytopathicity. Thus, *in vivo*, numerous genetic and biological variants of HIV can develop over time and coexist in a single individual. The significance of the genetic and biological changes in the immunopathogenesis of HIV infection is unclear at present. As is the case in infection with equine infectious anemia virus (Montelaro *et al.*, 1984), genetic variation in HIV may enable the virus to undergo antigenic drift and escape destruction by the immune response. Reitz *et al.* (1988) have recently reported on the generation of a neutralization-resistant variant of HIV after incubation of the parent virus in neutralizing antisera. The genetic change resulting in the neutralization-resistant phenotype was localized to a single nucleotide change in the *env* gene. The combination of immune pressure and genetic variability may result in the generation of viruses with increased virulence. In this regard, isolates with high replicative or cytopathic abilities appear to be found more frequently in patients with symptomatic HIV infection (Asjo *et al.*, 1986; Cheng-Mayer *et al.*, 1988).

D. HIV-2

A second human lentivirus, HIV-2 (previously designated LAV-2 or SBL-6669), was originally isolated from AIDS patients in West Africa and was shown to be antigenically distinct from the HIV that causes AIDS in the United States, Central Africa, and other parts of the world (Clavel *et al.*, 1986b; Albert *et al.*, 1987). With the discovery of HIV-2, the previously described isolates of HIV were designated HIV-1. Similar to HIV-1, HIV-2 infects $CD4^+$ cells and is found in patients with a syndrome that is clinically indistinguishable from AIDS. However, antisera to the HIV-2 env glycoprotein do not recognize HIV-1 (Clavel *et al.*, 1987; Albert *et al.*, 1987). In addition, there is no cross-reactivity in antibody-dependent cellular cytotoxicity (ADCC) between HIV-1 and HIV-2 (Ljunggren *et al.*, 1988b). HIV-1 and HIV-2 do, however, share cross-reactive epitopes of the core structural proteins (Brun-Vezinet *et al.*, 1987).

Molecular cloning and genetic analysis of the genome of HIV-2 has revealed that HIV-2 is a novel member of the human lentivirus family and is not an envelope variant of HIV-1 (Clavel et al., 1986a; Franchini et al., 1987a). The genome of HIV-2 contains coding regions analogous to the HIV-1 *tat, rev, vif,* and *vpr* genes. In HIV-2, the coding region for *nef* contains a large insertion in the amino terminus (Guyader et al., 1987). The HIV-1 *tat* gene has been shown to transactivate both the HIV-1 and HIV-2 LTRs to the same degree. However, HIV-2 *tat* transactivates the HIV-2 LTR to a greater extent than the HIV-1 LTR (Guyader et al., 1987; Arya et al., 1987). Whereas the two tat gene products are thought to act via a common mechanism, the differences in *trans*-activating efficiencies may be due to a requirement by HIV-2 *tat* for additional unique target sequences in the HIV-2 LTR (Emerman et al., 1987).

There are two major differences in the genomes of HIV-1 and HIV-2. Researchers have identified a novel gene, *vpx*, found only in HIV-2 and SIV that encodes for an immunogenic 14-kDa virion-associated protein. While its function is presently unknown, the vpx protein has been shown to bind to single-stranded nucleic acids *in vitro* and does not appear to be essential for virus infectivity or replication (Henderson et al., 1988; Yu et al., 1988; Kappes et al., 1988; Franchini et al., 1988). The second major genomic disparity between HIV-1 and HIV-2 is that the HIV-1-encoded vpu protein is not found in HIV-2-infected cells, nor does HIV-2 have the capacity to encode for the *vpu* protein (Cohen et al., 1988; Matsuda et al., 1988).

HIV-2 appears to possess the same degree of biological variability as HIV-1, including variation in the degree of *in vitro* cytopathic effects (Clavel et al., 1987). In this regard there have been two recent reports of strains of HIV-2 that replicate well in $CD4^+$ cells but do not cause any cytopathic effects (Evans et al., 1988; Kong et al., 1988).

III. Immunopathogenic Mechanisms

A. THE CD4–HIV INTERACTION

The interaction of HIV with the CD4 molecule that is present on the surface of the helper/inducer subset of T lymphocytes is the critical event in the pathogenesis of HIV infection (Fauci, 1987). Since the T4 cell plays a pivotal role in the induction of most immunological responses, HIV-induced damage to the T4 cell population results in the abrogation of a wide range of immune functions, ultimately leading to extreme immunosuppression and opportunistic diseases (Bowen et al., 1985).

As discussed in Section II,B, HIV binds with high affinity to the CD4 molecule via the env glycoprotein, gp120. In fact, the affinity of gp120 for CD4 is higher than that of the MHC class II molecule, the natural ligand of CD4 (Dalgleish et al., 1984; Klatzmann et al., 1984a; McDougal et al., 1986). It has been well documented that, in vitro, HIV-1 infectivity can be inhibited by the addition of soluble recombinant CD4 molecules (Smith et al., 1987; Fisher et al., 1988a; Hussey et al., 1988; Deen et al., 1988; Traunecker et al., 1988). HIV-infected cells can also be killed by soluble recombinant CD4 which has been conjugated to the A chain of the toxin ricin (Till et al., 1988). Recombinant gp120, CD4, or a monoclonal antibody to the gp120–CD4 binding site could abrogate this killing.

Using monoclonal antibodies to various regions of CD4, Sattentau et al. (1986) found that there are two discrete epitopes of CD4 that are critical for virus binding. The location of the HIV binding site on the CD4 molecule has been further confined to the amino-terminal half of the extracellular region of CD4 (Berger et al., 1988), a loop extending from amino acid residues 31–57 of the amino-terminal portion of CD4 (Mizukami et al., 1988), residues 37–53 (Jameson et al., 1988), residues 37–83 (Landau et al., 1988), residues 83–94 (J. D. Lifson et al., 1988), residues 42–49 (Peterson and Seed, 1988), and residues 48–51 and 121–123 (Clayton et al., 1988). Researchers have also noted that sequences in domain II of CD4, adjacent to the amino terminus, may encourage efficient gp120 binding by contributing to the three-dimensional structure of the binding site (Landau et al., 1988; Clayton et al., 1988).

Lasky et al. (1987) have shown by monoclonal antibody mapping that the carboxy-terminal region of the gp120 molecule is involved in binding to the CD4 receptor. In vitro mutagenesis analysis of this region of the gp120 resulted in the identification of a stretch of 12 amino acids (410–421) which are critical for gp120–CD4 binding, with decreased binding occurring following substitution of a single amino acid (417) in this region (Dowbenko et al., 1988). In addition, gp120 molecules with mutations in the amino terminus and central conserved domains of gp120 were unable to bind tightly to CD4, suggesting that regions outside the carboxy terminus are important for the high-affinity gp120–CD4 interaction (Dowbenko et al., 1988).

B. DEPLETION OF CD4+ CELLS

Infection of T4 lymphocytes with HIV in vitro results in widespread and rapid cell death (Popovic et al., 1984). Although the specific mechanisms by which HIV destroys T4 lymphocytes are not known at present, it has been postulated that HIV can exert its deleterious effects both directly and indirectly. One direct mechanism of cell killing may be the formation of microholes in the cell membrane, which is the result of intense virus budding (R. Leonard et al., 1988) (Fig. 3). It has also been suggested that the insertion of HIV env proteins into the cell membrane causes a change in cell membrane permeability to ions with subsequent increases in intracellular calcium levels. A rise in intracellular calcium has been shown to perturbate lipid synthesis and is associated with a loss of cell viability (Lynn et al., 1988).

Other direct mechanisms of cell killing involve the accumulation of unintegrated viral DNA in the cell cytoplasm (discussed in Section II,B) as well as the accumulation of high levels of heterodisperse RNAs containing repetitive sequences that do not contain long open reading frames (Koga et al., 1988). It has also been suggested that the binding of HIV env proteins to intracellular CD4 molecules may result in cell death (Hoxie et al., 1986). In support of this hypothesis, there have been several reports of a correlation between expression of the env gene and cytopathic effects on T4 cells (Sodroski et al., 1986c; Fisher et al., 1986b). In

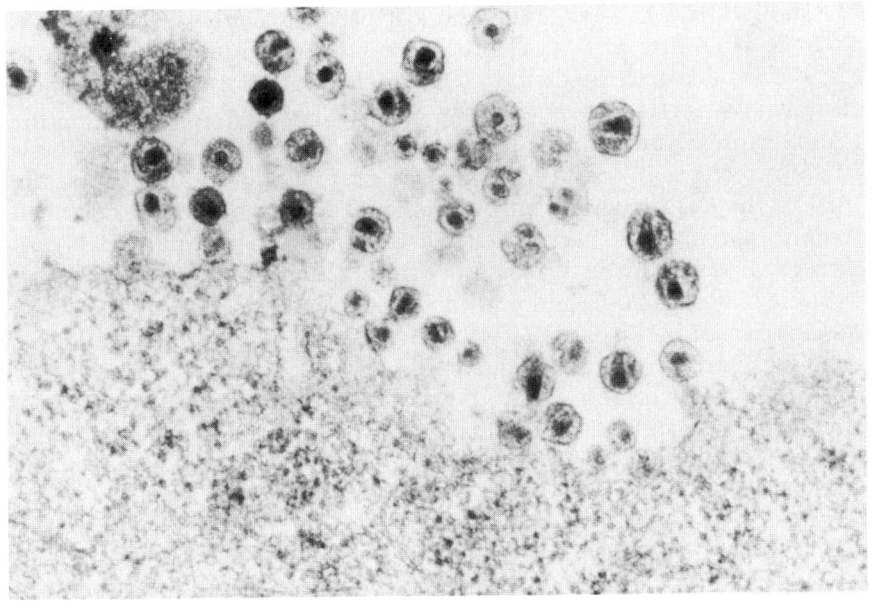

FIG. 3. Massive release of HIV particles from the extracellular membrane of T4 lymphocytes. [Reprinted with permission from Fauci, A. S. (1988). In *Human Retroviruses and Diseases They Cause* (J. P. Allain, R. C. Gallo, and L. Montagnier, eds.) p. 30. Princeton, N.J.: Excerpta Medica.]

addition, when HTLV-I-infected T4 or T8 cell clones were superinfected with HIV, only the T4 cells were killed (De Rossi et al., 1986). Since the virus that was produced from both the T4 and T8 cell clones was cytopathic for fresh T4 cells, these data provide additional evidence that the interaction of HIV and CD4 is important for cell killing.

Several indirect mechanisms of T4 cell destruction have been implicated in the pathogenesis of HIV infection. The dramatic depletion of T4 cells that occurs in AIDS patients may be the consequence of HIV infection of T4 cell precursors or cells which secrete factors that can stimulate the propagation of the entire lymphoid cell pool (Fauci, 1987). Another mechanism involves the generation of multinucleated giant cells, which results *in vitro* from the high-affinity binding of gp120 that is expressed on the surface of HIV-infected cells to CD4 molecules on neighboring uninfected T4 cells (Lifson et al., 1986a,b; Sodroski et al., 1986c; Yoffe et al., 1987). It is thought that these syncytia die soon after formation and contribute to the indirect cytopathic effects of HIV infection. However, experimental evidence from other investigators does not support the theory that syncytia formation is the major mechanism of cell death in HIV infection. Somasundaran and Robinson (1987) have shown that, *in vitro*, HIV can kill peripheral blood lymphocytes and a $T4^+$ cell line without syncytia formation. Similarly, R. Leonard *et al.* (1988) demonstrated that cells infected with a mutant HIV show substantial syncytia formation with little cell killing.

Autoimmune phenomena may also play a role in the pathogenesis of HIV infection. It has been hypothesized that the binding of soluble gp120 to the CD4 receptor on uninfected T4 cells may render the cell susceptible to immune clearance (Klatzmann and Gluckman, 1986). In this regard, several investigators have found that human anti-HIV sera were able to lyse gp120-bound normal T lymphocytes (Lyerly et al., 1987a) and inactivated HIV-coated $CD4^+$ cells (Katz et al., 1988) in an ADCC assay. In addition, it has recently been shown that $CD4^+$ T cells can effectively process soluble gp120, present the processed antigen to $CD4^+$ gp120-specific cytolytic clones, and be lysed by a CD4-dependent autocytolytic mechanism (Lanzavecchia et al., 1988; Siliciano et al., 1988) (Fig. 4).

Other investigators have reported that antibodies to normal helper T cells are present in the sera of patients with AIDS and AIDS-related complex (ARC) (Dorsett et al., 1985) as well as cytotoxic antibodies to lectin-stimulated or HIV-infected $CD4^+$ T cells (Stricker et al., 1987). These autoantibodies may result from a process of antigenic mimicry due to a proposed cross-reactivity between the HIV envelope and a portion of the MHC class II that is recognized by the CD4 molecule

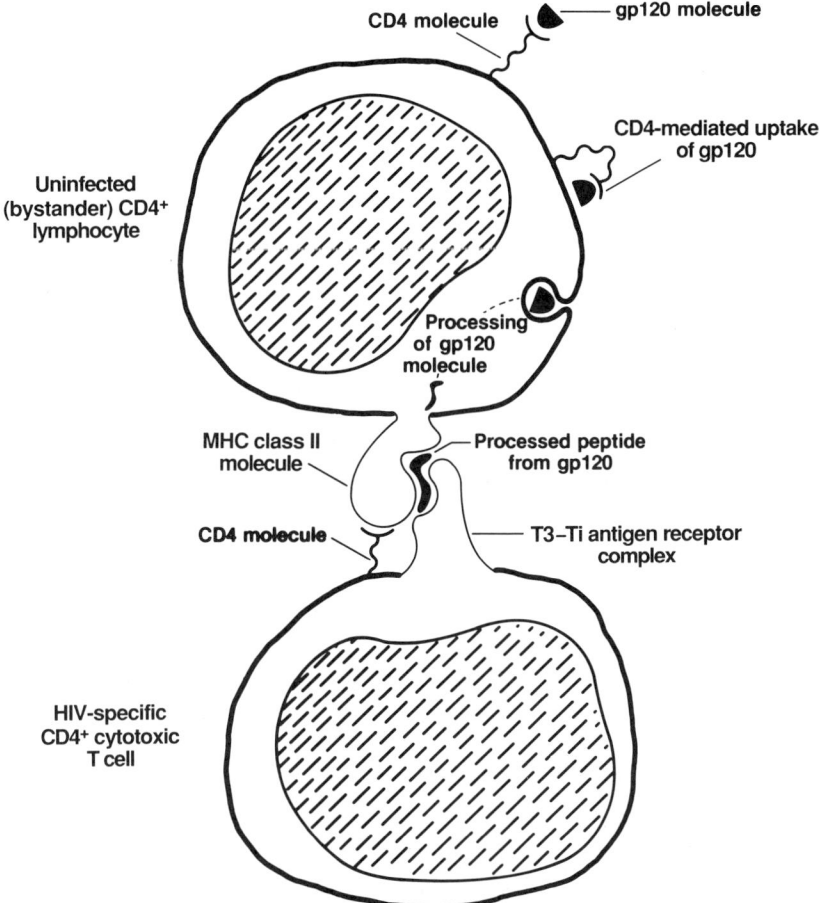

FIG. 4. Elimination of uninfected CD4+ T cells exposed to soluble gp120 by HIV-specific CD4+ cytotoxic T cells.

during normal cell–cell interactions (Ziegler and Stites, 1986). Golding et al. (1988) have identified a region of the HIV gp41 that is homologous to the MHC class II B-1 domain. Antibodies to the gp41 peptide are found in the sera of some AIDS patients and can bind to the MHC class II-derived peptide.

C. FUNCTIONAL ABNORMALITIES OF T4 CELLS

While long-term infection with HIV is characterized by a reduction in the absolute number of CD4+ cells, functional abnormalities of viable and normal-appearing cells have been noted at all stages of HIV infection. Prior to the discovery of HIV, investigators observed that T4$^+$ cells from AIDS patients were defective in their ability to induce B cells to secrete immunoglobulin and to respond to alloantigens (Lane et al., 1983; Gupta and Safai, 1983; Gupta et al., 1984). It was subsequently shown that lymphocytes of AIDS patients, while responding normally to mitogens, were defective in their ability to recognize and proliferate in response to soluble antigens (Lane et al., 1985; Shearer et al., 1986; Giorgi et al., 1987; Hoy et al., 1988). Abnormal T cell responses to soluble antigen were observed early in the course of HIV infection prior to a significant drop in T4 cell numbers (Lane et al., 1985; Fauci, 1987; Hoy et al., 1988). Studies of T cell responses in identical twins, in which one sibling had AIDS and the other was seronegative and healthy, demonstrated that the defective T cell response to soluble antigen was not due to abnormalities in antigen-presenting cells but was likely due to a functional defect of T4 lymphocytes (Fauci, 1987).

Defective T cell cloning efficiency is another measure of functional impairment of T4 lymphocytes that is observed in HIV infection (Margolick et al., 1985). Winkelstein et al. (1985, 1988) have shown that defective T cell colony formation and impaired expression of interleukin (IL)-2 receptors occurs throughout HIV disease, with a more profound defect apparent at later stages of illness. Other investigators have described a range of immunological defects in HIV-infected individuals, including defective antigen-induced IL-2 production (Antonen and Krohn, 1986), defective mitogen-induced IL-2 production (Creemers et al., 1986; Prince and John, 1987; H. E. Prince et al., 1988), and depressed HLA class I-restricted cytotoxic T lymphocyte (CTL) responses against cytomegalovirus (CMV) and influenza (Sheridan et al., 1984; Shearer et al., 1985; Rook et al., 1985). This latter defect is thought to be due primarily to T4 helper/inducer dysfunction, since *in vitro* CTL activity against CMV can be restored by the addition of IL-2 (Rook et al., 1983).

Suppression of *in vitro* lymphocyte activation of normal T cells has been shown to occur upon exposure to sera from AIDS patients (Cunningham-Rundles et al., 1983; Hennig and Tomar, 1984) or supernatants of peripheral blood mononuclear cells (PBMCs) from AIDS patients (Laurence et al., 1983). The inhibitory activity of AIDS sera occurred even when added several hours after phytohemagglutinin (PHA) stimulation of normal T cells and could be diluted out with normal serum. It is thought that the inhibitory factor(s) causes a decline in IL-2 receptor expression (Donnelly et al., 1987). It has recently been shown that serum-inhibitory factors are also present in HIV-infected individuals at earlier stages of infection, but are found to a greater degree in patients with low CD4 cell counts (Israel-Biet et al., 1988).

The qualitative immunological abnormalities observed in HIV-infected individuals can be mimicked in the *in vitro* situation. A progressive loss of response to soluble antigen prior to cell killing has been shown to occur after *in vitro* infection of T4 cells with HIV (Lyerly et al., 1986). Margolick et al. (1987) have demonstrated a striking inhibition of antigen-specific, lymphoproliferative responses and a lesser inhibition of mitogen-induced responses following noncytopathic exposure of PBMCs to HIV. Inhibition of T lymphocyte proliferative responses has also been demonstrated by exposure to formaldehyde-treated HIV-infected cells (Sandstrom et al., 1986), noninfectious ultraviolet-inactivated HIV (Amadori et al., 1988), purified natural HIV gp120 (Mann et al., 1987), recombinant HIV gp120 (Shalaby et al., 1987; Krowka et al., 1988), and synthetic peptides homologous to regions of gp41 (Chanh et al., 1988). Similarly in other retroviral systems, the immunosuppressive effects of a synthetic peptide (CSK-17) homologous to a region of the transmembrane protein of murine, feline, and HTLV-I and HTLV-II human retroviruses have been well documented (Cianciolo et al., 1985; Harrell et al., 1986; Mitani et al., 1987; Ogasawara et al., 1988).

There are several potential mechanisms to explain how HIV can cause a functional impairment of antigen-responsive T4 cells in the absence of cell infection. In the first case, HIV or its products may interfere with CD4-mediated monocyte–T cell interactions. The interaction of CD4 molecules on the surface of T4 cells with MHC class II molecules on the surface of monocytes is required for antigen-specific responses (Gay et al., 1987, 1988; Doyle and Strominger, 1987). Since the HIV gp120–CD4 interaction occurs with a very high affinity (Dalgleish et al., 1984; Klatzmann et al., 1984a; McDougal et al., 1986), the binding of HIV or free gp120 may prevent the MHC class II molecule from binding to CD4 and thus may block the antigen-specific response. The finding of normal mitogen-specific responses in HIV infection is consistent with this proposed mechanism, since mitogen stimulation is not dependent on the CD4–MHC class II interaction (Fauci, 1987). In addition, Diamond et al. (1988) have recently shown that HIV gp120 can specifically inhibit CD4 function in a murine T cell hybridoma which expresses human CD4.

The binding of HIV or its products to CD4 may also result in a postreceptor signal transduction defect that occurs following ligand binding at either the CD4 or antigen–receptor (CD3–Ti complex) level. In this regard it has been shown that membrane signaling in HIV-infected T cells was impaired when the cells were stimulated via the CD3–Ti complex (Gupta and Vayuvegula, 1987; Linette et al., 1988). Alternatively, some investigators have found a region of homology between HIV gp120 and IL-2 and have suggested that HIV gp120 can bind to the IL-2 receptor and interfere with IL-2 activity either directly or indirectly (Reiher et al., 1986). In support of this hypothesis, Krowka et al. (1988) showed that proliferative responses to CMV were inhibited by recombinant gp120 and that this inhibition could be completely overcome by the addition of IL-2.

A noncytopathic HIV infection of T4 cells may result in functional abnormalities in antigen-specific responses as a consequence of a decrease in CD4 expression on the cell surface. Decreased CD4 levels have been observed in cells infected with HIV *in vitro* (Folks et al., 1985; Hoxie et al., 1985) and are thought to result from several factors, including decreased steady-state levels of CD4-specific mRNA, inhibition of CD4 biosynthesis, reduced levels of immunoprecipitable CD4, and intracellular complexing of CD4 with gp120 (Hoxie et al., 1986; Stevenson et al., 1987; Yuille et al., 1988). A lack of expression of surface CD4 would prohibit the interaction of CD4 and MHC class II molecules that is required for antigen-specific responses.

In addition to decreases in CD4 levels, infection with HIV has been reported to down-regulate other cellular genes including surface T3, T8, and T11 markers, and IL-2 receptor expression (Stevenson et al., 1987). W. C. Greene et al. (personal communication) have also found decreased expression of the IL-2 gene. Down-regulation of IL-2 or IL-2 receptor gene expression may contribute to the functional defects for antigen-specific responses that require IL-2 for amplification.

While HIV or its proteins can convincingly suppress a variety of T4 cell functions, the virus may also have a stimulatory effect on these cells. It has recently been shown that HIV peptides from both the HIV *env* and *gag* regions can induce a substantial proliferative response in PBMCs in both $CD3^+$ and $CD3^-$ lymphocyte subpopulations (Nair et al., 1988). Similarly, other investigators have shown that native gp120 can activate resting $CD4^+$ lymphocytes and induce increased IL-2 receptor expression (Kornfeld et al., 1988). These findings suggest that HIV may suppress immune function by continually activating immune cells, thus making them less responsive to immune signals encountered during normal immune responses.

D. HIV Infection of Monocytes and Macrophages

Monocytes and macrophages are another class of cells that are infected by HIV. Infection may occur through phagocytosis of HIV particles or through attachment to the CD4 receptor that is present on the surface of monocyte/macrophages (Talle et al., 1983; Stewart et al., 1986; Crowe et al., 1987). Researchers have shown that HIV can infect established monocytic and promyelocytic cell lines (Levy et al., 1985a), peripheral blood monocytes (Ho et al., 1986; Nicholson et al., 1986; Gartner et al.,

1986b; Crowe et al., 1987), and alveolar macrophages (Salahuddin et al., 1986). HIV has also been cultured from or detected in monocyte/macrophages from the blood (Ho et al., 1986), lung (Gartner et al., 1986b), and brain (Gartner et al., 1986a,b; Koenig et al., 1986; Wiley et al., 1986; Vazeux et al., 1987) of HIV-infected individuals.

There are several important differences in the outcome of HIV infection of monocyte/macrophages and T4 cells. HIV infection of monocyte/macrophages appears to be persistent and does not result in significant cell death or syncytia formation that occurs after infection of T4 cells (Levy et al., 1985a; Ho et al., 1986; Nicholson et al., 1986; Salahuddin et al., 1986). In HIV-infected macrophages virus particles are often located within cytoplasmic vacuoles (Gartner et al., 1986b). Orenstein et al. (1988) have shown that HIV in infected monocytes predominantly buds and accumulates intracellularly within intracytoplasmic vesicles rather than from the plasma membrane. The relative lack of detectable extracellular reverse transcriptase activity in infected monocyte/macrophage cultures and the increase in such activity after freeze-thawing of the cells supports these findings (Gendelman et al., 1988). It has recently been found that intracellular or extracellular production of HIV is dependent on culture conditions and the state of differentiation of the cells. In differentiated cells of the monocytic lineage HIV replicates predominantly intracellularly; whereas in undifferentiated cells, virus budding occurs predominantly extracellularly (G. Poli, personal communication). If HIV is located within intracytoplasmic vesicles of macrophages *in vivo*, then sheltering from the immune response may occur.

Some investigators have reported that certain isolates of HIV display a specific tropism for monocyte/macrophages or T4 cells. HIV isolated from lung and brain macrophages of infected individuals was shown to infect macrophages more readily than T cells as compared with a standard tissue culture strain, HTLV-IIIb, which showed a markedly lower ability to infect monocyte/macrophages than T cells (Gartner et al., 1986b). HIV that was isolated from infected individuals onto both monocytes and lymphocyte cultures and passaged serially onto the homologous cells appeared to lose the ability to infect the heterologous cell type (Gendelman et al., 1988). It has also been reported that two distinct viruses isolated from the central nervous system of an AIDS patient and passaged in T cells had dissimilar cell tropism. One isolate could infect macrophages, whereas the other isolate infected only gliomas (Koyanagi et al., 1987). Recently, G. Poli (personal communication) has found that HIV from antibody-positive, T cell culture-negative individuals can be isolated onto primary macrophages. It is not clear at present whether certain strains of HIV display an "all-or-none" tropism for specific cells or whether the cell preferences are due to quantitative differences in levels of infectivity. Molecular cloning of HIV isolates with different cell tropisms and more sensitive tests for measuring the presence of virus in infected cells should provide additional information on this issue.

It has long been known that some of the functions of monocyte/macrophages in AIDS patients are abnormal. These defects include reductions in monocyte chemotaxis (Smith et al., 1984; Poli et al., 1985), monocyte-dependent T cell proliferation (Prince et al., 1985; Shannon et al., 1985), Fc receptor function (Bender et al., 1985), and C3 receptor-mediated clearance (Bender et al., 1987). In addition, impairment of certain monocyte/macrophage functions in asymptomatic, HIV-infected individuals has been reported (Braun et al., 1988). However, many of the functions of monocyte/macrophages, such as superoxide anion release, intracellular antimicrobicidal activity, monocyte-mediated tumoricidal activity, candidacidal activity, response to γ-interferon, and production of tumor necrosis factor (TNF), remain unaltered during HIV infection (Poli et al., 1985; Washburn et al., 1985; Murray et al., 1985, 1987; Kleinerman et al., 1985; Estevez et al., 1986; Nielsen et al., 1986; Haas et al., 1987). While IL-1 production and secretion is thought to be normal in AIDS patients (Poli et al., 1985; Enk et al., 1986), inhibitors of IL-1 may be present (Enk et al., 1986). Recently, Locksley et al. (1988) have demonstrated that *in vitro* HIV infection of human monocyte/macrophages results in the release of an IL-1-inhibitory activity.

HIV infection of monocyte/macrophages may also result in a down-regulation of cellular gene function, similar to that seen in the T cell system. In this regard Heagy et al. (1984) reported that monocytes from AIDS patients exhibited decreased expression of human MHC class II antigens. This finding is supported by *in vitro* experiments that showed that expression of human MHC class II antigens on a human promonocytic cell line was reduced following infection with HIV (Petit et al., 1987). However, Haas et al. (1987) found no difference in class II expression in AIDS patients' monocytes versus those of controls.

It has recently been observed that *in vitro* HIV infection of a human monocytic cell line caused a decline in accessory cell function (Petit et al., 1988). However, because of the low frequency of infected monocyte/macrophages in the peripheral blood of HIV-infected individuals (S. Schnittman, personal communication), it is unlikely that the functional defects observed in these cells are due to direct infection of monocyte/macrophages but rather to the deficiency of inductive signals from T cells. This is supported by the fact that the addition of exogenous γ-interferon can correct some of the defects in AIDS patients' monocytes

(Murray et al., 1984). Nonetheless, HIV infection of monocyte/macrophages may play an important role in the pathogenesis of AIDS. The sequestration of the virus within monocytes/macrophages implies that these infected cells may function as a reservoir of virus infection in the body, such as has been described in other lentivirus systems (Gendelman et al., 1985). The relative lack of extracellular budding virus may help explain why the HIV-specific immune response is unsuccessful in ridding the body of HIV. In addition, the infected monocyte/macrophage may be responsible for transporting HIV to the lung or the brain, resulting in neuropsychiatric problems (see Section IV,B, Fig. 5).

E. HIV INFECTION OF PRECURSOR CELLS

Hematological abnormalities, including leukopenia, anemia, thrombocytopenia, and myelodysplasia, have been found in the majority of AIDS patients under study (Spivak et al., 1984; Delacretaz et al., 1987). The myelodysplastic changes in HIV infection appear similar to those found in patients with myelodysplastic syndromes and thus suggest an involvement of hematopoietic progenitor cells in HIV infection (Schneider and Picker, 1985). Several investigators have examined hematopoietic progenitor cells of AIDS patients and have found evidence of defects in these cells. Donahue et al. (1987) reported that bone marrow progenitor cells from patients with AIDS or ARC were responsive to stimulating factors but the growth of the progenitors could be suppressed by anti-HIV antibodies in the serum of HIV-infected individuals. Inhibition of in vitro hematopoietic colony growth in the absence of sera has also been observed (Stella et al., 1987). Analysis of the proliferative capacity of granulocyte-macrophage (GM) progenitor cells from HIV-infected individuals revealed a significant inhibition of growth as compared to controls (Leiderman et al., 1987). In addition, conditioned media from the patient GM cells contained a unique 84-kDa glycoprotein that inhibited colony formation of control GM progenitors.

It has been hypothesized that the hematological abnormalities in AIDS are the result of HIV infection of bone marrow cells. Two studies support this hypothesis indirectly. One study showed that HIV-1 RNA is present in myeloid precursor cells from bone marrow samples of AIDS patients (Busch et al., 1986). The experiments reported by Donahue et al. (1987) (see above) suggest that bone marrow progenitor cells, like monocyte/macrophages, may be infected by HIV and may be resistant to its cytopathic effects. It is assumed that pathological effects occur only when anti-HIV antibody blocks the growth of infected progenitor cells by binding to virus-encoded proteins on the cell surface. Direct evidence for HIV infection of bone marrow progenitor cells was obtained by Folks

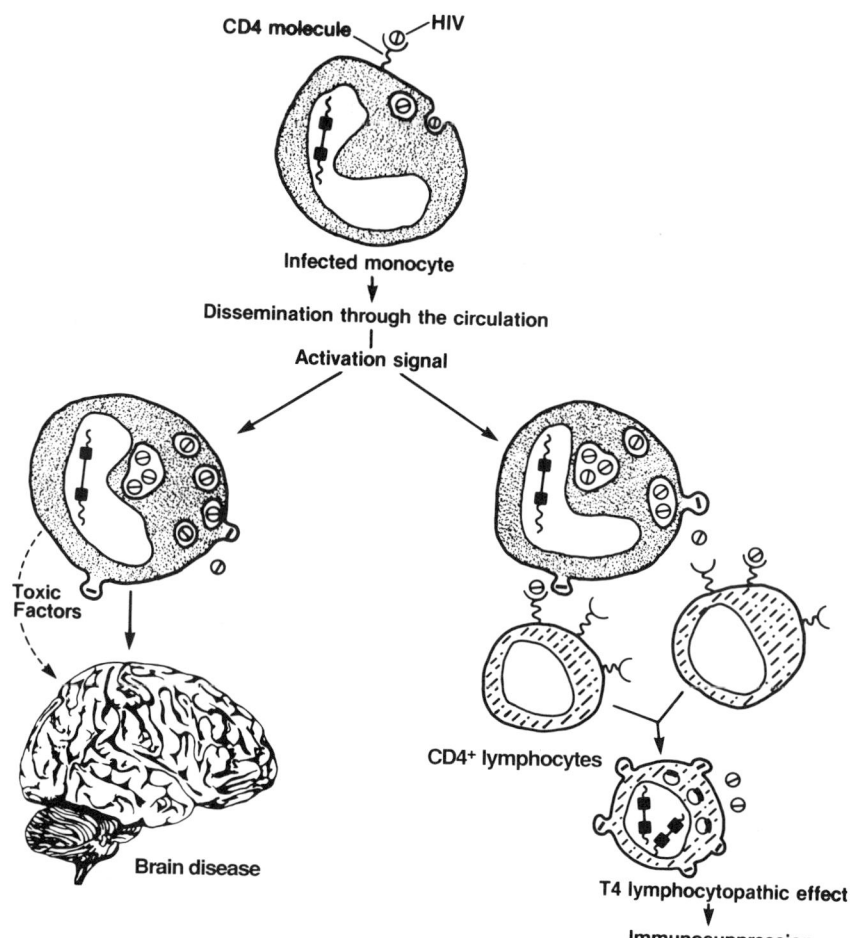

FIG. 5. The role of the monocyte in the propagation of HIV infection. [Reprinted with permission from Fauci, A. S. (1989) *Trans. Assoc. Am. Physicians* **101** (in press).]

et al. (1988b), using a new cell fractionation technique that allowed for the positive selection of virtually pure $CD34^+$ human bone marrow cells. After exposure *in vitro* to HIV-1, these myeloid progenitor cells were shown to be infected with HIV-1 in a manner similar to that seen in infection of monocyte/macrophages. In addition to establishing a noncytopathic infection in the bone marrow precursor cells, HIV was produced predominantly intracellularly, budding within cytoplasmic vesicles rather than from the cell surface. In many cases, the intracytoplasmic vesicles were packed with virions to the point that entire regions of the cytoplasm were displaced with HIV. It is unclear whether HIV infection of bone marrow precursors is responsible for the hematological abnormalities seen *in vivo*. However, these results suggest that the bone marrow may function as a reservoir of HIV infection in the body, differentiating into cells of the monocytoid lineage and spreading HIV throughout the body.

F. HIV Infection of Other Cell Types

The requirement for binding of HIV to the CD4 receptor during the initial stage of virus infection suggests that any cell in the body that expresses the CD4 receptor may be infected by HIV. Expression of CD4 mRNA has been demonstrated not only in T lymphocytes and macrophages but in B cells, neurons, and glial cells (Maddon *et al.*, 1986; Funke *et al.*, 1987). It has been shown that HIV can replicate in both established Epstein-Barr virus (EBV)-transformed (Montagnier *et al.*, 1984; Levy *et al.*, 1985a; Malkovsky *et al.*, 1988) and EBV$^-$ human B cell lines (Monroe *et al.*, 1988). Researchers have also successfully infected CD4$^+$ human colorectal (Adachi *et al.*, 1987) and human glial cell lines (Dewhurst *et al.*, 1987; Malkovsky *et al.*, 1988). Both latent and chronic HIV infections of glioma cell lines have been established with minimal cytopathic effects (Chiodi *et al.*, 1987; Dewhurst *et al.*, 1988). It has also recently been reported that HIV can infect neuroretinal (Pomerantz *et al.*, 1987) and cervical cells (Pomerantz *et al.*, 1988) *in vivo*.

Like monocytes and macrophages, CD4$^+$ epidermal Langerhans cells have been shown to be a target for HIV infection *in vivo* (Tschachler *et al.*, 1987). The observation that Ia$^+$ Langerhans cells are reduced in AIDS and ARC patients suggests that antigen presentation in the skin may be abnormal (Belsito *et al.*, 1984). In this regard, it has recently been reported that there is a negative correlation between the number of Langerhans cells in the epidermis of HIV-infected individuals and the stage of disease (Dreno *et al.*, 1988). Similarly, it has been shown that HIV can infect peripheral blood dendritic cells *in vitro* (Patterson and Knight, 1987). Peripheral blood dendritic cells from patients with AIDS or progressive persistent generalized lymphadenopathy displayed a deficiency in MHC class II antigen expression and in their ability to stimulate lymphocytes (Eales *et al.*, 1988). The precise contribution that these cells and the cells described above play in the pathogenesis of HIV infection remains to be determined.

G. ACTIVATION OF LATENT HIV INFECTION

1. Mitogens and Antigens

One of the hallmarks of HIV infection is the extended period that often elapses between initial infection with HIV and the clinical signs and symptoms of immunological deterioration. Viral replication, as measured by the detection of p24 antigenemia, is thought to occur early in the course of HIV infection and then decline concomitant with the onset of antibody production. Late in the course of disease, p24 antigen levels again rise and are usually sustained through the development of AIDS. However, small, intermittent bursts of p24 antigenemia can occur during the long, asymptomatic period of infection (H. C. Lane, personal communication). It has recently been reported that, in four HIV-infected individuals, the asymptomatic period was accompanied by a loss of p24 antigenemia as well as a loss of HIV-1 antibodies. Analyses of the PBMCs by polymerase chain reaction assays revealed the presence of the HIV-1 provirus in all four individuals in the absence of either virus or antibody production (Farzadegan et al., 1988). These studies suggest that the virus exists in vivo in either a true microbiologically latent form in which no virus expression can be detected or in a clinically latent form in which virus expression occurs at chronic, low levels (Rosenberg and Fauci, 1989) (Fig. 6).

A wide range of in vitro experiments have revealed several ways that latent or chronic, low-level HIV-infected cells can be activated to produce increased quantities of virus. The first successful attempts to isolate HIV from the blood of AIDS patients demonstrated that several different T cell activation signals, including PHA and IL-2 (Gallo et al., 1984; Levy et al., 1984; Barré-Sinoussi et al., 1985), were needed to boost virus replication to levels that were detectable by reverse transcriptase activity. PHA was also able to activate virus expression in long-term, non-HIV-producing T cell cultures from AIDS patients (Zagury et al., 1986). Similarly, augmentation of HIV expression in cell lines that were infected with HIV in vitro was observed following exposure of the cells to either 5-iodo-2′-deoxyuridine (Folks et al., 1986a,c) or 12-O-tetradecanoyl-phorbol-13-acetate (TPA) (Harada et al., 1986). Mitogenic activation signals also enhance HIV productivity in de novo infections of normal human lymphocytes in vitro (McDougal et al., 1985; Folks et al., 1986b). In this regard, a regulatory protein, rpt-1, that is selectively expressed in resting T4 cells, has recently been shown to down-regulate expression of the HIV LTR as well as the promoter region of the IL-2 receptor α chain (Patarca et al., 1988). Activation of resting T cells may thus

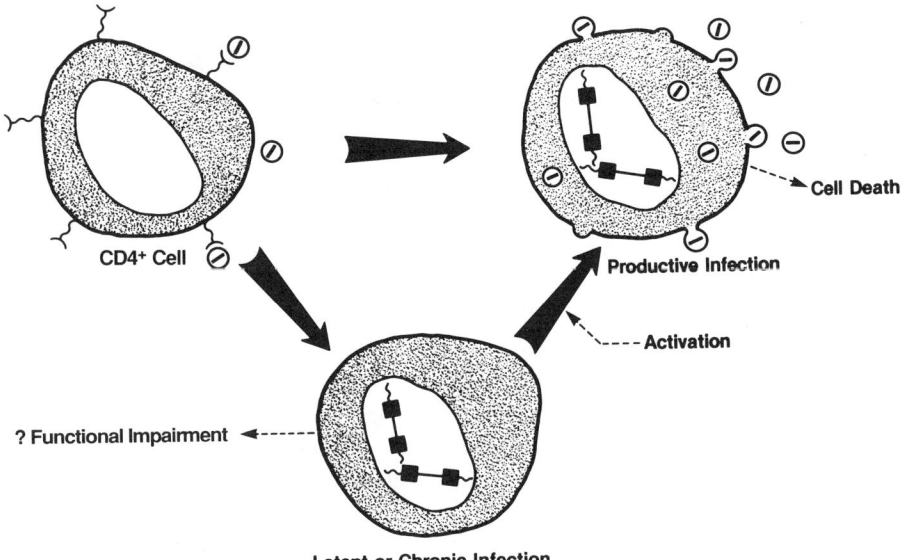

FIG. 6. HIV infection of CD4+ cells: conversion of latent to active infection. [Reprinted with permission from Fauci, A. S. (1989). *Adv. Allerg. Clin. Immunol.* (in press).]

result in suppression of rpt-1 and subsequent alleviation of the suppression of HIV expression.

To delineate the mechanism by which activating agents up-regulate HIV activity, investigators have examined the effects of these agents on the ability of the HIV LTR to regulate expression of an indicator gene, the chloramphenicol acetyltransferase (CAT) gene. These experiments have demonstrated that PMA- and PHA-induced up-regulation of HIV occurs by the induction of T cell activation factors that interact with two tandemly repeated core transcriptional enhancer elements on the HIV LTR (Nabel and Baltimore, 1987; Kaufman *et al.*, 1987; Tong-Starksen *et al.*, 1987; Siekevitz *et al.*, 1987; Dinter *et al.*, 1987). Further analyses have revealed that a T cell activation factor, NF$\varkappa$B (Nabel and Baltimore, 1987), binds to an upstream NF$\varkappa$B binding site and can activate *in vitro* transcription of the HIV promoter (Kawakami *et al.*, 1988). Another mitogen-inducible nuclear protein, HIVEN86A, has been shown to bind to both the HIV enhancer (Franza *et al.*, 1987) and related sequences in the 5'-regulatory region of the IL-2 receptor α gene (Bohnlein *et al.*, 1988).

Antigenic stimulation of T cells has also been shown to affect HIV expression. Using PBMCs from HIV⁻ donors, HIV was observed to replicate ten to 100 times more efficiently in those PBMCs that had been activated prior to infection by either tetanus toxoid or keyhole limpet hemocyanin (Margolick et al., 1987). Similarly, HIV has been shown to replicate to higher titer in peripheral blood leukocytes that had been stimulated prior to infection with noninfectious HTLV-I virions. An increase in HIV expression was also detected if the cells were exposed to HTLV-I antigens either during or after HIV infection (Zack et al., 1988).

2. Heterologous Viruses

One class of antigens that individuals often encounter *in vivo* are viral proteins from a wide range of human pathogens. AIDS patients in particular are often coinfected with herpesviruses, especially herpes simplex virus (HSV), CMV, and EBV (Quinnan et al., 1984; Quinn et al., 1987). It has been shown by a number of investigators that *in vitro* cotransfection of plasmids containing the immediate-early genes of HSV-1, CMV, and EBV, together with HIV LTR–CAT constructs, into a variety of cell types resulted in up-regulation of CAT expression (Gendelman et al., 1986; Rando et al., 1987; Davis et al., 1987; Kenney et al., 1988). Infection of cells transfected with HIV LTR–CAT constructs with HSV-1 also caused an increase in CAT activity (Mosca et al., 1987a).

These experiments suggest that heterologous viral genes can upregulate HIV expression in HIV-infected cells. This theory is supported by data by Ostrove et al. (1987) that show an increase in reverse transcriptase activity in the supernatant of cells that were cotransfected with an infectious clone of HIV and immediate-early genes of HSV-1. The relevance of this theory *in vivo*, however, depends on whether HIV and the heterologous virus can infect the same cell. In this regard, it has been shown that HSV can replicate in the major target cells for HIV infection: peripheral blood leukocytes (Nahmias et al., 1964; Rinaldo et al., 1978) and undifferentiated monocytes and macrophages (Kirchner, 1982). Coinfection of brain cells by CMV and HIV has also been reported *in vivo* in AIDS patients (Nelson et al., 1988). Another virus with a cell tropism similar to HIV is hepatitis B virus (HBV). It has recently been established that the HBV X protein can *trans*-activate the HIV LTR and cause a tenfold increase in CAT activity (Seto et al., 1988). A new member of the human herpesvirus family, HHV-6, has also been found to infect $CD4^+$ lymphocytes (Lusso et al., 1988b) and has been shown to stimulate expression of the HIV LTR (Lusso et al., 1989).

The mechanism of action of heterologous viral genes on the HIV LTR has been explored using deletion mutant analyses. Some researchers have presented evidence that the site on the HIV LTR that is involved in HSV-1-induced activation encompasses the three Sp1 transcription factor binding sites and does not include the *tat* responsive region, TAR (Mosca *et al.*, 1987b; Ostrove *et al.*, 1987). In contrast, other investigators have shown that HSV-1 may function by inducing a DNA-binding protein that binds to the NF$\varkappa$B core enhancer sequence (Gimble *et al.*, 1988). However, Nabel *et al.* (1988) suggest that HSV-1 early gene activation occurs independently of any specific site on the HIV LTR. In studies of adenovirus-induced activation of HIV, they found that the TATA sequences of HIV appear to be important. The HBV X protein appears to exert its effect through *cis*-acting elements in the upstream, enhancer, and TAR regions, which, in these experiments, are all required for *trans*-activation of the HIV LTR (Seto *et al.*, 1988).

In addition to a direct effect of heterologous viral proteins on several distinct regions of the HIV LTR, heterologous viruses may also activate HIV expression by causing a stress response in the HIV-infected cell. Valerie *et al.* (1988) have recently demonstrated that ultraviolet (UV) light and mitomycin C, agents which are known to cause stress responses in cells, can independently up-regulate CAT activity in cells transfected with an HIV LTR-CAT construct. Pretreatment of human T cell lines with UV light prior to HIV infection resulted in significantly earlier detection of virus as compared to the untreated controls. The authors also showed that exposure of HIV LTR-CAT-transfected cells to sunlight resulted in an increase in CAT activity. UV light activation of HIV expression in latently infected promonocytic cells has recently been shown by Stanley *et al.* (1989). Since activation of HIV expression in these cells occurred with UV light doses that reduced cell viability and impaired cell growth, the authors suggest that activation of virus expression results from the triggering of a cellular "SOS" repair response. Heat shock with exposure of chronically infected cell lines to temperatures of 41.3° C also resulted in induction of HIV expression (S. Stanley, personal communication).

3. Cytokines

Cytokines are another class of activating agents that may play an important role in stimulating a latent or low-level chronic HIV infection to productivity. Exposure of a chronically HIV-infected promonocytic cell line, U1 (Folks *et al.*, 1988a), to a PHA-induced supernatant containing multiple cytokines or to recombinant GM colony-stimulating factor (GMCSF) induced the cells to produce significantly higher levels of HIV than unexposed cells (Folks *et al.*, 1987). Induction of HIV expression by GMCSF and other cytokines has also been shown in acute

HIV infection of primary peripheral blood monocytes (Koyanagi et al., 1988). Similarly, Clouse et al. (1989a) have found that monokine-enriched, bacterial lipopolysaccharide (LPS)-induced supernatants from monocyte/macrophages were able to up-regulate virus expression in ACH-2 cells, a chronically HIV-infected T cell clone derived from A3.01 cells (Folks et al., 1985). It has also recently been found that supernatants from viral antigen-stimulated monocytes can induce HIV expression in both U1 and ACH-2 cells (Clouse et al., 1989b).

There is growing evidence that TNF-α, a monocyte-derived cytokine, may play an important role in the pathogenesis of HIV infection. Clouse et al. (1989a) have shown that the ability of LPS-induced monocyte supernatant to increase HIV expression can be completely eliminated by passing the supernatant over immunoaffinity gels specific for human TNF-α. Recent data by Folks et al. (1989) show that recombinant TNF-α and TNF-β can significantly augment HIV expression in ACH-2 cells, whereas a multitude of other cytokines, including IL-1, IL-2, IL-3, IL-4, platelet-derived growth factor, and γ-interferon, had little effect on HIV expression. Other HIV-infected cells that respond to TNF-α and TNF-β by increasing virus expression include U1 cells (G. Poli, personal communication) and MOLT-4 cells (Matsuyama et al., 1988), respectively. Increases in CAT activity were observed after TNF-α exposure of ACH-2 cells transfected with either HIV LTR–CAT alone or in combination with HIV tat, but not with HTLV-I LTR–CAT (Folks et al., 1989). Although the precise mechanism by which TNF-α influences HIV expression is not known, it appears to function by inducing the expression of specific DNA-binding proteins that bind to the NF$\varkappa$B sites on the HIV LTR (A. Rabson, personal communication).

The significance of TNF-α in the regulation of virus expression during HIV infection is unclear at present. However, it is known that TNF-α is produced in humans in response to naturally occurring infections (Cerami and Beutler, 1988). AIDS patients, in particular, have been shown to express high levels of TNF-α (>150 pg/ml) in their sera, whereas asymptomatic HIV-infected subjects expressed levels of TNF that were similar to normal controls (Lahdevirta et al., 1988). In vitro, concentrations of TNF-α as low as 50 pg/ml have been shown to up-regulate HIV expression in a chronically infected T cell line. In addition, these HIV-infected cells displayed a higher number of TNF receptors than did their uninfected counterparts, suggesting that HIV-infected cells may be more sensitive to TNF-α than are uninfected cells (Folks et al., 1989).

While exposure of uninfected promonocytic U937 cells to PMA results in a significant decrease in TNF receptors (Aggarwal and Eessalu, 1987), it has recently been shown that HIV-infected U1 cells exposed to PMA produce increased levels of TNF-α and TNF receptors. Addition of TNF-α to the PMA-stimulated U1 cells resulted in a synergistic increase of TNF-α secretion (G. Poli, personal communication). Although one report has shown that PBMCs from patients with AIDS or ARC are deficient in TNF production (Ammann et al., 1987), another study found that peripheral blood monocytes from AIDS patients spontaneously secreted high levels of TNF-α as compared to normal controls (Wright et al., 1988). Thus TNF-α production in response to opportunistic infections could accelerate the progression of HIV disease in symptomatic individuals in an autocrine/paracrine fashion. Since TNF-α is also known to function in the normal regulation of immune responses (Ruggiero et al., 1986; Kehrl et al., 1987), it may play a role in the gradual progression of HIV disease prior to the onset of opportunistic infection. The recent finding of TNF-α in the cerebrospinal fluid of patients with bacterial meningitis suggests that TNF-α may also up-regulate HIV expression in the brain (see Section IV,B) (Leist et al., 1988). Most recently, it has been demonstrated that IL-6 can induce HIV expression in chronically infected U1 cells and that IL-6 and GMCSF synergize with TNF-α in the induction of HIV expression in this cell line (G. Poli, personal communication).

IV. Neuropsychiatric Manifestations

A. HIV Infection of the Brain

Early in the course of the AIDS epidemic, it was noted that neurological complications were commonly found in AIDS patients and fell into several different categories including opportunistic diseases, such as toxoplasmosis, cryptococcal meningitis, or CMV encephalitis; CNS tumors; vascular problems; and undiagnosed CNS abnormalities (subacute encephalitis) (Snider et al., 1983). This latter category, also known as AIDS encephalopathy (Shaw et al., 1985) or AIDS–dementia complex, is found in approximately two thirds of AIDS patients who were examined neuropathologically at autopsy (Navia et al., 1986). In some cases symptoms of the AIDS–dementia complex may precede the development of opportunistic infections or may occur in the total absence of such infections (Navia and Price, 1987).

Evidence for HIV infection of the brain and CNS comes from a variety of studies. HIV DNA and HIV-specific RNA have been detected in the brains of both adult and pediatric AIDS cases (Shaw et al., 1985; Stoler et al., 1986). In addition, infectious HIV has been isolated from both the cerebrospinal fluid and the brain tissue of AIDS patients (Levy et al.,

1985b; Ho et al., 1985b; Gartner et al. 1986a). While some investigators have reported HIV infection *in vivo* in capillary endothelial cells (Wiley et al., 1986), oligodendroglial cells, and astrocytes (Epstein et al., 1984; Stoler et al., 1986; Gyorkey et al., 1987) as well as macrophages, it is generally thought that the predominant cell type in the brain that is infected with HIV is the macrophage (Koenig et al., 1986; Gabuzda et al., 1986; Gartner et al., 1986a; Vazeux et al., 1987; Meyenhofer et al., 1987).

Additional evidence for HIV infection of the brain comes from studies that demonstrate the synthesis of HIV-specific antibodies and antigens within the brain and their appearance in the cerebrospinal fluid of AIDS and ARC patients as well as in asymptomatically infected individuals (Resnick et al., 1985; Goudsmit et al., 1986, 1987; Gallo et al., 1988). HIV has also been isolated from the cerebrospinal fluid of asymptomatic individuals (Hollander and Levy, 1987; Resnick et al., 1988; Chiodi et al., 1988), suggesting that HIV can infect the CNS early in the course of disease and exist as a latent or chronic infection before the onset of neurological abnormalities.

B. Potential Mechanisms of Neuropathogenesis

The cause(s) of the neurological pathology in HIV infection is not known. Because the macrophage is most frequently found to be infected in the brain, it is thought that this cell plays an instrumental role in the neuropathogenesis of HIV infection through the release of cytokines or other factors that are either directly toxic to neurons or lead to inflammation (Fauci, 1988; Price et al., 1988). In this regard, it has recently been shown that neuropeptides can induce the release of IL-1, TNF-α, and IL-6 from human blood monocytes (Lotz et al., 1988). Based on the findings that TNF-α may function as an autocrine inducer of HIV expression (see Section III,G,3), it is possible that the release of TNF-α from HIV-infected macrophages results not only in damage to nearby cells but in an activation of HIV expression as well. HIV may also directly or indirectly stimulate astrocytes to produce cytotoxic factors similar to TNF-α (Robbins et al., 1987).

HIV may also cause brain cell abnormalities by interfering with the binding of neurotrophic factors. Preliminary data suggest that both HIV and SIV can inhibit the growth of sensory neurons in the presence of neuroleukin, a neurotropic factor for spinal and sensory neurons, but not in the presence of nerve growth factor (Lee et al., 1987). The inhibitory activity of HIV is thought to be due to gp120, which displays regions of sequence homology with neuroleukin. Similarly, it has recently been reported that gp120 can cause neuronal cell death by interfering with a neuropeptide transmitter, vasoactive intestinal peptide (Brenneman et al., 1988).

Another mechanism of HIV-induced neuropathology involves the upregulation of HIV expression by heterologous viruses (discussed in Section III,G,2). As previously mentioned, HIV and CMV have been reported to infect the same cells in the brain in AIDS patients (Nelson *et al.*, 1988) and thus may interact and enhance the pathogenesis of either virus. Autoimmune phenomena may also be responsible for some of the nervous system lesions associated with HIV (Johnson *et al.*, 1988). Finally, while direct evidence of HIV infection of neuronal cells has been lacking, the presence of CD4 message in neuronal cells (Funke *et al.*, 1987) raises the possibility that, under certain circumstances, HIV can directly infect neural tissue and potentially result in functional abnormalities or cell death. The case for direct HIV-induced cytopathicity in the brain is not supported by the finding that four of five HIV isolates from the brain were noncytocidal to T4 cells (Anand *et al.*, 1987).

V. Immune Response to HIV

While the nature of a protective immune response to HIV, or indeed its very existence, is currently unknown, substantial progress has been made in defining the various virus-specific humoral and cell-mediated responses. As discussed above, potentially deleterious immune responses in the form of HIV-specific antibody-dependent cellular cytotoxicity, anti-gp120-specific $CD4^+$ T cell killing, and autoantibodies have been implicated in the pathogenesis of HIV infection. However, it is presumed that the immune response against HIV may also influence the course of the disease in a beneficial way.

A. Humoral Response to HIV

1. General Characteristics

The existence of antibodies to HIV was noted early in the AIDS epidemic (Safai *et al.*, 1984; Brun-Vezinet *et al.*, 1984; Cheingsong-Popov *et al.*, 1984), and testing for such antibodies constitutes the basis for the HIV enzyme-linked immunosorbent assay. It was subsequently shown that the viral gp120 and gp160 env glycoproteins were the major proteins recognized by HIV-infected individuals at all stages of infection (Barin *et al.*, 1985; Allan *et al.*, 1985). Further studies show that approximately 50% of HIV-infected individuals produce nonneutralizing antibodies to a highly conserved, 15-amino acid region (504–518) of the carboxy terminus of gp120 (Palker *et al.*, 1987). Antibodies to the p24 core structural protein and to the gp41 transmembrane portion of the envelope have also been detected (Kalyanaraman *et al.*, 1984; Groopman *et al.*, 1986; Wang *et al.*, 1986). It has been shown that 100% of

HIV-infected individuals recognize a 12-amino acid immunodominant sequence (598–609) in gp41 (Gnann et al., 1987).

While a few investigators have reported that antibody levels to all HIV proteins either remain constant or decline as the disease progresses (Groopman et al., 1986; McDougal et al., 1987), the majority of studies suggest that the titer of antibodies to p24 are highest early in HIV infection and lowest at late stages of disease (Schupbach et al., 1985; Biggar et al., 1985; Lange et al., 1986; Pan et al., 1987; Cao et al., 1987; de Wolf et al., 1988), even in the presence of high levels of anti-env reactivity (Kenealy et al., 1987). This pattern was also observed in serial bleeds from the same individuals (Weber et al., 1987; Manca et al., 1987). It has been hypothesized that the decline in anti-p24 antibodies is due to an excess production of HIV core protein (Lange and Goudsmit, 1987).

An association between the presence of another anti-HIV antibody and asymptomatic disease has recently been shown by Klasse et al. (1988). They reported that antibodies to a portion of gp41 that shares sequence similarity to immunosuppressive peptides from the transmembrane proteins of other retroviruses were present in the majority of sera from healthy HIV-infected individuals and absent in sera from symptomatic patients. Similarly, antibodies to the HIV reverse transcriptase have been detected in infected individuals (Pan et al., 1987), have been shown to inhibit reverse transcriptase activity, and were negatively correlated with disease progression (Chatterjee et al., 1987; Laurence et al., 1987). Serial antibody tests performed on hemophiliacs for whom the date of initial seroconversion was known demonstrated that a decline in anti-gag or anti-pol antibodies precedes the development of AIDS by 1–4 years, as compared with non-AIDS cases (Ragni et al., 1988). It has also been shown that HIV can be more readily isolated from individuals who lack antibody to reverse transcriptase than from those who do not (Sano et al., 1987). In addition to antibody responses to HIV structural proteins, sera from some infected individuals have been shown to contain antibodies to HIV-regulatory proteins (Barone et al., 1986; Franchini et al., 1987b; Ranki et al., 1987; Strebel et al., 1988). It has been suggested that antibodies to rev appear most frequently in early symptomatic patients (Chanda et al., 1988).

The antibody isotypes that are produced against HIV vary according to the specific protein and the route of infection. IgG_1 appears to be the major isotype that is produced in response to HIV (Sundqvist et al., 1986; Klasse and Blomberg, 1987; Ljunggren et al., 1988a). Khalife et al. (1988) have shown that the antibody response to env is restricted to the IgG_1 subclass, whereas the response to gag and nef proteins includes IgG_1, IgM, IgA, and, in the case of gag, IgG_3. They also found that IgG_4 and IgE were present only in infected hemophiliacs.

2. Neutralizing Antibodies

Within the spectrum of antibodies that are produced against HIV, low titers of neutralizing antibodies have been detected in HIV-infected individuals (Robert-Guroff *et al.*, 1985; Weiss *et al.*, 1985; Ho *et al.*, 1985a). While several studies have found no significant correlation between neutralizing antibody titers and clinical status (Weber *et al.*, 1987; Prince *et al.*, 1987; Groopman *et al.*, 1987), other investigators have reported that neutralizing antibody titers are highest in HIV-infected individuals who are asymptomatic, as compared with those diagnosed with AIDS (Robert-Guroff *et al.*, 1985; Ho *et al.*, 1987b). Several studies have found that an increase in neutralization titers over time is associated with a stable clinical course (Wendler *et al.*, 1987; Ranki *et al.*, 1987) and that a decrease in neutralization titers was indicative of disease progression (Robert-Guroff *et al.*, 1988; Sei *et al.*, 1988).

Experimental stimulation of neutralizing antibodies to HIV was first achieved by inoculation of animals with either genetically engineered or purified natural gp120 (Lasky *et al.*, 1986; Robey *et al.*, 1986). Deglycosylated recombinant gp120 was also able to elicit neutralizing antibodies (Putney *et al.*, 1986; Krohn *et al.*, 1987). While it has been reported that the HIV p17 core protein may be a target for neutralizing antibodies (Sarin *et al.*, 1986), Matthews *et al.* (1986) have found that HIV-specific neutralizing antibodies react predominantly with the env glycoprotein, similar to that observed in other retroviral systems. It has also been demonstrated that antibodies to the immunodominant epitope of gp41 described in Section V,A,1 have neutralizing activity (Schrier *et al.*, 1988).

The gp120-specific neutralizing antibodies appear to be type specific in goats immunized with either recombinant or purified viral gp120 (Matthews *et al.*, 1986; Rusche *et al.*, 1987). However, group-specific neutralizing antibodies have been detected in human sera from HIV-infected individuals (Matthews *et al.*, 1986; Weiss *et al.*, 1986). Serological analyses of HIV-infected chimpanzees have shown that the neutralizing antibody response broadened over time to be group specific (Nara *et al.*, 1987a; Goudsmit *et al.*, 1988). However, no group-specific reactivity was seen after repeated immunizations of goats, horses, or chimpanzees with purified gp120 (Arthur *et al.*, 1987; Nara *et al.*, 1988).

Considerable effort has been devoted to identifying the type- and group-specific determinants for neutralization. Both humans and animals have been shown to generate type-specific neutralizing antibodies to a region of gp120 that encompasses amino acids 303–231, 307–330, and 296–331 (Palker *et al.*, 1988; Matsushita *et al.*, 1988; Goudsmit *et al.*, 1988). Type-specific neutralization of variants of a single isolate of HIV that differed by one amino acid at position 305 of gp120 has also been shown to occur (Looney et al., 1988). Neutralizing antibodies to this type-specific region do not inhibit gp120–CD4 binding (Skinner et al., 1988) and presumably interfere with HIV replication at a postreceptor binding stage.

Several studies have shown that type-specific antibodies that inhibit cell fusion are made in animals immunized with glycosylated gp120 (Putney et al., 1986; Rusche et al., 1987) or infected with HIV (Goudsmit et al., 1988). It has recently been shown that the target for fusion-blocking antibodies is the same as that for neutralizing antibodies, namely amino acids 307–330 of the env glycoprotein (Matsushita et al., 1988; Rusche et al., 1988). Since HIV can be transmitted by cell-to-cell fusion, the presence of antibodies that can block cell fusion is necessary for the control of the spread of HIV in vivo.

Whether neutralizing or fusion-blocking antibodies can inhibit HIV infection in vivo is the subject of considerable debate. The rapid mutations that occur in the HIV genome during replication (see Section II,C,2) may result in the creation of new viral strains that can escape neutralization. In fact, the very presence of neutralizing antibodies has been shown to select for HIV variants in vitro (Robert-Guroff et al., 1986) and for other lentiviruses in vivo (Montelaro et al., 1984). Other drawbacks in relying on neutralizing antibodies as the main line of defense against HIV infection have been seen in two experiments with chimpanzees. The presence of neutralizing antibodies in chimpanzees immunized with recombinant gp120 did not afford protection from subsequent challenge with HIV (Berman et al., 1988). Similarly, chimpanzees passively immunized with HIV immunoglobulin became infected after inoculation with HIV (A. M. Prince et al., 1988).

However, a recent study has shown that passive immunization of AIDS or ARC patients with pooled, high-titered plasma from healthy HIV-infected individuals resulted in the sustained elimination of p24 antigen in these patients (Karpas et al., 1988). At the same time, viral antibody titers increased to levels higher than expected from the immunization. Clearly, further research on the role of neutralizing antibodies in the prevention of HIV infection and disease progression is necessary, particularly for the development of an effective vaccine against HIV. In this regard, it has recently been reported that vaccination of HIV$^-$ volunteers with a vaccinia–env recombinant virus boosted with autologous, killed HIV-infected cells and recombinant gp160 resulted in the generation of high levels of group-specific neutralizing antibodies (Zagury et al., 1988).

3. ADCC

ADCC has been shown to play an important role in the control of several viral infections, including CMV infection in humans (Quinnan et al., 1982) and retroviral diseases in cats (de Noronha et al., 1978). Several investigators have reported that sera from HIV-infected individuals can mediate ADCC activity *in vitro*. When compared to healthy seropositive individuals, AIDS patients have been shown to have lower titers of ADCC antibodies (Rook et al., 1987; Ojo-Amaize et al., 1987; Ljunggren et al., 1987). While ADCC antibodies occur most often in the presence of neutralizing antibodies, no correlation in titers of these two antibody categories was found (Bottiger et al., 1988). Antibodies that mediate ADCC have been shown to react with target cells chronically infected with three divergent strains of HIV in a group-specific manner (Lyerly et al., 1987b). Several investigators have shown that the principal target for ADCC reactivity is gp120 (Lyerly et al., 1987b; Shepp et al., 1988). The transmembrane glycoprotein, gp41, has also been implicated as a target for ADCC (Blumberg et al., 1987).

Group-specific antibody-mediated complement-dependent cytotoxicity (ACC) of HIV-infected cells was observed in experimentally inoculated chimpanzees (Nara et al., 1987a) and correlated closely with the induction of neutralizing antibodies (Nara et al., 1987b). HIV-infected humans, on the other hand, exhibited no ACC, even in the presence of high-titered, group-specific neutralizing antibodies (Nara et al., 1987b). It is possible that the presence of ACC in HIV-infected chimpanzees is related to their apparent resistance to disease development after years of chronic HIV infection.

B. Cellular Responses to HIV

1. T Cell-Proliferative Responses

In many viral infections, T cell immunity plays a major role in eliminating virus-infected cells and in eliciting a memory antibody response. Group-specific T cell proliferation to gp120 and three different HIV isolates has been observed in goats immunized with native gp120 but not with deglycosylated proteins, and in chimpanzees and gibbon apes chronically infected with HIV (Krohn et al., 1987; Zarling et al., 1987; Lusso et al., 1988a). The infected apes also responded to recombinant gp160; purified, native p24; and a highly conserved region of gp120 (Lusso et al., 1988a). HIV-infected chimpanzees were shown to have strong T cell-proliferative responses to intact, purified HIV as well as natural gp120, recombinant gp120 and gp41, and p24 (Eichberg et al., 1987).

T cell-proliferative responses to HIV antigens have been reported in

HIV-infected individuals. One study detected responses in only nine of 40 subjects, responses being higher for asymptomatically HIV-infected patients than for diseased individuals (Wahren et al., 1987). A second study demonstrated that between 50 and 70% of HIV-infected individuals at all stages of infection responded to HIV antigens (Reddy et al., 1987). Whereas Krohn et al. (1987) have reported that no T cell-proliferative responses to gp120 were seen in HIV-infected people, other investigators have found that T cells from HIV-infected individuals display significant lymphocyte blastogenesis in response to p24 and gp120 (Wahren et al., 1987; Ahearne et al., 1988). Some of the discrepancy in these findings may result from the wide range of antigenic preparations used in the experiments.

It appears that a significant discordance exists between the antigenic regions of HIV that elicit neutralizing antibody and cellular responses, since it was shown that only the amino terminus of gp120 induced T cell-proliferative responses (Ahearne et al., 1988). These data have been confirmed through the isolation of two type-specific helper T cell clones specific for the amino-terminal half of gp120 (C. M. Walker et al., 1988). Although Ahearne et al. (1988) did not detect proliferative responses to gp41 or the carboxy terminus of gp120, it has been reported that T cells from approximately one quarter of HIV-infected patients undergo proliferation in response to an immunodominant epitope of gp41 (Schrier et al., 1988).

Since a vaccine that invokes both cellular and humoral responses will have a greater chance of affording protection from viral infection, researchers have been studying those regions of HIV that can elicit T cell responses. Using computer analyses, Cease et al. (1987) have identified two conserved regions of gp120 that, when injected into mice, resulted in the induction of lymph node proliferation to intact gp120. It was subsequently shown that approximately 60% of healthy volunteers who had been immunized with a vaccinia–*env* recombinant virus manifested a T cell-proliferative response to at least one of the peptides from these regions (Berzofsky et al., 1988).

2. Cell-Mediated Cytotoxicity

Along with neutralizing antibodies, ADCC, and ACC, virus-specific cytotoxic T lymphocytes (CTLs) are an important component of the immune response against viral infections. In animal models MHC-restricted cytotoxic responses were shown to be present in both gibbon apes and chimpanzees who had been chronically infected with HIV (Lusso et al., 1988a; Zarling et al., 1987). In mice CTL responses are directed primarily to a single immunodominant epitope on gp160 in conjunction with only one of four MHC class I molecules tested (Takahashi et al., 1988).

MHC-restricted HIV-specific CTLs have been detected in the peripheral blood, lungs, and cerebrospinal fluid of HIV-infected individuals (Walker et al., 1987; Plata et al., 1987; Sethi et al., 1988). Circulating CTLs were shown to be capable of killing env-, gag-, and pol-expressing target cells (B. D. Walker et al., 1987, 1988; Langlade-Demoyen et al., 1988; Nixon et al., 1988). A recent study has found that cloned CTLs can lyse cells expressing HIV reverse transcriptase as well as env proteins from highly divergent HIVs, suggesting that the epitope on gp120 that is recognized by CTLs is conserved (Koenig et al., 1988). This latter study also found that some of the CTL activity was non-MHC restricted.

CMC by non-T effector cells has been described in HIV-infected patients (Ruscetti et al., 1986), the highest levels of CMC occurring in asymptomatic seropositive individuals (Weinhold et al., 1988). The non-MHC-restricted CMC is effected by $CD16^+$ natural killer (NK) cells, directed at gp120-coated target cells, and augmented in the presence of IL-2. NK cell-mediated CMC against HIV has also been observed in unfractionated cells from both HIV-infected and uninfected individuals in the presence of IL-2 (Rook et al., 1985). The delineation of the role of both MHC-restricted and unrestricted CMC responses in the prevention of initial infection with HIV or in the progression of HIV-induced disease awaits further study.

3. Other Cellular Responses to HIV

Suppression of HIV replication by $CD8^+$ lymphocytes has been reported by Walker et al. (1986). They found that HIV reverse transcriptase activity substantially increased when $CD8^+$ cells were removed from cultured PBMCs from HIV-infected individuals. The addition of autologous $CD8^+$ cells suppressed both initial and ongoing virus replication in a dose-dependent manner and did not appear to act via a cytolytic mechanism.

VI. Summary and Conclusions

The successful control of HIV infection through either therapeutic agents or vaccines requires an extensive understanding of the agent itself and its pathogenesis. The fact that HIV is a member of the lentivirus subfamily of viruses was an immediate clue that the natural history of HIV infection would entail a lengthy latent period and disease progression, despite the generation of an immune response. Investigators have now characterized nine genes of HIV, including six regulatory genes which are thought to play an important role in the regulation of virus expression. The finding that the CD4 molecule is the receptor for HIV was instrumental in the recognition of the cell types, particularly T4 lymphocytes and monocyte/macrophages, that are infected by HIV *in vivo*. The rapid variation in the HIV genome that occurs during virus replication may impact on the ability of the virus to escape immune surveillance as well as the apparent differences in isolate specific cell tropism.

Although the exact processes by which HIV causes immunosuppression, neurological abnormalities, and other clinical manifestations are not known, it is clear that HIV can either kill T4 lymphocytes or render the cells functionally incompetent. Many studies have shown that the immunological abnormalities observed in HIV infection are not due solely to a depletion in $CD4^+$ cells but to interference with the proper functioning of these cells as a result of virus binding to CD4 or through down-regulation of cellular gene function. Since the $CD4^+$ T helper/inducer cell interacts with a myriad of other immune cells during the normal immune response, quantitative or qualitative changes in the T4 cell population have a pervasive effect on the immune system as a whole. Other cell types, such as monocyte/macrophages, bone marrow precursor cells, and Langerhans cells, may play an important part in the pathogenesis of HIV infection by functioning as reservoirs of HIV in the body and by infecting T4 cells during immune interactions.

The question of why infection with HIV results in a long and variable asymptomatic period has not yet been adequately answered. Clearly, suppression or activation of viral regulatory genes is involved in HIV expression. Agents that have been shown to up-regulate HIV expression include mitogens, specific antigens, heterologous viruses, and cytokines that are invoked during normal human immune responses. Cytokines, mitogens, and heterologous viral genes have all been shown to up-regulate HIV expression via a *trans*-activating mechanism that acts on the HIV promoter sequences and is mediated by the binding of specific DNA-binding proteins to the HIV LTR. Five separate cellular protein-binding regions of the HIV LTR have been identified, implying that up-regulation of HIV expression may occur through several distinct mechanisms (Garcia *et al.*, 1987). Activating agents may also up-regulate HIV expression by demethylating LTR enhancer sequences (Bednarik *et al.*, 1987). At the same time that agents may be activating HIV expression, HIV infection may be affecting cellular gene expression (Fig. 7).

Neurological abnormalities, commonly found in HIV infection, can present in either a latent or active form both with or without immunological impairment. The precise mechanisms whereby HIV

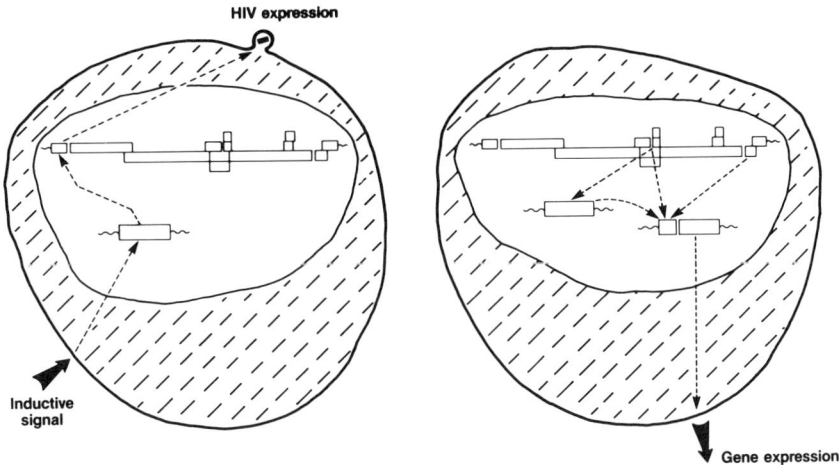

FIG. 7. The effect of inductive signals on the activation of HIV expression and the effect of HIV gene products on cellular gene expression. [Adapted with permission from Fauci, A. S. (1989). *Trans. Assoc. Am. Physicians* **101** (in press).]

induces a wide range of neurological dysfunction are not well understood. Some hypotheses include the elaboration of cytotoxic factors from HIV-infected macrophages in the brain, interference with neurological transmitters or neurotropic factors, direct infection of neuronal cells, synergism between HIV and opportunistic viruses in the CNS of AIDS patients, and autoimmune phenomena.

The role of the immune system in preventing or limiting infection with HIV is poorly understood. While many immune responses to HIV, such as the development of neutralizing antibodies, ADCC, ACC, and CTLs, have been delineated, the majority of HIV-infected individuals appear to follow an inexorable path to full-blown AIDS. The development of effective anti-HIV vaccines or immune system enhancers depends on a further understanding of a protective immune response.

Although many questions have been answered with unprecedented speed, a greater understanding of the complex interactions between HIV and its host are clearly needed in order to effectively treat active infections and prevent the acquisition of new infections and the progression of latent infection to active disease. Further research into the pathogenesis of HIV infection using both *in vitro* experiments and *in vivo* studies in novel small-animal models, such as the severe combined immunodeficiency and transgenic mouse models (Mosier *et al.*, 1988; McCune *et al.*, 1988a; J. M. Leonard *et al.*, 1988; Namikawa *et al.*, 1988), should continue to provide important insights for the control of AIDS in particular and other human diseases in general.

REFERENCES

Adachi, A., Koenig, S., Gendelman, H. E., Daugherty, D., Gattoni-Celli, S., Fauci, A. S., and Martin, M. A. (1987). *J. Virol.* **61**, 209.
Aggarwal, B. B., and Eessalu, T. E. (1987). *J. Biol. Chem.* **262**, 16450.
Ahearne, P. M., Matthews, M. J., Lyerly, H. K., White, G. C., Bolognesi, D., P., and Weinhold, K. J. (1988). *AIDS Res. Hum. Retroviruses* **4**, 259.
Ahmad, N., and Venkatesan, S. (1988). *Science* **241**, 1481.
Albert, J., Bredberg, U., Chiodi, F., Bottiger, B., Fenyo, E. M., Norrby, E., and Biberfeld, G. (1987). *AIDS Res. Hum. Retroviruses* **3**, 3.
Alizon, M., Sonigo, P., Barré-Sinoussi, F., Chermann, J. C., Tiollais, P., Montagnier, L., and Wain-Hobson, S. (1984). *Nature (London)* **312**, 757.
Alizon, M., Wain-Hobson, S., Montagnier, L., and Sonigo, P. (1986). *Cell (Cambridge, Mass.)* **46**, 63.
Allan, J. S., Coligan, J. E., Barin, F., McLane, M. F., Sodroski, J. G., Rosen, C. A., Haseltine, W. A., Lee, T. H., and Essex, M. (1985). *Science* **228**, 1091.
Amadori, A., Faulkner-Valle, G. P., De Rossi, A., Zanovello, P., Collavo, D., and Chieco-Bianchi, L. (1988). *Clin. Immunol. Immunopathol.* **46**, 3.
Ammann, A. J., Palladino, M. A., Volberding, P., Abrams, D., Martin, N. L., and Conant, M. (1987). *J. Clin. Immunol.* **7**, 481.
Anand, R., Siegal, F., Reed, C., Cheung, T., Forlenza, S., and Moore, J. (1987). *Lancet* **2**, 234.
Antonen, J., and Krohn, K. (1986). *Clin. Exp. Immunol.* **65**, 489.
Arthur, L. O., Pyle, S. W., Nara, P. L., Bess, J. W., Jr., Gonda, M. A., Kelliher, J. C., Gilden, R. V., Robey, W. G., Bolognesi, D. P., Gallo, R. C., and Fischinger, P. J. (1987). *Proc. Natl. Acad. Sci. U.S.A.* **84**, 8583.
Arya, S. K., and Gallo, R. C. (1986). *Proc. Natl. Acad. Sci. U.S.A.* **83**, 2209.
Arya, S. K., Guo, C., Josephs, S. F., and Wong-Staal, F. (1985). *Science* **229**, 69.
Arya, S. K., Beaver, B., Jagodzinski, L., Ensoli, B., Kanki, P. J., Albert, J., Fenyo, E. M., Biberfeld, G., Zagury, J. F., Laure, F., Essex, M., Norrby, E., Wong-Staal, F., and Gallo, R. C. (1987). *Nature (London)* **328**, 548.
Asjo, B., Morfeldt-Manson, L., Albert, J., Biberfeld, G., Karlsson, A., Lidman, K., and Fenyo, E. M. (1986). *Lancet* **2**, 660.
Barin, F., McLane, M. F., Allan, J. S., Lee, T. H., Groopman, J. E., and Essex, M. (1985). *Science* **228**, 1094.
Barone, A. D., Silva, J. J., Ho, D. D., Gallo, R. C., Wong-Staal, F. F., and Chang, N. T. (1986). *J. Immunol.* **137**, 669.
Barré-Sinoussi, F., Chermann, J. C., Rey, F., Nugeyre, M. T., Chamaret, S., Gruest, J., Dauguet, C., Axler-Blin, C., Vezinet-Brun, F., Rouzioux, C., Rozenbaum, W., and Montagnier, L. (1983). *Science* **220**, 868.
Barré-Sinoussi, F., Mathur-Wagh, U., Rey, F., Brun-Vezinet, F., Yancovitz, S. R., Rouzioux, C., Montagnier, L., Mildvan, D., and Chermann, J. C. (1985). *J. Am. Med. Assoc.* **253**, 1737.
Bedinger, P., Moriarty, A., von Borstel, R. C., 2nd, Donovan, N. J., Steimer, K. S., and Littman, D. R. (1988). *Nature (London)* **334**, 162.
Bednarik, D. P., Mosca, J. D., and Raj, N. B. (1987). *J. Virol.* **61**, 1253.
Belsito, D. V., Sanchez, M. R., Baer, R. L., Valentine, F., and Thorbecke, G. J. (1984). *N. Engl. J. Med.* **310**, 1279.

Bender, B. S., Frank, M. M., Lawley, T. J., Smith, W. J., Brickman, C. M., and Quinn. T. C. (1985). *J. Infect. Dis.* **152**, 409.
Bender, B. S., Bohnsack, J. F., Sourlis, S. H., Frank, M. M., and Quinn, T. C. (1987). *J. Clin. Invest.* **79**, 715.
Benn, S., Rutledge, R., Folks, T., Gold, J., Baker, L., McCormick, J., Feorino, P., Piot, P., Quinn, T., and Martin, M. (1985). *Science* **230**, 949.
Berger, E. A., Fuerst, T. R., and Moss, B. (1988). *Proc. Natl. Acad. Sci. U.S.A.* **85**, 2357.
Berman, P. W., Groopman, J. E., Gregory, T., Clapham, P. R., Weiss, R. A., Ferriani, R., Riddle, L., Shimasaki, C., Lucas, C., Lasky, L. A., and Eichberg, J. W. (1988). *Proc. Natl. Acad. Sci. U.S.A.* **85**, 5200.
Berzofsky, J. A., Bensussan, A., Cease, K. B., Bourge, J. F., Cheynier, R., Lurhuma, Z., Salaun, J. J., Gallo, R. C., Shearer, G. M., and Zagury, D. (1988). *Nature (London)* **334**, 706.
Biggar, R. J., Melbye, M., Ebbesen, P., Alexander, S., Nielsen, J. O., Sarin, P., and Faber, V. (1985). *Br. J. Med.* **291**, 997.
Blumberg, R. S., Paradis, T., Hartshorn, K. L., Vogt, M., Ho, D. D., Hirsch, M. S., Leban, J., Sato, V. L., and Schooley, R. T. (1987). *J. Infect. Dis.* **156**, 878.
Bohnlein, E., Lowenthal, J. W., Siekevitz, M., Ballard, D. W., Franza, B. R., and Greene, W. C. (1988). *Cell (Cambridge, Mass.)* **53**, 827.
Bolton, V., Pedersen, N. C., Higgins, J., Jennings, M., and Carlson, J. (1987). *J. Clin. Microbiol.* **25**, 1411.
Bottiger, B., Ljunggren, K., Karlsson, A., Krohn, K., Fenyo, E., Jondal, M., and Biberfeld, G. (1988). *Clin. Exp. Immunol.* **73**, 339.
Bowen, D. L., Lane, H. C., and Fauci, A. S. (1985). *Ann. Intern. Med.* **103**, 704.
Braun, D. P., Kessler, H., Falk, L., Paul, D., Harris, J. E., Blaauw, B., and Landay, A. (1988). *J. Clin. Immunol.* **8**, 486.
Brenneman, D. E., Westbrook, G. L., Fitzgerald, S. P., Ennist, D. L., Elkins, K. L., Ruff, M. R., and Pert, C. B. (1988). *Nature (London)* **335**, 639.
Brun-Vezinet, F., Rouzioux, C., Barre-Sinoussi, F., Klatzmann, D., Saimot, A. G., Rozenbaum, W., Christol, D., Gluckmann, J. C., Montagnier, L., and Chermann, J. C. (1984). *Lancet* **1**, 1253.
Brun-Vezinet, F., Rey, M. A., Katlama, C., Girard, P. M., Roulot, D., Yeni, P., Lenoble, L., Clavel, F., Alizon, M., Gadelle, S., Madjar, J. J., and Harzic, M. (1987). *Lancet* **1**, 128.
Busch, M., Beckstead, J., Gantz, D., and Vyas, G. (1986). *Blood* **68**, Suppl. 1, 122a.
Cao, Y., Valentine, F., Hojvat, S., Allain, J.-P., Rubinstein, P., Mirabile, M., Czelusniak, S., Leuther, M., Baker, L., and Friedman-Kien, A. E. (1987). *Blood* **70**, 575.
Cease, K. B., Margalit, H., Cornette, J. L., Putney, S. D., Robey, W. G., Ouyang, C., Streicher, H. Z., Fischinger, P. J., Gallo, R. C., DeLisi, C., and Berzofsky, J. A. (1987). *Proc. Natl. Acad. Sci. U.S.A.* **84**, 4249.
Centers for Disease Control (1989). *CDC HIV AIDS Surveillance Report, January 1989*, p. 1.
Cerami, A., and Beutler, B. (1988). *Immunol. Today* **9**, 28.
Chanda, P. K., Ghrayeb, J., and Wong-Staal, F. (1988). *AIDS Res. Hum. Retroviruses* **4**, 11.
Chanh, T. C., Kennedy, R. C., and Kanda, P. (1988). *Cell. Immunol.* **111**, 77.
Chatterjee, R., Rinaldo, C. R., Jr., and Gupta, P. (1987). *J. Clin. Immunol.* **7**, 218.
Cheingsong-Popov, R., Weiss, R. A., Dalgleish, A., Tedder, R. S., Shanson, D. C., Jeffries, D. J., Ferns, R. B., Briggs, E. M., Weller, I. V., Mitton, S., Adler, M. W.,

Farthing, C., Lawrence, A. G., Gazzard, B. G., Weber, J., Harris, J. R. W., Pinching, A. J., Craske, J., and Barbara, J. A. J. (1984). *Lancet* **2**, 477.
Cheng-Mayer, C., Seto, D., Tateno, M., and Levy, J. A. (1988). *Science* **240**, 80.
Chiodi, F., Fuerstenberg, S., Gidlund, M., Asjo, B., and Fenyo, E. M. (1987). *J. Virol.* **61**, 1244.
Chiodi, F., Albert, J., Olausson, E., Norkrans, G., Hagberg, L., Sonnerborg, A., Asjo, B., and Fenyo, E. M. (1988). *AIDS Res. Hum. Retroviruses* **4**, 351.
Chiu, I. M., Yaniv, A., Dahlberg, J. E., Gazit, A., Skuntz, S. F., Tronick, S. R., and Aaronson, S. A. (1985). *Nature (London)* **317**, 366.
Cianciolo, G. J., Copeland, T. D., Oroszlan, S., and Snyderman, R. (1985). *Science* **230**, 453.
Clavel, F., Guyader, M., Guetard, D., Salle, M., Montagnier, L., and Alizon, M. (1986a). *Nature (London)* **324**, 691.
Clavel, F., Guetard, D., Brun-Vezinet, F., Chamaret, S., Rey, M. A., Santos-Ferreira, M. O., Laurent, A. G., Dauguet, C., Katlama, C., Rouzioux, C., Klatzmann, D., Champalimaud, J. L., and Montagnier, L. (1986b). *Science* **233**, 343.
Clavel, F., Mansinho, K., Chamaret, S., Guetard, D., Favier, V., Nina, J., Santos-Ferreira, M. O., Champalimaud, J. L., and Montagnier, L. (1987). *N. Engl. J. Med.* **316**, 1180.
Clayton, L. K., Hussey, R. E., Steinbrich, R., Ramachandran, H., Husain, Y., and Reinherz, E. L. (1988). *Nature (London)* **335**, 363.
Clouse, K. A., Powell, D., Washington, I., Poli, G., Strebel, K., Farrar, W., Barstad, P., Kovacs, J., Fauci, A. S., and Folks, T. M. (1989a). *J. Immunol.* (in press).
Clouse, K. A., Robbins, P. B., Fornie, B., Ostrove, J. M., and Fauci, A. S. (1989b). *J. Immunol.* (in press).
Cohen, E. A., Terwilliger, E. F., Sodroski, J. G., and Haseltine, W. A. (1988). *Nature (London)* **334**, 532.
Creemers, P. C., O'Shaughnessy, M., and Boyko, W. J. (1986). *Immunology* **59**, 627.
Crowe, S., Mills, J., and McGrath, M. S. (1987). *AIDS Res. Hum. Retroviruses* **3**, 135.
Cunningham-Rundles, S., Michelis, M. A., and Masur, H. (1983). *J. Clin. Immunol.* **3**, 156.
Curran, J. W., Jaffe, H. W., Hardy, A. M., Morgan, W. M., Selik, R. M., and Dondero, T. J. (1988). *Science* **239**, 610.
Dahl, K., Martin, K., and Miller, G. (1987). *J. Virol.* **61**, 1602.
Dalgleish, A. G., Beverley, P. C., Clapham, P. R., Crawford, D. H., Greaves, M. F., and Weiss, R. A. (1984). *Nature (London)* **312**, 763.
Daniel, M. D., Letvin, N. L., King, N. W., Kannagi, M., Sehgal, P. K., Hunt, R. D., Kanki, P. J., Essex, M., and Desrosiers, R. C. (1985). *Science* **228**, 1201.
Davis, M. G., Kenney, S. C., Kamine, J., Pagano, J. S., and Huang, E. S. (1987). *Proc. Natl. Acad. Sci. U.S.A.* **84**, 8642.
Dayton, A. I., Sodroski, J. G., Rosen, C. A., Goh, W. C., and Haseltine, W. A. (1986). *Cell (Cambridge, Mass.)* **44**, 941.
Deen, K. C., McDougal, J. S., Inacker, R., Folena-Wasserman, G., Arthos, J., Rosenberg, J., Maddon, P. J., Axel, R., and Sweet, R. W. (1988). *Nature (London)* **331**, 82.
Delacrétaz, F., Perey, L., Schmidt, P. M., Chave, J. P., and Costa, J. (1987). *Virchows. Arch. A: Pathol. Anat. Histol.* **411**, 543.
de Noronha, F., Schafer, W., Essex, M., and Bolognesi, D. P. (1978). *Virology* **85**, 617.
De Rossi, A., Franchini, G., Aldovini, A., Del Mistro, A., Chieco-Bianchi, L., Gallo, R. C., and Wong-Staal, F. (1986). *Proc. Natl. Acad. Sci. U.S.A.* **83**, 4297.
Desrosiers, R. C., and Letvin, N. L. (1987). *Rev. Infect. Dis.* **9**, 438.
Dewhurst, S., Sakai, K., Bresser, J., Stevenson, M., Evinger-Hodges, M. J., and Volsky, D. J. (1987). *J. Virol.* **61**, 3774.

Dewhurst, S., Sakai, K., Zhang, X. H., Wasiak, A., and Volsky, D. J. (1988). *Virology* **162**, 151.
de Wolf, F., Lange, J. M., Houweling, J. T., Coutinho, R. A., Schellekens, P. T., Van der Noordaa, J., and Goudsmit, J. (1988). *J. Infect. Dis.* **158**, 615.
Diamond, D. C., Sleckman, B. P., Gregory, T., Lasky, L. A., Greenstein, J. L., and Burakoff, S. J. (1988). *J. Immunol.* **141**, 3715.
diMarzo Veronese, F., DeVico, A. L., Copeland, T. D., Oroszlan, S., Gallo, R. C., and Sarngadharan, M. G. (1985). *Science* **229**, 1402.
Dinter, H., Chiu, R., Imagawa, M., Karin, M., and Jones, K. A. (1987). *EMBO J.* **6**, 4067.
Donahue, R. E., Johnson, M. M., Zon, L. I., Clark, S. C., and Groopman, J. E. (1987). *Nature (London)* **326**, 200.
Donnelly, R. P., La Via, M. F., and Tsang, K. Y. (1987). *Clin. Exp. Immunol.* **68**, 488.
Dorsett, B., Cronin, W., Chuma, V., and Ioachim, H. L. (1985). *Am. J. Med.* **78**, 621.
Dougherty, J. P., and Temin, H. M. (1988). *J. Virol.* **62**, 2817.
Dowbenko, D., Nakamura, G., Fennie, C., Shimasaki, C., Riddle, L., Harris, R., Gregory, T., and Lasky, L. (1988). *J. Virol.* **62**, 4703.
Doyle, C., and Strominger, J. L. (1987). *Nature (London)* **330**, 256.
Dreno, B., Milpied, B., Bignon, J. D., Stalder, J. F., and Litoux, P. (1988). *Br. J. Dermatol.* **118**, 481.
Eales, L. J., Farrant, J., Helbert, M., and Pinching, A. J. (1988). *Clin. Exp. Immunol.* **71**, 423.
Eichberg, J. W., Zarling, J. M., Alter, H. J., Levy, J. A., Berman, P. W., Gregory, T., Lasky, L. A., McClure, J., Cobb, K. E., Moran, P. A., Hu, S.-L., Kennedy, R. C., Chanh, T. C., and Dreesman, G. R. (1987). *J. Virol.* **61**, 3804.
Emerman, M., Guyader, M., Montagnier, L., Baltimore, D., and Muesing, M. A. (1987). *EMBO J.* **6**, 3755.
Enk, C., Gerstoft, J., Müller, S., and Remvig, L. (1986). *Scand. J. Immunol.* **23**, 491.
Epstein, L. G., Sharer, L. R., Cho, E. S., Myenhofer, M., Navia, B., and Price, R. W. (1984). *AIDS Res.* **1**, 447.
Estevez, M. E., Ballart, I. J., Diez, R. A., Planes, N., Scaglione, C., and Sen, L. (1986). *Scand. J. Immunol.* **24**, 215.
Evans, L. A., McHugh, T. M., Stites, D. P., and Levy, J. A. (1987). *J. Immunol.* **138**, 3415.
Evans, L. A., Moreau, J., Odehouri, K., Legg, H., Barboza, A., Cheng-Mayer, C., and Levy, J. A. (1988). *Science* **240**, 1522.
Farzadegan, H., Polis, M. A., Wolinsky, S. M., Rinaldo, C. R., Jr., Sninsky, J. J., Kwok, S., Griffith, R. L., Kaslow, R. A., Phair, J. P., Polk, B. F., and Saah, A. J. (1988). *Ann. Intern. Med.* **108**, 785.
Fauci, A. S. (1987). *Clin. Res.* **35**, 503.
Fauci, A. S. (1988). *Science* **239**, 617.
Feinberg, M. B., Jarrett, R. F., Aldovini, A., Gallo, R. C., and Wong-Staal, F. (1986). *Cell (Cambridge, Mass.)* **46**, 807.
Fenyo, E. M., Morfeldt-Manson, L., Chiodi, F., Lind, B., von Gegerfelt, A., Albert, J., Olausson, E., and Asjo, B. (1988). *J. Virol.* **62**, 4414.
Fisher, A. G., Feinberg, M. B., Josephs, S. F., Harper, M. E., Marselle, L. M., Reyes, G., Gonda, M. A., Aldovini, A., Debouk, C., Gallo, R. C., and Wong-Staal, F. (1986a). *Nature (London)* **320**, 367.
Fisher, A. G., Ratner, L., Mitsuya, H., Marselle, L. M., Harper, M. E., Broder, S., Gallo, R. C., and Wong-Staal, F. (1986b). *Science* **233**, 655.
Fisher, A. G., Ensoli, B., Ivanoff, L., Chamberlain, M., Petteway, S., Ratner, L., Gallo, R. C., and Wong-Staal, F. (1987). *Science* **237**, 888.

Fisher, R. A., Bertonis, J. M., Meier, W., Johnson, V. A., Costopoulos, D. S., Liu, T., Tizard, R., Walker, B. D., Hirsch, M. S., Schooley, R. T., and Flavell, R. A. (1988a). *Nature (London)* **331**, 76.

Fisher, A. G., Ensoli, B., Looney, D., Rose, A., Gallo, R. C., Saag, M. S., Shaw, G. M., Hahn, B. H., and Wong-Staal, F. (1988b). *Nature (London)* **334**, 444.

Folks, T., Benn, S., Rabson, A., Theodore, T., Hoggan, M. D., Martin, M., Lightfoote, M., and Sell, K. (1985). *Proc. Natl. Acad. Sci. U.S.A.* **82**, 4539.

Folks, T., Powell, D. M., Lightfoote, M. M., Benn, S., Martin, M. A., and Fauci, A. S. (1986a). *Science* **231**, 600.

Folks, T., Kelly, J., Benn, S., Kinter, A., Justement, J., Gold, J., Redfield, R., Sell, K. W., and Fauci, A. S. (1986b). *J. Immunol.* **136**, 4049.

Folks, T. M., Powell, D., Lightfoote, M., Koenig, S., Fauci, A. S., Benn, S., Rabson, A., Daugherty, D., Gendelman, H. E., Hoggan, M. D., Venkatesan, S., and Martin, M. A. (1986c). *J. Exp. Med.* **164**, 280.

Folks, T. M., Justement, J., Kinter, A., Dinarello, C. A., and Fauci, A. S. (1987). *Science* **238**, 800.

Folks, T. M., Justement, J., Kinter, A., Schnittman, S., Orenstein, J., Poli, G., and Fauci, A. S. (1989). *Proc. Natl. Acad. Sci. U.S.A.* **86**, 2365.

Folks, T. M., Kessler, S. W., Orenstein, J. M., Justement, J. S., Jaffe, E. S., and Fauci, A. S. (1988b). *Science* **242**, 919.

Folks, T. M., Clouse, K. A., Justement, J., Rabson, A., Duh, E., Kehrl, J. H., and Fauci, A. S. (1989). *Proc. Natl. Acad. Sci. U.S.A.* (in press).

Franchini, G., Collalti, E., Arya, S. K., Fenyo, E. M., Biberfeld, G., Zagury, J. F., Kanki, P. J., Wong-Staal, F., and Gallo, R. C. (1987a). *AIDS Res. Hum. Retroviruses* **3**, 11.

Franchini, G., Robert-Guroff, M., Aldovini, A., Kan, N. C., and Wong-Staal, F. (1987b). *Blood* **69**, 437.

Franchini, G., Rusche, J. R., O'Keeffe, T. J., and Wong-Staal, F. (1988). *AIDS Res. Hum. Retroviruses* **4**, 243.

Franza, B. R., Jr., Josephs, S. F., Gilman, M. Z., Ryan, W., and Clarkson, B. (1987). *Nature (London)* **330**, 391.

Funke, I., Hahn, A., Rieber, E. P., Weiss, E., and Riethmüller, G. (1987). *J. Exp. Med.* **165**, 1230.

Gabuzda, D. H., Ho, D. D., de la Monte, S. M., Hirsch, M. S., Rota, T. R., and Sobel, R. A. (1986). *Ann. Neurol.* **20**, 289.

Gallo, P., De Rossi, A., Amadori, A., Tavolato, B., and Chieco-Bianchi, L. (1988). *AIDS Res. Hum. Retroviruses* **4**, 211.

Gallo, R. C., Salahuddin, S. Z., Popovic, M., Shearer, G. M., Kaplan, M., Haynes, B. F., Palker, T. J., Redfield, R., Oleske, J., Safai, B., White, G., Foster, P., and Markham, P. D. (1984). *Science* **224**, 500.

Garcia, J. A., Wu, F. K., Mitsuyasu, R., and Gaynor, R. B. (1987). *EMBO J.* **6**, 3761.

Gartner, S., Markovits, P., Markovitz, D. M., Betts, R. F., and Popovic, M. (1986a). *J. Am. Med. Assoc.* **256**, 2365.

Gartner, S., Markovits, P., Markovitz, D. M., Kaplan, M. H., Gallo, R. C., and Popovic, M. (1986b). *Science* **233**, 215.

Gay, D., Maddon, P., Seklay, R., Talle, M. A., Godfrey, M., Long, E., Goldstein, G., Chess, L., Axel, R., Kappler, J., and Marrack, P. (1987). *Nature (London)* **328**, 626.

Gay, D., Buus, S., Pasternak, J., Kappler, J., and Marrack, P. (1988). *Proc. Natl. Acad. Sci. U.S.A.* **85**, 5629.

Gendelman, H. E., Narayan, O., Molineaux, S., Clements, J. E., and Ghotbi, Z. (1985). *Proc. Natl. Acad. Sci. U.S.A.* **82**, 7086.

Gendelman, H. E., Phelps, W., Feigenbaum, L., Ostrove, J. M., Adachi, A., Howley, P. M., Khoury, G., Ginsberg, H. S., and Martin, M. A. (1986). *Proc. Natl. Acad. Sci. U.S.A.* **83**, 9759.

Gendelman, H. E., Orenstein, J. M., Martin, M. A., Ferrua, C., Mitra, R., Phipps, T., Wahl, L. A., Lane, H. C., Fauci, A. S., Burke, D. S., Skillman, D., and Meltzer, M. S. (1988). *J. Exp. Med.* **167**, 1428.

Gimble, J. M., Duh, E., Ostrove, J. M., Gendelman, H. E., Max, E. E., and Rabson, A. B. (1988). *J. Virol.* **62**, 4104.

Giorgi, J. V., Fahey, J. L., Smith, D. C., Hultin, L. E., Cheng, H. L., Mitsuyasu, R. T., and Detels, R. (1987). *J. Immunol.* **138**, 3725.

Gnann, J. W., Jr., Schwimmbeck, P. L., Nelson, J. A., Truax, A. B., and Oldstone, M. B. (1987). *J. Infect. Dis.* **156**, 261.

Golding, H., Robey, F. A., Gates, F. T., 3rd, Linder, W., Beining, P. R., Hoffman, T., and Golding, B. (1988). *J. Exp. Med.* **167**, 914.

Gonda, M. A., Wong-Staal, F., Gallo, R. C., Clements, J. E., Narayan, O., and Gilden, R. V. (1985). *Science* **227**, 173.

Gonda, M. A., Braun, M. J., Clements, J. E., Pyper, J. M., Wong-Staal, F., Gallo, R. C., and Gilden, R. V. (1986). *Proc. Natl. Acad. Sci. U.S.A.* **83**, 4007.

Gonda, M. A., Braun, M. J., Carter, S. G., Kost, T. A., Bess, J. W., Jr., Arthur, L. O., and Van der Maaten, M. J. (1987). *Nature (London)* **330**, 388.

Goudsmit, J., de Wolf, F., Paul, D. A., Epstein, L. G., Lange, J. M., Krone, W. J., Speelman, H., Wolters, E. C., Van der Noordaa, J., Oleske, J. M., Van Der Helm, H. J., and Coutinho, R. A. (1986). *Lancet* **2**, 177.

Goudsmit, J., Epstein, L. G., Paul, D. A., Van Der Helm, H. J., Dawson, G. J., Asher, D. M., Yanagihara, R., Wolff, A. V., Gibbs, C. J., Jr., and Gajdusek, D. C. (1987). *Proc. Natl. Acad. Sci. U.S.A.* **84**, 3876.

Goudsmit, J., Debouck, C., Meloen, R. H., Smit, L., Bakker, M., Asher, D. M., Wolff, A. V., Gibbs, C. J., Jr., and Gajdusek, D. C. (1988). *Proc. Natl. Acad. Sci. U.S.A.* **85**, 4478.

Groopman, J. E., Chen, F. W., Hope, J. A., Andrews, J. M., Swift, R. L., Benton, C. V., Sullivan, J. L., Volberding, P. A., Sites, D. P., Landesman, S., Gold, J., Baker, L., Craven, D., and Boches, F. S. (1986). *J. Infect. Dis.* **153**, 736.

Groopman, J. E., Benz, P. M., Ferriani, R., Mayer, K., Allan, J. D., and Weymouth, L. A. (1987). *AIDS Res. Hum. Retroviruses* **3**, 71.

Gupta, S., and Safai, B. (1983). *J. Clin. Invest.* **71**, 296.

Gupta, S., and Vayuvegula, B. (1987). *J. Clin. Immunol.* **7**, 486.

Gupta, S., Gillis, S., Thornton, M., and Goldberg, M. (1984). *Clin. Exp. Immunol.* **58**, 395.

Gurgo, C., Guo, H. G., Franchini, G., Aldovini, A., Collalti, E., Farrell, K., Wong-Staal, F., Gallo, R. C., and Reitz, M. S., Jr. (1988). *Virology* **164**, 531.

Guy, B., Kieny, M. P., Riviere, Y., Le Peuch, C., Dott, K., Girard, M., Montagnier, L., and Lecocq, J. P. (1987). *Nature (London)* **330**, 266.

Guyader, M., Emerman, M., Sonigo, P., Clavel, F., Montagnier, L., and Alizon, M. (1987). *Nature (London)* **326**, 662.

Gyorkey, F., Melnick, J. L., and Gyorkey, P. (1987). *J. Infect. Dis.* **155**, 870.

Haas, J. G., Riethmüller, G., and Ziegler-Heitbrock, H. W. (1987). *Scand. J. Immunol.* **26**, 371.

Hahn, B. H., Shaw, G. M., Arya, S. K., Popovic, M., Gallo, R. C., and Wong-Staal, F. (1984). *Nature (London)* **312**, 166.

Hahn, B. H., Shaw, G. M., Taylor, M. E., Redfield, R. R., Markham, P. D., Salahuddin,

S. Z., Wong-Staal, F., Gallo, R. C., Parks, E. S., and Parks, W. P. (1986). *Science* **232**, 1548.

Harada, S., Koyanagi, Y., Nakashima, H., Kobayashi, N., and Yamamoto, N. (1986). *Virology* **154**, 249.

Harrell, R. A., Cianciolo, G. J., Copeland, T. D., Oroszlan, S., and Snyderman, R. (1986). *J. Immunol.* **136**, 3517.

Haseltine, W. A. (1988). *J. AIDS* **1**, 217.

Heagy, W., Kelley, V. E., Strom, T. B., Mayer, K., Shapiro, H. M., Mandel, R., and Finberg, R. (1984). *J. Clin. Invest.* **74**, 2089.

Henderson, L. E., Sowder, R. C., Copeland, T. D., Benveniste, R. E., and Oroszlan, S. (1988). *Science* **241**, 199.

Hennig, A. K., and Tomar, R. H. (1984). *Clin. Immunol. Immunopathol.* **33**, 258.

Ho, D. D., Rota, T. R., and Hirsch, M. S. (1985a). *N. Engl. J. Med.* **312**, 649.

Ho, D. D., Rota, T. R., Schooley, R. T., Kaplan, J. C., Allan, J. D., Groopman, J. E., Resnick, L., Felsenstein, D., Andrews, C. A., and Hirsch, M. S. (1985b). *N. Engl. J. Med.* **313**, 1493.

Ho, D. D., Rota, T. R., and Hirsch, M. S. (1986). *J. Clin. Invest.* **77**, 1712.

Ho, D. D., Pomerantz, R. J., and Kaplan, J. C. (1987a). *N. Engl. J. Med.* **317**, 278.

Ho, D. D., Sarngadharan, M. G., Hirsch, M. S., Schooley, R. T., Rota, T. R., Kennedy, R. C., Chanh, T. C., and Sato, V. L. (1987b). *J. Virol.* **61**, 2024.

Hollander, H., and Levy, J. A. (1987). *Ann. Intern. Med.* **106**, 692.

Hoxie, J. A., Haggarty, B. S., Rackowski, J. L., Pillsbury, N., and Levy, J. A. (1985). *Science* **229**, 1400.

Hoxie, J. A., Alpers, J. D., Rackowski, J. L., Huebner, K., Haggarty, B. S., Cedarbaum, A. J., and Reed, J. C. (1986). *Science* **234**, 1123.

Hoxie, J. A., Rackowski, J. L., Haggarty, B. S., and Gaulton, G. N. (1988). *J. Immunol.* **140**, 786.

Hoy, J. F., Lewis, D. E., and Miller, G. G. (1988). *J. Infect. Dis.* **158**, 1071.

Hussey, R. E., Richardson, N. E., Kowalski, M., Brown, N. R., Chang, H. C., Siciliano, R. F., Dorfman, T., Walker, B., Sodroski, J., and Reinherz, E. L. (1988). *Nature (London)* **331**, 78.

Israel-Biet, D., Ekwalanga, M., Venet, A., Even, P., and Andrieu, J.-M. (1988). *Clin. Exp. Immunol.* **74**, 185.

Jameson, B. A., Rao, P. E., Kong, L. I., Hahn, B. H., Shaw, G. M., Hood, L. E., and Kent, S. B. (1988). *Science* **240**, 1335.

Johnson, R. T., McArthur, J. C., and Narayan, O. (1988). *FASEB J.* **2**, 2970.

Kalyanaraman, V. S., Cabradilla, C. D., Getchell, J. P., Narayanan, R., Braff, E. H., Chermann, J. C., Barre Sinoussi, F., Montagnier, L., Spira, T. J., Kaplan, J., Fishbein, D., Jaffe, H. W., Curran, J. W., and Francis, D. P. (1984). *Science* **225**, 321.

Kao, S. Y., Calman, A. F., Luciw, P. A., and Peterlin, B. M. (1987). *Nature (London)* **330**, 489.

Kappes, J. C., Morrow, C. D., Lee, S. W., Jameson, B. A., Kent, S. B., Hood, L. E., Shaw, G. M., and Hahn, B. H. (1988). *J. Virol.* **62**, 3501.

Karpas, A., Hill, F., Youle, M., Cullen, V., Gray, J., Byron, N., Hayhoe, F., Tenant-Flowers, M., Howard, L., Gilgen, D., Oates, J. K., Hawkins, D., and Gazzard, B. (1988). *Proc. Natl. Acad. Sci. U.S.A.* **85**, 9234.

Katz, J. D., Nishanian, P., Mitsuyasu, R., and Bonavida, B. (1988). *J. Clin. Immunol.* **8**, 453.

Kaufman, J. D., Valandra, G., Roderiquez, G., Bushar, G., Giri, C., and Norcross, M. A. (1987). *Mol. Cell. Biol.* **7**, 3759.

Kawakami, K., Scheidereit, C., and Roeder, R. G. (1988). *Proc. Natl. Acad. Sci. U.S.A.* **85**, 4700.
Kehrl, J. H., Alvarez-Mon, M., Delsing, G. A., and Fauci, A. S. (1987). *Science* **238**, 1144.
Kenealy, W., Reed, D., Cybulski, R., Tribe, D., Taylor, P., Stevens, C., Matthews, T., and Petteway, S. (1987). *AIDS Res. Hum. Retroviruses* **3**, 95.
Kenney, S., Kamine, J., Markovitz, D., Fenrick, R., and Pagano, J. (1988). *Proc. Natl. Acad. Sci. U.S.A.* **85**, 1652.
Keshet, E., and Temin, H. M. (1979). *J. Virol.* **31**, 376.
Khalife, J., Guy, B., Capron, M., Kieny, M. P., Ameisen, J. C., Montagnier, L., Lecocq, J. P., and Capron, A. (1988). *AIDS Res. Hum. Retroviruses* **4**, 3.
Kirchner, H. (1982). *Monogr. Virol.* **13**, 1.
Klasse, P. J., and Blomberg, J. (1987). *J. Infect. Dis.* **156**, 1026.
Klasse, P. J., Pipkorn, R., and Blomberg, J. (1988). *Proc. Natl. Acad. Sci. U.S.A.* **85**, 5225.
Klatzmann, D., and Gluckman, J. C. (1986). *Immunol. Today* **7**, 291.
Klatzmann, D., Champagne, E., Chamaret, S., Gruest, J., Guetard, D., Hercend, T., Gluckman, J. C., and Montagnier, L. (1984a). *Nature (London)* **312**, 767.
Klatzmann, D., Barre-Sinoussi, F., Nugeyre, M. T., Danquet, C., Vilmer, E., Griscelli, C., Brun-Vezinet, F., Rouzioux, C., Gluckman, J. C., Chermann, J. C., and Montagnier, L. (1984b). *Science* **225**, 59.
Kleinerman, E. S., Ceccorulli, L. M., Zwelling, L. A., Twilley, T., Herberman, R. B., Jacob, J., and Gelmann, E. P. (1985). *J. Clin. Oncol.* **3**, 1005.
Knight, D. M., Flomerfelt, F. A., and Ghrayeb, J. (1987). *Science* **236**, 837.
Koenig, S., Gendelman, H. E., Orenstein, J. M., Dal Canto, M. C., Pezeshkpour, G. H., Yungbluth, M., Janotta, F., Aksamit, A., Martin, M. A., and Fauci, A. S. (1986). *Science* **233**, 1089.
Koenig, S., Earl, P., Powell, D., Pantaleo, G., Merli, S., Moss, B., and Fauci, A. S. (1988). *Proc. Natl. Acad. Sci. U.S.A.* **85**, 8638.
Koga, Y., Lindstrom, E., Fenyo, E. M., Wigzell, H., and Mak, T. W. (1988). *Proc. Natl. Acad. Sci. U.S.A.* **85**, 4521.
Kohl, N. E., Emini, E. A., Schleif, W. A., Davis, L. J., Heimbach, J. C., Dixon, R. A., Scolnick, E. M., and Sigal, I. S. (1988). *Proc. Natl. Acad. Sci. U.S.A.* **85**, 4686.
Kong, L. I., Lee, S. W., Kappes, J. C., Parkin, J. S., Decker, D., Hoxie, J. A., Hahn, B. H., and Shaw, G. M. (1988). *Science* **240**, 1525.
Kornfeld, H., Cruikshank, W. W., Pyle, S. W., Berman, J. S., and Center, D. M. (1988). *Nature (London)* **335**, 445.
Koyanagi, Y., Miles, S., Mitsuyasu, R. T., Merrill, J. E., Vinters, H. V., and Chen, I. S. (1987). *Science* **236**, 819.
Koyanagi, Y., O'Brien, W. A., Zhao, J. Q., Golde, D. W., Gasson, J. C., and Chen, I. S. (1988). *Science* **241**, 1673.
Krohn, K., Robey, W. G., Putney, S., Arthur, L., Nara, P., Fischinger, P., Gallo, R. C., Wong-Staal, F., and Ranki, A. (1987). *Proc. Natl. Acad. Sci. U.S.A.* **84**, 4994.
Krowka, J., Stites, D., Mills, J., Hollander, H., McHugh, T., Busch, M., Wilhelm, L., and Blackwood, L. (1988). *Clin. Exp. Immunol.* **72**, 179.
Lahdevirta, J., Maury, C. P., Teppo, A. M., and Repo, H. (1988). *Am. J. Med.* **85**, 289.
Landau, N. R., Warton, M., and Littman, D. R. (1988). *Nature (London)* **334**, 159.
Lane, H. C., Masur, H., Edgar, L. C., Whalen, G., Rook, A. H., and Fauci, A. S. (1983). *N. Engl. J. Med.* **309**, 453.
Lane, H. C., Depper, J. M., Greene, W. C., Whalen, G., Waldmann, T. A., and Fauci, A. S. (1985). *N. Engl. J. Med.* **313**, 79.

Lange, J., and Goudsmit, J. (1987). *Lancet* 1, 448.
Lange, J. M. A., Coutinho, R. A., Krone, W. J. A., Verdonck, L. F., Danner, S. A., Van der Noordaa, J., and Goudsmit, J. (1986). *Br. J. Med.* 292, 228.
Langlade-Demoyen, P., Michel, F., Hoffenbach, A., Vilmer, E., Dadaglio, G., Garicia-Pons, F., Mayaud, C., Autran, B., Wain-Hobson, S., and Plata, F. (1988). *J. Immunol.* 141, 1949.
Lanzavecchia, A., Roosnek, E., Gregory, T., Berman, P., and Abrignani, S. (1988). *Nature (London)* 334, 530.
Lasky, L. A., Groopman, J. E., Fennie, C. W., Benz, P. M., Capon, D. J., Dowbenko, D. J., Nakamura, G. R., Nunes, W. M., Renz, M. E., and Berman, P. W. (1986). *Science* 233, 209.
Lasky, L. A., Nakamura, G., Smith, D. H., Fennie, C., Shimasaki, C., Patzer, E., Berman, P., Gregory, T., and Capon, D. J. (1987). *Cell (Cambridge, Mass.)* 50, 975.
Laure, F., Leonard, R., Mbayo, K., Lurhuma, Z., Kayembe, N., Brechot, C., Sarin, P. S., Sarngadharan, M., Wong-Staal, F., Gallo, R. C., and Zagury, D. (1987). *AIDS Res. Hum. Retroviruses* 3, 343.
Laurence, J., Gottlieb, A. B., and Kunkel, H. G. (1983). *J. Clin. Invest.* 72, 2072.
Laurence, J., Saunders, A., and Kulkosky, J. (1987). *Science* 235, 1501.
Ledbetter, J. A., Evans, R. L., Lipinski, M., Cunningham-Rundles, C., Good, R. A., and Herzenberg, L. A. (1981). *J. Exp. Med.* 153, 310.
Lee, M. R., Ho, D. D., and Gurney, M. E. (1987). *Science* 237, 1047.
Lee, T. H., Coligan, J. E., Allan, J. S., McLane, M. F., Groopman, J. E., and Essex, M. (1986). *Science* 231, 1546.
Leider, J. M., Palese, P., and Smith, F. I. (1988). *J. Virol.* 62, 3084.
Leiderman, I. Z., Greenberg, M. L., Adelsberg, B. R., and Siegal, F. P. (1987). *Blood* 70, 1267.
Leist, T. P., Frei, K., Kam-Hansen, S., Zinkernagel, R. M., and Fontana, A. (1988). *J. Exp. Med.* 167, 1743.
Leonard, J. M., Abramczuk, J. W., Pezen, D. S., Rutledge, R., Belcher, J. H., Hakim, F., Shearer, G., Lamperth, L., Travis, W., Fredrickson, T., Notkins, A. L., and Martin, M. A. (1988). *Science* 242, 1665.
Leonard, R., Zagury, D., Desportes, I., Bernard, J., Zagury, J. F., and Gallo, R. C. (1988). *Proc. Natl. Acad. Sci. U.S.A.* 85, 3570.
Letvin, N. L., Daniel, M. D., Sehgal, P. K., Desrosiers, R. C., Hunt, R. D., Waldron, L. M., MacKey, J. J., Schmidt, D. K., Chalifoux, L. V., and King, N. W. (1985). *Science* 230, 71.
Levy, J. A., Hoffman, A. D., Kramer, S. M., Landis, J. A., Shimabukuro, J. M., and Oshiro, L. S. (1984). *Science* 225, 840.
Levy, J. A., Shimabukuro, J., McHugh, T., Casavant, C., Stites, D., and Oshiro, L. (1985a). *Virology* 147, 441.
Levy, J. A., Shimabukuro, J., Hollander, H., Mills, J., and Kaminsky, L. (1985b). *Lancet* 2, 586.
Lifson, A. R., Rutherford, G. W., and Jaffe, H. W. (1988). *J. Infect. Dis.* 158, 1360.
Lifson, J. D., Reyes, G. R., McGrath, M. S., Stein, B. S., and Engleman, E. G. (1986a). *Science* 232, 1123.
Lifson, J. D., Feinberg, M. B., Reyes, G. R., Rabin, L., Banapour, B., Chakrabarti, S., Moss, B., Wong-Staal, F., Steimer, K. S., and Engleman, E. G. (1986b). *Nature (London)* 323, 725.
Lifson, J. D., Hwang, K. M., Nara, P. L., Fraser, B., Padgett, M., Dunlop, N. M., and Eiden, L. E. (1988). *Science* 241, 712.

Linette, G. P., Hartzman, R. J., Ledbetter, J. A., and June, C. H. (1988). *Science* **241**, 573.
Ljunggren, K., Bottiger, B., Biberfeld, G., Karlson, A., Fenyo, E. M., and Jondal, M. (1987). *J. Immunol.* **139**, 2263.
Ljunggren, K., Broliden, P.-A., Morfeldt-Manson, L., Jondal, M., and Wahren, B. (1988a). *Clin. Exp. Immunol.* **73**, 343.
Ljunggren, K., Chiodi, F., Biberfeld, G., Norrby, E., Jondal, M., and Fenyo, E. M. (1988b). *J. Immunol.* **140**, 602.
Locksley, R. M., Crowe, S., Sadick, M. D., Heinzel, F. P., Gardner, K. D., Jr., McGrath, M. S., and Mills, J. (1988). *J. Clin. Invest.* **82**, 2097.
Looney, D. J., Fisher, A. G., Putney, S. D., Rusche, J. R., Redfield, R. R., Burke, D. S., Gallo, R. C., and Wong-Staal, F. (1988). *Science* **241**, 357.
Lotz, M., Vaughan, J. H., and Carson, D. A. (1988). *Science* **241**, 1218.
Luciw, P. A., Potter, S. J., Steimer, K., Dina, D., and Levy, J. A. (1984). *Nature (London)* **312**, 760.
Luciw, P. A., Cheng-Mayer, C., and Levy, J. A. (1987). *Proc. Natl. Acad. Sci. U.S.A.* **84**, 1434.
Lusso, P., Markham, P. D., Ranki, A., Earl, P., Moss, B., Dorner, F., Gallo, R. C., and Krohn, K. J. (1988a). *J. Immunol.* **141**, 2467.
Lusso, P., Markham, P. D., Tschachler, E., diMarzo Veronese, F., Salahuddin, S. Z., Ablashi, D. V., Pahwa, S., Krohn, K., and Gallo, R. C. (1988b). *J. Exp. Med.* **167**, 1659.
Lusso, P., Ensoli, B., Markham, P. D., Ablashi, D. V., Salahuddin, S. Z., Tschachler, E., Wong-Staal, F., and Gallo, R. C. (1989). *Nature (London)* **337**, 370.
Lyerly, H. K., Weinhold, K. J., Cohen, O. J., and Bolognesi, D. P. (1986). *Surg. Oncol.* **37**, 404.
Lyerly, H. K., Matthews, T. J., Langlois, A. J., Bolognesi, D. P., and Weinhold, K. J. (1987a). *Proc. Natl. Acad. Sci. U.S.A.* **84**, 4601.
Lyerly, H. K., Reed, D. L., Matthews, T. J., Langlois, A. J., Ahearne, P. A., Petteway, S. R., Jr., and Weinhold, K. J. (1987b). *AIDS Res. Hum. Retroviruses* **3**, 409.
Lynn, W. S., Tweedale, A., and Cloyd, M. W. (1988). *Virology* **163**, 43.
Maddon, P. J., Dalgleish, A. G., McDougal, J. S., Clapham, P. R., Weiss, R. A., and Axel, R. (1986). *Cell (Cambridge, Mass.)* **47**, 333.
Maddon, P. J., McDougal, J. S., Clapman, P. R., Dalgleish, A. G., Jamal, S., Weiss, R. A., and Axel, R. (1988). *Cell* **54**, 865.
Malkovsky, M., Philpott, K., Dalgleish, A. G., Mellor, A. L., Patterson, S., Webster, A. D., Edwards, A. J., and Maddon, P. J. (1988). *Eur. J. Immunol.* **18**, 1315.
Manca, N., diMarzo Veronese, F., Ho, D. D., Gallo, R. C., and Sarngadharan, M. G. (1987). *Eur. J. Epidemiol.* **3**, 96.
Mann, D. L., Lasane, F., Popovic, M., Arthur, L. O., Robey, W. G., Blattner, W. A., and Newman, M. J. (1987). *J. Immunol.* **138**, 2640.
Mann, D. L., Read-Connole, E., Arthur, L. O., Robey, W. G., Wernet, P., Schneider, E. M., Blattner, W. A., and Popovic, M. (1988). *J. Immunol.* **141**, 1131.
Mann, J. M., Chin, J., Piot, P., and Quinn, T. (1988). *Sci. Am.* **259**, 82.
Margolick, J. B., Volkman, D. J., Lane, H. C., and Fauci, A. S. (1985). *J. Clin. Invest.* **76**, 709.
Margolick, J. B., Volkman, D. J., Folks, T. M., and Fauci, A. S. (1987). *J. Immunol.* **138**, 1719.
Matsuda, Z., Chou, M. J., Matsuda, M., Huang, J. H., Chen, Y. M., Redfield, R., Mayer, K., Essex, M., and Lee, T. H. (1988). *Proc. Natl. Acad. Sci. U.S.A.* **85**, 6968.

Matsushita, S., Robert-Guroff, M., Rusche, J., Koito, A., Hattori, T., Hoshino, H., Javaherian, K., Takatsuki, K., and Putney, S. (1988). *J. Virol.* **62**, 2107.
Matsuyama, T., Hamamoto, Y., Kobayashi, S., Kurimoto, M., Minowada, J., Kobayashi, N., and Yamamoto, N. (1988). *Med. Microbiol. Immunol.* **177**, 181.
Matthews, T. J., Langlois, A. J., Robey, W. G., Chang, N. T., Gallo, R. C., Fischinger, P. J., and Bolognesi, D. P. (1986). *Proc. Natl. Acad. Sci. U.S.A.* **83**, 9709.
McClure, M. O., Marsh, M., and Weiss, R. A. (1988). *EMBO J.* **7**, 513.
McCune, J. M., Namikawa, R., Kaneshima, H., Shultz, L. D., Lieberman, M., and Weissman, I. L. (1988a). *Science* **241**, 1632.
McCune, J. M., Rabin, L. B., Feinberg, M. B., Lieberman, M., Kosek, J. C., Reyes, G. R., and Weissman, I. L. (1988b). *Cell (Cambridge, Mass.)* **53**, 55.
McDougal, J. S., Mawle, A., Cort, S. P., Nicholson, J. K., Cross, G. D., Scheppler-Campbell, J. A., Hicks, D., and Sligh, J. (1985). *J. Immunol.* **135**, 3151.
McDougal, J. S., Kennedy, M. S., Sligh, J. M., Cort, S. P., Mawle, A., and Nicholson, J. K. (1986). *Science* **231**, 382.
McDougal, J. S., Kennedy, M. S., Nicholson, J. K., Spira, T. J., Jaffe, H. W., Kaplan, J. E., Fishbein, D. B., O'Malley, P., Aloisio, C. H., Black, C. M., Hubbard, M., and Reimer, C. B. (1987). *J. Clin. Invest.* **80**, 316.
Meyenhofer, M. F., Epstein, L. G., Cho, E. S., and Sharer, L. R. (1987). *J. Neuropathol. Exp. Neurol.* **46**, 474.
Miller, R. H. (1988). *Science* **239**, 1420.
Mitani, M., Cianciolo, G. J., Snyderman, R., Yasuda, M., Good, R. A., and Day, N. K. (1987). *Proc. Natl. Acad. Sci. U.S.A.* **84**, 237.
Mizukami, T., Fuerst, T. R., Berger, E. A., and Moss, B. (1988). *Proc. Natl. Acad. Sci. U.S.A.* **85**, 9273.
Monroe, J. E., Calender, A., and Mulder, C. (1988). *J. Virol.* **62**, 3497.
Montagnier, L., Gruest, J., Chamaret, S., Dauguet, C., Axler, C., Guetard, D., Nugeyre, M. T., Barre-Sinoussi, F., Chermann, J. C., Brunet, J. B., Klatzmann, D., and Gluckman, J. C. (1984). *Science* **225**, 63.
Montelaro, R. C., Parekh, B., Orrego, A., and Issel, C. J. (1984). *J. Biol. Chem.* **259**, 10539.
Mosca, J. D., Bednarik, D. P., Raj, N. B., Rosen, C. A., Sodroski, J. G., Haseltine, W. A., and Pitha, P. M. (1987a). *Nature (London)* **325**, 67.
Mosca, J. D., Bednarik, D. P., Raj, N. B., Rosen, C. A., Sodroski, J. G., Haseltine, W. A., Hayward, G. S., and Pitha, P. M. (1987b). *Proc. Natl. Acad. Sci. U.S.A.* **84**, 7408.
Mosier, D. E., Gulizia, R. J., Baird, S. M., and Wilson, D. B. (1988). *Nature (London)* **335**, 256.
Muesing, M. A., Smith, D. H., Cabradilla, C. D., Benton, C. V., Lasky, L. A., and Capon, D. J. (1985). *Nature (London)* **313**, 450.
Muesing, M. A., Smith, D. H., and Capon, D. J. (1987). *Cell (Cambridge, Mass.)* **48**, 691.
Murray, H. W., Rubin, B. Y., Masur, H., and Roberts, R. B. (1984). *N. Engl. J. Med.* **310**, 883.
Murray, H. W., Gellene, R. A., Libby, D. M., Rothermel, C. D., and Rubin, B. Y. (1985). *J. Immunol.* **135**, 2374.
Murray, H. W., Scavuzzo, D., Jacobs, J. L., Kaplan, M. H., Libby, D. M., Schindler, J., and Roberts, R. B. (1987). *J. Immunol.* **138**, 2457.
Nabel, G., and Baltimore, D. (1987). *Nature (London)* **326**, 711.
Nabel, G. J., Rice, S. A., Knipe, D. M., and Baltimore, D. (1988). *Science* **239**, 1299.
Nahmias, A. J., Kibrick, S., and Rosan, R. C. (1964). *J. Immunol.* **93**, 69.

Nair, M. P., Pottathil, R., Heimer, E. P., and Schwartz, S. A. (1988). *Proc. Natl. Acad. Sci. U.S.A.* **85**, 6498.
Namikawa, R., Kaneshima, H., Lieberman, M., Weissman, I. L., and McCune, J. M. (1988). *Science* **242**, 1684.
Nara, P. L., Robey, W. G., Arthur, L. O., Asher, D. M., Wolff, A. V., Gibbs, C. J., Jr., Gajdusek, D. C., and Fischinger, P. J. (1987a). *J. Virol.* **61**, 3173.
Nara, P. L., Robey, W. G., Gonda, M. A., Carter, S. G., and Fischinger, P. J. (1987b). *Proc. Natl. Acad. Sci. U.S.A.* **84**, 3797.
Nara, P. L., Robey, W. G., Pyle, S. W., Hatch, W. C., Dunlop, N. M., Bess, J. W., Jr., Kelliher, J. C., Arthur, L. O., and Fischinger, P. J. (1988). *J. Virol.* **62**, 2622.
Navia, B. A., and Price, R. W. (1987). *Arch. Neurol. (Chicago)* **44**, 65.
Navia, B. A., Jordan, B. D., and Price, R. W. (1986). *Ann. Neurol.* **19**, 517.
Nelson, J. A., Reynolds-Kohler, C., Oldstone, M. B., and Wiley, C. A. (1988). *Virology* **165**, 286.
Nicholson, J. K., Cross, G. D., Callaway, C. S., and McDougal, J. S. (1986). *J. Immunol.* **137**, 323.
Nielsen, H., Kharazmi, A., and Faber, V. (1986). *Scand. J. Immunol.* **24**, 291.
Nixon, D. F., Townsend, A. R., Elvin, J. G., Rizza, C. R., Gallwey, J., and McMichael, A. J. (1988). *Nature (London)* **336**, 484.
Ogasawara, M., Cianciolo, G. J., Snyderman, R., Mitani, M., Good, R. A., and Day, N. K. (1988). *J. Immunol.* **141**, 614.
Ojo-Amaize, E. A., Nishanian, P., Keith, D. E., Jr., Houghton, R. L., Heitjan, D. F., Fahey, J. L., and Giorgi, J. V. (1987). *J. Immunol.* **139**, 2458.
Orenstein, J. M., Meltzer, M. S., Phipps, T., and Gendelman, H. E. (1988). *J. Virol.* **62**, 2578.
Ostrove, J. M., Leonard, J., Weck, K. E., Rabson, A. B., and Gendelman, H. E. (1987). *J. Virol.* **61**, 3726.
Palker, T. J., Matthews, T. J., Clark, M. E., Cianciolo, G. J., Randall, R. R., Langlois, A. J., White, G. C., Safai, B., Snyderman, R., Bolognesi, D. P., and Haynes, B. F. (1987). *Proc. Natl. Acad. Sci. U.S.A.* **84**, 2479.
Palker, T. J., Clark, M. E., Langlois, A. J., Matthews, T. J., Weinhold, K. J., Randall, R. R., Bolognesi, D. P., and Haynes, B. F. (1988). *Proc. Natl. Acad. Sci. U.S.A.* **85**, 1932.
Pan, L. Z., Cheng-Mayer, C., and Levy, J. A. (1987). *J. Infect. Dis.* **155**, 626.
Patarca, R., Freeman, G. J., Schwartz, J., Singh, R. P., Kong, Q. T., Murphy, E., Anderson, Y., Sheng, F. Y., Singh, P., Johnson, K. A., Guarnagia, S. M., Durfee, T., Blattner, F., and Cantor, H. (1988). *Proc. Natl. Acad. Sci. U.S.A.* **85**, 2733.
Patterson, S., and Knight, S. C. (1987). *J. Gen. Virol.* **68**, 1177.
Pedersen, N. C., Ho, E. W., Brown, M. L., and Yamamoto, J. K. (1987). *Science* **235**, 790.
Peterlin, B. M., Luciw, P. A., Barr, P. J., and Walker, M. D. (1986). *Proc. Natl. Acad. Sci. U.S.A.* **83**, 9734.
Peterson, A., and Seed, B. (1988). *Cell (Cambridge, Mass.)* **54**, 65.
Petit, A. J., Terpstra, F. G., and Miedema, F. (1987). *J. Clin. Invest.* **79**, 1883.
Petit, A. J., Tersmette, M., Terpstra, F. G., de Goede, R. E., van Lier, R. A., and Miedema, F. (1988). *J. Immunol.* **140**, 1485.
Plata, F., Autran, B., Martins, L. P., Wain-Hobson, S., Raphael, M., Mayaud, C., Denis, M., Guillon, J. M., and Debre, P. (1987). *Nature (London)* **328**, 348.
Poiesz, B. J., Ruscetti, F. W., Gazdar, A. F., Bunn, P. A., Minna, J. D., and Gallo, R. C. (1980). *Proc. Natl. Acad. Sci. U.S.A.* **77**, 7415.

Poiesz, B. J., Ruscetti, F. W., Reitz, M. S., Kalyanaraman, V. S., and Gallo, R. C. (1981). *Nature (London)* **294**, 268.
Poli, G., Bottazzi, B., Acero, R., Bersani, L., Rossi, V., Introna, M., Lazzarin, A., Galli, M., and Mantovani, A. (1985). *Clin. Exp. Immunol.* **62**, 136.
Pomerantz, R. J., Kuritzkes, D. R., de la Monte S.M., Rota, T. R., Baker, A. S., Albert, D., Bor, D. H., Feldman, E. L., Schooley, R. T., and Hirsch, M. S. (1987). *N. Engl. J. Med.* **317**, 1643.
Pomerantz, R. J., de la Monte S. M., Donegan, S. P., Rota, T. R., Vogt, M. W., Craven, D. E., and Hirsch, M. S. (1988). *Ann. Intern. Med.* **108**, 321.
Popovic, M., Sarngadharan, M. G., Read, E., and Gallo, R. C. (1984). *Science* **224**, 497.
Preston, B. D., Poiesz, B. J., and Loeb, L. A. (1988). *Science* **242**, 1168.
Price, R. W., Brew, B., Sidtis, J., Rosenblum, M., Scheck, A. C., and Cleary, P. (1988). *Science* **239**, 586.
Prince, A. M., Pascual, D., Kosolapov, L. B., Kurokawa, D., Baker, L., and Rubinstein, P. (1987). *J. Infect. Dis.* **156**, 268.
Prince, A. M., Horowitz, B., Baker, L., Shulman, R. W., Ralph, H., Valinsky, J., Cundell, A., Brotman, B., Boehle, W., Rey, F., Piet, M., Reesink, H., Lelie, N., Tersmette, M., Miedema, F., Barbosa, L., Nemo, G., Nastala, C. L., Allan, J. S., Lee, D. R., and Eichberg, J. W. (1988). *Proc. Natl. Acad. Sci. U.S.A.* **85**, 6944.
Prince, H. E., and John, J. K. (1987). *Clin. Exp. Immunol.* **67**, 59.
Prince, H. E., Moody, D. J., Shubin, B. I., and Fahey, J. L. (1986). *J. Clin. Immunol.* **5**, 21.
Prince, H. E., Kleinman, S. H., Maino, V. C., and Jackson, A. L. (1988). *J. Clin. Immunol.* **8**, 114.
Putney, S. D., Matthews, T. J., Robey, W. G., Lynn, D. L., Robert-Guroff, M., Mueller, W. T., Langlois, A. J., Ghrayeb, J., Petteway, S. R., Jr., Weinhold, K. J., Fischinger, P. J., Wong-Staal, F., Gallo, R. C., and Bolognesi, D. P. (1986). *Science* **234**, 1392.
Quinn, T. C., Piot, P., McCormick, J. B., Feinsod, F. M., Taelman, H., Kapita, B., Stevens, W., and Fauci, A. S. (1987). *J. Am. Med. Assoc.* **257**, 2617.
Quinnan, G. V., Jr., Kirmani, N., Rook, A. H., Manischewitz, J. F., Jackson, L., Moreschi, G., Santos, G. W., Saral, R., and Burns, W. H. (1982). *N. Engl. J. Med.* **307**, 7.
Quinnan, G. V., Jr., Masur, H., Rook, A. H., Armstrong, G., Frederick, W. R., Epstein, J., Manischewitz, J. F., Macher, A. M., Jackson, L., Ames, J., Smith, H. A., Parker, M., Pearson, G. R., Parillo, J., Mitchell, C., and Straus, S. E. (1984). *J. Am. Med. Assoc.* **252**, 72.
Rabson, A. B. (1988). *In* "AIDS: Pathogenesis and Treatment" (J. A. Levy, ed.), p. 231. Dekker, New York.
Rabson, A. B., and Martin, M. A. (1985). *Cell (Cambridge, Mass.)* **40**, 477.
Ragni, M. V., O'Brien, T. A., Reed, D., Spero, J. A., and Lewis, J. H. (1988). *AIDS Res. Hum. Retroviruses* **4**, 223.
Rando, R. F., Pellett, P. E., Luciw, P. A., Bohan, C. A., and Srinivasan, A. (1987). *Oncogene* **1**, 13.
Ranki, A., Weiss, S. H., Valle, S. L., Antonen, J., and Krohn, K. J. (1987). *Clin. Exp. Immunol.* **69**, 231.
Ratner, L., Haseltine, W., Patarca, R., Livak, K. J., Starcich, B., Josephs, S. F., Doran, E. R., Rafalski, J. A., Whitehorn, E. A., Baumeister, K., Ivanoff, L., Petteway, S. R., Jr., Pearson, M. L., Lautenberger, J. A., Papas, T. S., Ghrayeb, J., Chang, N. T., Gallo, R. C., and Wong-Staal, F. (1985). *Nature (London)* **313**, 277.

Reddy, M. M., Englard, A., Brown, D., Buimovici-Klien, E., and Grieco, M. H. (1987). *J. Infect. Dis.* **156**, 374.
Reiher, W. E., 3rd, Blalock, J. E., and Brunck, T. K. (1986). *Proc. Natl. Acad. Sci. U.S.A.* **83**, 9188.
Reinherz, E. L., and Schlossman, S. F. (1980). *Cell (Cambridge, Mass.)* **19**, 821.
Reinherz, E. L., Kung, P. C., Goldstein, G., and Schlossman, S. F. (1979). *Proc. Natl. Acad. Sci. U.S.A.* **76**, 4061.
Reitz, M. S., Jr., Wilson, C., Naugle, C., Gallo, R. C., and Robert-Guroff, M. (1988). *Cell (Cambridge, Mass.)* **54**, 57.
Resnick, L., diMarzo Veronese, F., Schupbach, J., Tourtellotte, W. W., Ho, D. D., Muller, F., Shapshak, P., Vogt, M., Groopman, J. E., Markham, P. D., and Gallo, R. C. (1985). *N. Engl. J. Med.* **313**, 1498.
Resnick, L., Berger, J. R., Shapshak, P., and Tourtellotte, W. W. (1988). *Neurology* **38**, 9.
Rice, A. P., and Mathews, M. B. (1988). *Nature (London)* **332**, 551.
Rinaldo, C. R., Jr., Richter, B. S., Black, P. H., Callery, R., Chess, L., and Hirsch, M. S. (1978). *J. Immunol.* **120**, 130.
Robbins, D. S., Shirazi, Y., Drysdale, B. E., Lieberman, A., Shin, H. S., and Shin, M. L. (1987). *J. Immunol.* **139**, 2593.
Robert-Guroff, M., Brown, M., and Gallo, R. C. (1985). *Nature (London)* **316**, 72.
Robert-Guroff, M., Reitz, M. S., Jr., Robey, W. G., and Gallo, R. C. (1986). *J. Immunol.* **137**, 3306.
Robert-Guroff, M., Goedert, J. J., Naugle, C. J., Jennings, A. M., Blattner, W. A., and Gallo, R. C. (1988). *AIDS Res. Hum. Retroviruses* **4**, 343.
Roberts, J. D., Bebenek, K., and Kunkel, T. A. (1988). *Science* **242**, 1171.
Robey, W. G., Arthur, L. O., Matthews, T. J., Langlois, A., Copeland, T. D., Lerche, N. W., Oroszlan, S., Bolognesi, D. P., Gilden, R. V., and Fischinger, P. J. (1986). *Proc. Natl. Acad. Sci. U.S.A.* **83**, 7023.
Rook, A. H., Masur, H., Lane, H. C., Frederick, W., Kasahara, T., Macher, A. M., Djeu, J. Y., Manischewitz, J. F., Jackson, L., Fauci, A. S., and Quinnan, G. V., Jr. (1983). *J. Clin. Invest.* **72**, 398.
Rook, A. H., Manischewitz, J. F., Frederick, W. R., Epstein, J. S., Jackson, L., Gelmann, E., Steis, R., Masur, H., and Quinnan, G. V., Jr. (1985). *J. Infect. Dis.* **152**, 627.
Rook, A. H., Lane, H. C., Folks, T., McCoy, S., Alter, H., and Fauci, A. S. (1987). *J. Immunol.* **138**, 1064.
Rosen, C. A., Sodroski, J. G., and Haseltine, W. A. (1985). *Cell (Cambridge, Mass.)* **41**, 813.
Rosen, C. A., Sodroski, J. G., Goh, W. C., Dayton, A. I., Lippke, J., and Haseltine, W. A. (1986). *Nature (London)* **319**, 555.
Rosenberg, Z. F., and Fauci, A. S. (1989). *AIDS Res. Hum. Retroviruses* **5**, 1.
Ruggiero, V., Tavernier, J., Fiers, W., and Baglioni, C. (1986). *J. Immunol.* **136**, 2445.
Ruscetti, F. W., Mikovits, J. A., Kalyanaraman, V. S., Overton, R., Stevenson, H., Stromberg, K., Herberman, R. B., Farrar, W. L., and Ortaldo, J. R. (1986). *J. Immunol.* **136**, 3619.
Rusche, J. R., Lynn, D. L., Robert-Guroff, M., Langlois, A. J., Lyerly, H. K., Carson, H., Krohn, K., Ranki, A., Gallo, R. C., Bolognesi, D. P., Putney, S. D., and Matthews, T. J. (1987). *Proc. Natl. Acad. Sci. U.S.A.* **84**, 6924.
Rusche, J. R., Javaherian, K., McDanal, C., Petro, J., Lynn, D. L., Grimaila, R., Langlois, A., Gallo, R. C., Arthur, L. O., Fischinger, P. J., Bolognesi, D. P., Putney, S. D., and Matthews, T. J. (1988). *Proc. Natl. Acad. Sci. U.S.A.* **85**, 3198.

Saag, M. S., Hahn, B. H., Gibbons, J., Li, Y. X., Parks, E. S., Parks, W. P., and Shaw, G. M. (1988). *Nature (London)* **334**, 440.
Sadaie, M. R., Benter, T., and Wong-Staal, F. (1988). *Science* **239**, 910.
Safai, B., Sarngadharan, M. G., Groopman, J. E., Arnett, K., Popovic, M., Sliski, A., Schupbach, J., and Gallo, R. C. (1984). *Lancet* **1**, 1438.
Sakai, K., Dewhurst, S., Ma, X. Y., and Volsky, D. J. (1988). *J. Virol.* **62**, 4078.
Salahuddin, S. Z., Rose, R. M., Groopman, J. E., Markham, P. D., and Gallo, R. C. (1986). *Blood* **68**, 281.
Samuel, K. P., Seth, A., Konopka, A., Lautenberger, J. A., and Papas, T. S. (1987). *FEBS Letts.* **218**, 81.
Sanchez-Pescador, R., Power, M. D., Barr, P. J., Steimer, K. S., Stempien, M. M., Brown-Shimer, S. L., Gee, W. W., Renard, A., Randolph, A., Levy, J. A., Dina, D., and Luciw, P. A. (1985). *Science* **227**, 484.
Sandström, E. G., Andrews, C., Schooley, R. T., Byington, R., and Hirsch, M. S. (1986). *Clin. Immunol. Immunopathol.* **40**, 253.
Sano, K., Lee, M. H., Morales, F., Nishanian, P., Fahey, J., Detels, R., and Imagawa, D. T. (1987). *J. Clin. Microbiol.* **25**, 2415.
Sarin, P. S., Sun, D. K., Thornton, A. H., Naylor, P. H., and Goldstein, A. L. (1986). *Science* **232**, 1135.
Sattentau, Q. J., Dalgleish, A. G., Weiss, R. A., and Beverley, P. C. (1986). *Science* **234**, 1120.
Schneider, D. R., and Picker, L. J. (1985). *Am. J. Clin. Pathol.* **84**, 144.
Schrier, R. D., Gnann, J. W., Jr., Langlois, A. J., Shriver, K., Nelson, J. A., and Oldstone, M. B. (1988). *J. Virol.* **62**, 2531.
Schupbach, J., Haller, O., Vogt, M., Luthy, R., Joller, H., Oelz, O., Popovic, M., Sarngadharan, M. G., and Gallo, R. C. (1985). *N. Engl. J. Med.* **312**, 265.
Sei, Y., Tsang, P. H., Roboz, J. P., Sarin, P. S., Wallace, J. I., and Bekesi, J. G. (1988). *J. Clin. Immunol.* **8**, 464.
Sethi, K. K., Näher, H., and Stroehmann, I. (1988). *Nature (London)* **335**, 178.
Seto, E., Yen, T. S., Peterlin, B. M., and Ou, J. H. (1988). *Proc. Natl. Acad. Sci. U.S.A.* **85**, 8286.
Shalaby, M. R., Krowka, J. F., Gregory, T. J., Hirabayashi, S. E., McCabe, S. M., Kaufman, D. S., Stites, D. P., and Ammann, A. J. (1987). *Cell. Immunol.* **110**, 140.
Shannon, K., Cowan, M. J., Ball, E., Abrams, D., Volberding, P., and Ammann, A. J. (1985). *J. Clin. Immunol.* **5**, 239.
Shaw, G. M., Hahn, B. H., Arya, S. K., Groopman, J. E., Gallo, R. C., and Wong-Staal, F. (1984). *Science* **226**, 1165.
Shaw, G. M., Harper, M. E., Hahn, B. H., Epstein, L. G., Gajdusek, D. C., Price, R. W., Navia, B. A., Petito, C. K., O'Hara, C. J., Groopman, J. E., Cho, E.-S., Oleske, J. M., Wong-Staal, F., and Gallo, R. C. (1985). *Science* **227**, 177.
Shearer, G. M., Salahuddin, S. Z., Markham, P. D., Joseph, L. J., Payne, S. M., Kriebel, P., Bernstein, D. C., Biddison, W. E., Sarngadharan, M. G., and Gallo, R. C. (1985). *J. Clin. Invest.* **76**, 1699.
Shearer, G. M., Bernstein, D. C., Tung, K. S., Via, C. S., Redfield, R., Salahuddin, S. Z., and Gallo, R. C. (1986). *J. Immunol.* **137**, 2514.
Shepp, D. H., Chakrabarti, S., Moss, B., and Quinnan, G. V., Jr. (1988). *J. Infect. Dis.* **157**, 1260.
Sheridan, J. F., Aurelian, L., Donnenberg, A. D., and Quinn, T. C. (1984). *J. Clin. Immunol.* **4**, 304.

Siekevitz, M., Josephs, S. F., Dukovich, M., Peffer, N., Wong-Staal, F., and Greene, W. C. (1987). *Science* **238**, 1575.
Siliciano, R. F., Lawton, T., Knall, C., Karr, R. W., Berman, P., Gregory, T., and Reinherz, E. L. (1988). *Cell (Cambridge, Mass.)* **54**, 561.
Skinner, M. A., Langlois, A. J., McDanal, C. B., McDougal, J. S., Bolognesi, D. P., and Matthews, T. J. (1988). *J. Virol.* **62**, 4195.
Smith, D. H., Byrn, R. A., Marsters, S. A., Gregory T., Groopman, J. E., and Capon, D. J. (1987). *Science* **238**, 1704.
Smith, P. D., Ohura, K., Masur, H., Lane, H. C., Fauci, A. S., and Wahl, S. M. (1984). *J. Clin. Invest.* **74**, 2121.
Snider, W. D., Simpson, D. M., Nielsen, S., Gold, J. W., Metroka, C. E., and Posner, J. B. (1983). *Ann. Neurol.* **14**, 403.
Sodroski, J., Patarca, R., Rosen, C., Wong-Staal, F., and Haseltine, W. (1985). *Science* **229**, 74.
Sodroski, J., Goh, W. C., Rosen, C., Dayton, A., Terwilliger, E., and Haseltine, W. (1986a). *Nature (London)* **321**, 412.
Sodroski, J., Goh, W. C., Rosen, C., Tartar, A., Portetelle, D., Burny, A., and Haseltine, W. (1986b). *Science* **231**, 1549.
Sodroski, J., Goh, W. C., Rosen, C., Campbell, K., and Haseltine, W. A. (1986c). *Nature (London)* **322**, 470.
Somasundaran, M., and Robinson, H. L. (1987). *J. Virol.* **61**, 3114.
Spivak, J. L., Bender, B. S., and Quinn, T. C. (1984). *Am. J. Med.* **77**, 224.
Stanley, S. K., Folks, T. M., and Fauci, A. S. (1989). *J. Immunol.* (in press).
Starcich, B., Ratner, L., Josephs, S. F., Okamoto, T., Gallo, R. C., and Wong-Staal, F. (1985). *Science* **227**, 538.
Starcich, B. R., Hahn, B. H., Shaw, G. M., McNeely, P. D., Modrow, S., Wolf, H., Parks, E. S., Parks, W. P., Josephs, S. F., Gallo, R. C., and Wong-Staal, F. (1986). *Cell (Cambridge, Mass.)* **45**, 637.
Stein, B. S., Gowda, S. D., Lifson, J. D., Penhallow, R. C., Bensch, K. G., and Engleman, E. G. (1987). *Cell (Cambridge, Mass.)* **49**, 659.
Stella, C. C., Ganser, A., and Hoelzer, D. (1987). *J. Clin. Invest.* **80**, 286.
Stevenson, M., Zhang, X. H., and Volsky, D. J. (1987). *J. Virol.* **61**, 3741.
Stewart, S. J., Fujimoto, J., and Levy, R. (1986). *J. Immunol.* **136**, 3773.
Stoler, M. H., Eskin, T. A., Benn, S., Angerer, R. C., and Angerer, L. M. (1986). *J. Am. Med. Assoc.* **256**, 2360.
Strebel, K., Daugherty, D., Clouse, K., Cohen, D., Folks, T., and Martin, M. A. (1987). *Nature (London)* **328**, 728.
Strebel, K., Klimkait, T., and Martin, M. A. (1988). *Science* **241**, 1221.
Stricker, R. B., McHugh, T. M., Moody, D. J., Morrow, W. J., Stites, D. P., Shuman, M. A., and Levy, J. A. (1987). *Nature (London)* **327**, 710.
Sundqvist, V. A., Linde, A., Kurth, R., Werner, A., Helm, E. B., Popovic, M., Gallo, R. C., and Wahren, B. (1986). *J. Infect. Dis.* **153**, 970.
Takahashi, H., Cohen, J., Hosmalin, A., Cease, K. B., Houghten, R., Cornette, J. L., DeLisi, C., Moss, B., Germain, R. N., and Berzofsky, J. A. (1988). *Proc. Natl. Acad. Sci. U.S.A.* **85**, 3105.
Takeuchi, Y., Nagumo, T., and Hoshino, H. (1988). *J. Virol.* **62**, 3900.
Talle, M. A., Rao, P. E., Westberg, E., Allegar, N., Makowski, M., Mittler, R. S., and Goldstein, G. (1983). *Cell. Immunol.* **78**, 83.
Terwilliger, E., Burghoff, R., Sia, R., Sodroski, J., Haseltine, W., and Rosen, C. (1988). *J. Virol.* **62**, 655.

Till, M. A., Ghetie, V., Gregory, T., Patzer, E. J., Porter, J. P., Uhr, J. W., Capon, D. J., and Vitetta, E. S. (1988). *Science* **242**, 1166.
Tong-Starksen, S. E., Luciw, P. A., and Peterlin, B. M. (1987). *Proc. Natl. Acad. Sci. U.S.A.* **84**, 6845.
Traunecker, A., Luke, W., and Karjalainen, K. (1988). *Nature (London)* **331**, 84.
Tschachler, E., Groh, V., Popovic, M., Mann, D. L., Konrad, K., Safai, B., Eron, L., diMarzo Veronese, F., Wolff, K., and Stingl, G. (1987). *J. Invest. Dermatol.* **88**, 233.
U.S. Public Health Service (1988). *Public Health Rep.* **103**, 10.
Valerie, K., Delers, A., Bruck, C., Thiriart, C., Rosenberg, H., Debouck, C., and Rosenberg, M. (1988). *Nature (London)* **333**, 78.
Varmus, H. (1988). *Science* **240**, 1427.
Vazeux, R., Brousse, N., Jarry, A., Henin, D., Marche, C., Vedrenne, C., Mikol, J., Wolff, M., Michon, C., Rozenbaum, W., Bureau, J.-F., Montagnier, L., and Brahic, M. (1987). *Am. J. Pathol.* **126**, 403.
von Briesen, H., Becker, W. B., Henco, K., Helm, E. B., Gelderblom, H. R., Brede, H. D., and Rubsamen-Waigmann H. (1987). *J. Med. Virol.* **23**, 51.
Wahren, B., Morfeldt-Mansson, L., Biberfeld, G., Moberg, L., Sonnerborg, A., Ljungman, P., Werner, A., Kurth, R., Gallo, R., and Bolognesi, D. (1987). *J. Virol.* **61**, 2017.
Wain-Hobson, S., Sonigo, P., Danos, O., Cole, S., and Alizon, M. (1985). *Cell (Cambridge, Mass.)* **40**, 9.
Walker, B. D., Chakrabarti, S., Moss, B., Paradis, T. J., Flynn, T., Durno, A. G., Blumberg, R. S., Kaplan, J. C., Hirsch, M. S., and Schooley, R. T. (1987). *Nature (London)* **328**, 345.
Walker, B. D., Flexner, C., Paradis, T. J., Fuller, T. C., Hirsch, M. S., Schooley, R. T., and Moss, B. (1988). *Science* **240**, 64.
Walker, C. M., Moody, D. J., Stites, D. P., and Levy, J. A. (1986). *Science* **234**, 1563.
Walker, C. M., Steimer, K. S., Rosenthal, K. L., and Levy, J. A. (1988). *J. Clin. Invest.* **82**, 2172.
Wang, J. J., Steel, S., Wisniewolski, R., and Wang, C. Y. (1986). *Proc. Natl. Acad. Sci. U.S.A.* **83**, 6159.
Washburn, R. G., Tuazon, C. U., and Bennett, J. E. (1985). *J. Infect. Dis.* **151**, 565.
Weber, J. N., Clapham, P. R., Weiss, R. A., Parker, D., Roberts, C., Duncan, J., Weller, I., Carne, C., Tedder, R. S., Pinching, A. J., and Cheingsong-Popov, R. (1987). *Lancet* **1**, 119.
Weinhold, K. J., Lyerly, H. K., Matthews, T. J., Tyler, D. S., Ahearne, P. M., Stine, K. C., Langlois, A. J., Durack, D. T., and Bolognesi, D. P. (1988). *Lancet* **1**, 902.
Weiss, R. A., Clapham, P. R., Cheingsong-Popov, R., Dalgleish, A. G., Carne, C. A., Weller, I. V., and Tedder, R. S. (1985). *Nature (London)* **316**, 69.
Weiss, R. A., Clapham, P. R., Weber, J. N., Dalgleish, A. G., Lasky, L. A., and Berman, P. W. (1986). *Nature (London)* **324**, 572.
Weller, S. K., Joy, A. E., and Temin, H. M. (1980). *J. Virol.* **33**, 494.
Wendler, I., Beinzle, U., and Hunsmann, G. (1987). *AIDS Res. Hum. Retroviruses* **3**, 157.
Wiley, C. A., Schrier, R. D., Nelson, J. A., Lampert, P. W., and Oldstone, M. B. (1986). *Proc. Natl. Acad. Sci. U.S.A.* **83**, 7089.
Willey, R. L., Rutledge, R. A., Dias, S., Folks, T., Theodore, T., Buckler, C. E., and Martin, M. A. (1986). *Proc. Natl. Acad. Sci. U.S.A.* **83**, 5038.
Winkelstein, A., Klein, R. S., Evans, T. L., Dixon, B. W., Holder, W. L., and Weaver, L. D. (1985). *J. Immunol.* **134**, 151.
Winkelstein, A., Kingsley, L. A., Klein, R. S., Lyter, D. W., Evans, T. L., Rinaldo,

C. R., Jr., Weaver, L. D., Machen, L. L., and Schadle, R. C. (1988). *Clin. Exp. Immunol.* **71**, 417.
Wong-Staal, F., Shaw, G. M., Hahn, B. H., Salahuddin, S. Z., Popovic, M., Markham, P., Redfield, R., and Gallo, R. C. (1985). *Science* **229**, 759.
Wong-Staal, F., Chanda, P. K., and Ghrayeb, J. (1987). *AIDS Res. Hum. Retroviruses* **3**, 33.
Wright, C. M., Felber, B. K., Paskalis, H., and Pavlakis, G. N. (1986). *Science* **234**, 988.
Wright, S. C., Jewett, A., Mitsuyasu, R., and Bonavida, B. (1988). *J. Immunol.* **141**, 99.
Yoffe, B., Lewis, D. E., Petrie, B. L., Noonan, C. A., Melnick, J. L., and Hollinger, F. B. (1987). *Proc. Natl. Acad. Sci. U.S.A.* **84**, 1429.
Yu, X. F., Ito, S., Essex, M., and Lee, T. H. (1988). *Nature (London)* **335**, 262.
Yuille, M. A. R., Hugunin, M., John, P., Peer, L., Sacks, L. V., Poiesz, B. J., Tomar, R. H., and Silverstone, A. E. (1988). *J. AIDS* **1**, 131.
Zack, J. A., Cann, A. J., Lugo, J. P., and Chen, I. S. (1988). *Science* **240**, 1026.
Zagury, D., Bernard, J., Leonard, R., Cheyneir, R., Feldman, M., Sarin, P. S., and Gallo, R. C. (1986). *Science* **231**, 850.
Zagury, D., Bernard, J., Cheynier, R., Desportes, I., Leonard, R., Fouchard, M., Reveil, B., Ittele, D., Lurhuma, Z., Mbayo, K., Wane, J., Salaun, J.-J., Goussard, B., Dechazal, L., Burny, A., Nara, P., and Gallo, R. C. (1988). *Nature (London)* **332**, 728.
Zarling, J. M., Eichberg, J. W., Moran, P. A., McClure, J., Sridhar, P., and Hu, S. L. (1987). *J. Immunol.* **139**, 988.
Ziegler, J. L., and Stites, D. P. (1986). *Clin. Immunol. Immunopathol.* **41**, 305.

This article was accepted for publication on 22 February 1989.

The Obese Strain of Chickens: An Animal Model with Spontaneous Autoimmune Thyroiditis

GEORG WICK, HANS PETER BREZINSCHEK, KAREL HÁLA, HERMANN DIETRICH, HUGO WOLF, AND GUIDO KROEMER*

Institute for General and Experimental Pathology, University of Innsbruck Medical School, and the Immunoendocrinology Research Unit, Austrian Academy of Sciences, A-6020 Innsbruck, Austria

I. Introduction

Autoimmune diseases (AID) that are experimentally induced in primarily normal animals by appropriate immunization with antigens with or without adjuvants have greatly contributed to our insight into the natural history of this large group of diseases. By this means, experimental AID can be produced in animals of many different species and in nearly every organ. As a matter of fact, even induction of systemic murine lupus by immunization of normal mice with antiidiotypic antibodies to human antinuclear antibodies carrying the so-called idiotype 16.6 has recently been successfully achieved (Mendlovic et al., 1988). Prototypes of organ-specific experimentally induced AID, e.g., experimental autoimmune encephalomyelitis (EAE) (Paterson, 1966), are often considered a model for human multiple sclerosis, and experimental autoimmune thyroiditis (EAT) (Witebsky and Rose, 1956; Rose and Witebsky, 1956; Weigle, 1980) was originally deemed to be a model for human Hashimoto thyroiditis (Roitt et al., 1956). Although there is no question that certain of these experimental AID closely mimic their human counterparts, animal models with spontaneously developing AID, i.e., without the necessity of experimental manipulation, certainly resemble human AID more closely. The best known and some other promising animal models with spontaneously developing AID are listed in Table I.

Chickens of the obese strain (OS) develop a spontaneous autoimmune thyroiditis (SAT) that closely resembles human Hashimoto thyroiditis in all clinical, endocrinological, histopathological, and immunological

---

* Present address: Institut d'Embryologie Cellulaire et Moléculaire, Centre National de la Recherche Scientifique et du Collège de France, F-94736 Nogent-sur-Marne, France.

TABLE I
SOME ANIMAL MODELS FOR SPONTANEOUS AID

	Reference
Autoimmune hemolytic anemia, systemic lupus erythematosus, glomerulonephritis, pneumonitis	
NZB mice	Bielschowsky et al. (1959)
(NZB × NZW)F_1 mice	Helyer and Howie (1963); Dixon (1979)
MRL/l (lrp) mice	Murphy (1981)
BXSB (yaa) mice	Murphy (1981)
C3H/HeJ (gld) mice	Murphy and Roths (1979)
C57BL/6 moth-eaten (me) mice	Shultz and Green (1976)
Thyroiditis	
Obese strain (OS) chicken	Cole (1966); Cole et al. (1968)
Dog	Lewis and Schwartz (1971)
Buffalo (Buf) rat	Silverman and Rose (1975)
Mastomys	Solleved et al. (1982)
Mink disease (glomerulonephritis, arteritis, orchitis)	
Aleutian mink disease	Lodmell and Portis (1981)
Diabetes mellitus	
BB Wistar (BB/W) rat	Nakhooda et al. (1977)
Chinese hamster	Gerritsen and Blanks (1970)
Obese (ob) mice	Coleman and Hummel (1967)
Cutaneous amelanosis	
Delayed amelanosis (DAM) chicken	Lamont and Smyth (1981)
Scleroderma	
University of California at Davis (UCD 200) chicken	Gershwin et al. (1981)

aspects (Cole et al., 1970; Wick et al., 1974, 1981, 1982a, 1985; Rose et al., 1976). The OS was discovered and developed over 30 years ago (Van Tienhoven and Cole, 1962; Cole, 1966; Cole et al., 1968), and the present review will attempt to summarize the data that have been obtained in studies of this model by various groups. The fact that this disease occurs in an avian species has several advantages. These include the now classical anatomical division of the avian immune system into B and T cell dependent portions facilitating separate experimental manipulation of humoral and cellular immune responses. Further advantages are the extramaternal development, thus easy accessibility of the avian embryo, and the availability of a large number of offspring from one pair of parents, thus accumulation of convenient numbers of animals for immunogenetic work and statistical analyses. The chicken major histocompatibility complex (MHC) class I antigens are expressed in high density on the surface of erythrocytes, thus allowing for histocompatibility typing by simple hemagglutination procedures (Hála, 1977). Finally, avian erythrocytes are nucleated and constitute a convenient source for large amounts of DNA for molecular biological studies. The most important advantage of the OS model is perhaps that severe SAT already develops in the second or third week after hatching, as compared to the long lag period in other animal species with spontaneous AID, e.g., murine lupus (Theofilopoulos and Dixon, 1985).

Working with chickens as experimental animals, however, also includes certain disadvantages, such as the considerably higher costs of breeding and raising them as compared to rodents, and the relatively long generation time of 6-7 months. Some of these problems are briefly mentioned in the next section.

Furthermore, there are relatively few inbred strains available for immunogenetic studies, and the chicken MHC is less well characterized than that of humans, mice, or rats. Finally, only few monoclonal antibodies (Mabs) are available for phenotypic and functional analyses of lymphoid and nonlymphoid cells involved in the immune reaction of birds.

II. Development of the Strain—Breeding Requirements

The OS is a white Leghorn line that was originally developed at Cornell University, Ithaca, New York, from the special Cornell C strain (CS) in the late 1950s and was first described by Cole (1966). Historically, symptoms for hypothyroidism, such as small body weight, cold sensitivity, increased amounts of subcutaneous fat deposits, and delayed sexual maturation, were first clinically observed in a few (<1%) female CS chickens of this closed-bred colony. These phenotypically OS dams were mated with normal CS sires, and after three generations (1955-1957) of selective breeding the percentage of female chickens with the obese trait was raised to 10%. Several breeding populations were then selected based on this scheme, with respect to the phenotypic hypothyroid trait, and in 1958 the first sires were also found which showed the described signs of hypothyroidism. From this time on only dams and sires which expressed the described obese trait were selected for the parental population. The chronological emergence of the phenotypic signs of hypothyroidism is shown in Table II.

The OS flock in the Central Laboratory Animal Facilities of the Medical School, University of Innsbruck, Austria, derived from a nucleus

TABLE II
INCIDENCE OF THE OBESE-HYPOTHYROID TRAIT IN THE COURSE OF SELECTIVE BREEDING[a]

Generation	Year	No. of sires	No. of dams	Males		Females	
				No.	Obese (%)[b]	No.	Obese (%)[b]
1	1959	4	38	244	14	273	58
2	1960	5	43	334	25	355	70
3	1961	5	60	313	50	357	81
4	1962	4	50	376	67	328	88
5	1963	5	67	493	76	498	83
6	1965	6	42	238	83	289	93
7	1967	8	64	283	83	246	92
8	1969	8	72	390	89	380	93
9	1970	5	55	355	90	326	93
10	1971	8	64	352	93	343	94
11	1972	8	72	423	83	407	91
12	1974	8	72	451	97	441	97
13	1976	8	72	455	96	471	97
14	1978	8	72	396	98	338	99

[a] From Wick et al. (1981).
[b] Percentage of animals with phenotypic symptoms of hypothyroidism.

provided by Cole in 1970 and is separated more than 18 generations from the original OS population at Cornell University. Due to a limited number of appropriate animal rooms, only a relatively small colony of selected OS birds can be maintained every year as a breeding population. These limitations, which may also apply to other potential users of this model, necessitate the implementation of rigorous selection criteria for maintaining suitable parental generations which guarantee sufficient numbers of offspring. Only those dams and sires are selected which distinctly show the phenotypic hallmarks of OS and are typed as homozygous at the MHC (B locus in chickens). Additional selection criteria include serological analyses [thyroglobulin autoantibodies (Tg-AAbs)] and the production of sufficient numbers of eggs and high-quality semen for every individual OS bird.

The hypothyroid status of OS chickens essentially determines the housing and breeding schemes for parental birds. Specific requirements have to be fulfilled to establish a colony of this animal model and to maintain it successfully for several generations. This goal can only be accomplished if rigid precautions for adequate housing and breeding procedures are efficiently implemented.

A. Housing of OS Chickens

During the first 3 weeks after hatching, the usual housing conditions for newly hatched and growing chickens are used. Room temperatures of 28–30°C, adequate age-related space, a controlled day–night rhythm, and standard hygienic procedures (cleaning and disinfection programs, etc.) are offered to all chickens.

As adequate feed for the first 3 days after hatching, bruised corn and quartz sand are given to the chickens as a starter food. Then a commercial, age-related food is given as described elsewhere (Dietrich, 1989). To prevent functional failures due to the hypothyroidism of the OS chicken, the food of the parents is supplemented with protamone (i.e., iodinated casein, Agri-Tech, Kansas City, Missouri) for metabolizing T3 and T4; 100 g of protamone is carefully mixed with 1000 kg of food (100 ppm) by the food supplier. Alternatively, pure thyroxine (T4) can be used. In this case a premix of 1 g of T4 per kg of food is prepared and mixed with 4000 kg of food to a final thyroxine concentration of 250 μg/kg of food (Sundick et al., 1979). Fresh drinking water is offered by an automatic nipple system.

Due to their hypothyroid trait and thus cold sensitivity of 4- to 5-week-old OS chickens, the room temperature is kept at 26–28°C during the growth period. For adult OS birds the room temperature is reduced to 22–24°C and retained in this range during the production period.

Male and female OS birds are housed individually from the age of 10–12 weeks on, preferably using cages that provide considerably more floor space per bird than commercially available batteries.

B. Breeding of OS Chickens

The selection procedure of parental OS birds is based on a two-step classification schedule. In the first step 10-week-old male and female chickens are classified phenotypically with respect to body weight, feather structure, and comb and wattle development (see Section III,A). Serological determination of Tg-AAbs and analysis for the MHC haplotype (Hála, 1977) complete this first selection procedure. All appropriate OS birds are raised to the age of 20 weeks and are then reselected in a second classification step for the expression of the typical OS phenotype (Fig. 1). Moreover, for every individually housed OS dam the day of the first egg laying as well as egg weights and the number of layed eggs are recorded. For every OS sire the quality and quantity of the ejaculate are determined to confirm the accuracy of the selection for suitable parental birds.

Offspring of selected OS sires and dams destined as experimental birds or as the next breeding population are produced using artificial

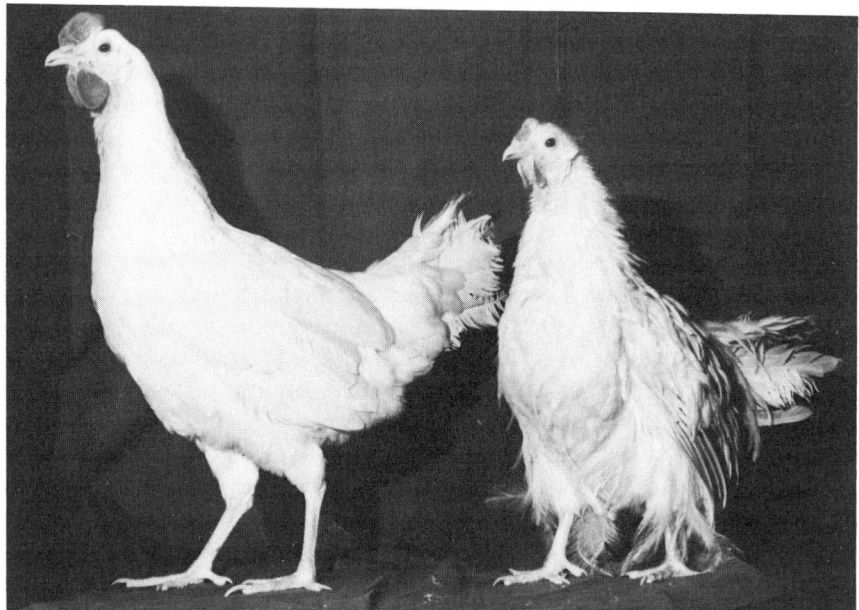

FIG. 1. Twenty-week-old female OS chicken (right) and age-matched normal white Leghorn (NWL) control (left). Note the phenotypic characteristics of the OS bird, such as smaller body size; small comb; long, silky feathers; and a ruffled appearance due to cold sensitivity.

insemination. Freshly collected, undiluted semen aliquots of 0.1–0.3 ml are gently placed into the uterus of selected hens by 1-ml syringes twice a week. The productivity of males and females is recorded for each bird. Eggs are collected daily; marked with the wing tag number of the dam, the MHC genotype, and the collecting date; and stored in a cooler at 16°C maximally for 2 weeks. During the incubation time, standardized temperature and relative humidity are observed. Hatched chickens are marked by two wing tags fixed in both wing webs and comb dubbed. Hatching date, wing tag numbers, and haplotypes of both parents are recorded. For security reasons all animals are MHC typed at the age of 4 weeks.

III. Clinical and Histopathological Characteristics

A. CLINICAL SYMPTOMS

The characteristic clinical features of hypothyroidism appear only 3–5 weeks after hatching and become more pronounced thereafter (Fig. 1). One such feature is small body size, albeit relatively high body weight due to subcutaneous and abdominal fat deposits (hence the name). Further symptoms include a soft, pliable skin; long silky feathers; small combs; lipemic serum; delayed sexual maturity; poor egg-laying ability; low fertility of eggs; and sensitivity to temperatures below 20°C (Cole et al., 1970). These symptoms can also be reproduced experimentally in normal chickens by pharmacological thyroidectomy (Van Tienhoven and Cole, 1962) and can be reversed by diet supplementation with thyroid hormones, as mentioned in Section II,A. Chickens possess two completely separated lobes of thyroid glands, each adjacent to the most caudal thymus lobe and firmly attached to the carotid arteries at the base of the neck. The thyroid glands first become grossly enlarged during the phase of maximal influx of mononuclear cells due to the attempt to compensate for the loss of functional thyroid tissue. After complete infiltration and destruction of thyroid glands have taken place, there is a significant reduction in size, up to complete atrophy ("burnt-out" thyroids) in older birds to an extent that it may be difficult to localize them during autopsy.

Thus far, involvement of other organs—in addition to the thyroids—in the autoimmune process has not been described in the OS chicken in spite of the fact that AAbs against nonthyroid antigens, both organ specific and systemic, have been demonstrated in this strain in rather high frequency (Khoury et al., 1982; Aichinger et al., 1984). As discussed in Section V, the reason for this seems to be that, for the development of SAT, an abnormal function of the immune system *and* a genetically determined susceptibility of the target organ to the autoimmune attack are essential prerequisites (Wick et al., 1986). In the case of SAT in the OS chicken, this predisposing susceptibility of the target organ has been proven by appropriate cross-breeding experiments between OS and healthy, inbred normal white Leghorn (NWL) chickens (see Section VIII,B).

General investigations on the pathophysiology of nonthyroid metabolic functions in the OS chicken are still scarce. Blood sugar, serum concentration of total lipids, total glycerol, cholesterol, and phosphatides were determined (Rudas et al., 1972). As expected on the basis of the characteristically lipemic serum, significantly increased serum lipid concentrations were found at the ages of 1, 5, 8, and 15 weeks. A single intravenous injection of heparin in a dose which prolongs bleeding time had no "clearing effect" on serum lipids of OS birds. Insulin, given subcutaneously for 4 days, had no effect on blood sugar but decreased the serum phosphatides and total lipid concentrations. The short-term administration of high doses of thyroxine significantly lowered the serum levels of total lipids, cholesterol, phosphatides, and total glycerol, thus supporting the notion that the hypothyroid state is the cause of the hyperlipidemia in this strain. These findings were later corroborated by Raheja et al. (1986), who found that OS chickens have significantly increased insulin/glucagon ratios and suggested that these could cause hyperlipidemia and obesity in these birds.

B. HISTOPATHOLOGY

1. Thyroid Glands

The histopathological changes of the thyroid glands in OS chickens have been studied in detail by conventional (Cole, 1966; Kite et al., 1969; Wick et al., 1970a) and electron microscopy (Wick and Graf, 1972) as well as by immunohistochemical techniques (Wick et al., 1970d). The thyroids become infiltrated by mononuclear cells just 1-2 weeks after hatching, and at the age of 3-4 weeks animals of both sexes display severe, often complete infiltration. The process of infiltration starts multifocally around capillaries and venules, then shows signs of confluence, and finally results in complete disruption of the thyroid architecture and replacement of the thyroid tissue by infiltrating mononuclear cells. The degree of SAT is arbitrarily graded according to an originally established scoring schedule (Kite et al., 1969), where 1+ corresponds to the involvement of up to 25% of the total histological cross-section, 2+ represents 25-50%, 3+ represents 50-75%, and 4+ corresponds to 75% to total thyroid infiltration (Fig. 2). Sundick and co-workers (1980) propagated a more accurate system using planimetric evaluation of the degree of thyroid infiltration.

In fully blown SAT both small and large lymphoid cells, abundant numbers of plasma cells, and many macrophages can be distinguished. A hallmark of SAT that is only paralleled in human Hashimoto thyroiditis, but not in EAT, is the presence of many well-developed germinal centers (Fig. 2d). At early stages of the disease the vessels are engorged with lymphoid cells, and electron-microscopic analysis showed migration of these through the vessel walls into the perivascular space.

As far as the nature of the infiltrating cells is concerned, original studies have emphasized the salient feature of plasma cells and immunoglobulin (Ig)-producing B cells in early stages of the disease. It is especially noteworthy that, in addition to the already mentioned germinal centers, B cells and plasma cells are also found in the immediate vicinity of thyroid follicles and even between thyroid epithelial cells (TECs), a process called

FIG. 2. Thyroid glands of 4-week-old OS chickens with different degrees of lymphoid infiltration. (a) 1+, up to 25% of cross-section occupied by mononuclear cell infiltrate; (b) 2+, 25-50% involved; (c) 3+, 50-75%; (d) 4+, 75% to total infiltration (note germinal centers). Hematoxylin-eosin stain was used; magnification ×27.

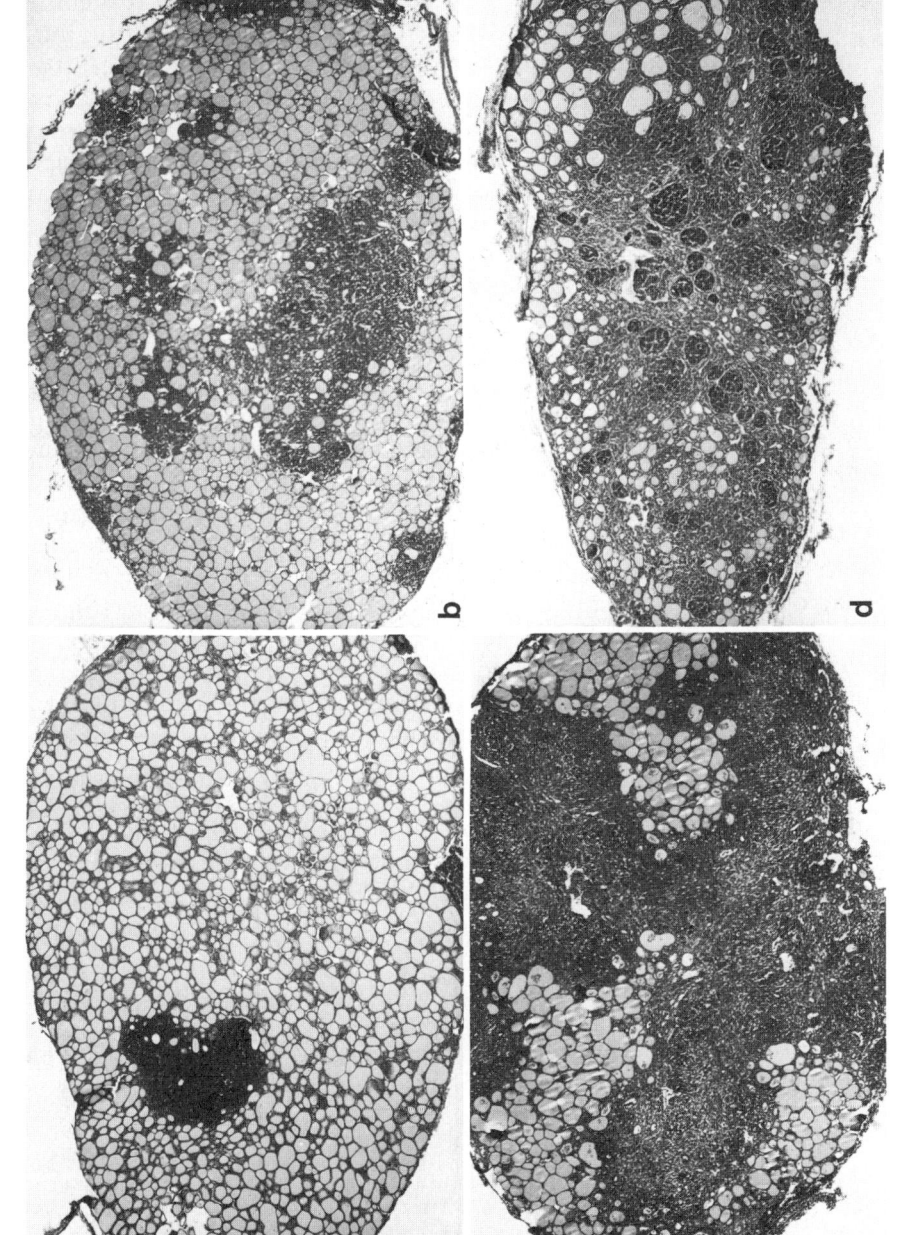

peripolesis (Wick and Graf, 1972). With the advent of new reagents for the identification of subpopulations of mononuclear cells, the initial events of infiltration could be scrutinized in more detail. Thus, it was possible to exactly identify the very first mononuclear cells that arrived in the thyroid glands as T cells that express interleukin-2 (IL-2) receptors on their surface (Hála et al., 1986). Although B cells participate in the process at an early stage, IL-2 receptor-positive T cells clearly precede them. A more accurate identification of the exact nature of these T cells will now be possible by the use of newly developed Mabs against the avian analogs of CD3 (Chen et al., 1986), CD4, and CD8 (Chan et al., 1988). Studies with these and Mabs against the chicken α/β (Chen et al., 1988; Cihak et al., 1988) and γ/δ (Sowder et al., 1988) T cell receptors are under way.

In later, more severe phases of thyroid infiltration, macrophages also invade the thyroid epithelial lining and can be found in the lumen of many follicles that are in a stage of degeneration. TECs which are in close contact with mononuclear cells show severe signs of disintegration (Wick and Graf, 1972) and, in the case of peripolesis, this is associated with disruption of the follicular lining, necrosis, and sloughing of TECs, macrophages, and lymphoid cells into the follicular lumen (Fig. 3). Finally, the follicles collapse, and often attempts at TEC regeneration, albeit unsuccessful, can be observed. Granulocytes are rare in all stages of the disease and TECs packed with mitochondria corresponding to the oncocytes (Hürthle cells) in Hashimoto disease have not been observed in SAT.

The degenerative changes of TECs can be found not only after onset of mononuclear cell infiltration but also in the thyroid glands of newly hatched chickens. They consist of formation of vacuoles in single TECs or even in whole follicles (Wick and Graf, 1972). These alterations are focal and seem to be due to the vertical transfer of antithyroid (mainly anti-Ig) antibodies from the mother hen via the egg yolk into the chick. Granular deposits of complement-fixing Tg-AAbs have been described along the follicular basement membrane in the thyroid glands of OS embryos and newly hatched chicks (Katz et al., 1981; Kofler et al., 1983). As discussed in Section IV,A, the presence of such antibodies may not cause but may accelerate the onset of SAT.

The different composition of the cellular infiltrates in the thyroids of animals with EAT as opposed to OS chickens with SAT has been compared in detail (Wick and Burger, 1971). One characteristic feature of SAT as compared to EAT is the self-limiting nature of the latter, which never entails complete destruction of the thyroid, and thus clinical symptoms of hypothyroidism.

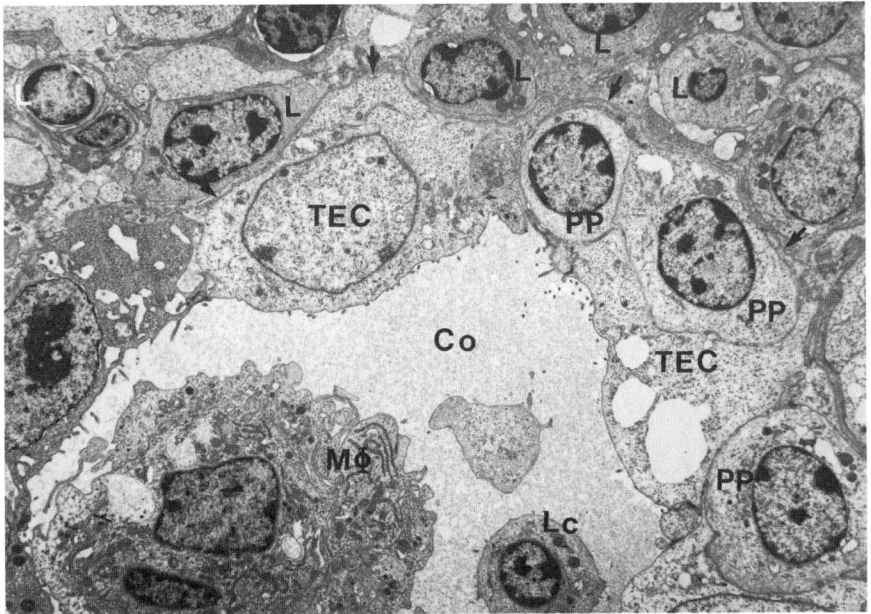

Fig. 3. Thyroid gland of a 4-week-old OS chicken showing destruction of a follicle by lymphoid cells penetrating between thyroid epithelial cells (TECs) [(PP (peripolesis)]. A macrophage (MΦ) and a lymphocyte (Lc) have merged into the follicular lumen. TECs are characterized by villi extending into colloid (Co), partly showing degenerative vacuoles. Lymphoid cells (L) are in the infiltrate surrounding the follicles. ↑, Follicular basement membrane. Magnification ×3575.

Two additional features, characteristic for chickens in general, have to be mentioned in this context. First, small foci of lymphoid cells are commonly found in different endocrine organs, including the thyroid glands. Such foci do occur in both NWL and OS chickens (Wick et al., 1970c). An experienced pathologist can easily distinguish them from "real" minimal infiltration, because these foci are well secluded and show no signs of penetration between thyroid follicles, and follicular damage cannot be observed in their vicinity. A second, more intriguing feature is the following: Chickens have 14 thymus lobes, seven on each side of the neck adjacent to the jugular veins, and the thyroid glands are in close contact with the most caudal thymus lobe. This last thymus lobe often lacks the cortex in the area abutting the thyroid gland, so that the medulla seems to come into direct contact with the latter, often only separated from it by a very thin connective tissue layer. A process tentatively called thymus–thyroid barrier breakdown can often be observed in the OS chicken (Wick et al., 1970b,c), where this connective tissue layer is destroyed and mononuclear cells seem to penetrate directly from the thymus into the thyroid gland, a phenomenon that has never been observed in NWL controls. This observation is one of the many problems that still need in-depth morphological and functional elucidation in this animal model, since it may play a crucial role at the beginning of the infiltration process.

2. Other Organs

The only clinical symptoms in the OS chicken are those associated with hypothyroidism. As will be mentioned in Section IV,A, the sera of OS chickens, however, also contain AAbs against a variety of other nonthyroid antigens (Wick et al., 1970d; Khoury et al., 1982; Aichinger et al., 1984). Despite this fact, strong mononuclear cell infiltration has not been found in organs other than the thyroid gland, and clinical symptoms of systemic AIDs are also absent in this animal model. However, it has to be emphasized that a detailed histopathological analysis of different organs known to be particularly prone to AIDs, such as the gonads and the adrenals, is still lacking in the OS chicken and may be a worthwhile subject of investigation.

3. Central and Peripheral Lymphoid Organs

The central and peripheral lymphoid organs of OS chickens show characteristic changes. In their bursa a marked thickening and branching of the basement membrane can be found separating the cortex from the medulla of the bursal follicles (Wick and Graf, 1972). The puzzling changes often, but not always, observed in the last thymus lobe have already been mentioned; the other lobes show no salient histopathological alterations. Germinal centers are constantly absent in the medulla of the upper six lobes of the thymus, but in the case of the above-mentioned breakdown of the thymus–thyroid barrier, the transition zone between the last thymus lobe and the thyroid gland seems to be a predilection site for the emergence of germinal centers (Wick et al., 1970c). Quantitative analysis of the proportional content of T and B cells in thymus, spleen, and peripheral blood revealed increased numbers of B cells in all of these organs, as discussed in Section IV,B (Albini and Wick, 1974).

IV. Humoral and Cellular Immune Reactions

A. HUMORAL IMMUNE REACTIONS

OS sera contain AAbs against thyroid antigens in a frequency of over 90%. The first antibodies that had been demonstrated in the strain were Tg-AAbs (Cole et al., 1968), but antibodies against microsomal antigens and T3 and T4 are also present. Tg-AAbs can be detected with a variety of methods including passive hemagglutination, double diffusion in gel, complement fixation, immunofluorescence, radioimmunometric techniques (Pontes de Carvalho et al., 1980), and enzyme-linked immunosorbent assays (Kofler et al., 1984). Tg-AAbs of IgG class clearly predominate over IgM antibodies. In the first stages of the disease, the titer of IgG Tg-AAbs correlates well with the severity of SAT. Later, i.e., in chickens with burnt-out thyroid glands, Tg-AAbs may, however, disappear.

This latter observation prompted us to determine whether the presence of the autoantigen, i.e., Tg, was necessary for the development and persistence of Tg-AAbs or whether such antibodies could also result from polyclonal activation. This point was studied by assessing the influence of neonatal thyroidectomy on the development of Tg-AAbs in OS chickens. As demonstrated in Table III (Pontes de Carvalho et al., 1982), Tg-AAbs fail to develop in the absence of the autoantigen. Furthermore, Tg-AAb production depends on the presence of an intact thymus, since depletion of T cells in OS chickens by neonatal thymectomy plus treatment with a highly specific turkey anti-chicken T cell serum prevents the formation of Tg-AAbs (Pontes de Carvalho et al., 1981; see also Table VII). It is noteworthy in this context that mammalian antibodies against

TABLE III
Effect of Neonatal Thyroidectomy on Tg-AAb Formation in OS Chickens[a]

Experiment	Treatment	Tg-AAb Incidence[b]	Titer ($\log_2$) of positive sera (mean ± SD)
1 (10 weeks after Tdx)	Tdx	0/5	<1
		$p = 0.01$[c]	
	None	18/25	3.8 ± 2.9
2 (9 weeks after Tdx)	Tdx	1/15	3
		$p = 0.02$[c]	
	Sham-Tdx	11/24	5.0 ± 2.4
	None	5/12	4.6 ± 1.9
3 (7 weeks after Tdx)	Tdx	3/13[d]	2.0 ± 1.0
		$p = 0.04$[c]	
	Sham-Tdx	11/16	3.7 ± 2.8

[a] Tdx, Thyroidectomy. (Modified from Pontes de Carvalho et al., 1982.)
[b] Number of animals with Tg-AAbs (passive hemagglutination) per total number in the group.
[c] p values were calculated by Fisher's exact probability test.
[d] Two of these chickens had thyroid remnants.

chicken T cells are not active in an avian system *in vivo*, presumably because they cannot bind avian complement. Tg-AAbs show a strict organ specificity and a limited species specificity. Thus, strong reactions can be obtained with Tg of other avian species, but cross-reactions with mammalian Tg are very rare and, if present, are rather weak (Wick and Burger, 1971).

At the present time in their natural history, OS chickens already start to produce Tg-AAbs during the second week of life and extremely high titers can be obtained 4–5 weeks after hatching. There is, however, a significant transfer of IgG Tg-AAbs from the mother hen via the yolk into the newly hatched OS chick. AAbs can be demonstrated not only in the serum of the embryo and the chick but also as granular deposits along their thyroid follicular basement membranes. Codistribution of complement with these IgG deposits has been shown in double-immunofluorescence tests. Furthermore, elution experiments with low pH buffers have been performed to prove that these immune complexes contain Tg as the relevant autoantigen (Katz *et al.*, 1981; Kofler *et al.*, 1983).

As will be discussed later, the first cells that seem to mediate the development of SAT are T cells that express IL-2 receptors (Hála *et al.*, 1986). The presence of Tg-AAbs only seems to have an accelerating effect on the disease process (Jaroszewski *et al.*, 1978). The fact that Tg-AAbs can already be found in the serum of OS embryos and newly hatched chickens as well as deposited *in situ* in the thyroid gland is therefore important for the early development of the disease. In chickens without circulating Tg-AAbs, SAT also emerges, but considerably later, i.e., 20–40 weeks after hatching (Hála, 1988), and less severe. This was one of the reasons that, in earlier publications on the pathogenesis of SAT, more emphasis was given to humoral as opposed to cellular effector mechanisms. As detailed in Section VI,A, the prominent role of effector T cells could only be studied later, when appropriate reagents, transfer systems, Mabs for identification of various subpopulations of mononuclear cells, and appropriate *in vitro* cell culture techniques had been developed for the chicken system. Attempts to identify the sites of Tg-AAb production in central and peripheral lymphoid organs, notably bursa, spleen, and the infiltrated thyroids themselves, were hampered by the lack of success in establishing a plaque-forming cell assay with chicken Tg-coated sheep red blood cells (SRBCs) (Kofler and Wick, 1979).

Tg-AAb-producing B cells, plasma cells, and germinal centers could be detected by immunofluorescence only in the infiltrated thyroid glands (Kofler and Wick, 1978) but not in the spleen, bone marrow, medulla of the thymus, bursa of Fabricius, and Harderian glands. (The Harderian gland is the lacrimal gland for the nictitating membrane—the "third eyelid"—of the chicken. It becomes populated by B cells, which then differentiate into mature plasma cells in the third week after hatching. The Harderian gland thus is a unique site where pure B cells home in the periphery. These B cells are capable of strong antibody production.) Some of the Tg-AAb$^+$ plasma cells in the thyroids were found in peripolesis, i.e., within the thyroid follicular epithelial cell lining (Schauenstein and Wick, 1974). To investigate whether all germinal centers in the thyroid glands of OS chickens produce Tg-AAbs, OS chickens were immunized with bovine serum albumin (BSA) and their thyroids were studied for BSA antibody-producing cells. Interestingly, a considerable number of the thyroidal germinal centers were found to produce such antibodies, thus underlining the notion that the heavily infiltrated thyroids of OS chickens are, so to speak, transformed into a peripheral lymphoid organ that is capable of production of AAbs as well as antibodies against exogenous antigens.

In more recent experiments we successfully stimulated peripheral blood lymphocytes (PBLs) of OS chickens to Tg-AAb production *in vitro*, thus proving that extrathyroidal synthesis of these AAbs actually occurs (Tempelis *et al.*, 1987). OS chickens also showed significantly higher counts of Tg binding (Tg-coated SRBC rosette-forming) cells in spleen, thymus, and peripheral blood as compared to NWL controls (Richter *et al.*, 1975b; Richter and Wick, 1975). This phenomenon is also found with PBLs of human Hashimoto disease patients and clearly precedes the emergence of the classical serological hallmarks of this disease (Perrudet-Badoux and Frei, 1969; Roberts *et al.*, 1973; Urbaniak *et al.*, 1973; Richter *et al.*, 1978). Attempts to demonstrate AAbs to the second colloid antigen in the sera of OS chickens were so far unsuccessful (Wick *et al.*, 1970d).

Nilsson *et al.* (1971) reported the occurrence of AAbs to T4 in 16% of OS chickens aged 1 week to 16 months, and the titer of these antibodies seemed to correlate well with the overall Tg-AAb titer, i.e., sera with high Tg-AAb titers were likely to also contain AAbs to T4. There was, however, no correlation between the severity of SAT and the presence of T4 AAbs. Later, Brown *et al.* (1985) showed AAbs to T3 and T4 (2.9% and 18%, respectively), also in the sera of adult female CS chickens. Again, these AAbs correlated well with the presence of Tg-AAbs. Similar to the situation in patients with thyroid disease (Moroz *et al.*, 1983), some of these T3 and T4 AAbs showed restricted heterogeneity of their mobility in electrophoretic-autoradiographic assays.

A further parallel of OS chickens to patients with Hashimoto thyroiditis is the presence of AAbs against microsomal antigens in both instances, an observation never described for EAT. AAbs to thyroid microsomal antigens were first demonstrated in about 10% of OS sera by Khoury et al. (1982), and later with more refined technique in 26% of all OS sera by Aichinger et al. (1984). In the course of these studies, analyses for nonthyroid AAbs were also performed, and both organ-specific and non-organ-specific AAbs were found in considerable percentages. The organ-specific varieties included AAbs against proventricular parietal cells, exocrine and endocrine (islets of Langerhans) constituents of the pancreas, the adrenal cortex, the parathyroid gland, and striated muscle. While such organ-specific AAbs were only rarely observed in the sera of inbred or outbred healthy NWL chickens, non-organ-specific AAbs, such as antinuclear antibodies, AAbs against mitochondria, smooth muscle antigens, and reticular fibers occurred in both OS and NWL chickens, often even in higher frequency in the latter. Furthermore, Neu et al. (1984) described "natural" hemagglutinins in chickens directed against MHC class IV antigens which, however, were also of equal frequency in OS and NWL birds.

The reason for the high incidence of non-organ-specific AAbs in both OS and NWL strains is not known. One possibility may be that viral infections lead to polyclonal stimulation of the immune system, resulting in the formation of various kinds of AAbs without pathological consequences. On the other hand, such AAbs may also play a physiological role, acting as transporters of breakdown products of cells and tissues (Grabar, 1975). In any case thus far we and others did not find any pathological correlate of nonthyroid organ-specific AAbs, e.g., no signs of Addison-like disease or diabetes. However, this point still needs additional histopathological and functional investigations before final statements can be made.

Luster et al. (1977) evaluated the serum concentrations of the three known classes of avian immunoglobulins in OS and CS chickens and found significantly lower values, sometimes even a complete lack, of IgA in OS birds. This selective IgA deficiency, which was paralleled by elevated IgM concentrations, is especially interesting in view of the known higher frequency of AIDs in humans under these circumstances (Horowitz and Hong, 1975).

In conclusion, OS chickens show a general autoimmune hyperreactivity of the B cell system, but concomitant organ lesions or systemic manifestation were only observed in the thyroid gland. As will be discussed in Section VII,A, several explanations may be put forward for this hyperreactivity, including a quantitative and/or qualitative alteration of the balance between helper and suppressor cells. If this were true, one would expect to find a general hyperreactivity of the humoral and cellular immune systems that is not confined to autoantigens. Data for such a generalized hyperreactivity of the humoral immune system include the observation of increased titers of natural antibodies to sheep and rabbit RBCs (Richter et al., 1975a) and high numbers of PBLs forming SRBC rosettes in OS as compared to age-matched NWL controls. In addition, Kite et al. (1979) have demonstrated higher hemagglutination titers in OS birds actively immunized with SRBCs as compared to NWL chicks, but this observation could not be confirmed in our laboratory.

B. Cellular Immune Reactions

During the first decade of investigations on the effector mechanisms of SAT, emphasis was put on the B cell system and the role of AAbs. The reasons for this were manifold, but the most striking argument for this hypothesis was that early SAT did not develop in OS birds that had been bursectomized *in ovo* or at the time of hatching (Wick et al., 1970a). In contrast, neonatal thymectomy entailed the development of the most severe, i.e., generally 4+, SAT (Wick et al., 1970b; Welch et al., 1973). In these experiments the histopathological and serological analyses were usually performed at the age of 7 weeks, i.e., at an early stage after hatching. The conclusion from these observations was that B cells and their products, e.g., Tg-AAbs, were instrumental for thyroid gland damage and that early removal of the thymus somehow resulted in the "abolition of the self-recognition control mechanism" (suppressor T cells were not known at that time) and thus led to the most severe disease. This concept was further supported by studying a unique combination of experimental models, viz. OS chickens with SAT and a simultaneous adjuvant-induced EAE. For this purpose, EAE was induced in either 7-week-old untreated or neonatally bursectomized or thymectomized OS birds and the effect of these treatments was assessed at the age of 12 weeks (Wick and Steiner, 1972a,b). The spontaneously developing thyroiditis and the experimentally induced autoimmune lesions of the central nervous system behaved completely independently: While bursectomized OS chickens developed only mild SAT, if at all, the severity of EAE was unaffected by this manipulation. In contrast, neonatal thymectomy again entailed very severe SAT but prevented the development of EAE, thus apparently pointing to a different pathogenesis of the spontaneous and experimentally induced AIDs.

Additional support for a preponderant role of B cells in the natural history of SAT came from the results of a quantitative analysis of the proportional content of B and T cells in the peripheral blood and the central and peripheral lymphoid organs of OS chickens as compared to NWL controls. A chronological study using specific polyclonal xenoantibodies for the enumeration of B and T cells in the peripheral blood, the thymus, and the spleen showed significantly higher proportional numbers of B cells in suspensions from these organs in the OS as compared to those of age-matched normal controls. Further analysis of these B cells showed that they were mainly μ-carrying cells (Albini and Wick, 1974).

Novak et al. (1978) determined the content of lymphocytes with IgG-Fc receptors in bursa, bone marrow, spleen, thymus, and embryonic liver of OS and normal chickens and found a significant increase of such cells in the OS spleen soon after hatching. Thunold et al. (1981) demonstrated a high number of IgG Fc receptor-positive cells in the thyroid infiltrate.

Based on the assumption of a possible central role of B cells in the development of SAT, OS chickens were treated with injections of turkey anti-B cell (ABS) or anti-T cell sera (ATS) as a possible way for selective immunosuppression. SAT was significantly suppressed by ABS, but ATS had only a slight protective effect (Wick et al., 1971). As this ATS treatment was first not combined with neonatal thymectomy, complete depletion of peripheral T cells was not to be expected and the slight suppressive effect was attributed to the elimination of the apparently minor T cell population within the infiltrate of the OS thyroid glands.

In addition to all of these observations pointing to a general hyperreactivity of the B cell system and perhaps also an important role of B cells in the pathogenesis of SAT, data on an increased reactivity of the T cell-dependent portion of the immune system emerged already in the early stages of investigations in the OS. These studies centered around the issue of a possible altered T cell responsiveness, against both autologous and exogenous antigens. Thus, Kite et al. (1979) showed that 3- to 6-week-old OS chickens were considerably more resistant to Rous sarcoma virus-induced tumors than CS chickens.

Delayed-type hypersensitivity to Tg has been demonstrated by skin tests in OS chickens in a preliminary study by Welch and Kite (1971), but these authors were not able to correlate these reactions with the incidence and the severity of SAT in the limited number of chickens used in these experiments.

Scanes et al. (1976) and Jaroszewski et al. (1978) reported reduced size, weight, and total cell number of OS lymphoid organs—in particular, the thymus, the bursa, and the blood. The significance of these findings in terms of the pathogenesis of SAT is not clear, but the most likely explanation is that the reduced cellularity was a consequence of the severe thyroiditis and, therefore, reduced levels of thyroid hormones.

Jakobisiak et al. (1976) studied the T cell reactivity of OS chicks in terms of the median survival time of skin grafts from donors matched with the recipient at the MHC (*B* locus in chickens). They did not find any difference in the median survival time of $B^{13}B^{13}$ (old nomenclature B^1B^1) transplants on $B^{13}B^{13}$ CS and OS recipients, but a significant difference was found when the recipients were thymectomized and skin grafted at hatching. Under these conditions OS chickens rejected their transplants significantly faster than did CS birds. The authors explained their observations by an abnormal composition of thymus cells or the presence of abnormal thymus-derived suppressor cells in the OS recipients. The fact that thymectomy did not prolong skin graft survival was attributed to a postulated acceleration of thymic development in OS chicks, thus resulting in a greater effector/suppressor T cell ratio in the periphery at the time of hatching as compared to CS controls. Possible criticisms of these conclusions include the fact that they did not consider minor histocompatibility antigen differences, which are known to be of relatively greater importance in chickens as compared to mammalian systems. Furthermore, the data did not take into account the possibility that the function of the suppressor cell system depends not only on the suppressor cells themselves but also on the target cells to be suppressed.

In the course of studies aimed at the elucidation of various effector mechanisms that may contribute to the development of SAT, Boyd and Wick (1980) developed microcytotoxicity assays utilizing ^{51}Cr-labeled chicken (C) RBCs coated with Tg (Tg-CRBCs) by tannic acid to determine Tg-specific direct cellular cytotoxicity (DCC) elicited by OS lymphocytes. Tg-CRBCs presensitized with OS sera containing high-titer Tg-AAbs were used as targets for antibody-dependent cell-mediated cytotoxicity (ADCC); tannic acid only-treated CRBCs served as specificity controls for DCC and as targets for spontaneous cellular cytotoxicity (SCC) toward surface-modified "normal" cells (Boyd and Wick, 1981). These experiments showed that Tg-specific cytotoxic cells exist in the OS bird, and thus perhaps present an effector mechanism in SAT, which is discussed later. This DCC seems to be unrelated to the presence and the titer of circulating Tg-AAbs. In contrast to DCC, there was no overall difference in ADCC between the OS and normal chickens when the two strains were considered as a whole. A chronological analysis, however, revealed that ADCC was significantly reduced in the peripheral blood of young OS birds, followed by a later elevation above the levels in normal control chickens. SCC activity was identical in OS and normal chickens throughout all age groups (Wick et al., 1982a,b).

The reason for this early decrease in peripheral blood ADCC reactivity is not known, but K cells may be involved initially in the destruction of the thyroid and therefore appear depleted in the periphery. This hypothesis is supported by the above-mentioned relatively high content of IgG Fc receptor-positive cells in the infiltrated thyroid gland (Thunold et al., 1981).

As a next experimental step, the responsiveness of PBLs and spleen cells of OS and NWL control chickens against the T cell mitogens concanavalin A (Con A) and phytohemagglutinin (PHA) was evaluated. The most dramatic and also most consistent results were obtained using an optimized method with Con A-coated CRBCs (Kroemer et al., 1984). OS chickens were found to exhibit significantly elevated mitogenic responses as compared to cells from NWL controls or CS chickens, the normal mother strain from which the OS has originally been developed (Table IV) (Schauenstein et al., 1985). This difference was observed throughout ontogeny to 15 months of age. Interestingly, spleen cells from 17- and 20-day OS and NWL embryos did not show any response to Con A-coated CRBCs, but a marked spontaneous proliferation (i.e., without mitogens) of OS spleen cells was noted in the late embryonic and early posthatching periods. This significantly increased spontaneous proliferation was not paralleled by an increase in total cell numbers in the spleen.

From the data discussed so far, it was concluded that PBLs and spleen cells of OS chickens were hyperreactive in a variety of test systems, including mitogen assays. In addition, development of the most severe SAT in neonatally thymectomized chicks pointed to the possibility of an increased helper–inducer/suppressor T cell ratio and/or activity as a possible reason for this generalized hyperreactivity of the B and T cell system in this strain. A possible explanation for the SAT-aggravating effect of neonatal thymectomy was an abnormal behavior of T cells, resulting in a precocious emigration of helper T cells to the periphery during ontogeny (Rose et al., 1976), and a concomitant relative accumulation of suppressor T cells in the thymus. Neonatal thymectomy would thus make an abnormally increased helper/suppressor T cell activity in the periphery even more prominent. Alternatively, there may be a functional defect of thymus-derived suppressor cells.

To study this question, Boyd et al. (1989) performed cell mixture experiments in which the reactivity of suboptimal PBL concentrations (Boyd et al., 1985) from OS or normal chickens was assessed in mitogen stimulation tests or DCC, ADCC, and SCC assays with or without added autologous thymocytes. Since PBLs always gave strong reactions in these assay systems, while thymocytes were only weakly reactive, any suppressive effect found in the mixtures could be attributed to an effect of the thymocyte population. These experiments clearly showed a lack of suppressor activity in suspensions of OS thymuses, as compared to those of NWL controls. This suppressive effect was not only observed when

TABLE IV
PROLIFERATIVE RESPONSE OF OS AND NWL LYMPHOCYTES TO Con A-COATED RBLs[a]

Age	Origin of cells	Strain	n	^{125}I UdR uptake (cpm ± SEM) with RBCs	with MRCs[b]	Stimulation index
Embryonic						
Day 17	Spleen	NWL	5	5570 ± 1431	3896 ± 2401	0.7
		OS	7	22,539 ± 9567	17,357 ± 7451[c]	0.8
Day 20	Spleen	NWL	5	9758 ± 3748	5375 ± 2136	0.5
		OS	6	23,901 ± 6150[c]	13,601 ± 2591[c]	0.6
After hatching						
1 day	Spleen	NWL	10	587 ± 183	660 ± 148	1.1
		OS	18	4758 ± 3544[c]	7105 ± 4750[c]	1.5
8 days	Spleen	NWL	7	664 ± 189	5393 ± 1904	8.1
		OS	15	1705 ± 227[c]	19,766 ± 5020[c]	11.6
14 days	Spleen	NWL	11	1632 ± 151	9732 ± 1364	6.0
		OS	15	2327 ± 192[c]	21,314 ± 1704[c]	9.2
21 days	Peripheral blood	NWL	9	211 ± 12	6304 ± 1502	29.8
		OS	8	367 ± 38[c]	18,671 ± 2048[c]	50.8
11 months	Peripheral blood	NWL	6	291 ± 4	5978 ± 1899	20.5
		OS	6	333 ± 17	36,679 ± 3056[c]	110.5
15 months	Peripheral blood	NWL	6	115 ± 10	12,089 ± 2783	105.3
		OS	6	125 ± 13	39,784 ± 5607[c]	318.3

[a] From Schauenstein et al., 1985.
[b] MRC, Mitogen-coated red blood cell.
[c] Significantly ($p < 0.01$) different from respective value of NWL cells.

cell suspensions were mixed but also when the supernatant of thymus cells was added to the PBL indicator cells.

OS spleen cells, thymus cells, and PBLs, furthermore, exhibit a numeric defect in strongly peanut agglutination-positive cells that are able to selectively suppress T cell responses (Schauenstein et al., 1983).

The hyperreactivity of peripheral OS lymphoid cells is, however, not only due to a deficiency in suppressor activity, but also to an intrinsically increased production of IL-2 (Fig. 4) (Schauenstein et al., 1985). In addition, the elevated response of OS T lymphocytes was manifested by an increased expression of IL-2 receptors, because Con A-stimulated lymphocytes of OS birds were significantly more effective than were those from normal controls in absorbing IL-2 activity from conditioned media of stimulated spleen cells. These functional data were later substantiated by fluorescence-activated cell sorter analyses, using a murine monoclonal antibody against the chicken IL-2 receptor (Schauenstein et al., 1987b).

Coculture experiments showed that OS and NWL splenocytes contain the same percentage of Con A-activatable T lymphocytes, i.e., cells which are able to express IL-2 receptors and thus acquire their ability to

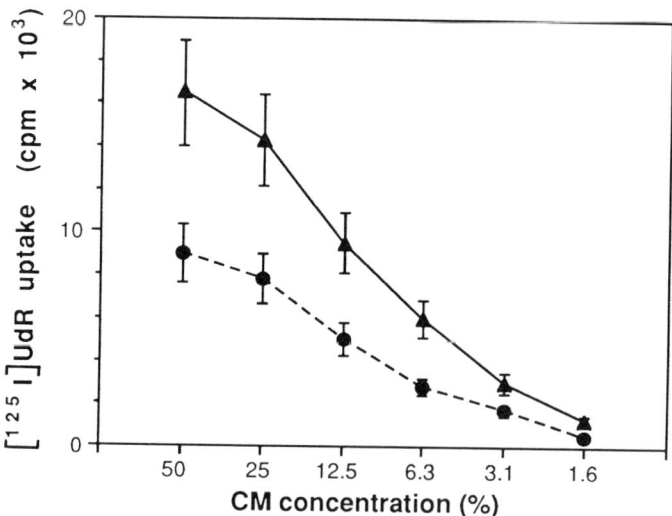

FIG. 4. IL-2 activity of different concentrations of conditioned medium (CM) of PBLs from 11-month-old OS (▲) and NWL (●) chickens cultured and harvested after 24-hour incubation. IL-2 activity was assayed in a proliferation assay with purified Con A blasts, as described by Kroemer et al. (1984). (Adapted from Schauenstein et al., 1985, with permission.)

proliferate with IL-2 (Kroemer et al., 1987; Schauenstein et al., 1987a). Approximately 25% of splenocytes from both strains express the IL-2 receptor recognized by a Mab after short-term (4- to 8-hour) Con A stimulation. Finally, enumeration of cells in the S phase showed that the enhanced proliferation of OS T lymphocytes was restricted not only to the *in vitro* response to Con A and PHA but was also a phenomenon that occurs *in vivo* (Kroemer et al., 1988a).

The various aspects of humoral and cellular hyperreactivity will again be mentioned in Section VII in the context of the discussion of altered immunoregulation in the OS.

In recent years we focused our interest on the thymus in a different area, viz. addressing the question of *where* the process of self-recognition may take place. In this respect our interest was caught by an unusual population of cellular complexes, the thymic nurse cells (TNCs). TNCs are large epithelial cells that contain numerous (e.g., in the mouse, up to 100–200) completely intact T cells engulfed in plasma membrane-lined vacuoles. In this specialized microenvironment, developing T cells come into close contact with MHC class I and class II antigens of the epithelial cells. TNCs were first described in the thymuses of mice and humans (Wekerle and Ketelsen, 1980; Wekerle et al., 1980), and we have shown that TNCs—as expected—also exist in chickens, but generally contain only about four T cells (Boyd et al., 1984). A comparative chronological study revealed a profound deficiency of these cells in OS as compared to NWL chickens: OS thymuses contained only about half the number of TNCs found in NWL thymuses, and OS TNCs contained only about half as many intra-TNC lymphocytes (TNC-Ls). In addition, TNCs became potentially more important with respect to the development of spontaneous AID in the OS by the results of subsequent functional studies of TNC-Ls (Wick and Oberhuber, 1986). In short, TNC-Ls from immunocompetent young normal inbred chickens elicited a graft-versus-host (GVH) reaction in allogeneic recipient embryos and even led to a GVH-like reaction in syngeneic recipients, thus pointing to the possibility that TNCs are a "school" for allo- and autoreactive T lymphocytes. Recent, still unpublished studies were aimed at studying the TNC-L phenotype and functional characteristics of normal chickens in more detail (Pennington et al., 1989). We showed that TNCs are a site for T cell differentiation and most probably for positive selection for MHC class I and class II restriction. Studies to verify a putative role of these TEC–lymphocyte complexes in the hyperreactivity of OS chickens in general, and their autoreactivity in particular, are now under way.

In summary, OS chickens display a significant hyperreactivity of the B and T cell-dependent portions of the immune system against exogenous and autologous antigens as well as an increased response to T cell mitogens. The autoimmune responses are not limited to thyroid antigens, and AAbs against a variety of nonthyroid autoantigens have also been observed. The generalized hyperreactivity of the immune system in this strain seems to be based on a disturbed balance between helper and suppressor T cell activity as manifested, e.g., by a decreased suppressive activity of OS thymocytes on the mitogen response of autologous PBLs as compared to NWL controls, and an increased production of IL-2 by OS spleen cells and PBLs. A possible role of a deficiency of TNCs for the heightened reactivity against exogenous and autologous antigens is still under investigation.

V. Altered Thyroid Function—Target Organ Defect

The clinical symptoms of hypothyroidism were the first that Cole observed in some female birds of a closed flock of the CS in the late 1950s that then served as a nucleus for the subsequent development of the OS by selective breeding (Cole et al, 1970). As mentioned above and detailed in Section VII,B,3, sex hormones may modulate the onset and final outcome of the disease, but are not essential for the development of SAT. Nevertheless, the OS is a very convenient test model for assessment of the therapeutic potency of various androgen analogs which retained their immunosuppressive properties without the unwanted concomitant endocrinological side effects (Wick et al., 1989). The clinical symptoms of hypothyroidism described in Section III,A, such as small body size, lipemic serum, and low fertility are the same as those observed in propylthiouracil-treated normal chickens and can be prevented or reversed by appropriate hormonal (e.g., T3, T4, iodinated casein) substitution. Newcomer (1973) showed that ^{131}I thyroid incorporation and ^{131}I serum clearance by the thyroid were inversely correlated with the severity of lymphocytic infiltration of the thyroid glands. In addition to the hypothyroidism-inducing effect of the severe lymphoid infiltration, AAbs against T3 and T4 are also contributing to this functional defect (Nilsson et al., 1971; Brown et al., 1985).

When the thyroid function of OS chicks was evaluated before the onset of SAT in OS embryos and newly hatched chicks, Sundick and Wick (1974) made the surprising observation that OS chicks injected with ^{131}I had a 20-hour uptake that was about double the value for CS controls and also significantly higher than in outbred NWL chicks. This finding was puzzling for several reasons, especially because the increased uptake and organification of iodine into Tg did not result in increased serum levels of T3 and T4 (Sundick et al., 1980). It was thus hypothesized that the elevated ^{131}I uptake by OS thyroid glands was an intrinsic property of the thyroid gland itself and was not due to elevated secretion of pituitary thyroid-stimulating hormone (TSH). This was the first indication of the possible existence of a primary alteration of the target organ for SAT, in addition to the already well-described abnormal function of the OS immune system. In further studies OS and normal thyroid glands from 16-day embryos were then transplanted onto the chorioallantoic membranes of 9-day normal chick embryos, and 6 days later the 20-hour ^{131}I uptake of the transplants was determined. The results confirmed our hypothesis, because OS embryonic thyroids exhibited a significantly higher uptake of ^{131}I compared to the controls, although both transplants were, of course, under the influence of the same pituitary gland, and thus TSH stimulation by the recipient embryo (Sundick and Wick, 1976).

Earlier, albeit preliminary (Van Tienhoven and Cole, 1962) comparisons of the gonadotropic and thyrotropic potency of pituitary extracts from OS versus normal egg-laying hens have already suggested that the deficiency of thyroxine is not due to a lack of TSH. Later, Sundick et al. (1979) asked the question of whether OS thyroid glands also function in the absence of pituitary TSH, i.e., similar to the autonomous thyroid function in some patients with goiter (Peter et al., 1985). For this purpose, OS and normal chickens were fed a high dose of T4 for 2-3 weeks, starting on the day of hatching, in order to suppress the pituitary secretion of TSH. To eliminate interference by circulating Tg-AAbs and AAbs against T3 and T4 as well as mononuclear cell infiltration of the thyroid gland, some of the OS and control chickens were, in addition, immunosuppressed at the time of hatching. T4 serum levels were tested by radioimmunoassay and were found to be very high in all strains, as expected. All chicks were then injected with ^{131}I and were again tested for the 20-hour thyroid isotope uptake. OS thyroid glands, especially those in which the development of SAT had been prevented by immunosuppression, showed a significant degree of autonomous function, supporting our hypothesis. Surprisingly, the greatest autonomy was found in thyroids of CS chickens, which are known to develop neither SAT nor Tg-AAbs. It was thus hypothesized that the autonomous function of the thyroid gland may be one of the risk factors leading to SAT development, but only in concert with an appropriate immune system abnormality. Thus, the OS chicken and chickens of its progenitor CS strain have an intrinsic abnormality of thyroid function, reflected by significantly higher uptake of iodine and increased iodotyrosine coupling in the presence of serum T4 levels which are sufficient to suppress these functions in control chickens. This poor suppressibility thus does not seem to be due to persistent pituitary TSH secretion, because OS and

CS chickens show normal serum and thyroidal T3 and T4 levels on regular feed (Sundick et al., 1979).

One possibility for this very high thyroid function in T4-suppressed OS and CS chickens might have been the presence of thyroid-stimulating immunoglobulins. To test for this, newly hatched chicks were first immunosuppressed with cyclophosphamide (2 mg/day for the first 4 days) to eliminate antibody responses (Sundick et al., 1980) and then fed T4 and analyzed 2 weeks later for 20-hour thyroidal ^{131}I uptake. OS and CS thyroids again incorporated significantly more ^{131}I than did normal controls. Hence, cyclophosphamide treatment had no suppressive effect on thyroid function but even resulted in doubling of the TSH-independent uptake of ^{131}I, thus proving that the previously described autonomy in CS chickens was not due to thyroid-stimulating immunoglobulins.

Another possibility was that OS and CS pituitary glands did not appropriately respond to the feedback control by high levels of T4. To examine this, OS (or CS) and NWL thyroid glands were simultaneously transplanted into the wing webs of newly hatched (OS × NWL)F_1 recipients (Livezey and Sundick, 1980). These recipients were maintained on a T4-supplemented diet. At 4 weeks of age the recipients were injected with ^{131}I and the transplanted thyroids were harvested 20 hours later for the assessment of isotope uptake. The results indicated that OS and CS thyroid lobes again had a significantly greater ^{131}I uptake than did normal thyroids when exposed to an environment with very low TSH. When the same experiments were repeated with recipients kept on normal feed (i.e., no T4 supplementation), the differences between the OS, CS, and normal thyroids became even more significant.

In conclusion, OS and CS thyroid glands show a significantly increased thyroid function under T4 suppression as compared to normal chickens. This hyperfunction is either completely autonomous, i.e., independent of TSH, or due to a hyperresponsiveness to very low TSH levels.

Further support for an abnormality of the thyroid gland came from experiments by Truden et al. (1983), who examined another functional parameter, viz. the capacity of TEC cultures to proliferate *in vitro*. These authors demonstrated that thyroid epithelial cells derived from OS embryos incorporated significantly less [^{3}H]thymidine and showed significantly slower doubling times than did CS cells (26 versus 18 hours). In addition, it was found that OS thyroid epithelial cells were not able to condition their own culture medium: Supplementation of conditioned media from CS thyroid cultures restored the normal growth and DNA synthesis of OS cells. So far, the cause for this reduced proliferation of OS TECs has not been further studied, but several possibilities have been discussed, such as the influence of an endogenous or exogenous virus, genetically programmed defects of the TECs, and an altered responsiveness to TSH.

The concerted data substantiated the hypothesis that an intrinsic thyroid abnormality exists in the OS chicken that may be a prerequisite for the development of SAT. Genetic analyses of this hypothetical target organ defect are discussed in detail in Section VIII. A series of further experiments in various laboratories was, therefore, aimed to further elucidate the puzzle of the nature of such a thyroid defect, in addition to those features described above (i.e., increased ^{131}I uptake, autonomous function not suppressible by high doses of T4, and decreased growth rate of OS thyroid cells *in vitro* with insufficient release of growth-promoting autocrine factors).

Other possibilities for potential disease-promoting thyroid abnormalities include an abnormal composition and thus immunogenicity of OS Tg, a primary aberrant expression of MHC class II antigens by TECs, and the role of viruses.

The pivotal role of Tg as an autoantigen in SAT was discussed in Section IV,A. Sanker *et al.* (1983) showed that tolerization of OS chickens with Tg at the time of hatching entailed a significant prevention of SAT development and Tg-AAb production, thus elegantly proving that immunoreactivity against this antigen is not just a secondary phenomenon not related to the disease process. In a very crucial set of experiments with possible importance for the human situation, Bagchi *et al.* (1985) suggested that an excess of dietary iodine may promote the development of autoimmune thyroiditis. In their experiments diet supplementation with iodine led to a dose-dependent, significant increase in the numbers of CS chickens, the clinically normal OS progenitor strain, with thyroiditis, Tg-AAbs, and AAbs against T3 and T4. An important control in these experiments was the demonstration that this dietary regimen had no influence on the capacity of CS chickens to produce antibodies against an exogenous antigen, i.e., SRBCs. These results were interpreted as providing direct experimental evidence that the excessive consumption of iodine in some parts of the world, including the United States, may be responsible for the increased incidence of autoimmune thyroiditis in these regions.

In subsequent studies Sundick *et al.* (1987) investigated the hypothesis that highly iodinated Tg might be significantly more immunogenic than is Tg containing fewer iodine atoms. To this end, Tg with high (HI-Tg) or low iodine (LI-Tg) content was purified from CS chickens fed a high- or low-iodine diet and injected intravenously into normal chickens without adjuvants. Animals immunized with HI-Tg produced a much higher titer of Tg antibodies, which also reacted better with HI-Tg than with LI-Tg, thus supporting this hypothesis.

The next question was, of course, whether the degree of iodination of Tg in OS thyroids could be identified as a possible factor for the induction of SAT. In marked contrast with the iodine-induced Tg antibodies in NWL, the Tg-AAbs in the sera of OS chickens were found to be independent of dietary iodine intake.

This conclusion had already been reached by Pontes de Carvalho et al. (1982), who showed that Tg-AAbs from OS chickens react equally well with Tg derived from OS and NWL donors. Further support for a normal composition of OS Tg came from detailed biochemical analyses that showed no difference in iodine and sugar content between OS and NWL Tg, with the exception of a higher value for fucose in NWL Tg (Table V). Murine Mabs against chicken Tg or against evolutionary conserved hormogenic sites of mammalian and avian Tg have also not revealed any difference between OS and NWL Tg. The only difference that was found in preliminary studies was a change in the sedimentation pattern upon ultracentrifugation over sucrose gradients (Wick et al., 1986). We observed a higher degree of heterogeneity of OS Tg manifested in a significantly increased 7 S peak in addition to the classical 19 S peak for normal Tg. These Tg preparations were derived from pooled thyroid glands of 1-day-old chicks, i.e., before overt lymphoid infiltration in the OS. The results were interpreted as a possibly higher susceptibility of OS Tg to disintegrate into the smaller 7 S subunits or even a defect in Tg synthesis.

TABLE V
CARBOHYDRATE CONTENT OF DIFFERENT Tg PREPARATIONS[a]

Carbohydrate (μmol/100 mg)	Human Tg	Chicken Tg (3 weeks)[b]	
		NWL	OS
Fucose	2.2	15.0	2.4
Mannose	11.6	18.1	20.5
Galactose	6.6	6.1	9.5
N-Acetylglucosamine	13.6	9.0	11.1
N-Acetylsialic acid	4.2	6.7	6.2

[a] Tg was prepared by column chromatography of thyroid saline extracts on Sepharose S300 (Shulman et al., 1967). For the determination of sugars, the procedure of Chambers and Clamp (1971), with some modification, was followed. R. Fischer-Colbrie, Department of Pharmacology, University of Innsbruck, Austria, kindly performed gas chromatographic carbohydrate determinations.

[b] OS chickens were hormonally (testosterone) bursectomized in ovo to prevent early SAT development.

More recently, we have reinvestigated this phenomenon, keeping in mind, that due to the constant rigid selective breeding procedure, a few scattered foci of mononuclear cells can already occasionally be found in the thyroids of OS chickens during the first week after hatching. In this case proteolytic enzymes may have been released by the infiltrating cells, which then may have cleaved the Tg molecule into smaller subunits either *in vivo* or during the *in vitro* purification process. We are currently probing this possibility by comparing OS and NWL Tg derived from chicks that had been hormonally bursectomized *in ovo* by treating 3-day embryos with testosterone, a procedure that has been shown to prevent or delay the development of SAT (Cole *et al.*, 1970).

A further possibility for a thyroid-related event that may trigger SAT development would be a primary "aberrant" expression of MHC class II antigens by TECs. Such an expression of MHC class II antigens has been described on TECs of human patients with Graves' disease by Bottazzo *et al.* (1983) and Hanafusa *et al.* (1983) and in Hashimoto thyroiditis by these and other authors (Aichinger *et al.*, 1985; Weetman *et al.*, 1985). However, with respect to the possible functional role of this expression, there is still considerable controversy: Some groups postulate that MHC class II antigens occur *before* lymphoid infiltration and that TECs may therefore act as antigen-presenting cells in the initial phase of autoimmune thyroiditis, while others—including ourselves—consider this a secondary phenomenon that does not trigger the disease but may contribute to its perpetuation. The OS chicken model is an optimal subject for the study of this question, because SAT development can be followed chronologically from the incipient to the most severe stages. We first investigated this question on frozen, unfixed sections of thyroid glands from OS and normal chickens and showed that MHC class II antigens (B-L in the chicken) are only expressed in the neighborhood of infiltrating T cells and not before infiltration or in uninfiltrated areas (Wick *et al.*, 1984). It was concluded, in analogy to the human disease, that γ-interferon produced by the first T cells that arrive in the thyroid gland induces this aberrant B-L expression. Unfortunately, at that time Mabs against chicken T cell subsets were not yet available and the helper-inducer nature of these first cells coming into close contact with the thyroid epithelium therefore could not yet be identified, in contrast to the findings in human tissues (Aichinger *et al.*, 1985).

To further study the possible effect of γ-interferon on the expression of MHC class II antigens on OS TECs, the following experiments were performed (Wick *et al.*, 1987): Epithelial cells were prepared from OS and NWL thyroids from chickens less than 2 weeks of age and cultured *in vitro* in a medium supplemented with TSH but without IL-2. Using this procedure, the TECs could be propagated, but any residual lymphocytes (from beginning infiltration or blood contamination) did not survive. After 3 days of culture aliquots of TECs were removed and tested for the expression of B-L in indirect immunofluorescence, using a monoclonal antibody against a nonpolymorphic epitope of the chicken MHC class II framework determinants.

As shown in Table VI, unstimulated OS and NWL TECs were negative for Ia-like determinants. However, following stimulation with chicken interferon for 48–72 hours, OS TECs expressed B-L in a higher percentage and considerably earlier than control cells, thus pointing to a lower threshold of the former to the induction of MHC class II expression by γ-interferon. Similar experiments performed with adrenal and kidney cell suspensions showed that this phenomenon is thyroid specific. If small amounts of B-L antigens, which are not detectable by conventional immunohistochemical methods, are synthesized by TECs must still be clarified by more sensitive methods, such as *in situ* hybridization with appropriate cDNA probes that are now available for different chains of the chicken Ia-like molecules.

Finally, a virus infection may be responsible for the increased susceptibility of the thyroid gland to the autoimmune attack. Bacterial and viral infections have been proposed, and even sometimes proven, as possible causes for the development of AIDs. Their effect could be exerted via polyclonal activation, circumventing the requirement of T cell help (Esquivel *et al.*, 1977), antigenic mimicry (Notkins and Prabhakar, 1986), and "altered self" (Weigle, 1978; Rose *et al.*, 1988), an alteration of the immune system itself. The development of autoimmune thyroiditis as a sequel of infections has been exemplified in rabbits after immunization with a group A streptococcal vaccine (Tonooka *et al.*, 1978) and in chickens infected with the Rous-associated virus type 7 (RAV-7) (Carter *et al.*, 1983). This latter observation is of special interest in the present context because RAV-7-infected chickens showed histopathological hallmarks of thyroiditis that exactly paralleled those found in the OS, e.g., a large number of well-developed germinal centers. In addition to Tg-AAbs, the sera of these birds also contained AAbs against nonthyroid antigens and showed a certain degree of lesions in such organs as the pancreas. In the OS, data on a possible virus involvement in the development of SAT are still limited. Early in the history of the strain Zeigel *et al.* (1970) published serological and electron-microscopic data arguing against a viral factor involvement in the pathogenesis. Later, in a more detailed electron-microscopic study, C-type particles were found in TECs of OS but not NWL chickens (Wick and Graf, 1972). In recent years our interest has focused on the possible role of endogenous viruses

TABLE VI
LOWERED THRESHOLD OF OS TECs FOR γ-INTERFERON-INDUCED B-L EXPRESSION[a]

Strain	No. of animals	B-L$^+$ cells (%)								
		72 hours without IFN			48 hours + IFN			72 hours + IFN		
		TECs	Adr.	Kid.	TECs	Adr.	Kid.	TECs	Adr.	Kid.
CB	5–10	Neg.	Neg.	Neg.	4	2	1	10	5	8
OS	5–10	Neg.	Neg.	Neg.	24	6	4	30	6	7

[a]Data were compiled from Wick et al. (1987) and from two additional experiments. Age of donors was 7–10 days. Preculture of thyroid epithelial cells (TECs) for 3 days in Dulbecco's modified essential medium containing 2 IU/ml of TSH [also for adrenal (Adr.) and kidney (Kid.) cells], 10% fetal calf serum, and 50 μg/ml of gentamicin (Schering Corp., Berlin, FRG) without γ-interferon (IFN), followed by 3 days 10 IU/ml of chicken γ-IFN. Neg., Negative results.

(*ev*s) as possible factors contributing to the emergence of AIDs in general and SAT in particular. The chicken is particularly well suited for such studies because *ev*s have first been described in this species and 21 *ev* loci have been identified in various chicken strains in the past (Smith *et al.*, 1986). As a matter of fact, all domestic chickens harbor endogenous retroviral genes related to the avian leukosis complex of viruses (Rovigatti and Astrin, 1983; Coffin, 1982; Hayward and Neel, 1981; Robinson, 1978). These *ev* genes can remain inactive or they may be expressed as viral proteins or particles. The expression of these genes can influence the outcome of exogenous avian leukosis virus infections, but so far no beneficial role of *ev*s has been demonstrated that may confer a selective advantage to those birds that possess certain *ev*s. However, integrated *ev*s can act as insertional mutagens by means of their long terminal repeats (LTRs) and thus influence the expression of host genes via *cis* or *trans* mechanisms (Nusse, 1986; Grindley *et al.*, 1987).

In view of a potential role of such *ev* loci for SAT pathogenesis, careful study of OS *ev* patterns was therefore deemed of interest. For this purpose, DNA from various chicken strains, including the OS, was isolated from the nucleated erythrocytes using standard techniques, digested with restriction endonucleases, and analyzed by Southern blotting using a nick-translated, cloned Rous sarcoma virus (pSRA-2) DNA as a probe. Different restriction enzymes give characteristic *ev* patterns with this approach. Thus, *Sac*I cleaves near the 5' LTR of *ev*s, supplying a unique virus cell function fragment for each *ev*, corresponding to their random integration in the host genome. DNA from birds of inbred strains with previously characterized *ev* patterns was used for the identification of new *ev*s.

A representative *ev* Southern blot pattern is shown in Fig. 5. The birds investigated in this experiment included OS chickens homozygous for the B^{13}, B^{15}, or B^5 MHC haplotypes, B^{13} CS chickens, and several well-characterized inbred strains with different other B haplotypes. It can be seen in the figure that chickens of each strain afforded a characteristic banding pattern, and these bands could be identified with the help of the control DNA preparations. However, there was one band migrating slightly faster than *ev* 2 that was only found in the OS but never in any other strain. This band has in the meantime been identified as a new *ev* locus tentatively called *ev* 22 (Ziemiecki *et al.*, 1988). Recent genetic analyses described below have shown that *ev* 22 is not linked to the MHC and that the presence of *ev* 22 is also not an essential factor for the development of SAT, but may have a modulating role in connection with a disturbed immune endocrine feedback loop in this strain, which possibly contributes to the general hyperreactivity of the immune system (Kroemer *et al.*, 1988b).

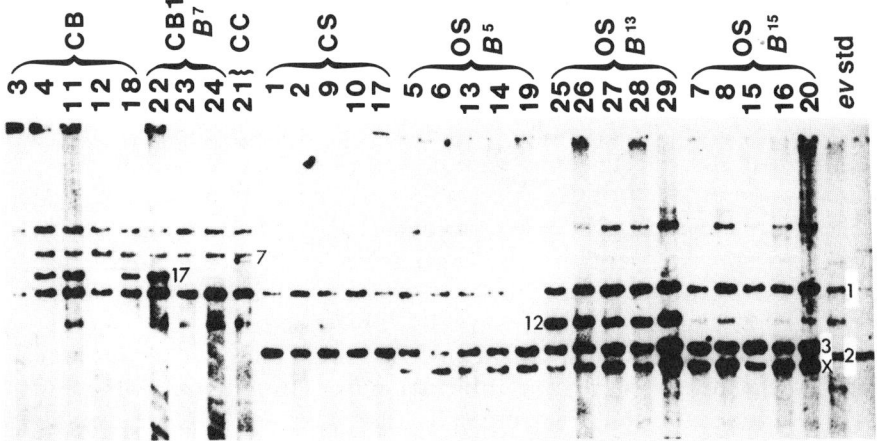

FIG. 5. Endogenous virus (*ev*) pattern in different strains of chickens. DNA was isolated from chicken erythrocyte nuclei, digested with restriction endonuclease *Sac*I, size separated on a 0.8% agarose gel, and transferred to GeneScreen plus. The filter was hybridized with ^{32}P nick-labeled pSRA-2, washed, and exposed to Kodak XAR-5 film with intensifying screen. DNA containing known *ev* loci were kindly provided by Barbara Baker, Eugene J. Smith, Eric H. Humphries, and Stephan H. Hughes. *ev* 1, 2, and 3 are indicated at the right of the figure. The numbers and letters above indicate codes of different chickens and the respective strain of inbred NWL (CB, CB.I-B7, CC), the CS and OS sublines (OS B^5, OS B^{13}, OS B^{15}). X, restriction fragment migrating slightly faster than the *ev* 2 reference band and referred to as *ev* 22. (From Ziemiecki *et al.*, 1988, with permission.)

VI. Potential Effector Mechanisms

A. Relative Role of the B and T Cell Lineages for SAT

The first studies concerning the effector mechanisms operative in SAT were designed to elucidate the relative contribution of the humoral and cellular mechanisms. As mentioned in Section IV,B, surgical bursectomy either *in ovo* on day 18 of incubation or posthatching resulted in a decrease in the frequency and the severity of SAT (Wick *et al.*, 1970a). Similarly, hormonal bursectomy by application of androgen into OS embryos on the third or twelfth day of incubation prevented the development of SAT until at least 3 months of age (Cole *et al.*, 1968), and chemical bursectomy by neonatal cyclophosphamide treatment postponed the beginning of infiltration for several weeks (Kroemer *et al.*, 1985a). In contrast, neonatal thymectomy of OS chicks not only failed to ameliorate SAT but actually resulted in more severe thyroid infiltration (Wick *et al.*, 1970b), possibly due to the removal of suppressive T cells. For this reason, in the 1970s SAT was classified as predominantly B cell-dependent as opposed to T-cell dependent autoimmunity, e.g., EAT (Jankovic et al., 1965; Wick et al., 1974), and the contribution of T cells to SAT was thought to be negligible.

However, Pontes de Carvalho et al. (1981) had shown that thyroiditis and the formation of Tg-AAbs were prevented when neonatal thymectomy was combined with the injection of a specific turkey anti-chicken T cell serum to completely deplete peripheral T lymphocytes (Table VII). These experiments were the first indication that T cells might also promote SAT or regulate its appearance, but they did not provide direct evidence that T cells were effector cells. The absence of AAbs against the thymus-dependent antigen Tg could be explained by a lack of T cell help, but the absence of thyroid infiltration by mononuclear cells could have been due to the absence of either T effector cells or Tg-AAbs capable of mediating ADCC.

Later, when Mabs against various lymphocyte subpopulations of the chicken became available, analysis of the thyroid-infiltrating lymphocytes (TILs) in the OS revealed them to be made up of a majority of mature T cells and a minority of B cells (Kroemer et al., 1985a). Moreover,

TABLE VII
EFFECT OF THYMECTOMY AND HIGH-DOSE TURKEY ANTI-CHICKEN T-CELL SERUM ON THE DEVELOPMENT OF SPONTANEOUS THYROID AUTOIMMUNITY[a]

Group	Treatment[b]	Thyroid infiltration		Tg-AAb	
		Incidence[c]	Degree (mean ± SD)	Incidence[d]	Titer (mean ± SD)[e]
I	None	12/15	1.1 ± 1.0	7/16	1.1 ± 1.8
II	NS	5/5	1.4 ± 0.5	3/5	1.0 ± 1.0
III	ATS	4/4	1.3 ± 0.5	2/5	0.8 ± 1.3
IV	Tx	8/8	1.4 ± 0.7	4/8	1.1 ± 1.4
V	Tx + NS	6/8	1.0 ± 0.8	5/8	1.0 ± 0.9
VI	Tx + ATS	1/8	0.1 ± 0.4	0/7	0

[a] Data are from Pontes de Carvalho et al. (1981).
[b] Thymectomies (Tx) were performed during the first 24 hours after hatching. A total volume of 3 ml anti-chicken T-cell serum (ATS) or normal turkey serum (NS) was given to each chicken intraperitoneally: 0.5 ml on days 2, 4, 10, and 14 and 1.0 ml on day 6 after hatching. The experiment was terminated on day 21.
[c] Number of animals with thyroiditis per total number in the group.
[d] Number of animals with Tg-AAbs (passive hemagglutination) per total number in the group.
[e] Mean $\log_2$ (hemagglutination titer) ± SD.

isolated TILs exhibited high proliferative responses to the T cell-specific mitogens PHA and Con A. Neonatal cyclophosphamide treatment of OS B^{13} chicks entailed a complete disappearance of the B cells and plasma cells within the TILs and selectively abrogated their response to the B cell-specific mitogen LPS. Such B lymphocyte-depleted TILs were, nevertheless, capable of transferring autoimmune thyroiditis when injected into MHC-compatible CS recipients (Table VIII). Through this procedure non-antibody-mediated transfer of the disease was demonstrated for the first time, as the CS recipients developed severe thyroid infiltration but showed no circulating Tg-AAbs (Kroemer et al., 1985a). These data pointed to the predominance of T effector cell mechanisms over humoral factors for the initiation of SAT. This view was corroborated by recent morphological studies in which T lymphoblasts were shown to be the very first cells invading the thyroid gland in the OS (Hála et al., 1986). In fully blown disease about 20% of the TILs express neither surface Ig nor a marker specific for mature T cells, CH1 (Kroemer et al., 1985a), and could be identified as macrophages (often in peripolesis), granulocytes, or non-B, non-T lymphocytes. Since destruction of the macrophage system of the OS by repeated injection of silica particles during the early posthatching period did not affect SAT (G. Kroemer

TABLE VIII
ADOPTIVE TRANSFER OF THYROIDITIS AND Tg-AAb PRODUCTION IN CS CHICKENS[a]

Cells injected	No. of CS recipients	Thyroid infiltration (mean ± SEM; %)	Log_2 anti-Tg titer (mean ± SEM; %)
OS TILs	18	81 ± 15[b]	4.5 ± 1.0[b]
OS TILs from CP-treated recipients[c]	4	71 ± 6[b]	0 ± 0
OS PBLs	4	20 ± 5	0 ± 0
OS splenocytes	18	26 ± 5	0.3 ± 0.3
OS thymocytes	7	26 ± 10	0 ± 0
CS splenocytes or no cells	27	15 ± 7	0 ± 0

[a] Thyroid-infiltrating lymphocytes (TILs) derived from untreated or chemically bursectomized [cyclophosphamide (CP)] OS $B^{13}B^{13}$ birds or control cell suspensions (2- to 5-week-old donors) were injected intravenously into 2- to 7-day-old, 750 rad-irradiated Cornell strain (CS) chicks (3.5-5 × 10^7 cells per recipient). The percentage of infiltrated thyroid area and the Tg-AAb passive hemagglutination titers were determined after 2-3 weeks. (Data are from Kroemer et al., 1985a.)

[b] Significantly different from control data ($p < 0.01$; Student's t test).

[c] TILs from CP-treated OS animals contained less than 0.3% B cells and no detectable plasma cells.

and G. Wick, unpublished observations), the relative contribution of macrophages to the initial phases of thyroid destruction appears to be of secondary importance.

Further transfer experiments revealed the abnormalities in T cell lineage of the OS rather than in the B cell system. Injection of OS but not CS thymocytes induced thyroidits in thymectomized CS recipients (Livezey et al., 1981), whereas CS and OS bursa cells were equally effective in restoring Tg-AAb production and thyroiditis in bursectomized OS chicks.

An unexpected result, intriguing at first sight, was the finding that treatment of OS embryos with intra-yolk sac injections of cyclosporine A (CsA) resulted in significantly more severe SAT and significantly higher frequency and titers of Tg-AAbs in these chickens 3 weeks after hatching, as compared to sham-treated OS controls (Wick et al., 1982b). These results were perhaps the first indication that CsA may also affect suppressor T cells. In the meantime, similar observations were made in adjuvant arthritis (Kaibara et al., 1983) and in diabetic rats (Iwakiri et al., 1987), thus pointing to possible hazards of CsA as therapy for certain AIDs. As a matter of fact, Jenkins et al. (1988) have recently suggested that CsA may interfere with the deletion of cells bearing self-reactive α/β T cell receptors in the thymus.

B. B CELLS AND AABs

As mentioned above, Tg-AAbs are characteristic features of SAT present in most OS chickens older than 3 weeks and showing a significant relationship with the severity of the disease. Furthermore, the particular pathogenetic relevance of Tg-AAbs is suggested by the fact that neonatal tolerization with Tg prevents the development of SAT (Sanker et al., 1983).

In vivo transfer of high-titer OS serum to recipients without the putative "thyroid defect" of the OS chicken has consistently failed to induce thyroiditis. This was found regardless of the application scheme employed, with cross-circulation in OS/NWL parabionts (Sundick et al., 1973), or injection of Tg-AAbs containing OS sera into NWL embryos (Rose et al., 1971) or into neonatally thymectomized (suppressor T cell-depleted) NWL chicks, although the OS antibody caused immune complex formation in recipient thyroids (Sundick and Wick, 1974). In contrast, OS sera induced thyroiditis when injected into newly hatched NWL recipients, in which one of the thyroid lobes had been surgically damaged by incision at hatching (Pontes de Carvalho, quoted by Wick et al., 1982a). Moreover, high-titer OS sera were able to induce severe thyroiditis in individuals of a low-responder OS family (Jaroszewski et al., 1978) and also lead to severe disease in a significant percentage of

(OS × CB)F_1 × OS backcrosses (Neu et al., 1985), thus providing conclusive evidence for a role of Tg-AAbs as an effector mechanism.

Immunofluorescence analysis using the double-wavelength technique with fluorescein isothiocyanate (FITC)-labeled anti-chicken Ig and tetramethylrhodamin isothiocyanate (TRITC)-conjugated Tg localized Tg-AAb-producing cells exclusively in the thyroid (Kofler and Wick, 1978) but not in the bursa or the peripheral lymphoid organs. Accordingly, isolated TILs were much more effective in inducing Tg-AAb produciton in an *in vivo* transfer system as compared to PBLs or splenocytes from the same donors (Kroemer et al., 1985a; see also Table VIII). Within the infiltrated thyroid, Tg-AAbs are formed both in germinal centers and in plasma cells and B lymphocytes scattered in interstitium or even in peripolesis. Moreover, Tg-AAbs can be transferred from the mother OS hen via the egg yolk into the embryo and the newly hatched chick (Kofler et al., 1983).

As to the mechanism by which Tg-AAbs may damage the thyroid, evidence for direct, complement mediated cytotoxicity is available. However, ADCC has also been demonstrated by using an *in vitro* ^{51}Cr-release microtoxicity assay, in which CRBCs first coated with purified chicken Tg and then presensitized with Tg-AAbs were exposed to PBLs (Boyd and Wick, 1980). No functional data concerning antimicrosomal AAbs are so far available for the OS chicken.

C. T Cells

Immunohistochemical analysis has demonstrated that the majority of TILs are T cells (Kroemer et al., 1985a), particularly among the cells in close apposition to TECs (Thunold et al., 1981). Moreover, a high proportion of these T cells are activated, MHC class II antigen- and IL-2 receptor-positive lymphoblasts. As discussed for AAb-secreting B cells, autoreactive T effector cells are also concentrated within TILs as revealed by comparison to thymic, splenic, and blood lymphocytes in an adoptive transfer system (Kroemer et al., 1985a).

Cytotoxic T lymphocytes capable of lysing Tg-coated CRBCs via DCC were detected in the circulation of OS chickens, even in very young animals, but not in normal controls. The notion that DCC might represent a probable effector mechanism in SAT is supported by its quantitative correlation with the responder state of different OS sublines (Wick et al., 1982a).

VII. Disturbed Immunoregulation

During the past few years evidence has accumulated for disturbed immunoregulation in the OS at two levels: (1) abnormalities intrinsic to the immune system and (2) endocrinological disturbances and aberrations in the bilateral interaction between the immune and the endocrine systems. The latter may contribute as extrinsic factors to the OS phenotype, thus corroborating the current notion that immunoregulation is not confined to the immune system but may involve mutual interactions with the neuroendocrine communication network (Kroemer et al., 1988d). In this section, the relative role of SAT and the functional interrelationship of various intrinsic or extrinsic dysregulations will be discussed.

A. DYSREGULATION INTRINSIC TO THE IMMUNE SYSTEM OF THE OS

As mentioned in Section VI,A, transfer experiments between MHC-compatible OS and CS chickens suggest a primary aberration of the T but not B cell lineage in the former. Moreover, OS chickens produce AAbs against various nonthyroid autoantigens (Khoury et al., 1982; Aichinger et al., 1984) and exhibit increased cellular and humoral responses to exogenous antigens (Wick et al., 1974; Kite et al., 1979), which suggest general rather than specific immunoregulatory defects underlying antithyroid autoimmune responses. Consequently, our laboratory has undertaken considerable efforts to explore general malfunctions of the OS T cell regulatory system using polyclonal T cell activation by mitogens as an *in vitro* model.

1. In Vitro T Cell Mitogen Hyperreactivity

Functional investigations *in vitro* revealed that OS peripheral lymphocytes (PBLs and splenocytes) exhibit elevated responses to the two T cell-stimulatory lectins, Con A (Kite et al., 1979; Schauenstein et al., 1985; Kroemer et al., 1985b) and PHA (Kroemer et al., 1988a). This phenomenon was observed irrespective of the mitogen dose, the cell concentration, the length of incubation (12–72 hours), and whether soluble or matrix-bound lectins were used as stimulators (Schauenstein et al., 1985). As mentioned in Section IV,B, the uptake of radioactive DNA precursors, in the presence as well as the absence of T cell mitogens was elevated in the OS as compared to outbred (NWL), closed-bred (CS), and inbred (CB, K) normal controls (see Table IV). In addition, the stimulation index was constantly increased in the OS. Con A hyperresponsiveness of the OS started even before the development of SAT, persisted throughout ontogeny, and was not affected by administration of exogenous thyroxine. Moreoever, induction of hypothyroidism in NWL controls by *in vivo* treatment with the thyrostatic drug propylthiouracil did not modulate Con A responsiveness (Kroemer et al., 1985b), thus excluding that the Con A hyperreactivity of the OS might be a consequence of thyroid dysfunction. Mitogen-driven proliferation was invariably increased in several OS families differing in the severity of thyroid infiltration and in all OS sublines homozygous for various MHC haplotypes (B^5, B^{13}, B^{15}), thus arguing against MHC linkage of this phenomenon (Schauenstein et al., 1985). Interestingly, OS splenocytes and PBLs have an increased capacity to adsorb FITC-labeled Con A (Kroemer et al., 1988a). In contrast, no aberrations were found in the Con A adsorption by OS thymocytes, which also hyperrespond to Con A (Boyd et al., 1985), and in the PHA-binding capacity of OS cells (Kroemer et al., 1988a). Thus, the apparent polyclonal T cell hyperreactivity in vivo (vide infra) and the hyperproliferation of OS lymphocytes in response to the tumor promoter phorbolmyristic acetate in combination with the calcium ionophore ionomycin (Kroemer et al., 1988b), exclude that increased mitogen responses of OS lymphocytes might be an in vitro artifact due to an elevated expression of lectin receptors.

To elucidate the mechanism of Con A hyperreactivity, cocultures of OS lymphocytes and NWL or CS controls were performed in communicating chambers, which prevent direct contact between the respective responder cells but allow the mutual exchange of conditioned media. Free diffusion of soluble immunoregulatory factors between OS and control PBLs did not abrogate the differences in Con A response (Schauenstein et al., 1987a). However, this protocol completely abolished the difference in Con A-driven proliferation between OS and NWL splenocytes (Kroemer et al., 1985b). This suggested that Con A hyperresponse of OS splenocytes might be due to differences in the production of regulatory cytokines, rather than to shifts in the responder cell population, and pointed to entirely different mechanisms of mitogen hyperreactivity operative in OS spleen and peripheral blood (Schauenstein et al., 1987b).

2. IL-2 Production and IL-2 Receptor Expression in the OS

In contrast to earlier reports favoring an "IL-2 defect" in autoimmunity (reviewed by Kroemer et al., 1986), OS T cells exhibit increased production of, and response to, IL-2. Regardless of the age of the donors, i.e., before and during the manifestation of SAT, Con A-stimulated peripheral OS T cells secrete at least two times more IL-2 than do those of normal control strains, when stimulated for 18 hours (Schauenstein et al., 1985; Kroemer et al., 1987). When cells are incubated for a longer period, the relative difference in IL-2 production between control and OS cells tends to augment for one order of magnitude, since the lymphokine is released by OS lymphocytes in a protracted fashion (Kroemer et al., 1987). A strong positive correlation between mitogen response and IL-2 secretion in individual splenocyte cultures suggested a determining role of the IL-2 concentration in the quantitative outcome of Con A stimulation. Accordingly, IL-2 production tended to increase during the first 3 months of life, as did the mitogen response. Moreover, acquisition of mitogen responsiveness and the capacity to produce IL-2 during ontogeny developed in parallel in the first 3-6 days after hatching, in both OS and NWL birds (Schauenstein et al., 1985). Semipurified IL-2 was able to elevate the Con A response of NWL splenocytes, but not PBLs, suggesting that the T cell mitogen hyperresponse of OS splenocytes might be functionally related to IL-2 hypersecretion (Kroemer et al., 1985; Schauenstein et al., 1987a).

Characterization of the kinetics of IL-2 receptor expression, using a Mab (INNCh16) directed against the chicken homolog of the β chain (L chain, p55, Tac antigen) of the mammalian high-affinity α/β heterodimeric IL-2 receptor (Hála et al., 1986; Schauenstein et al., 1988), confirmed the notion of divergent mechanisms for OS splenocyte and PBL hyperproliferation. As expected from the results of coculture experiments, OS and NWL splenocytes contain the same percentage of Con A-activatable T lymphocytes, i.e., cells which are able to express IL-2 receptor and thus acquire the ability to proliferate with IL-2. In both strains about 20% of splenocytes express IL-2 receptors upon short-term (4- and 8-hour) Con A stimulation. OS PBLs, in contrast, contain about twice as many Con A-activatable cells (40%) as do NWL PBLs. The IL-2 receptor density on a per-cell basis, determined by immunofluorescence, was the same in 4-hour Con A-stimulated OS and NWL splenocytes or PBLs. However, after prolonged stimulation (>36 hours) OS splenic Con A blasts markedly differed from their NWL counterparts: OS lymphocytes displayed an increased capacity to absorb IL-2 (Schauenstein et al., 1985), elevated binding of INNCh16, and an enhanced proliferative response to IL-2 (Schauenstein et al., 1988). All of these abnormalities were not observed with PBL blasts and are secondary to the altered cytokine concentrations in the culture supernatant, since the difference in the reactivity toward IL-2 disappeared when OS and control splenocytes were cocultured in communicating chambers. Interestingly, lymphokine hyperreactivity is not unique to OS splenic blasts. As discussed in Section V, OS TECs are also significantly more sensitive to the MHC class II (B-L) antigen-inducting effect of chicken γ-interferon as compared to normal thyrocytes (Wick et al., 1987). Thus, the OS exhibits both elevated lymphokine production and increased responses in several in vitro systems.

Morphological and functional characterization of lymphocytes infiltrating the OS thyroid gland strongly suggests the involvement of

IL-2 and IL-2 receptor-positive cells in SAT: (1) Immunohistological analysis (Fig. 6) of OS thyroid glands revealed that IL-2 receptor-positive T lymphoblasts are among the very first cells to invade the target organ (Hála et al., 1986). Only with the aggravation of thyroid infiltration does the portion of INNCh16$^+$ cells decline from nearly 100% to about 10% among intrathyroidal T lymphocytes, still a high proportion as compared to OS spleen or peripheral blood, each of which contains less than 1% of IL-2 receptor-positive cells (Kroemer et al., 1985a). This is probably due to the loss of the IL-2 receptor, which is only transiently expressed on activated T cells (Schauenstein et al., 1987b). (2) TILs from 4-week-old OS donors effectively respond to PHA or Con A, thus pointing to an intact lymphokine cascade at the site of the inflammatory process. (3) Local IL-2 production in the thyroid gland is suggested by spontaneous IL-2 production *in vitro* by freshly isolated TILs. Similarly, TILs not preactivated with mitogen mount high proliferative responses to IL-2 *in vitro* (Kroemer et al., 1985a).

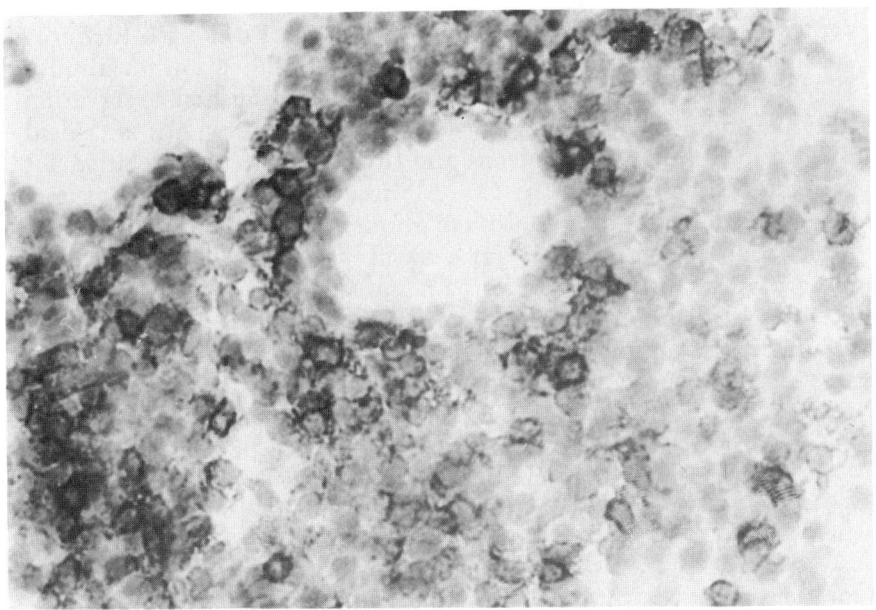

FIG. 6. IL-2 receptor expression on early thyroid-infiltrating lymphocytes. A frozen, unfixed thyroid section of a 10-day-old OS animal was stained with the chicken IL-2 receptor-specific Mab INNCh16 and a goat anti-mouse Ig peroxidase conjugate. (From Hála et al., 1986, with permission.)

These results, together with cosegregation of OS-like IL-2 hypersecretion with foci of lymphoid infiltration in the thyroid gland of (OS × CB)F_2 birds (*vide infra*), prompted us to postulate that IL-2 may play an important role in the etiopathogenesis of SAT (Kroemer *et al.*, 1986, 1989b).

3. In Vivo Hyperreactivity of OS T Lymphocytes and Further T Cell Abnormalities

In accordance with our *in vitro* findings, OS chickens exhibit signs of marked T cell hyperfunction *in vivo*, including increased antiviral responses (Kite *et al.*, 1979), allotransplant rejections (Jakobisiak *et al.*, 1976), and GVH reactions (Wick *et al.*, 1974). Pulse labeling of freshly isolated lymphocytes and cytofluorometric cell cycle analysis revealed that the thymus and spleen, but not the bursa, of OS embryos and newly hatched chicks contain elevated percentages of cells in the S phase of the cell cycle (Kroemer *et al.* 1988a). Double-staining experiments demonstrated that the elevated number of S phases in the spleen of the OS was due to a hyperproliferation of T cells, but not B cells. In this context it is noteworthy that stimulation of OS PBLs with *Escherichia coli* lipopolysaccharide, similarly revealed no indication for abnormal B cell proliferation *in vitro* (G. Kroemer, unpublished observations).

Hyperproliferating T lymphocytes may not remain *in situ* since neither the overall cellularity of spleens and thymuses nor their relative T cell content are increased in the OS (Albini and Wick, 1974). To the contrary, OS spleens and thymuses are smaller in size than are healthy controls (Scanes *et al.*, 1976; Jaroszewski *et al.*, 1978). Thus, further abnormalities in lymphopoiesis and/or cellular turnover have to be postulated in the OS. For example, the elevated T cell replication in OS thymuses and spleens could entail an increased emigration of T cells and therefore could account for the enhanced percentage of functional T lymphocytes in OS peripheral blood.

Similarly, a speculative explanation for the observed discrepancy between a normal or even supraphysiological thymic suppressor cell activity, as evident, e.g., by the capacity of thymocytes to block mitogen or cytotoxic responses of autologous PBLs (R. L. Boyd and G. Wick, unpublished observations; Wick *et al.*, 1982a), and low peripheral immunosuppression in the OS may be due to a delayed emigration of thymic suppressor cells to the periphery (Rose *et al.*, 1981). In accordance with this, thymectomized OS, but not normal chickens, exhibit accelerated skin graft rejection (Jakobisiak *et al.*, 1976).

In addition to an overall decrease in thymic cellularity, OS chickens show selective deficiency of a special population of thymus cells, the TNCs (Boyd et al., 1984), as mentioned in Section IV,B. The mechanisms of T cell hyperreactivity observed in different lymphoid cell populations of OS chickens are summarized in Table IX.

4. Defects in the Mononuclear Phagocytic System

Supernatants of cultured splenocytes and PBLs as well as normal chicken serum contain a factor of monocyte/macrophage origin, which interferes with the uptake of [^{3}H]thymidine or its analog 5-[^{125}I]-2-deoxyuridine into proliferating cells and which was identified as cold thymidine (Kroemer et al., 1985b, 1987, 1988c), the functional significance of which remains to be established. Interestingly, circulating monocytes produce normal levels of thymidine, whereas sessile macrophages from OS spleens are deficient in this respect and OS sera contained less thymidine than did control sera. Thymectomy, adoptive transfer of thymocytes and concentrated Con A supernatants, as well as correction of endocrine abnormalities did not normalize the thymidine concentration in OS sera, which points to a primary rather than a secondary abnormality of the OS macrophage. In addition, phagocytes of OS chicks show an elevated oxidative burst activity: compared to NWL controls, OS thymocytes or splenocytes exhibit a two- to 20-fold luminol-dependent chemiluminescence both in the absence of stimulatory agents

TABLE IX
DIFFERENT MECHANISMS OF T CELL HYPERREACTIVITY OPERATIVE IN OS THYMUS, PBLs, SPLEEN, AND TILs[a]

	Thymus	Spleen	PBLs	TILs
Con A- or PHA-driven proliferation	↑	↑	↑	—
Spontaneous proliferation	↑	↑	(↑)[b]	—
Con A-induced IL-2 production	ND	↑	↑	—
Spontaneous IL-2 secretion	ND	ND	ND	↑
Con A-activatable cells	ND	—	↑	ND
IL-2 receptor + cells	—	—	—	↑
Overall cellularity	↓	↓	—	
Con A-binding capacity	—	↑	↑	ND

[a] Arrows indicate significant increase or decrease of the parameters as compared to the respective control group (NWL or CS cells for OS thymocytes, splenocytes, and PBLs, OS PBLs for TILs). —, No difference; ND, not determined. All comparisons were done with 1- to 4-week-old chickens. (Data are from Kroemer et al., 1988e.)
[b] ( ), Weak.

and in the presence of zymosan and phorbolmyristic acetate. This phenomenon could be observed both prior to and during SAT development of SAT (H. Wolf, unpublished observations). Finally, OS macrophages express more MHC class II (B-L) antigen than do normal controls (G. Wick, unpublished observations).

B. DYSREGULATION EXTRINSIC TO THE IMMUNE SYSTEM OF THE OS

The notion that the quantitative outcome of an immune response is subject to endocrine—above all, glucocorticoid-mediated—regulation has recently been corroborated by experimental data showing a negative feedback mechanism by which the concentration of glucocorticoids, in turn, is regulated by immunological stimuli in several mammalian systems. We therefore investigated whether static and/or dynamic alterations in the glucocorticoid tonus might be present in the OS.

1. Decreased Basal Glucocorticoid Tonus in the OS

The glucocorticoid tonus, defined as the hormonally active corticosteroid concentration, is the combined result of corticosterone (CN) secretion by the suprarenal cortex and the production of corticosteroid-binding globulin (CBG), the transport protein for CN, by hepatocytes. CN bound to CBG is hormonally inactive and only the small unbound fraction of plasma CN is freely available to penetrate into intracellular compartments and to exert its pleiotropic effects via CN receptors. Whereas total CN plasma levels did not differ between OS and NWL animals, plasma CBG concentrations were constantly elevated in OS chicks over those of NWL controls (Faessler *et al.*, 1986a). This CBG elevation was found irrespective of sex and at every age investigated, i.e., before, during, and after the onset of SAT. Since OS-derived CBG had the same affinity and specificity spectra as NWL CBG (Faessler *et al.*, 1988a), its increase in plasma concentration must entail diminished biologically active (i.e., free) plasma CN. This decreased basal CN tonus of the OS is neither functionally compensated for by CN receptor upregulation in lymphoid cells nor by a hyperfunction of the postreceptive machinery mediating the CN effect. In OS bursa, thymus, or spleen cells no abnormality in CN receptivity, association, dissociation, and sedimentation constants or steroid binding spectra of CN receptors could be detected (Faessler *et al.*, 1986b). Moreover, OS and control splenocytes were equally susceptible to the suppressive effect of CN on the mitogen-driven proliferation (Faessler *et al.*, 1986a).

In view of the widespread effect of glucocorticoids on the immune system, it is interesting to speculate which disturbances in the OS chicken might be due to a diminished CN tonus. Glucocorticoids are well known to regulate the cellularity of lymphoid organs (del Rey et al., 1984), suppress the production of a variety of lymphokines, including IL-1 (Snyder and Unanue, 1982; Knudsen et al., 1987), IL-2 (Gillis et al., 1979a), and γ-interferon (Arya et al., 1984), inhibit cytotoxic and proliferative responses of T lymphocytes (Gillis et al., 1979b), suppress the B cell activation process (Bowen and Fauci, 1984), or reduce MHC class II antigen expression (Aberer et al., 1984). Raising the unbound fraction of glucocorticoids in the OS chicken by subcutaneous administration of cortisol during the first 4 weeks after hatching inhibited the development of SAT and simultaneously corrected Con A hyperreactivity and IL-2 hypersecretion (Faessler et al., 1986a), but did not decrease the size of OS lymphoid organs. This set of data suggested that defects intrinsic to the immune system on the one hand and diminished CN activity on the other hand may be functionally linked to each other.

2. Deficient Glucocorticoid Tonus in Response to Immunological Stimuli

Antigenic challenge leads to a transient increase in serum glucocorticoids in normal mice (Besedovsky et al., 1975), rats (Waterston, 1970), and chickens (Schauenstein et al., 1987a), with a peak at 3–6 days, i.e., coincident with that of the humoral immune response. This phenomenon appears to be the mechanism responsible for "sequential antigenic competition," viz. the impaired ability to respond to a second, unrelated antigen administered several days after the first (Besedovsky et al., 1979). Since the suppressive effect of corticosteroids primarily concerns the inductive phase of lymphocyte activation but has little effect on the growth factor-dependent proliferation of preactivated lymphocytes (Gillis et al., 1979a), CN may ensure the maintenance of immune specificity by suppression of less specific lymphocyte clones that are coelicited in the course of the immune response. According to current understanding, the elevation of glucocorticoids after immunization is due to the production of glucocorticoid-inducing cytokines by antigen-responsive cells of the immune system. Recombinant murine IL-1 (Besedovsky et al., 1986) and human IL-1 (Uehara et al., 1987) induce the transcription of the gene coding for proopiomelanocortin, the precursor of the adrenocorticotropic hormone (ACTH, or corticotropin) in pituitary cells either directly (Bernton et al., 1987) or indirectly by triggering hypothalamic neurons, which release corticotropin-releasing factor (Sapolsky et al., 1987; Berkenbosch et al., 1987; Uehara et al., 1987). Further candidates for glucocorticoid-inducing factors (GIFs) are IL-2, which has been reported to stimulate ACTH release in the human system (Lotze et al., 1985; Brown et al., 1987), and ACTH-like factors produced by stimulated immune cells, which, in contrast to IL-1 and IL-2, would act directly on the adrenal cortex (Smith *et al.*, 1982, 1986). CN, secreted due to a direct or indirect stimulation of the suprarenal cortex, may then inhibit immune function, thus completing a feedback control loop (Fig. 7).

Interestingly, the autoimmunity-prone OS chickens lack the physiological elevation in serum CN when immunized with xenogeneic RBCs (Schauenstein *et al.*, 1987a). Since systemic autoimmunity in mammals has been associated with defective production of IL-1 and other cytokines *in vitro* (Linker-Israeli *et al.*, 1983; Bocchieri *et al.*, 1985), we initially suspected that OS chickens were deficient in the generation of GIFs. However, conditioned media of Con A-stimulated OS splenocytes and NWL control supernatants were equally effective in eliciting an ephemeric increase in serum levels of CN when injected into NWL chickens. In contrast, OS chickens were hyporesponsive to GIFs because injection of GIFs containing supernatants elicited significantly lower CN peaks than in their normal counterparts (Schauenstein *et al.*, 1987a).

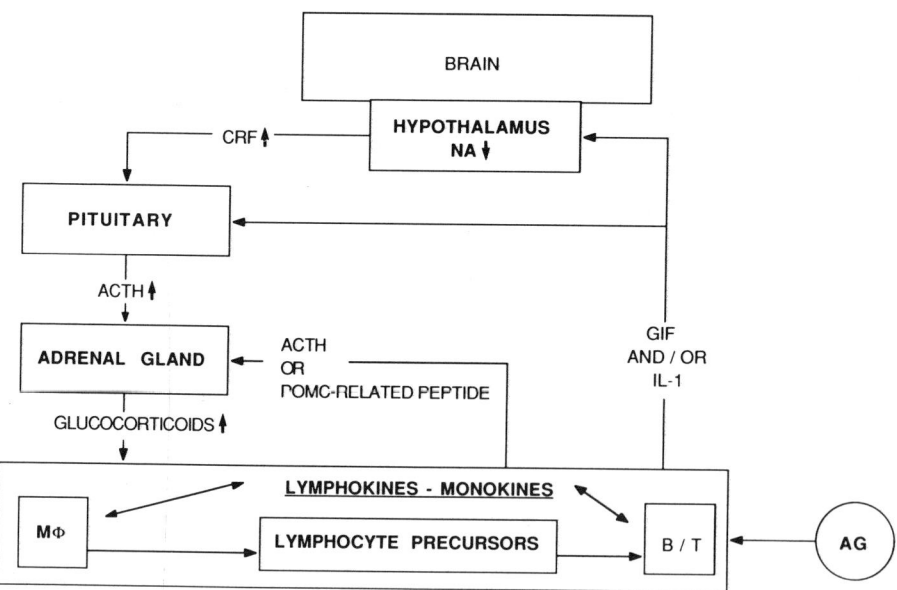

FIG. 7. Immunoendocrine feedback loop. MΦ, Macrophage; AG, antigen; B, B lymphocyte; T, T lymphocyte; GIF, glucocorticoid-inducing factor; IL-1, interleukin-1; NA, noradrenaline; CRF, corticotropin-releasing factor; ACTH, adrenocorticotropic hormone; POMC, proopiomelanocortin.

To elucidate the mechanism of this GIF hyporesponsiveness in the OS chicken, we decided to characterize the chemical nature and mode of action of GIFs. GIF responses in NWL chicks could be completely blocked by dexamethasone administration, which suppresses ACTH production (Jingami et al., 1985), indicating that GIFs in the chicken do not stimulate CN release by acting directly on the adrenal gland (Brezinschek et al., 1989). This raised the question of whether the defect in GIF responsiveness was located in the hypothalamo-pituitary area, which might result in insufficient ACTH production, or in the adrenal gland, which might be incapable of responding to the ACTH stimulus. Injection of the synthetic ACTH analog Synacthen (Liba-Geigy, Basel, Switzerland) provoked an equal increase in serum CN levels in OS and NWL chickens, indicating normal adrenal cortex function in OS chickens. Therefore, their GIF hyporesponsiveness is probably due to a defect within the hypothalamo-hypophyseal axis. The diminished CN response to GIF does not, however, reflect a general inability of the OS chickens to deal with stress, since they respond normally to unspecific stressors, e.g., restraining for 5 minutes. Molecular sieve and anion-exchange chromatography revealed GIFs to be a 16- to 18-kDa basic protein. GIF activity could be separated from IL-2 and coeluted with a protein that in immunoblots reacts with a polyclonal antiserum against human IL-1β and a Mab specific for a common determinant of human IL-1α and β. Subsequent affinity chromatography over an IL-1 antibody column allowed the separation of two GIF activities, one being retained by the column and sensitive to repeated freezing and thawing, the other in the unbound fraction and more stable (Brezinschek et al., 1989). We are presently investigating whether the OS is hyporesponsive to both types of GIF.

To explore the relevance of the immune signal–GIF–CN axis for immune reactivity, we designed the following experiment: Concentrated GIF was injected intravenously into OS and NWL chickens, followed by repeated blood sampling. Concomitantly with the CN peak appearing 1 hour after GIF application, a decrease of Con A responses by PBLs was observed. As expected, this suppression was much less pronounced in OS birds (Fig. 8) (Schauenstein et al., 1987a).

Our concerted findings indicate that in OS chickens a reduction of the dynamic and static CN tonus occurs, which might facilitate the initiation of "forbidden" immune reactions in terms of a "derepression" of immune function. The defect in glucocorticoid-mediated immunoregulation in the OS is twofold, involving (1) a decreased basal CN tonus due to an elevation of plasma CBG and (2) an impaired CN rise in response to antigenic stimulation due to a defect in the hypothalamo-pituitary system, which fails to secrete ACTH in response to a normally produced GIF.

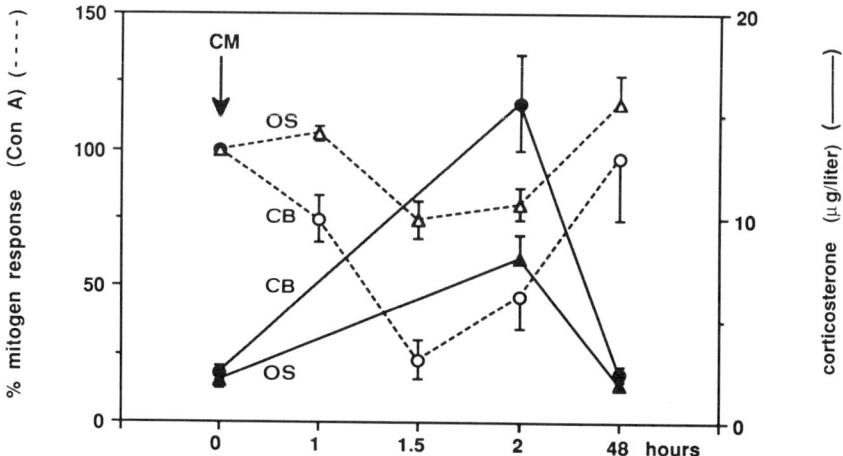

FIG. 8. Effect of cytokine-induced corticosterone elevation on the reactivity of lymphocytes. CM, Conditioned medium. Results are expressed as means ± SEM. (From Schauenstein et al., 1987a, with permission.)

3. Sex Steroids and SAT

A prominent characteristic of most systemic as well as organ-specific autoimmune diseases is a female preponderance, claimed to be due to differences in the levels of sex steroids (Grossman, 1984). Accordingly, when the OS was first established, only female animals developed SAT (Cole, 1966). As mentioned in Section II, this female predominance later disappeared as a result of selective breeding, and SAT was already manifested in a sexually immature, hormonally still "neutral" young age. As for CN, no differences between age- and sex-matched prepubertal OS and NWL birds were detected in testosterone, estradiol, and progesterone plasma levels (Faessler et al., 1988b). In contrast to mammals, chicken serum is devoid of a sex hormone-binding globulin, which implicates that the sex steroid concentration in birds actually reflects real hormone bioavailability. Moreover, affinity, binding capacity, or steroid binding spectra of receptors for the different classes of sex steroids did not differ (Faessler et al., 1986b). Interestingly, immunization with SRBCs not only increased CN plasma levels in NWL chickens, but concomitantly modulated testosterone serum concentrations, although in an inverse direction and without a significant difference between OS and healthy control chickens (Faessler et al., 1988b). These results suggest that, in contrast to the glucocorticoid tonus, the androgen tonus as well as its modulation by immune signals are normal in the OS.

Androgens modulate immune functions and suppress the development of experimentally induced and genetically transmitted AID (Roubinian *et al.*, 1978; Okayasu *et al.*, 1981), including SAT (Gause and Marsh, 1986). In view of the potential clinical use of androgens or androgenlike substances in immunosuppressive therapy, the mechanism by which testosterone attenuates SAT was studied. Repeated administration of a pharmacological testosterone dose (1 mg/100 g of body weight) during the posthatching period resulted in a significant reduction of both thyroid infiltration and circulating Tg-AAbs in addition to a pseudopubertas precox (Faessler *et al.*, 1988b). Since chicken thyroids are devoid of sex hormone receptors, SAT prevention is probably more related to an immunomodulation rather than to a direct effect on the target organ. Immunosuppression by testosterone affects the B rather than the T cell lineage, since androgen treatment provokes a complete involution of bursal parenchyma and reduced circulating B cells (Glick, 1964), but does not alter thymic cellularity or *in vitro* Con A responses by peripheral T cells (Faessler *et al.*, 1988b). Since immature bursal lymphoid cells and mature spleen cells lack detectable androgen receptors, the suppression of Tg-AAb production and the reduction in blood B lymphocytes cannot be attributed to a direct effect of testosterone on lymphocytes. Bursal involution is most likely due to a direct effect on bursal epithelial cells that express high quantities of androgen receptors. Interestingly, CBG levels were significantly depressed upon testosterone application, pointing to an elevated CN tonus that may exert additional indirect immunoregulatory effects. Moreover, high testosterone levels may compete for CN binding sites on CBG (Faessler *et al.*, 1988b), which could further elevate free, hormonally active glucocorticoid concentrations.

Preliminary data (H. Dietrich, R. Faessler, and G. Wick, unpublished observations) suggest that estradiol, but not progesterone, also significantly modulates SAT. In estradiol-treated OS chicks the only alteration among those parameters investigated (i.e., T cell mitogen responses, distribution of lymphocyte subsets, cellularity and morphology of lymphoid organs, endocrine parameters) was a profound decrease in CBG plasma levels. This underlines the possible role of free glucocorticoid levels in SAT development.

VIII. Genetics

A. Role of the MHC (*B* Locus)

1. General Remarks

The basis for the successful development of the OS chicken from the CS mother strain by selective breeding was the hereditary nature of SAT (Cole, 1966). The polygenic character of this trait was proven by means of appropriate cross-breeding of OS with NWL chickens (Cole, 1966).

Based on the data of such cross-breedings and adoptive transfer studies, Rose et al. (1976) and Wick et al. (1979) proposed that at least three genetic loci are involved in the regulation of SAT: (1) MHC genes, (2) non-MHC genes coregulating the immunological hyperreactivity, and (3) genes coding for a target organ susceptibility to autoimmune effector mechanisms. Further analyses of the genetic control of SAT were done using crosses of OS and CS chickens (Bacon et al., 1981) and of OS birds with the highly inbred normal CB line (Neu et al., 1985, 1986).

The relationship between the MHC, originally characterized as blood group locus B (Briles et al., 1950), and SAT in OS chickens was described by Bacon et al. (1974) and by Wick et al. (1979) and has recently been summarized by Hála (1988).

The serological analysis of MHC haplotypes in OS chickens revealed the occurrence of three haplotypes in this strain (Bacon et al., 1973): B^1, B^3, and B^4 [on the basis of the new internationally accepted nomenclature (Briles et al., 1982) these were renamed B^{13}, B^{15}, and B^5, respectively]. For functional analysis of MHC haplotypes, these authors used skin grafts (Schierman and Nordskog, 1961) and as a second test system GVH reactivity, which is also under the control of the MHC (Jaffe and McDermid, 1962).

The relative importance of the MHC haplotype for the development of SAT became evident from the following experiments of Bacon et al. (1974). Assessing the development of SAT in the progeny of B^5B^{13} families, these authors observed most the severe lymphoid infiltration of thyroid glands in animals carrying the B^{13} haplotype (thyroid glands from homozygous animals were infiltrated to a greater extent than were those of heterozygous chickens). Mild thyroid infiltration was detected in B^5B^5 animals. In another series of experiments chickens possessing the haplotype B^{15} (Bacon, 1976) had more severe infiltration than did B^{13} chickens. In studies by Wick et al. (1979) performed in an OS colony that had been separated from the original flock for nearly 10 years, the haplotypes B^{13} and B^5 were associated with the most severe disease, while B^{15} chickens suffered only very mild thyroiditis. The same association was observed between the presence of certain MHC haplotypes and the frequency and the titer of Tg-AAbs (Bacon et al., 1974; Wick et al., 1979). These controversial results suggested the existence of additional non-MHC genes involved in the regulation of the disease.

The importance of non-MHC loci for the development of SAT emerged from breeding experiments with sublines with identical MHC haplotypes selected for high and low levels of Tg-AAbs (Boyd et al., 1983). These studies afforded data similar to those obtained by Bacon et al. (1978), Rose et al. (1978), and Bacon and Rose (1979) with three OS sublines with the identical B haplotype. In these experiments, the same haplotype (B^5B^5) was associated with severe disease in one subline and mild disease in another. The authors concluded that the B haplotype might influence the pathogenesis of SAT differently in each subline (Bacon et al., 1978). Segregation of non-MHC genes (Wick et al., 1979) or qualitative differences between the B^5 haplotypes in these sublines (Rose et al., 1978) were considered possible explanations for this different responsiveness.

To further address the latter possibility, the genetic make-up of the Innsbruck OS colony was studied with the help of mixed-lymphocyte reaction, GVH reaction, and serological analyses for all OS haplotypes (B^5, B^{13}, and B^{15}) (Hála, 1988). Within the limits of these methods, we did not observe any inconsistencies in groups of chickens with a given haplotype. Subsequently, we used restriction fragment-length polymorphism (RFLP) analyses to further probe for possible MHC microheterogeneities among chickens with the same haplotype (Fig. 9). For this purpose, BamHI-digested DNA was hybridized to a cDNA probe (Bourlet et al., 1988) corresponding to the $\beta 2$ domain of the B-L class II gene. DNA of B^5B^5 and $B^{13}B^{13}$ animals analyzed in this way showed characteristic RFLP patterns for both haplotypes without differences among chickens with an identical haplotype. However, Southern blots

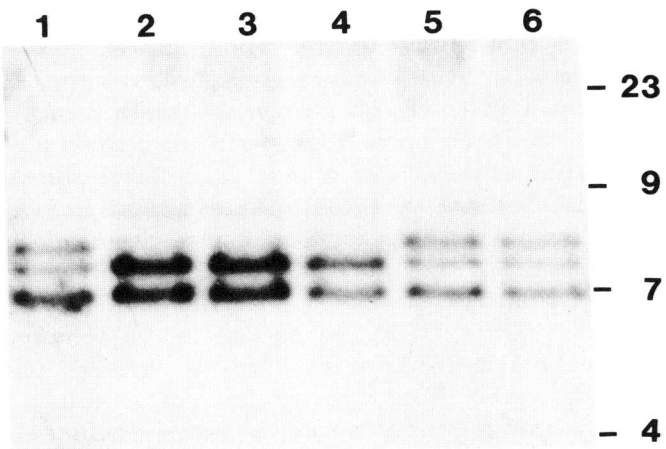

FIG. 9. Restriction fragment-length polymorphism analysis of DNA from six $B^{15}B^{15}$ OS chickens. DNA from RBC nuclei was digested with restriction enzyme BamHI. Blots were hybridized with the ^{32}P-labeled p232 probe for the chicken MHC class II β chain (Bourlet et al., 1988). HindIII-digested λ phage DNA was used as a size marker (right). Note two different RFLP patterns in these MHC-identical chickens.

with BamHI-digested DNA from $B^{15}B^{15}$ OS chickens revealed two RFLP patterns (Hála et al., 1989). This heterogeneity among serologically identical B haplotypes might perhaps explain high and low responders (with respect to SAT and Tg-AAbs) among such animals (Rose et al., 1978; Boyd et al., 1983).

How the MHC influences SAT development and which gene(s) within, or linked to, the MHC might be important for the natural history of this disease are not yet clear. Among the MHC genes with identified products (B-F, class I antigens; B-L, class II antigens; and B-G, class IV antigens, the latter expressed only on RBCs) (Pink et al., 1977), B-L genes are the best candidates for regulators of immune responses against different exogenous antigens (Guenther et al., 1974; Balcarová et al., 1974) and therefore are also the best candidates for regulation of the autoimmune reactions in OS chickens. However, a possible role of additional MHC genes, without known products or function (Guillemot et al., 1988), cannot be excluded.

2. Analysis of the Genetic Basis of SAT by Means of Crosses of OS with Outbred Chickens

The genetic background of OS chickens was first analyzed by crossbreeding with the CS, i.e., the OS mother strain, established in 1935 (Van Tienhoven and Cole, 1962). In subsequent, more detailed experiments randomly selected CS dams carrying B^6, B^{13}, or B^{15} were mated with B^5, B^{13}, or B^5B^5 OS sires (Bacon et al., 1977). Half of the F_1 hybrid offspring showed thyroid infiltration (at least 1+). In addition, differences in SAT severity were observed regardless of the haplotype. For instance, in CS females, the haplotype B^5 together with B^{15} was associated with a high frequency of SAT (83% of F_1 animals showed lymphoid infiltration of the thyroid glands), but B^5B^6 F_1 hybrids were free of thyroiditis. In this F_1 progeny a positive correlation emerged among Tg-AAb titers, thyroid pathology, and clinical phenotype, irrespective of the genotype (B^5B^5, B^6B^6, and B^5B^6). However, homozygous B^{15} chickens developed more severe disease than did B^{13} homozygotes.

From the B^6B^{15} (OS × CS)F_1 generation, 440 F_2 chickens were derived and Tg-AAb and thyroid infiltration was recorded at 7 weeks of age (Bacon et al., 1981). The proportion of chickens with SAT varied significantly between families from different sires, although a possible influence of the MHC haplotype was only observed in B^6 homozygotes, but not in B^6B^{15} heterozygotes and B^{15} homozygotes. These authors concluded that the influence of the B complex on the genetic susceptibility for SAT is more evident in animals with limited susceptibility at other loci.

3. Analysis of the Genetic Basis of SAT by Means of Crosses of OS with Normal Inbred Chickens

Early genetic analyses had determined SAT as a polygenic disease controlled by rather few genes (Cole, 1966; Rose et al., 1976; Wick et al., 1979). It was reasoned that in such a case, i.e., the development of SAT being under the control of several genes, these may also segregate within a normal, healthy population. However, their frequency in an outbred population would be so low that the probability for accumulation in one single individual with resulting disease would also be very low. Since there are at present no means to identify such genes directly, one could only study their effect via the assessment of the disease itself. To eliminate further complications in the interpretation of data due to undetectable differences between animals from different families and generations, we therefore resorted to the highly inbred CB strain as a reference line.

This inbred line, founded in England in 1933, is now — after more than 50 generations of brother × sister matings (for a review, see Hála, 1987) — syngeneic and homozygotic at practically all loci. The CB line may, of course, share some of the *obese* alleles with the OS, but there is at least no difference among individual CB animals and one can repeat crossing experiments with animals with a homogenous genetic background.

The results of our experiments (Neu et al., 1985, 1986; Kroemer et al., 1989) are summarized in Table X. Assuming a simple Mendelian inheritance, we postulated the existence of different genetic control mechanisms for the heightened immune responsiveness and the target organ sensitivity in the OS, respectively.

It seemed that the reactivity of the immune system against Tg is regulated by one (maximally two), probably dominant, gene(s). F_1 hybrids produce Tg-AAbs (Neu et al., 1986), but no substantial thyroid infiltration was recorded in these birds. In the first backcross generation we observed severe ($\geq 2+$) infiltration in about 5% of all chickens and in about one quarter of all F_2 chickens with significant (more than 10% of the thyroid cross-section affected) lymphoid infiltration. From this fraction of afflicted animals, one can calculate the number of genes (one or two genes) involved in the regulation of target organ sensitivity to the autoimmune attack. All of these calculations are, of course, only valid for the combination of the OS and inbred CB lines.

B. Genetic Control of the Target Organ Sensitivity

As mentioned in Section V, the thyroid gland of OS chickens shows a series of intrinsic functional abnormalities, such as an increased ^{131}I

TABLE X
Tg-AABs AND THYROID INFILTRATION IN BACKCROSS GENERATION AND F_1 HYBRIDS[a]

Cross	Age (wk)	No. of animals	Tg-AAb ELISA (% pos.)	Tg-AAb Precipitation (% pos.)	Animals with thyroiditis (%)[b]				
					4+	3+	2+	1+	−
(CB × OS)F_1 × CB	10	10	0	0					100
	21	8	25	0					100
	40–50	3	67	33				(33)	67
(CB × OS)F_1 × OS	14	26	46	23	4		15	31	50
	17–22	9	67	67			22	33	45
	105	5	60	60		20	20		60
(OS × CB)F_2	15	19	47	16				21	79
	16	126	ND	18		8[c]		16[c]	76[c]
	40–50	11	75	42			25	17	58

[a] ELISA, Enzyme-linked immunosorbent assay; pos., positive; ND, not done. [From Neu et al. (1986) and Kroemer et al. (1989a).]
[b] Infiltration of thyroid gland: 1+, up to 25% of the histological section infiltrated; 2+, 25–50% infiltration; 3+, 50–75% infiltration; 4+, 75% to total infiltration.
[c] Classified according to a different scoring schedule for SAT, i.e., percentage of the infiltrated area of thyroid cross-sections: below 10% infiltration, 10–40% infiltration, and more than 40% infiltration.

uptake, resistance to T4 suppression, and decreased *in vitro* proliferation of TECs.

The augmented capacity for ^{131}I uptake in the OS was analyzed in crosses between OS (with high ^{131}I uptake) and inbred CB chickens (with low ^{131}I uptake), suppressed by the presence of T4 in the diet. (OS × CB)F$_1$ hybrids showed low ^{131}I uptake, like CB chickens, and the (OS × CB)F$_1$ × OS backcross generation segregated into two groups, one each of low and high iodine uptake. It was concluded that this functional trait is encoded by one recessive gene (Neu *et al.*, 1985). Further genetic analyses, discussed in the next section, revealed that this gene is neither linked to the MHC nor associated with thyroid infiltration.

Another OS thyroid abnormality is its susceptibility to passively transferred Tg-AAbs (Jaroszewski *et al.*, 1978). Similar observations were made by Neu *et al.* (1985), using (OS × CB)F$_1$ hybrids and (OS × CB)F$_1$ × OS backcrosses. From the number of animals with significant infiltration after passive transfer of Tg-AAbs ($\geq 2+$), we concluded that this susceptibility is encoded by approximately three genes, at least one of them recessive.

C. GENETIC ANALYSIS OF SAT-ASSOCIATED DYSFUNCTIONS

In addition to the above-mentioned investigations of a possible role of the MHC in the development of SAT, we recently performed further, more extensive studies with several hundred chickens concerning the thyroidal and extrathyroidal endocrinological, immunological, virological, and clinical characteristics of hybrids of the OS and CB strain to (1) further define the number of genes contributing to SAT-associated aberrations, (2) unravel their possible functional relationship, which could be reflected by genetic linkage (Kroemer *et al.*, 1988b, 1989b), and (3) weigh the relative contributions of these abnormalities to the generation of SAT.

1. Mode of Inheritance of OS-Specific Functional Disturbances

OS-like PBL hyperproliferation to Con A-coated erythrocytes is inherited by all (OS × CB)F$_1$ and (F$_1$ × OS) and by 50% of the (F$_1$ × CB) backcross animals, suggesting control by a single autosomal dominant gene. Interestingly, the (F$_1$ × CB) backcross high responders tended to group themselves in the lower range of their OS ancestors, suggesting additional modulatory genetic influences determining Con A hyperresponsiveness. The elevated proliferative response of OS lymphocytes to Con A segregated from the MHC but was associated with supranormal proliferation with PHA. Thus, MHC-associated genes and different genetic systems for Con A and PHA reactivity, which determine the magnitude of mitogen responsiveness in normal chickens (Morrow and Abplanalp, 1982; Pink and Vainio, 1983; Frederickson and Gilmour, 1983), are not involved in OS T cell hyperreactivity.

IL-2 hypersecretion, elevated percentages of circulating potential IL-2 responders, and increased proliferative Con A responses cosegregated in the (F_1 × CB) backcross generation. Similarly, PBL and splenocyte responses to Con A exhibited a high degree of correlation, although different regulatory defects have been implicated in the Con A hyperreactivity of both cell populations (Schauenstein et al., 1987b). Thus, the T cell hyperreactivity of the OS chicken constitutes one block of genetically and/or functionally linked characteristics. Whereas the increased percentage of Con A-activatable PBLs was fully expressed in (F_1 × CB) backcross high responders, IL-2 secretion by these animals did not reach the OS levels, although it always exceeded the CB average. This might explain why the mitogen response of (F_1 × CB) backcross high responders, on average, is lower than in the OS.

Similar to T cell hyperreactivity, the OS in vivo hyporesponse to the CN-inducing effect of cytokine preparations is controlled by one autosomal dominant gene not linked to the MHC. However, this disturbed immunoendocrine communication segregated from the Con A high-responder phenotype in the (F_1 x CB) backcross generation, indicating functional and genetic independence of these two aberrations. Unexpectedly, GIF hyporesponsiveness cosegregated with the OS-specific endogenous virus ev 22. At present, we do not know whether this genetic phenomenon reflects a coincidental vicinity of the ev 22 locus and the gene regulating GIF responses or a functional relationship between these two OS-specific characteristics.

The decreased thymidine concentration in OS sera, which may be attributed to a functional macrophage defect, is also an MHC-independent autosomal dominant trait and segregates from both T cell hyperreactivity and ev 22 in (F_1 × CB) backcrosses (Kroemer et al., 1988c).

Neu et al. (1985) have shown that the increased iodine uptake by the OS thyroid is controlled by a recessive gene. More recent analysis (Kroemer et al., 1989b) confirmed this finding and revealed its MHC independence.

OS-like high plasma CBG levels were not found among (OS × CB)F_1 hybrids or (F_1 × CB) backcrosses, but were encountered among about half of the (F_1 × OS) backcross generation of either the $B^{15}B^{15}$ or $B^{12}B^{15}$ haplotype, indicating that the decreased basal glucocorticoid tonus of the OS is controlled by one recessive locus independent of the MHC. No association was found between high CBG levels and high iodine uptake into the thyroid, indicating independence of these two endocrinological abnormalities.

From these data, it was concluded that five independent genes code for the different regulatory disturbances studied. Three separate autosomal dominant loci code for (1) the whole complex of T cell hyperreactivity, (2) hypothymidinemia, and (3) *ev 22*, which cosegregates with the *in vivo* hyporesponsiveness to the glucocorticoid-inducing effect of cytokines. Two autosomal recessive genes determine independently from each other (4) the altered iodine metabolism and (5) the abnormal ratio between free CN and that bound to CBG.

2. Associations of Functional Disturbances with SAT in OS × CB Hybrids

To elucidate the etiopathogenic relevance of the above-described abnormalities, we studied their genetics in conjunction with thyroid pathology and serological analysis in (OS × CB)F_1, F_2, and backcross generations. If one or several putative etiological agents were indispensable for SAT development, any animal afflicted with SAT should carry this/these feature(s). Such an immunological or endocrinological abnormality would constitute an essential factor in the pathogenesis of SAT. In addition, nonessential functional abnormalities may influence the onset and/or severity of SAT. Such a modulatory factor should become apparent by a statistically significant correlation between SAT severity (or time of onset) and occurrence of the respective pathogenetic change in (OS × CB)F_2 animals.

As discussed above, none of the (OS × CB)F_1 or (F_1 × CB) backcrosses, about half of the (F_1 × OS) backcrosses, and one quarter of the (OS × CB)F_2 generation developed a significant ($\geq 1+$) (*vide supra*) thyroid infiltration, thus suggesting that only a single recessive gene governs the decision as to whether SAT develops or not, although disease severity follows a more complex pattern of inheritance. For the calculation of the number of genes regulating SAT severity, it is important to clearly characterize and define the borderline between healthy and affected animals. Accepting a low degree of lymphoid infiltration of the thyroid gland as a criterion for unequivocal disease results in a higher frequency of positive animals and a lower number of genes calculated to be responsible for SAT. On the other hand, considering only severe infiltration ($>2+$) means fewer animals classified as affected and a higher number of genes controlling the disease (Neu *et al.*, 1986).

Therefore, either of the two recessively inherited endocrinological disorders of the OS—namely, elevated thyroidal iodine uptake and increased CBG production—seemed possible candidates for the putative major SAT gene. However, these two features did not cosegregate with the occurrence of SAT in ($F_1 \times CB$) backcrosses, and SAT developed in chickens with normal CBG levels and iodine uptake. This proved that these two endocrine dysfunctions are not essential for SAT.

A possible impact of the dominantly inherited features was assessed in (OS × CB)F_2 crosses. Even severe thyroiditis (>40% of thyroid parenchyma replaced by lymphoid infiltration) occurred in F_2 birds with T cell responses or thymidine levels in the normal CB range and devoid of ev 22, thus ruling out an essential role of these abnormalities on SAT as well. Interestingly, development of small foci of thyroid infiltration, which occasionally are also found in the CB control group, positively correlated with high Con A response.

Altogether, these data (summarized in Table XI) indicate that none of the five genetically determined OS-specific abnormalities studied is a *conditio sine qua non* for the development of SAT. Among these traits, only CBG levels and T cell responses so far have been shown to modulate the degree of thyroid infiltration, as previously reported for sex, MHC,

TABLE XI
Genetic Analysis of Functional Abnormalities in the OS Chicken[a]

Parameter	Percentage (no. of positive/total investigated) of animals with "OS-like" characteristics in			
	(OS × CB)F_1	(F_1 × CB)Bc	(F_1 × OS)Bc	(OS × CB)F_2
Hyperresponse to Con A[b]	100 (42/42)	41 (64/158)	100 (29/29)	73 (92/126)
IL-2 hypersecretion[b]	100 (35/35)	55 (11/20)	ND	73 (91/125)
Con A-activatable PBLs[b]	100 (9/9)	52 (21/40)	100 (17/17)	81 (43/53)
Hyporesponse to GIF[c]	100 (11/11)	55 (11/20)	ND	ND
ev 22[c]	100 (6/6)	50 (38/76)	100 (17/17)	ND
Elevated CBG	0 (0/20)	0 (0/20)	47 (21/44)	21 (28/136)
Thyroidal iodine uptake	0 (0/11)	ND	42 (43/102)	ND
Decreased serum thymidine	100 (9/9)	56 (10/18)	ND	ND

[a] Con A, Concanavalin A; IL-2, interleukin-2; ND, not determined; PBLs, peripheral blood leukocytes; GIF, glucocorticoid-inducing factor; CBG, corticosteroid-binding globulin; ev 22, OS-specific endogenous virus 22; Bc, backcross. [Data were compiled from Neu et al. (1985) and Kroemer et al. (1988b,c).]
[b,c] Cosegregation of the respective parameters.

and MHC-linked immune response genes (Hála, 1988). The question remains as to why aberrations that appear to have little, or even no, apparent influence on the development of SAT, e.g., the abnormal iodine metabolism of the OS, are found in all OS sublines. A speculative explanation for this observation would be that these features once contributed as coetiological factors to SAT and that, as reported for the female sex, their pathogenetic role has been superceded in importance by other factors during the three-decade selection process to which this closed-bred chicken strain has been subjected.

We have therefore put forward the concept that the genes involved in the genetic control of SAT can be divided into two categories: essential and modulating genes (Wick et al., 1987; Hála, 1988). From our last experiments, discussed in this section (Kroemer et al., 1989a), it is evident that we are not yet able to identify the essential genes. The majority of all analyzed traits characteristic for the OS chicken seem to depend on the activity of modulating genes. The classical example of such a modulating factor is sex. In the OS chicken, in which thyroid infiltration already occurs 2 weeks after hatching, sex is now without any apparent influence. However, in an inbred population of chickens (Cole, 1966) or in humans (i.e., patients with Hashimoto disease) a strong prevalence for females exists.

IX. Conclusion

OS chickens already develop SAT during the first few weeks of life. This disease closely resembles human Hashimoto thyroiditis with respect to clinical symptoms, histopathology, and cellular and humoral immune function. Thyroid glands of OS chickens become severely infiltrated by mononuclear cells and the occurrence of numerous germinal centers is a characteristic histological hallmark of the disease. Autoimmune thyroid destruction leads to thyroid hormone deficiency that entails the development of hypothyroid symptoms, such as small body size; massive subcutaneous and abdominal fat deposits (hence the name); lipid serum; long, silky feathers; small combs; cold sensitivity; low fertility; and poor hatching ability. Originally, these symptoms were found only in females, but after several decades of selective breeding, both sexes are now affected to the same extent. The hypothyroid state of these birds necessitates thyroid hormone supplementation for successful breeding and propagation of the strain.

The serum of OS chickens contains AAbs to Tg, microsomal antigens, and T3 and T4. Tg-AAb formation is not due to polyclonal activation, but requires the presence of the autoantigen. The infiltrated thyroid itself has been identified as the major Tg-AAb-producing organ and can also be the site of the formation of antibodies against exogenous antigens. Complement-binding Tg-AAbs are vertically transferred from the mother hen via the egg yolk into the newly hatched chick, where they seem to play an accelerating role in SAT development. In addition to AAbs against thyroid antigens, OS chickens also produce AAbs against a variety of other organ-specific and non-organ-specific antigens, albeit with significantly lower frequency and titers, and without concomitant histopathological or functional lesions, such as Addison-like disease or diabetes mellitus.

With the advent of appropriate functional *in vitro* assays for avian systems and the development of Mabs against different chicken leukocyte markers, the natural history of SAT could be followed more closely. It became clear that the first thyroid-infiltrating cells were T cells that express a high density of IL-2 receptors. Depletion of peripheral T cells by neonatal thymectomy plus injections of turkey anti-chicken T cell antibodies (mammalian antibodies are not active *in vivo* in avian systems) prevented Tg-AAb development and thyroid infiltration. Together with the demonstration of Tg-specific cytotoxic T cells and the successful elicitation of thyroiditis in histocompatible CS recipients by transfer of B cell-depleted OS TILs, these results proved the essential primary role of T cells in SAT development. Further functional studies revealed a general hyperreactivity of the OS immune system against autoantigens, and also against exogenous antigens, such as xenogeneic RBCs and Rous sarcoma virus-induced tumors, as well as the T cell mitogens Con A and PHA. This hyperreactivity is reflected by a significantly higher production of IL-2 by OS PBLs and spleen cells as compared to various normal strains. Together with the results of genetic experiments that showed a positive correlation between OS IL-2 hypersecretion and thyroid infiltration, these observations prompted us to postulate an important role for increased IL-2 production in the etiopathogenesis of SAT. In addition to lymphoid cells, OS macrophages also reveal signs of hyperreactivity, such as an elevated oxidative burst activity.

Coculture experiments of autologous thymus cells and PBLs demonstrated a suppressor defect in the OS thymus as a factor intrinsic to the immune system that significantly contributes to the overall immunological hyperreactivity in this strain. It has been hypothesized that a significant deficiency of TNCs in OS chickens may be relevant for the observed altered immunoregulation. TNCs are large complexes consisting of single thymic epithelial cells that contain several intact thymocytes enclosed within membrane-lined intracytoplasmic vacuoles, where they may undergo the MHC self-recognition process.

In addition, factors extrinsic to the immune system that also affect immunoregulation have been found to be altered in the OS. Thus, OS chickens display a significantly decreased glucocorticoid tonus due to an increased serum concentration of corticosteroid-binding globulin and therefore markedly decreased free, metabolically active glucocorticoids. Furthermore, OS chickens show a malfunctioning immunoendocrine feedback loop in the sense that injections of SRBCs or conditioned media from mitogen-stimulated spleen cells do not result in the normally occurring surge of CN in the blood. This disturbed endogenous glucocorticoid response, which is mainly, but not exclusively, mediated by the action of IL-1 via the hypothalamic–pituitary–adrenal axis, is due neither to a deficiency or functional abnormality of IL-1 nor to altered ACTH release by the pituitary or an insufficient adrenal response. This interesting immunoendocrine defect has so far been localized to an altered responsiveness of the hypothalamus to peripheral stimuli, or of the pituitary to corticotropin-releasing factor.

The OS model has been proven to serve as an apt subject for the assessment of the therapeutic effects of new immunosuppressive drugs, notably steroid hormone analogs.

Transfer experiments and cross-breeding studies between OS and the highly inbred normal CB strain revealed that both the autoimmune hyperreactivity and a primary, genetically determined target organ susceptibility are required for fully blown SAT. Various functional abnormalities of OS thyroid glands were demonstrated, such as increased ^{131}I uptake preceding thyroid infiltration, autonomous thyroid function not suppressible by high doses of T4, and a decreased growth rate of OS TECs *in vitro* with insufficient release of growth-promoting autocrine factors. However, although these abnormalities may contribute to SAT severity, none of them seems to be essential for SAT development. Further investigations of possible etiological factors have not revealed any abnormality of OS Tg. Furthermore, no primary aberrant expression of MHC class II antigens on OS TECs was found. OS TECs do, however, show a lower threshold for γ-interferon-induced MHC class II expression than do those of normal chickens. This lower threshold was found for thyroid cells but not for similarly treated cell suspensions from other organs, i.e., the adrenal gland and the kidney.

Studies of the possible role of viruses led to the discovery of a new endogenous virus locus (*ev* 22) that seems to be specific for the OS. The presence of this *ev* 22 band in Southern blots of OS DNA digests correlates significantly with the decreased CN response to conditioned media injections. Whether this correlation has any pathophysiological significance remains to be elucidated.

Genetic analyses aimed at identifying the number and the nature of genes contributing to SAT led to the hypothesis of essential and modulating genes. Statistical analyses of SAT frequency in the offspring of crosses between OS and CB chickens point to the existence of a single, essential recessive autosomal "thyroid susceptibility" gene that has not been identified so far. Up to now, we were not yet able to identify the modulating genes, although possible candidates might be those regulating CBG levels and T cell hyperresponse. Other genes that may exert a modulating effect to different degrees are those determining macrophage hyperfunction; $ev\ 22$, which cosegregates with the altered glucocorticoid response to cytokines *in vivo*, the altered iodine metabolism of the thyroid; and MHC-linked immune response genes.

Acknowledgments

This work has been supported by grants from the Austrian Research Council (Project S-41/05; G. W.), the Jubliäumsfonds of the Austrian National Bank (Project 2784; G. W.) and the Austrian Ministry of Science and Research (K. H.). G. K. is the recipient of Erwin-Schrödinger fellowship No. J0307, awarded by the Austrian Research Council. We thank Reinhard Kofler for critical review, Pia-Ulrike Müller, Monika Ginzel, and Ruth Pfeilschifter-Resch for many years of competent technical assistance, the staff of our Central Laboratory Animal Facilities for efficient and thoughtful care of the chicken colonies, Ilona Atzinger for photography and artwork, and Gertrude Lechner for help in the preparation of this manuscript.

References

Aberer, W., Stingl, L., Pogantsch, S., and Stingl, G. (1984). *J. Immunol.* **133**, 792.
Aichinger, G., Kofler, H., Diaz-Merida, O., and Wick, G. (1984). *Clin. Immunol. Immunopathol.* **32**, 57.
Aichinger, G., Fill, H., and Wick, G. (1985). *Lab. Invest.* **52**, 132.
Akahoshi, T., Oppenheim, J. J., and Matsushima, K. (1988). *J. Exp. Med.* **167**, 924.
Albini, B., and Wick, G. (1974). *Nature (London)* **249**, 653.
Arya, S. K., Wong-Staal, F., and Gallo, R. C. (1984). *J. Immunol.* **133**, 273.
Bacon, L. D. (1976). *Fed. Proc. Fed. Am. Soc. Exp. Biol.* **35**, 713.
Bacon, L. D., and Rose, N. R. (1979). *Proc. Natl. Acad. Sci. U.S.A.* **76**, 1435.
Bacon, L. D., Kite, J. H., and Rose, N. R. (1973). *Transplantation* **16**, 591.
Bacon, L. D., Kite, J. H., and Rose, N. R. (1974). *Science* **186**, 274.
Bacon, L. D., Sundick, R. S., and Rose, N. R. (1977). *In* "Avian Immunology" (A. A. Benedict, ed.), p. 305. Plenum, New York.
Bacon, L. D., Cole, R. K., Polley, C. R., and Rose, N. R. (1978). *In* "Genetic Control of Autoimmune Disease" (N. R. Rose, P. E. Bigazzi, and N. L. Warner, eds.), p. 259. Elsevier/North-Holland, New York.
Bacon, L. D., Polley, C. R., Cole, R. K., and Rose, N. R. (1981). *Immunogenetics* **12**, 339.
Bagchi, N., Brown, T. R., Urdanivia, E., and Sundick, R. S. (1985). *Science* **230**, 325.
Balcarová, J., Derka, J., Hála, K., and Hraba, T. (1974). *Folia Biol. (Prague)* **20**, 346.
Berkenbosch, F., van Oers, J., del Rey, A., Tilders, F., and Besedovsky, H. O. (1987). *Science* **238**, 524.

Bernton, E. W., Beach, J. E., Holaday, J. W., Smallridge, R. C., and Fein, H. G. (1987). *Science* **238**, 519.
Besedovsky, H. O., Sorkin, E., Keller, M., and Mueller, J. (1975). *Proc. Soc. Exp. Biol. Med.* **150**, 466.
Besedovsky, H. O., del Rey, A., and Sorkin, E. (1979). *Clin. Exp. Immunol.* **37**, 106.
Besedovsky, H. O., del Rey, A., Sorkin, E., and Dinarello, C. A. (1986). *Science* **233**, 652.
Bielschowsky, M., Helyer, B. J., and Howie, J. B. (1959). *Proc. Univ. Otago Med. Sch.* **37**, 9.
Bocchieri, M. H., Smith, J. B., Jr., Smith, J. B., Staruch, M. J., and Wood, D. D. (1985). *Clin. Exp. Immunol.* **62**, 622.
Bottazzo, G. F., Pujol-Borrell, R., and Hanafusa, T. (1983). *Lancet* **2**, 1115.
Bourlet, Y., Béhar, G., Guillemot, F., Fréchin, N., Billault, A., Chaussé, A.-E., Zoorob, R., and Auffray, C. (1988). *EMBO J.* **7**, 1031.
Bowen, D. L., and Fauci, A. S. (1984). *J. Immunol. Methods* **35**, 233.
Boyd, R. L., and Wick, G. (1980). *Proc. Serono Symp.* **33**, 199.
Boyd, R. L., Cole, R. K., and Wick, G. (1983). *Immunol. Commun.* **12**, 263.
Boyd, R. L., Oberhuber, G., Hála, K., and Wick, G. (1984). *J. Immunol.* **132**, 718.
Boyd, R. L., Hála, K., and Wick, G. (1985). *J. Immunol.* **135**, 3039.
Boyd, R. L., Hála, K., and Wick, G. (1989). Submitted for publication.
Brezinschek, H. P., Faessler, R., Klocker, H., Kroemer, G., Scone, R., Dietrich, H., Jakober, R., and Wick, G. (1989). Submitted for publication.
Briles, W. E., McGibbon, W. H., and Irwin, M. R. (1950). *Genetics* **35**, 633.
Briles, W. E., Bumstead, N., Ewert, D. L., Gilmour, D. G., Gogusev, J., Hála, K., Koch, C., Longenecker, B. M., Nordskog, A. W., Pink, J. R. L., Schierman, L. W., Simonsen, M., Toivanen, A., Toivanen, P., Vainio, O., and Wick, G. (1982). *Immunogenetics* **15**, 441.
Brown, S. L., Smith, L. R., and Blalock, J. E. (1987). *J. Immunol.* **139**, 3181.
Brown, T. R., Bagchi, N., and Sundick, R. S. (1985). *J. Immunol.* **134**, 3845.
Carter, J. K., Ow, C. L., and Smith, R. E. (1983). *Infect. Immun.* **39**, 410.
Chambers, R. E., and Clamp, J. R. (1971). *Biochem. J.* **125**, 1009.
Chan, M. M., Chen, C. H., Ager, L. L., and Cooper, M. D. (1988). *J. Immunol.* **140**, 2133.
Chen, C.-L. H., Cihak, J., Ager, L. L., Gartland, G. L., and Cooper, M. D. (1986). *J. Exp. Med.* **164**, 375.
Chen, C.-L.H., Cihak, J., Loesch, U., and Cooper, M. D. (1988). *Eur. J. Immunol.* **18**, 539.
Cihak, J., Loems Ziegler-Heitbrock, H. W., Trainer, H., Schranner, I., Merkenschlager, M., and Loesch, U. (1988). *Eur. J. Immunol.* **18**, 533.
Coffin, J. M. (1982). In "Molecular Biology of Tumor Viruses: RNA Tumor Viruses" (R. A. Weiss *et al.*, eds), 2nd ed., p. 1108. Cold Spring Harbor Lab., Cold Spring Harbor, New York.
Cole, R. K. (1966). *Genetics* **53**, 1021.
Cole, R. K., Kite, J. H., Jr., and Witebsky, E. (1968). *Science* **160**, 1357.
Cole, R. K., Kite, J. H., Jr., Wick, G., and Witebsky, E. (1970). *Poult. Sci.* **49**, 840.
Coleman, D. L., and Hummel, H. P. (1967). *Diabetologia* **3**, 238.
del Rey, A., Besedovsky, H. O., and Sorkin, E. (1984). *J. Immunol.* **133**, 572.
Dietrich, H. (1989). *Lab. Anim.* (in press).
Dixon, F. J. (1979). *Am. J. Pathol.* **97**, 10.
Esquivel, P. S., Rose, N. R., and Kong, Y.-C. (1977). *J. Exp. Med.* **145**, 1250.

Faessler, R., Schauenstein, K., Kroemer, G., Schwarz, S., and Wick, G. (1986a). *J. Immunol.* **136**, 3657.
Faessler, R., Schwarz, S., Dietrich, H., and Wick, G. (1986b). *J. Steroid Biochem.* **24**, 405.
Faessler, R., Dietrich, H., Kroemer, G., Schwarz, S., Brezinschek, H. P., and Wick, G. (1988a). *J. Steroid Biochem.* **30**, 375.
Faessler, R., Dietrich, H., Kroemer, G., Boeck, G., Brezinschek, H. P., and Wick, G. (1988b). *J. Autoimmun.* **1**, 97.
Frederickson, T. L., and Gilmour, D. G. (1983). *J. Immunol.* **130**, 3528.
Gause, W. C., and Marsh, J. A. (1986). *Clin. Immunol. Immunopathol.* **39**, 464.
Gerritsen, G. C., and Blanks, M. C. (1970). *Diabetologia* **6**, 177.
Gershwin, M. E., Abplanalp, J. J., Castles, R. M., Ikeda, J., van de Water, J., Eklund, J., and Haynes, D. (1981). *J. Exp. Med.* **153**, 1640.
Gillis, S. D., Crabtree, G. R., and Smith, K. A. (1979a). *J. Immunol.* **123**, 1624.
Gillis, S. D., Crabtree, G. R., and Smith, K. A. (1979b). *J. Immunol.* **123**, 1632.
Glick, B. (1964). In "The Thymus in Immunology" (R. A. Good and A. E. Gabrielson, eds.), p. 343. Harper & Row, New York.
Grabar, P. (1975). *Clin. Immunol. Immunopathol.* **4**, 453.
Grindley, T., Soriano, P., and Jaenisch, R. (1987). *Trends Genet.* **2**, 162.
Grossman, C. J. (1984). *Endocr. Rev.* **5**, 435.
Guenther, E., Balcarová, J., Hála, K., Rüde, E., and Hraba, T. (1974). *Eur. J. Immunol.* **4**, 548.
Guillemot, F., Billault, A., Pourquié, O., Béhar, G., Chaussé, A.-M., Zoorob, R., Kreibich, G., and Auffray, C. (1988). *EMBO J.* **7**, 2775.
Hála, K. (1977). In "The Major Histocompatibility System in Man and Animals" (D. Goetze, ed.), p. 291. Springer-Verlag, Berlin and New York.
Hála, K. (1987). In "Avian Immunology: Basis and Practice" (A. Toivanen and P. Toivanen, eds.), Vol. 2, p. 85. CRC Press, Boca Raton, Florida.
Hála, K. (1988). *Immunobiology* **177**, 354.
Hála, K., Schauenstein, K., Neu, N., Kroemer, G., Wolf, H., Boeck, G., and Wick, G. (1986). *Eur. J. Immunol.* **16**, 1331.
Hála, K., Sgonc, R., Auffray, C., and Wick, G. (1989). In "Proceedings of Avian Immunology Meeting" (B. S. Bhogal, ed.). Liss, New York (in press).
Hanafusa, T., Chiovato, L., Doniach, D., Pujol-Borrell, P., Russell, G. C. G., and Bottazzo, G. F. (1983). *Lancet* **2**, 1111.
Hayward, W. S., and Neel, B. G. (1981). *Curr. Top. Microbiol. Immunol.* **103**, 218.
Helyer, B. J., and Howie, J. B. (1963). *Nature (London)* **197**, 197.
Horowitz, S., and Hong, R. (1975). In "Immunodeficiency in Man and Animals" (D. Bergsma, ed.), p. 129. Sinauer Associates, Sunderland, Massachusetts.
Iwakiri, R., Nagafuchi, S., Kounone, E., Nakano, S., Koya, T., Nakayama, M., Nakamura, M., and Niko, Y. (1987). *Experentia* **43**, 324.
Jaffe, W., and McDermid, E. M. (1962). *Science* **137**, 984.
Jakobisiak, M., Sundick, R. S., Bacon, L. D., and Rose, N. R. (1976). *Proc. Natl. Acad. Sci. U.S.A.* **73**, 2877.
Jankovic, B. D., Isvaneski, M., Popeskovic, L., and Mitrovic, K. (1965). *Int. Arch. Allergy Appl. Immunol.* **26**, 18.
Jaroszewski, I., Sundick, R. S., and Rose, N. R. (1978). *Clin. Immunol. Immunopathol.* **10**, 95.
Jenkins, M. K., Schwartz, R. H., and Pardoll, D. M. (1988). *Science* **241**, 1655.
Jingami, H., Matsukura, S., Numa, S., and Imura, H. (1985). *Endocrinology (Baltimore)* **117**, 1314.

Kaibara, N., Hotokebuchi, T., Takagashi, K., and Katsuki, I. (1983). *J. Exp. Med.* **158**, 2007.
Katz, D. V., Kite, J. H., and Albini, B. (1981). *J. Immunol.* **126**, 2296.
Khoury, E. L., Bottazzo, G. F., Pontes de Carvalho, L. C., Wick, G., and Roitt, I. M. (1982). *Clin. Exp. Immunol.* **49**, 273.
Kite, H. J., Wick, G., Twarog, B., and Witebsky, E. (1969). *J. Immunol.* **103**, 1331.
Kite, H. J., Tyler, J., and Pascale, J. (1979). *Immunopathol. Int. Convoc. Immunol. 6th, 1978*, p. 96.
Knudsen, P. J., Dinarello, C. A., and Strom, T. B. (1987). *J. Immunol.* **139**, 4129.
Kofler, H., Kofler, R., Wolf, H., and Wick, G. (1983). *Immunobiology* **164**, 390.
Kofler, H., Kofler, R., Wolf, H., Mueller, P.-U., and Wick, G. (1984). *J. Immunol. Methods* **69**, 243.
Kofler, R., and Wick, G. (1978). *Z. Immunitaets forsch.* **154**, 88.
Kofler, R., and Wick, G. (1979). *Folia Biol. (Prague)* **25**, 337.
Kroemer, G., Schauenstein, K., and Wick, G. (1984). *J. Immunol. Methods* **73**, 273.
Kroemer, G., Sundick, R. S., Schauenstein, K., Hála, K., and Wick, G. (1985a). *J. Immunol.* **135**, 2452.
Kroemer, G., Schauenstein, K., Neu, N., Stricker, K., and Wick, G. (1985b). *J. Immunol.* **135**, 2458.
Kroemer, G., Schauenstein, K., and Wick, G. (1986). *Immunol. Today* **7**, 199.
Kroemer, G., Schauenstein, K., Dietrich, H., Faessler, R., and Wick, G. (1987). *J. Immunol.* **138**, 2104.
Kroemer, G., Boeck, G., Schauenstein, K., Hilchenbach, M., Faessler, R., and Wick, G. (1988a). *Dev. Comp. Immunol.* **12**, 363.
Kroemer, G., Faessler, R., Hála, K., Boeck, G., Schauenstein, K., Brezinschek, H. P., Neu, N., Dietrich, H., Jakober, R., and Wick, G. (1988b). *Eur. J. Immunol.* **18**, 1499.
Kroemer, G., Klocker, H., Faessler, R., Sachsenmaier, W., and Wick, G. (1988c). *Immunol. Invest.* **17**, 243.
Kroemer, G., Brezinschek, H. P., Faessler, R., Schauenstein, K., and Wick, G. (1988d). *Immunol. Today* **9**, 163.
Kroemer, G., Faessler, R., and Wick, G. (1988e). *Concepts Immunopathol.* **5**, 106.
Kroemer, G., Faessler, R., Kuehr, T., Dietrich, H., Neu, N., Hála, K., and Wick, G. (1989). *Clin. Immunol. Immunopathol.* (in press).
Lamont, S. J., and Smyth, J. R., Jr. (1981). *Clin. Immunol. Immunopathol.* **21**, 407.
Lewis, R. M., and Schwartz, R. S. (1971). *J. Exp. Med.* **134**, 417.
Linker-Israeli, M., Bakke, A. C., Kitridou, R. C., Gendler, S., Gillis, S., and Horwitz, D. A. (1983). *J. Immunol.* **130**, 2651.
Livezey, M. D., and Sundick, R. S. (1980). *Gen. Comp. Endocrinol.* **41**, 243.
Livezey, M. D., Sundick, R. S., and Rose, N. R. (1981). *J. Immunol.* **127**, 1469.
Lodmell, D. L., and Portis, J. L. (1981). In "Immunologic Defects in Laboratory Animals" (M. E. Gershwin and B. Merchant, eds.), Vol. 2, p. 39. Plenum, New York.
Lotze, M. T., Matory, Y. L., Ettinghausen, S. E., Rayner, A. A., Sharrow, S. O., Seipp, C. A. Y., Custer, M. C., and Rosenberg, S. A. (1985). *J. Immunol.* **135**, 2865.
Luster, M. I., Bacon, L. D., Rose, N. R., and Leslie, G. A. (1977). *Cell. Immunol.* **32**, 417.
Mendlovic, S., Brocke, S., Shoenfeld, Y., Ben-Bassat, M., Meshorer, A., Bakimer, R., and Mozes, E. (1988). *Proc. Natl. Acad. Sci. U.S.A.* **85**, 2260.
Moroz, L. A., Meltazer, S. J., and Bastomsky, C. H. (1983). *J. Clin. Endocrinol. Metab.* **54**, 1009.

Morrow, R. P., and Abplanalp, H. (1982). *Immunogenetics* **13**, 189.
Murphy, E. D. (1981). In "Immunologic Defects in Laboratory Animals" (M. E. Gershwin and Merchant, eds.), Vol. 2, p. 143. Plenum, New York.
Murphy, E. D., and Roths, J. B. (1979). *Arthritis Rheum.* **22**, 1188.
Nakhooda, A. F., Like, A. A., Chappel, C. I., Murray, F. T., and Martiss, E. B. (1977). *Diabetes* **26**, 100.
Neu, N., Hála, K., and Wick, G. (1984). *Immunogenetics* **19**, 269.
Neu, N., Hála, K., Dietrich, H., and Wick, G. (1985). *Clin. Immunol. Immunopathol.* **37**, 397.
Neu, N., Hála, K., Dietrich, H., and Wick, G. (1986). *Int. Arch. Allergy Appl. Immunol.* **80**, 168.
Newcomer, W. S. (1973). *Gen. Comp. Endocrinol.* **21**, 322.
Nilsson, L. A., Rose, N. R., and Witebsky, E. (1971). *J. Immunol.* **107**, 997.
Notkins, A. L., and Prabhakar, B. S. (1986). *Ann. N.Y. Acad. Sci.* **475**, 123.
Novak, J. S., Bacon, L. D., and Rose, N. R. (1978). *Immunol. Commun.* **7**, 621.
Nusse, R. (1986). *Trends Genet.* **2**, 244.
Okayasu, I., Kong, Y. I. M., and Rose, N. R. (1981). *Clin. Immunol. Immunopathol.* **20**, 240.
Paterson, P. Y. (1966). *Adv. Immunol.* **5**, 131.
Penninger, J., Hála, K., and Wick, G. (1989). Submitted for publication.
Perrudet-Badoux, A., and Frei, P. C. (1969). *Clin. Exp. Immunol.* **5**, 117.
Peter, H. J., Gerber, H., Studer, H., and Smeds, S. (1985). *J. Clin. Invest.* **76**, 1992.
Pink, J. R. L., and Vainio, O. (1983). *Eur. J. Immunol.* **13**, 571.
Pink, J. R. L., Dröge, W., Hála, K., Miggiano, C., and Ziegler, A. (1977). *Immunogenetics* **5**, 203.
Pontes de Carvalho, L. C., Roitt, I. M., and Wick, G. (1980). *J. Immunol. Methods* **39**, 15.
Pontes de Carvalho, L. C., Wick, G., and Roitt, I. M. (1981). *J. Immunol.* **126**, 750.
Pontes de Carvalho, L. C., Templeman, J., Wick, G., and Roitt, I. M. (1982). *J. Exp. Med.* **155**, 1255.
Raheja, K. L., Linscher, W. G., and Patel, D. G. (1986). *Horm. Metab. Res.* **18**, 153.
Richter, E., and Wick, G. (1975). *J. Immunol.* **114**, 757.
Richter, E., Sundick, R., and Wick, G. (1975a). *Z. Immunitaetsforsch., Exp. Klin. Immunol.* **149**, 61.
Richter, E., Wick, G., and Schauenstein, K. (1975b). *Eur. J. Immunol.* **5**, 554.
Richter, E., Wick, G., Zambelis, N., Ludwig, H., and Schernthaner, G. (1978). *Clin. Immunol. Immunopathol.* **11**, 178.
Roberts, I. M., Wittingham, S., and Mackay, I. R. (1973). *Lancet* **1**, 936.
Robinson, H. R. (1978). *Curr. Top. Microbiol. Immunol.* **83**, 1.
Roitt, I. M., Doniach, D., Campbell, D. N., and Hudson, R. V. (1956). *Lancet* **2**, 820.
Rose, N. R., and Witebsky, E. (1956). *J. Immunol.* **76**, 417.
Rose, N. R., Kite, J. H., Flanagan, T. D., and Witebsky, E. (1971). *Cell. Interact. Immune Response Int. Convoc. Immunol. 2nd, 1970*, p. 264.
Rose, N. R., Bacon, L. D., and Sundick, R. S. (1976). *Transplant. Rev.* **31**, 264.
Rose, N. R., Bacon, L. D., Sundick, R. S., and Briles, W. E. (1978). In "Animal Models of Comparative and Developmental Aspects of Immunity and Disease" (M. E. Gershwin and E. L. Cooper, eds.), p. 143. Pergamon, New York.
Rose, N. R., Kong, Y. M., Okayasu, I., Giraldo, A. A., Beisel, K., and Sundick, R. S. (1981). *Immunol. Rev.* **55**, 299.
Rose, N. R., Herskowitz, A., Neumann, D. A., and Neu, N. (1988). *Immunol. Today* **9**, 117.

Roubinian, J. R., Talal, N., Greenspan, J. S., Goodman, J. R., and Siiteri, P. K. (1978). *J. Exp. Med.* **147**, 1568.
Rovigatti, V. G., and Astrin, S. M. (1983). *Curr. Top. Microbiol. Immunol.* **103**, 1.
Rudas, B., Wick, G., and Cole, R. K. (1972). *J. Endocrinol.* **55**, 609.,
Sanker, A. J., Sundick, R. S., and Brown, T. R. (1983). *J. Immunol.* **131**, 1252.
Sanker, A. J., Clark, C. R., and Sundick, R. S. (1985). *J. Immunol.* **135**, 281.
Sapolsky, R., Rivier, C., Yamamoto, G., Plotsky, P., and Vale, W. (1987). *Science* **238**, 522.
Scanes, C. G., Gales, L., Harvey, S., Chadwick, A., and Newcomer, W. S. (1976). *Gen. Comp. Endocrinol.* **30**, 419.
Schauenstein, K., and Wick, G. (1974). *Clin. Exp. Immunol.* **17**, 637.
Schauenstein, K., Globerson, A., Rosenberg, M., Sharon, N., and Wick, G. (1983). *Cell. Immunol.* **80**, 288.
Schauenstein, K., Kroemer, G., Sundick, R. S., and Wick, G. (1985). *J. Immunol.* **134**, 872.
Schauenstein, K., Faessler, R., Dietrich, H., Schwarz, S., Kroemer, G., and Wick, G. (1987a). *J. Immunol.* **139**, 1830.
Schauenstein, K., Kroemer, G., Boeck, G., Rossi, K., Hála, K., and Wick, G. (1987b). *Immunobiology* **175**, 226.
Schauenstein, K., Kroemer, G., Hála, K., Boeck, G., and Wick, G. (1988). *Dev. Comp. Immunol.* **12**, 823.
Schierman, L. W., and Nordskog, A. W. (1961). *Science* **134**, 1008.
Shulman, S., Mates, G., and Bronson, P. (1967). *Biochim. Biophys. Acta* **147**, 208.
Shultz, L. D., and Green, M. C. (1976). *J. Immunol.* **116**, 936.
Silverman, D. A., and Rose, N. R. (1975). *J. Immunol.* **114**, 145.
Smith, E. M., Meyer, W. J., and Blalock, J. E. (1982). *Science* **218**, 1311.
Smith, E. M., Morill, A. C., Meyer, W. J., and Blalock, J. E. (1986). *Nature (London)* **322**, 881.
Snyder, D. S., and Unanue, E. R. (1982). *J. Immunol.* **129**, 1803.
Solleved, H. A., Coolen, J., Hollander, C. F., and Zurcher, C. (1982). *Clin. Immunol. Immunopathol.* **25**, 179.
Sowder, J. T., Chen, C.-L. H., Ager, L. L., Chan, M. M., and Cooper, M. D. (1988). *J. Exp. Med.* **167**, 315.
Sundick, R. S., and Wick, G. (1974). *Clin. Exp. Immunol.* **18**, 127.
Sundick, R. S., and Wick, G. (1976). *J. Immunol.* **116**, 1319.
Sundick, R. S., Bloom, S. E., and Kite, J. H. (1973). *Clin. Exp. Immunol.* **14**, 437.
Sundick, R. S., Bagchi, N., Livezey, M. D., Brown, T. R., and Mack, R. E. (1979). *Endocrinology (Baltimore)* **105**, 493.
Sundick, R. S., Livezey, M. D., and Rose, N. R. (1980). *Thyroid Res. 8 [eight], Proc. Int. Thyroid Congr., 8th, 1980* p. 773.
Sundick, R. S., Herdegen, D. M., Brown, T. R., and Bagchi, N. (1987). *Endocrinology (Baltimore)* **120**, 2078.
Tempelis, C. H., Schauenstein, K., and Wick, G. (1987). *Clin. Exp. Immunol.* **67**, 477.
Theofilopoulos, A. N., and Dixon, F. J. (1985). *Adv. Immunol.* **37**, 269.
Thunold, S., Schauenstein, K., Wolf, H., Thunhold, K. S., and Wick, G. (1981). *Scand. J. Immunol.* **14**, 145.
Tonooka, N., Leslie, G. A., Green, M. A., and Olson, J. C. (1978). *Am. J. Pathol.* **92**, 681.
Truden, J. L., Sundick, R. S., Levine, S., and Rose, N. R. (1983). *Clin. Immunol. Immunopathol.* **29**, 294.

Uehara, A., Gottschall, P. E., Dahl, R. R., and Arimura, A. (1987). *Endocrinology (Baltimore)* **121**, 1580.
Urbaniak, S. J., Torrigiani, G., and Allison, A. C. (1973). *Clin. Exp. Immunol.* **15**, 345.
Van Tienhoven, A., and Cole, R. K. (1962). *Anat. Rec.* **142**, 111.
Waterston, R. H. (1970). *Science* **170**, 1108.
Weetman, A. P., Volkman, D. J., Burman, K. P., Gerrard, T. L., and Fauci, A. S. (1985). *J. Clin. Endocrinol. Metab.* **61**, 817.
Weigle, W. O. (1978). *In* "Autoimmunity: Genetic, Immunologic, Virologic and Clinical Aspects" (N. Talal, ed.), p. 141. Academic Press, New York.
Weigle, W. O. (1980). *Adv. Immunol.* **30**, 159.
Wekerle, H., and Ketelson, U.-P. (1980). *Nature (London)* **283**, 402.
Wekerle, H., Ketelson, U.-P., and Ernst, M. (1980). *J. Exp. Med.* **151**, 925.
Welch, P. C., and Kite, J. H. (1971). *Fed. Proc. Fed. Am. Soc. Exp. Biol.* **30**, 306.
Welch, P. C., Rose, N. R., and Kite, J. H. (1973). *J. Immunol.* **110**, 575.
Wick, G., and Burger, H. (1971). *Z. Immunitaetsforsch. Exp. Klin. Immunol.* **142**, 54.
Wick, G., and Graf, J. (1972). *Lab. Invest.* **27**, 400.
Wick, G., and Oberhuber, G. (1986). *Eur. J. Immunol.* **16**, 855.
Wick, G., and Steiner, R. (1972a). *J. Immunol.* **109**, 471.
Wick, G., and Steiner, R. (1972b). *J. Immunol.* **109**, 1031.
Wick, G., Kite, J. H., Cole, R. K., and Witebsky, E. (1970a). *J. Immunol.* **104**, 45.
Wick, G., Kite, J. H., and Witebsky, E. (1970b). *J. Immunol.* **104**, 54.
Wick, G., Kite, J. H., and Witebsky, E. (1970c). *J. Immunol.* **104**, 344.
Wick, G., Witebsky, E., Kite, J. H., and Beutner, E. H. (1970d). *Clin. Exp. Immunol.* **7**, 173.
Wick, G., Kite, J. H., and Cole, R. K. (1971). *Int. Arch. Allergy Appl. Immunol.* **40**, 603.
Wick, G., Sundick, R. S., and Albini, B. (1974). *Clin. Immunol. Immunopathol.* **3**, 272.
Wick, G., Gundolf, R., and Hála, K. (1979). *J. Immunogenet.* **6**, 177.
Wick, G., Boyd, R., Hála, K., Pontes de Carvalho, L., Kofler, R., Mueller, P.-U., and Cole, R. K. (1981). *Curr. Top. Microbiol. Immunol.* **91**, 109.
Wick, G., Boyd, R. L., Hála, K., Thunhold, S., and Kofler, H. (1982a). *Clin. Exp. Immunol.* **47**, 1
Wick, G., Mueller, P.-U., Schwarz, S. (1982b). *Eur. J. Immunol.* **12**, 877.
Wick, G., Hála, K., Wolf, H., Boyd, R. L., and Schauenstein, K. (1984). *Mol. Immunol.* **21**, 1259.
Wick, G., Moest, J., Schauenstein, K., Kroemer, G., Dietrich, H., Ziemiecki, A., Faessler, R., Neu, N., and Hála, K. (1985). *Immunol. Today* **6**, 359.
Wick, G., Hála, K., Wolf, H., Ziemiecki, A., Sundick, R. S., Stoeffler-Meilicke, M., and DeBaets, M. (1986). *Immunol. Rev.* **94**, 113.
Wick, G., Krömer, G., Neu, N., Faessler, R., Ziemiecki, A., Mueller, R. G., Ginzel, M., Béládi, I., Kuehr, T., and Hála, K. (1987). *Immunol. Lett.* **16**, 249.
Wick, G., Dietrich, H., Kroemer, G., Faessler, R., Brezinschek, H. P., and Schuurs, A. H. (1989). *In* "Progress in Autoimmunity" (P. L. Bigazzi, G. Wick, and K. Wicher, eds.). Dekker, New York (in press).
Witebsky, E., and Rose, N. R. (1956). *J. Immunol.* **76**, 408.
Zeigel, R. F., Barron, A. L., Kite, J. H., and Witebsky, E. (1970). *Avian Dis.* **14**, 617.
Ziemiecki, A., Kroemer, G., Mueller, R. G., Hála, K., and Wick, G. (1988). *Arch. Virol.* **100**, 267.

This article was accepted for publication on 1 February 1989.

Index

A

Acquired immune deficiency syndrome
  HIV infection and, 377, 413, 414
  activation, 398, 400, 403
  etiological agent, 378, 379, 384
  immune response, 405-409
  immunopathogenic mechanism, 388-391, 394, 395, 397
  neuropsychiatric manifestations, 403-405
  natural killer cells and, 285, 302, 303
Acquired immune deficiency syndrome-dementia complex, 377, 403
Acquired immune deficiency syndrome-related complex
  immune response, 408
  immunopathogenic mechanism, 388, 395, 397, 403
  neuropsychiatric manifestations, 404
Adaptive immunity, natural killer cells and, 291-295
Adenosine triphosphate, HIV infection and, 382
Adhesins, antigen-presenting cells and, 61
Adrenocorticotropic hormone
  natural killer cells and, 268, 269
  spontaneous autoimmune thyroiditis and, 477, 479, 493
Aging, CD5 B cell and, 122, 123
Allergic disease, immunoglobulin E biosynthesis and, 1
  antibody response, 7, 29, 30, 38
  binding factors, 13
Amino acids
  antigen-presenting cells and, 60, 66, 89
  CD5 B cell and, 145, 146
  HIV infection and, 386, 405-408
  immunoglobulin E biosynthesis and, 15-17, 20, 39
Androgens, spontaneous autoimmune thyroiditis and, 480, 481

Antibodies
  antigen-presenting cells and
    antigen presentation, 68, 73, 75
    antigen processing, 92
    APC-T cell binding, 95, 97, 99
    cell surface, 57-59, 61, 62
    immunogeneity, 102, 103
    interaction with T cells, 93
    T cell-dependent antibody responses, 81-86
    T cell growth, 100, 101
    tissue distribution, 49, 50, 53, 57
  CD5 B cell and, 161, 162
    Ig gene expression, 150-154, 157, 158
    lineage, 129
    marker for activation, 127
    physiology, 130, 131, 133, 135-137, 139, 140
    primordial immune network, 159-161
    surface antigen, 143, 144
  HIV infection and
    immune response, 405-410
    immunopathogenic mechanism, 388, 389, 393, 395, 398
    neuropsychiatric manifestations, 404
  immunoglobulin E biosynthesis and, 1
    binding factors, 12, 14, 15, 17, 19, 21-23, 25, 28
    response, 1-12
    response suppression, 28-39
  natural killer cells and, 189
    adaptive immunity, 292-294
    alteration, 300
    antimicrobial activity, 286-288
    cell-mediated cytotoxicity, 190, 196
    congenital defects, 224
    cytotoxicity, 249-251, 254, 257-259, 261
    differentiation, 231, 233
    effector mechanisms, 235, 237, 238, 240, 241, 243-248
    hematopoiesis, 274, 275, 277, 281
    identification, 196, 198

501

malignant expansion, 227–229
surface phenotype, 201, 202, 204–213
tissue distribution, 221
spontaneous autoimmune thyroiditis and, 433, 492
  altered thyroid function, 460
  disturbed immunoregulation, 479
  histopathology, 442
  humoral immune reactions, 444, 445, 447, 479
  potential effector mechanisms, 468
Antibody-dependent cell-mediated cytotoxicity
  HIV infection and, 384, 388, 405, 410, 413
  natural killer cells and, 189, 190
    antimicrobial activity, 285
    cytotoxicity, 251, 253, 258
    effector mechanisms, 241–243
    genetic control, 222
    malignant expansion, 227, 228
    reproduction, 271, 272
    surface phenotype, 204, 212, 213
  spontaneous autoimmune thyroiditis and, 451, 452, 466, 469
Antibody-mediated complement-dependent cytotoxicity, HIV infection and, 409, 410, 413
Antigen-presenting cells, 45–47, 105
  antigen presentation, 64
    allogeneic MHC products, 73–76
    H-Y antigens, 80
    Mls stimulation, 76–79
    protein, 65–73
    TNP-modified syngeneic cells, 79, 80
    viral antigens, 80, 81
  antigen processing
    B cells, 89, 90
    dendritic cells, 90, 91
    MHC-peptide complexes, 87–89
    MHC products, 92
  APC-T cell binding, 95–99
  autoimmunity, 104, 105
  cell surface, 57
    CD5 leukocyte common antigen, 60, 61
    integrins, 61
    MHC products, 57–60
    receptors, 62–64
  immunogeneity, 101–104
  immunoglobulin E biosynthesis and, 27, 28, 33, 37, 39
  interaction with T cells, 92–94

T cell-dependent antibody responses
  B cells, 81, 82, 84–86
  dendritic cells, 83
  helper T cell subsets, 83, 84
T cell growth, 99–101
tissue distribution
  circulation, 54–57
  delayed-type hypersensitivity, 57
  life span, 49, 50
  lymphoid organs, 50–52
  nonlymphoid organs, 52–54
  origin, 47–49
Antigens
  CD5 B cell and, 117, 118, 120, 161
    bone marrow transplantation, 129
    genetic influence, 148
    Ig gene expression, 150, 151, 155, 156, 158
    lineage, 129
    malignancies, 123, 124
    marker for activation, 125, 126
    ontogeny, 122
    physiology, 131, 133–136, 138–143
    primordial immune network, 159–161
    surface, 143–147
  HIV infection and
    activation, 398, 400, 402
    etiological agent, 378, 380, 383, 384
    immune response, 408–410
    immunopathogenic mechanism, 388, 390–392, 394, 397
    neuropsychiatric manifestations, 404
  immunoglobulin E biosynthesis and, 1
    antibody response, 3–6, 8, 10, 11
    antibody response suppression, 28, 29, 31–39
    binding factors, 12, 14, 15, 21, 23–28
  natural killer cells and, 187–190
    adaptive immunity, 292, 293, 295
    alterations, 302
    antimicrobial activity, 288, 289
    CNS, 266
    congenital defects, 226
    differentiation, 232, 233
    effector mechanisms, 235, 237–240, 247, 248
    genetic control, 222
    hematopoiesis, 273, 275, 281, 282
    lymphokine production, 264
    malignant expansion, 227
    regulation, 257, 259, 261

reproduction, 271, 272
surface phenotype, 200–212
tissue distribution, 221
spontaneous autoimmune thyroiditis and, 433, 435, 491, 492
altered thyroid function, 461, 462
cellular immune reactions, 450, 452, 455, 456
clinical symptoms, 439
disturbed immunoregulation, 470, 476, 477, 479
genetics, 484
histopathology, 444
humoral immune reactions, 444, 448
potential effector mechanisms, 469
Antimicrobial activity, natural killer cells and, 282–291
Antitumor activity, natural killer cells and, 295–300
Antiviral activity, natural killer cells and, 282–288
ATPase, antigen-presenting cells and, 53, 54
Autoantibodies
CD5 B cell and, 133–135
Ig gene expression, 150, 155, 157, 158
physiology, 130–136
primordial immune network, 159
spontaneous autoimmune thyroiditis and, 491, 492
altered thyroid function, 456, 457, 459, 462
cellular immune reactions, 449
clinical symptoms, 439
humoral immune reactions, 444, 446–448
potential effector mechanisms, 466, 468, 469
Autoantigens, spontaneous autoimmune thyroiditis and, 491, 492
cellular immune reactions, 456, 459
disturbed immunoregulation, 470
humoral immune reactions, 445, 446, 448
Autoimmune diseases
CD5 B cell and, 148–150
spontaneous autoimmune thyroiditis and, 433–435
altered thyroid function, 462, 464
cellular immune reactions, 449, 455
disturbed immunoregulation, 481
histopathology, 444
humoral immune reactions, 448
potential effector mechanisms, 468

Autoimmune thyroiditis, *see* Spontaneous autoimmune thyroiditis
Autoimmunity, antigen-presenting cells and, 104, 105
Autologous plaque-forming B cell response, natural killer cells and, 300, 301

B

B cell growth factor
CD5 B cell and, 119, 140, 141
natural killer cells and, 265
B cell lymphomas, CD5 B cell and
Ig gene expression, 150–152, 154
malignancies, 123–125
B cells
antigen-presenting cells and, 45, 47, 87
antigen presentation, 66–70, 72–76, 78, 79
antigen processing, 88–90, 92–94
APC-T cell binding, 95, 97–99
cell surface, 57, 59, 61–64
immunogeneity, 103, 104
T cell-dependent antibody responses, 81–86
T cell growth, 99–101
tissue distribution, 48–51, 53–57
CD5, *see* CD5 B cell
HIV infection and, 390, 397
immunoglobulin E biosynthesis and
antibody response, 5–12
antibody response suppression, 28
binding factors, 13, 19–23
natural killer cells and, 188, 199
adaptive immunity, 291
alterations, 300
congenital defects, 225, 226
differentiation, 230
effector mechanisms, 255, 264
hematopoiesis, 281
malignant expansion, 228
surface phenotype, 201, 209, 211
spontaneous autoimmune thyroiditis and, 434, 492
cellular immune reactions, 449, 450, 452, 455
histopathology, 440, 444
humoral immune reactions, 446–448
B lymphoblasts, natural killer cells and, 292
B lymphocytes
antigen-presenting cells and, 45, 46
antigen presentation, 72

cell surface, 57–64
immunogeneity, 101
T cell growth, 99
tissue distribution, 47–57
CD5 B cell and, 117–120, 161
bone marrow transplantation, 129, 130
Ig gene expression, 150, 152
lineage, 128, 129
malignancies, 125
marker for activation, 125–128
ontogeny, 121, 122
physiology, 131, 133, 134, 136–138
primordial immune network, 160
surface antigen, 143, 147
natural killer cells and, 225, 232
spontaneous autoimmune thyroiditis and, 467, 469, 481
Bacteria
antigen-presenting cells and, 87
CD5 B cell and, 160
HIV infection and, 402
natural killer cells and, 216, 224, 235, 263, 289
spontaneous autoimmune thyroiditis and, 462
Bone marrow
antigen-presenting cells and, 45, 47, 48, 81
CD5 B cell and
aging, 122
anatomic localization, 120, 121
lineage, 128
malignancies, 124
physiology, 132, 142
primordial immune network, 161
transplantation, 129, 130
HIV infection and, 395–397
natural killer cells and, 188, 201
adaptive immunity, 292
antimicrobial activity, 289, 290
antitumor activity, 298
differentiation, 229–233
effector mechanisms, 234, 235, 263, 265
hematopoiesis, 272–283
reproduction, 270, 271
tissue distribution, 219, 221
spontaneous autoimmune thyroiditis and, 446, 450
Bradykinin, immunoglobulin E biosynthesis and, 18, 25

C

Calcium
CD5 B cell and, 127, 144, 145
HIV infection and, 387
immunoglobulin E biosynthesis and, 26
natural killer cells and, 291
cytotoxicity, 249–251, 253, 254, 261
effector mechanisms, 241, 244, 245
lymphokines, 265, 266
spontaneous autoimmune thyroiditis and, 471
Calmodulin, natural killer cells and, 249
Cancer, natural killer cells and, 297–300
Carbohydrate
immunoglobulin E biosynthesis and, 15–17
natural killer cells and, 207, 241
spontaneous autoimmune thyroiditis and, 460
CD4 cells
antigen-presenting cells and
antigen presentation, 64, 75, 80
cell surface, 57
immunogeneity, 102
interaction with T cells, 93, 94
T cell-dependent antibody responses, 83, 84, 86
tissue distribution, 50
HIV infection and
depletion, 386–389
etiological agent, 379, 382, 384, 385
immune response, 405, 408
immunopathogenic mechanism, 385, 386, 389–392, 394
neuropsychiatric manifestations, 405
CD5 antigen, natural killer cells and, 227
CD5 B cell, 117, 118, 161, 162
aging, 122, 123
anatomic localization, 120, 121
autoimmune diseases, 148–150
bone marrow transplantation, 129, 130
definition, 118–120
genetic influence, 147, 148
Ig gene expression
lymphomas, 150–152
malignancies, 152–159
lineage, 128, 129
malignancies, 123–125
marker for activation, 125–128

ontogeny, 121, 122
physiology
    autoantibody production, 130-136
    helper B cells, 137-141
    monocytoid features, 141-143
    primordial immune network, 159-161
    surface antigen, 143-147
CD5 cells, antigen-presenting cells and, 47, 55, 63
CD8 cells, antigen-presenting cells and
    antigen presentation, 64, 75, 80, 81
    antigen processing, 92
    immunogeneity, 102
CD11 antigen, natural killer cells and, 291
    congenital defects, 224
    differentiation, 234
    effector mechanisms, 245, 246
    hematopoiesis, 281
    malignant expansion, 226
    surface phenotype, 207, 208
CD16 antigen, natural killer cells and, 188, 189
    adaptive immunity, 291, 295
    alterations, 302
    antimicrobial activity, 288, 289
    antitumor activity, 298
    CNS, 267
    congenital defects, 224
    cytotoxicity, 249, 257, 258, 261
    differentiation, 233, 234
    effector mechanisms, 237, 242, 244, 247
    genetic control, 222, 223
    hematopoiesis, 275, 279
    lymphokines, 265
    morphology, 218
    reproduction, 271
    surface phenotype, 201-206, 208
    tissue distribution, 219, 220
CD18 antigen, natural killer cells and, 207, 224
cDNA
    CD5 B cell and, 145-147, 154
    immunoglobulin E biosynthesis and, 16-18, 21
    natural killer cells and, 209
    spontaneous autoimmune thyroiditis and, 462, 483
Cell-mediated cytotoxicity
    HIV infection and, 410, 411
    natural killer cells and, 189-196

Central nervous system
    HIV infection and, 378, 413
    immunopathogenic mechanism, 393
    neuropsychiatric manifestations, 403, 404
    natural killer cells and, 266-269
Chediak-Higashi syndrome, natural killer cells and, 224, 225, 299
Chemiluminescence, natural killer cells and, 263, 266
Cholesterol, spontaneous autoimmune thyroiditis and, 439
Chromatin, natural killer cells and, 214
Chromosomes
    CD5 B cell and, 132, 148, 157
    HIV infection and, 380
    natural killer cells and, 227, 228, 231
Chronic lymphocytic leukemia
    CD5 B cell and
        aging, 123
        autoimmune diseases, 150
        Ig gene expression, 153-159
        malignancies, 123, 124
        physiology, 136, 140, 141
        surface antigen, 146, 147
    natural killer cells and, 298
Clones
    antigen-presenting cells and, 45
    antigen presentation, 65, 66, 68-71, 73
    antigen processing, 91, 92
    APC-T cell binding, 95, 99
    cell surface, 61, 62
    immunogeneity, 102, 103
    interaction with T cells, 94
    T cell-dependent antibody responses, 83
    T cell growth, 99
    tissue distribution, 48, 49
    CD5 B cell and
        aging, 122
        Ig gene expression, 151, 152, 154, 156, 158
        physiology, 133, 134, 136, 140, 142
        surface antigen, 146
    HIV infection and, 400, 411
        etiological agent, 380, 385
        immunopathogenic mechanism, 388, 390, 394
    immunoglobulin E biosynthesis and
        antibody response, 6, 7, 10-12
        antibody response suppression, 33, 39
        binding factors, 13, 15-18, 20, 21, 27

natural killer cells and, 188, 199, 291
  cytotoxicity, 252
  differentiation, 231, 234
  effector mechanisms, 240, 243,
    245-248, 254, 264, 265
  hematopoiesis, 273, 274, 277, 279
  malignant expansion, 228
  morphology, 217
  surface phenotype, 202, 204-207, 209,
    210, 212
  spontaneous autoimmune thyroiditis and,
    464, 477
Collagenase, antigen-presenting cells and, 52
Complete Freund's adjuvant, immunoglobulin E biosynthesis and, 2-5, 14, 24
Conacanavalin A, antigen-presenting cells
  and, 84, 100
Conalbumin, immunoglobulin E
  biosynthesis and, 11
Concanavalin A
  CD5 B cell and, 121
  immunoglobulin E biosynthesis and, 15,
    18-20
  spontaneous autoimmune thyroiditis
    and, 492
    cellular immune reactions, 452-455
    disturbed immunoregulation, 470-473,
      475, 477-479
    genetics, 487, 488, 490
    potential effector mechanisms, 467
Corticosteroid-binding globulin, 492, 494
  genetics, 488-490
  immunoregulation, 476, 479, 481
Corticosteroids, spontaneous autoimmune
  thyroiditis and, 477
Corticosterone, spontaneous autoimmune
  thyroiditis and, 493
  disturbed immunoregulation, 476-481
  genetics, 488, 489
Corticotropin-releasing factor
  natural killer cells and, 268, 269
  spontaneous autoimmune thyroiditis
    and, 493
Cross-reactive idiotypes, CD5 B cell and,
  150, 151, 153-158
Cyclic AMP, natural killer cells and,
  249, 250
Cycloheximide, antigen-presenting cells
  and, 59
Cysteine, immunoglobulin E biosynthesis
  and, 17

Cytokines
  antigen-presenting cells and, 47, 104
  antigen presentation, 72
  cell surface, 63
  immunogeneity, 103
  T cell growth, 100
  tissue distribution, 53
  CD5 B cell and, 120
  marker for activation, 127
  physiology, 139, 142
  surface antigen, 145
  HIV infection and, 401-404
  natural killer cells and, 241, 263, 265, 266
  spontaneous autoimmune thyroiditis
    and, 494
    disturbed immunoregulation, 471,
      477, 478
    genetics, 488, 489
Cytolytic T lymphocytes, CD5 B cell and,
  144, 145
Cytomegalovirus, HIV infection and
  immune response, 409
  immunopathogenic mechanism, 390,
    392, 400
  neuropsychiatric manifestations, 392,
    403, 405
Cytoplasm
  antigen-presenting cells and
  antigen presentation, 81
  antigen processing, 87
  cell surface, 60
  T cell growth, 101
  tissue distribution, 48, 51
  CD5 B cell and, 144-146
  HIV infection and, 393, 396, 397
  immunoglobulin E biosynthesis and, 4,
    20, 21
  natural killer cells and, 197
    congenital defects, 225
    effector mechanisms, 249, 253, 262
    morphology, 214
Cytotoxic T lymphocytes
  antigen-presenting cells and, 73, 79-61
  antigen processing, 92
  immunogeneity, 104
  HIV infection and, 390, 410, 411, 413
  natural killer cells and, 187, 188, 196,
    283, 295, 302
    congenital defects, 225
    cytotoxicity, 252-254
    differentiation, 229, 232

effector mechanisms, 241, 245, 246
hematopoiesis, 282
reproduction, 272
surface phenotype, 208, 211

D

Delayed-type hypersensitivity
  antigen-presenting cells and, 57, 104
  natural killer cells and, 226
  spontaneous autoimmune thyroiditis and, 450
Dendritic cells, antigen-presenting cells and, 45–47, 87, 104, 105
  antigen presentation, 71, 72, 74–76, 78–81
  antigen processing, 88–92
  APC-T cell binding, 95–97, 99
  cell surface, 57–64
  immunogeneity, 101–104
  interaction with T cells, 93, 94
  T cell-dependent antibody responses, 83, 84, 86
  T cell growth, 99–101
  tissue distribution, 47–57
Diabetes
  natural killer cells and, 301
  spontaneous autoimmune thyroiditis and, 448, 468, 492
Differentiation
  antigen-presenting cells and, 48, 83, 84
  CD5 B cell and, 117, 118, 123, 125
    physiology, 139, 141, 142
  HIV infection and, 379, 393
  immunoglobulin E biosynthesis and
    antibody response, 8, 9, 11
    binding factors, 12, 13, 21, 23
  natural killer cells and, 188, 198
    adaptive immunity, 291, 292, 294
    congenital defects, 225
    effector mechanisms, 235, 239
    hematopoiesis, 272, 276
    morphology, 216
    surface phenotype, 201, 205, 208
    in vitro, 232–234
    in vivo, 229–232
  spontaneous autoimmune thyroiditis and, 447
Dinitrophenyl, immunoglobulin E biosynthesis and, 28

Dinitrophenyl-Asc, immunoglobulin E biosynthesis and, 3–5
Dinitrophenyl-KLH, immunoglobulin E biosynthesis and
  antibody response, 5, 6
  antibody response suppression, 29, 31, 33, 34, 37
Dinitrophenyl-OVA, immunoglobulin E biosynthesis and
  antibody response, 5
  antibody response suppression, 28–30, 32–34, 37
  binding factors, 12, 14
Dinitrophenyl-Rag, immunoglobulin E biosynthesis and, 4
Direct cellular cytotoxicity, spontaneous autoimmune thyroiditis and, 451, 452, 469
DNA
  antigen-presenting cells and, 75
  antigen processing, 92
  APC-T cell binding, 95–97
  T cell growth, 99–101
  CD5 B cell and, 161
    Ig gene expression, 152, 154–156
    marker for activation, 127
    physiology, 131, 133, 134, 136, 137
  HIV infection and
    etiological agent, 380, 382
    immunopathogenic mechanism, 387, 401, 402
    neuropsychiatric manifestations, 403
  immunoglobulin E biosynthesis and, 17
  natural killer cells and, 209, 235, 253, 254
  spontaneous autoimmune thyroiditis and, 435, 493
    altered thyroid function, 458, 464
    disturbed immunoregulation, 470
    genetics, 483, 484

E

Effector cells, natural killer cells and, 196, 302
  antimicrobial activity, 286, 287
  hematopoiesis, 273, 274, 277, 280
Effector mechanisms
  natural killer cells and, 234, 235
    cytotoxicity, 248–254
    lymphokines, 262–266

receptors, 242–248
regulation, 254–262
target cells, 235–242
spontaneous autoimmune thyroiditis and, 446, 449, 465–469
Electron microscopy
 antigen-presenting cells and
  antigen processing, 91
  interaction with T cells, 94
  tissue distribution, 51, 52, 57
 natural killer cells and, 218
 spontaneous autoimmune thyroiditis and, 440, 462
Endocytosis
 antigen-presenting cells and
  antigen presentation, 64, 67, 68, 71, 81
  antigen processing, 87–91
  immunogeneity, 102
  tissue distribution, 51
 HIV infection and, 379
Epithelium, antigen-presenting cells and, 54
Epitopes
 antigen-presenting cells and, 60, 62, 63
 CD5 B cell and, 155
 HIV infection and, 384, 386
  immune response, 407, 410, 411
 natural killer cells and, 221, 245, 247
 spontaneous autoimmune thyroiditis and, 462
Epstein-Barr virus
 antigen-presenting cells and, 63, 99
 CD5 B cell and, 136
 HIV infection and, 397, 400
 natural killer cells and, 224, 227, 267, 283, 292
Erythrocytes, immunoglobulin E biosynthesis and, 8, 12, 19
Experimental autoimmune encephalomyelitis, 433, 449
Experimental autoimmune thyroiditis, 433, 440, 442, 447

F

Fatty acids, natural killer cells and, 249
FcεR, immunoglobulin E biosynthesis and
 antibody response, 8, 9
 binding factors, 12, 15, 17, 19–23
Feedback, spontaneous autoimmune thyroiditis and, 476, 478
Fibronectin, antigen-presenting cells and, 61
Fluorescence
 antigen-presenting cells and, 86, 94
 CD5 B cell and, 118, 127
 natural killer cells and, 198, 213, 219
 spontaneous autoimmune thyroiditis and, 454
Fluorescence microscopy, CD5 B cell and, 149

G

G reactive protein, natural killer cells and, 246, 247
Genetics, spontaneous autoimmune thyroiditis and, 481–491
Glucagon, spontaneous autoimmune thyroiditis and, 440
Glucocorticoid-inducing factors, spontaneous autoimmune thyroiditis and, 477–479, 488
Glucocorticoids
 CD5 B cell and, 145
 immunoglobulin E biosynthesis and, 24
 spontaneous autoimmune thyroiditis and, 493, 494
  disturbed immunoregulation, 476, 477, 479, 480
  genetics, 488, 489
Glycoprotein
 antigen-presenting cells and, 92
 CD5 B cell and, 118, 146
 HIV infection and, 378, 395
  immune response, 405, 407–409
 natural killer cells and, 298
  antimicrobial activity, 286, 287
  effector mechanisms, 237, 248
  morphology, 218
  surface phenotype, 207
Glycosylation, immunoglobulin E biosynthesis and, 16, 17, 20, 23, 25, 26
Glycosylation-enhancing factor, immunoglobulin E biosynthesis and, 32, 36, 38
 binding factors, 23, 25, 26, 27
Glycosylation-inhibiting factor, immunoglobulin E biosynthesis and, 32–39
 binding factors, 23–27
Golgi apparatus, natural killer cells and, 214, 216, 303
Graft-versus-host disease
 CD5 B cell and, 129, 130

natural killer cells and, 231, 280–282
spontaneous autoimmune thyroiditis and, 455, 474, 482, 483

H

Hay fever, immunoglobulin E biosynthesis and, 1, 28
Hemagglutinin, spontaneous autoimmune thyroiditis and, 435, 445, 488, 489
Hematopoietic cells
  HIV infection and, 395
  natural killer cells and, 187, 198, 303
    differentiation, 233
    effector mechanisms, 235
    malignant expansion, 228
    surface phenotype, 201, 212
HNK-1, natural killer cells and, 291, 292
  CNS, 266
  differentiation, 234
  effector mechanisms, 257
  genetic control, 222
  hematopoiesis, 275
  malignant expansion, 226
  morphology, 218
  surface phenotype, 206, 207
  tissue distribution, 221
Homologous restriction factor, natural killer cells and, 252, 254
Hormones
  natural killer cells and, 299
    reproduction, 269, 270
  spontaneous autoimmune thyroiditis and, 491, 493
    altered thyroid function, 456, 461
    cellular immune reactions, 450
    clinical symptoms, 439
    disturbed immunoregulation, 476, 480, 481
    potential effector mechanisms, 465
Human immunodeficiency virus, 377, 378, 411–414
  etiological agent, 378
    genome, 380–384
    HIV-2, 384, 385
    life cycle, 379, 380
  immune response, 405
    cellular response, 409–411
    humoral response, 405–409
  immunoglobulin E biosynthesis and, 22

  immunopathogenic mechanism, 397
    activation, 398–403
    CD4 cell depletion, 386–389
    CD4-HIV interaction, 385, 386
    macrophages, 392–395
    monocytes, 392–395
    precursor cells, 395–397
    T4 cells, 389–392
  natural killer cells and, 302, 303
  neuropsychiatric manifestations
    brain, 403, 404
    mechanisms, 404, 405
Human leukocyte antigen, natural killer cells and, 198, 223
Human T cell leukemia lymphoma virus (HTLV), HIV infection and
  etiological agent, 378
  immunopathogenic mechanism, 388, 391, 393, 400, 402
Human T lymphotropic virus (HTLV)
  immunoglobulin E biosynthesis and, 21
  natural killer cells and, 229
Humoral immune reactions, spontaneous autoimmune thyroiditis and, 444–449, 491
Humoral mechanisms, spontaneous autoimmune thyroiditis and, 465–470
Humoral response, HIV infection and, 405–410
Hybridization
  antigen-presenting cells and, 65–67, 70, 71, 87
  CD5 B cell and, 134
  immunoglobulin E biosynthesis and, 17
  natural killer cells and
    genetic control, 223
    hematopoiesis, 273, 274, 280
    surface phenotype, 204, 209
  spontaneous autoimmune thyroiditis and
    altered thyroid function, 462
    genetics, 483, 484, 486–491
Hybridomas
  antigen-presenting cells and, 65, 68–70, 77
    antigen processing, 87
    T cells, 86, 93
  CD5 B cell and, 159
    Ig gene expression, 151, 152, 156
    physiology, 133–135, 138
  HIV infection and, 391
  immunoglobulin E biosynthesis and
    antibody response, 8, 32, 33, 35–39
    binding factors, 13, 15, 17, 18, 21, 25–27

Hydroxyurea, natural killer cells and, 230, 231, 283
Hyperlipidemia, spontaneous autoimmune thyroiditis and, 440
Hypersensitivity, antigen-presenting cells and, 104, 105
Hypothalamus, natural killer cells and, 266
Hypothyroidism, spontaneous autoimmune thyroiditis and
  altered thyroid function, 456
  breeding, 435–437
  clinical symptoms, 438
  disturbed immunoregulation, 470
  histopathology, 442, 444

I

Ia molecules, immunoglobulin E biosynthesis and, 9, 23, 27
Immunization
  antigen-presenting cells and, 67, 72, 86, 94
  HIV infection and, 407–410
  immunoglobulin E biosynthesis and
    antibody response, 2–6, 8, 9
    antibody response suppression, 30–32, 36
    binding factors, 14, 15, 23
  natural killer cells and, 282, 292, 293
  spontaneous autoimmune thyroiditis and, 433
Immunofluorescence
  CD5 B cell and, 118
    Ig gene expression, 153, 157
    lineage, 129
    marker for activation, 127
  immunoglobulin E biosynthesis and, 4, 8, 19, 21
  natural killer cells and, 211
  spontaneous autoimmune thyroiditis and, 445, 446, 462
Immunogeneity, antigen-presenting cells and, 101–105
Immunoglobulin, *see also* specific immunoglobulin
  antigen-presenting cells and
    antigen presentation, 66–70
    antigen processing, 89, 90
    cell surface, 62–64
    immunogeneity, 103

  interaction with T cells, 93
  tissue distribution, 47
  CD5 B cell and, 161, 162
    gene expression, 150–159
    genetic influence, 148
    lineage, 128
    malignancies, 123
    physiology, 137, 138, 140–142
    surface antigen, 143, 146
  HIV infection and, 390, 406, 408
  natural killer cells and, 203, 292–294
  spontaneous autoimmune thyroiditis and
    altered thyroid function, 458
    cellular immune reactions, 452
    histopathology, 440
    humoral immune reactions, 445, 446, 448
    potential effector mechanisms, 469
Immunoglobulin A
  antigen-presenting cells and, 52, 53
  biosynthesis and, 7, 19
  CD5 B cell and, 138
Immunoglobulin D
  antigen-presenting cells and, 48
  biosynthesis and, 7, 19
  CD5 B cell and, 121, 122
Immunoglobulin E, antigen-presenting cells and, 63
Immunoglobulin E biosynthesis, 1
  antibody response, 1–3
    B cells, 7–12
    T cells, 8, 10–12
    in vitro, 3–7
  antibody response suppression, 28
    anti-IL-4, 31
    antigens, 28–30
    GIF, 32–35
    interferon-γ, 31, 32
    T cell hybridomas, 36–39
  binding factors
    biological activities, 12–15
    FcϵRII structure, 19–22
    formation, 22–28
    physicochemical properties, 15–19
Immunoglobulin E-potentiating factor, 5
Immunoglobulin G
  antigen-presenting cells and, 62, 67, 85
  biosynthesis and
    antibody response, 2–11, 31, 32
    binding factors, 12, 19, 27
  CD5 B cell and, 132, 134, 136, 144

natural killer cells and, 189, 293
    cell-mediated cytotoxicity, 190, 196
    cytotoxicity, 249, 256
    effector mechanisms, 237, 243–245, 247, 248
    malignant expansion, 227
    surface phenotype, 201, 202, 212
Immunoglobulin H, CD5 B cell and, 129, 161
Immunoglobulin M
    antigen-presenting cells and, 48, 85
    biosynthesis and, 4, 6, 7, 9–11
    CD5 B cell and, 129
        physiology, 130–133, 135, 136
    natural killer cells and, 207, 292, 293
Infectious mononucleosis, natural killer cells and, 224
Inhibition
    antigen-presenting cells and, 69, 77
    CD5 B cell and, 161
    HIV infection and
        etiological agent, 379
        immune response, 406, 408
        immunopathogenic mechanism, 386, 390–392, 394, 395
    immunoglobulin E biosynthesis and
        antibody response, 7, 9, 33, 39
        binding factors, 12, 19, 23–25
    natural killer cells and, 298
        adaptive immunity, 291–294
        antimicrobial activity, 284, 287–290
        CNS, 268, 269
        cytotoxicity, 249, 253, 254, 257, 259
        effector mechanisms, 237, 238, 240, 242, 243, 245–247
        hematopoiesis, 273, 274, 276–280
        morphology, 218
    spontaneous autoimmune thyroiditis and, 477
Insulin, spontaneous autoimmune thyroiditis and, 440
Integrins, antigen-presenting cells and, 61, 97
Interdigitating cell, antigen-presenting cells and, 50–52
Interferon, see also specific interferon
    HIV infection and, 394, 402
    natural killer cells and
        adaptive immunity, 291, 293–295
        alterations, 300, 301, 303
        antimicrobial activity, 283–290
        antitumor activity, 295, 298
        cell-mediated cytotoxicity, 195, 196
        CNS, 269
        congenital defects, 225, 226
        cytotoxicity, 250, 251, 254–260, 262
        differentiation, 229, 233, 234
        effector mechanisms, 235, 237, 238, 241–244
        genetic control, 222–224
        hematopoiesis, 274, 277–280, 283
        identification, 198
        lymphokines, 264–266
        reproduction, 271
        surface phenotype, 201
        tissue distribution, 219
    spontaneous autoimmune thyroiditis and, 493
        altered thyroid function, 461–463
        disturbed immunoregulation, 472, 477
Interferonα, immunoglobulin E biosynthesis and, 9
Interferonγ
    antigen-presenting cells and, 59, 83, 97
    immunoglobulin E biosynthesis and
        antibody response, 9, 10, 12, 31, 32
        binding factors, 22–24
Interleukin-1
    antigen-presenting cells and, 64, 99–101, 103
    CD5 B cell and, 142, 143, 145, 146
    HIV infection and, 394, 404
    immunoglobulin E biosynthesis and, 22
    natural killer cells and, 233, 262, 266
    spontaneous autoimmune thyroiditis and, 477, 478, 493
Interleukin-2
    antigen-presenting cells and, 75
        cell surface, 63–65
        T cells, 84, 86, 100
        tissue distribution, 53, 55
    CD5 B cell and, 144, 145, 161
    HIV infection and, 390, 392, 398, 399, 411
    immunoglobulin E biosynthesis and
        antibody response, 10, 11, 36, 37
        binding factors, 22
    natural killer cells and, 189, 292
        adaptive immunity, 294, 295
        antitumor activity, 295, 296, 298
        cell-mediated cytotoxicity, 196
        congenital defects, 226
        cytotoxicity, 250, 252, 253, 257–262
        differentiation, 231–234
        effector mechanisms, 235, 237, 238, 242–244, 247

genetic control, 222, 223
hematopoiesis, 280
identification, 199
lymphokines, 264, 265
malignant expansion, 228
surface phenotype, 206, 207, 209
tissue distribution, 221
spontaneous autoimmune thyroiditis
 and, 492
 altered thyroid function, 461
 cellular immune reactions, 454–456
 disturbed immunoregulation, 471–474, 479
 genetics, 488
 histopathology, 442
 humoral immune reactions, 446
Interleukin-3
 immunoglobulin E biosynthesis and, 10, 22
 natural killer cells and, 232, 233, 266, 277, 278
Interleukin-4
 antigen-presenting cells and, 75, 84, 100
 cell surface, 59, 63, 64
 immunogeneity, 103
 CD5 B cell and, 120
 immunoglobulin E biosynthesis and
  antibody response, 6–12, 31
  binding factors, 13, 21–23
 natural killer cells and, 233, 262
Interleukin-5
 antigen-presenting cells and, 63, 64, 103
 immunoglobulin E biosynthesis and, 9, 10
Interleukin-6
 antigen-presenting cells and, 64, 100, 103
 HIV infection and, 403, 404
Iodine, spontaneous autoimmune thyroiditis and
 altered thyroid function, 456, 459, 460
 genetics, 487–490
Irradiation, natural killer cells and, 291, 295
 differentiation, 229–232
 effector mechanisms, 260, 261
 hematopoiesis, 273, 274, 276

K

Kallikrein, immunoglobulin E biosynthesis and, 25
Keyhole limpet hemocyanin
 antigen-presenting cells and, 66, 69, 70
 T cells, 86, 97, 99
 HIV infection and, 400
 immunoglobulin E biosynthesis and, 6, 14, 34, 35
Kidney
 antigen-presenting cells and, 76
 CD5 B cell and, 134
 immunoglobulin E biosynthesis and, 16
 natural killer cells and, 187, 282
 spontaneous autoimmune thyroiditis and, 462, 493

L

Laminin, natural killer cells and, 246
Langerhans cells, antigen-presenting cells and, 71–73, 75
 antigen processing, 90–92
 APC-T cell binding, 96, 97
 cell surface, 57, 59, 62, 63
 immunogeneity, 102
 interaction with T cells, 94
 T cell growth, 100
 tissue distribution, 50, 51, 53–57
Large granular lymphocyte, 188, 222, 283, 295
 congenital defects, 226
 cytotoxicity, 250, 253, 257
 differentiation, 231, 234
 effector mechanisms, 248
 hematopoiesis, 275, 276, 278
 identification, 197–199
 lymphokines, 262, 263
 malignant expansion, 226–228
 morphology, 214, 216–218
 reproduction, 271
 surface phenotype, 204, 205, 208, 211, 213
 tissue distribution, 219–221
Large granular lymphocyte lymphocytosis, 227–229, 275, 276, 279
Lectin
 antigen-presenting cells and, 99, 100
 immunoglobulin E biosynthesis and, 15–20
 natural killer cells and, 241, 250, 261, 286
 spontaneous autoimmune thyroiditis and, 470, 471
Lentivirus, HIV infection and, 395, 411
 etiological agent, 378, 384, 385
Leu-7 antigen, natural killer cells and, 275, 291, 292
 CNS, 266

congenital defects, 225
differentiation, 234
genetic control, 222
malignant expansion, 226
morphology, 218
surface phenotype, 206, 207
tissue distribution, 220, 221
Leu-19 antigen, natural killer cells and, 289, 293, 294, 302
CNS, 266, 267
differentiation, 233, 234
reproduction, 271
surface phenotype, 205, 206
Leukemia
CD5 B cell and, 123, 124
bone marrow transplantation, 129, 130
Ig gene expression, 153, 154, 156, 157
physiology, 136, 140, 141, 143
surface antigen, 147
immunoglobulin E biosynthesis and, 20
natural killer cells and, 190, 199, 298
congenital defects, 227
differentiation, 231
effector mechanisms, 238, 262
hematopoiesis, 276, 277
malignant expansion, 226
surface phenotype, 205
Leukocyte common antigen, antigen-presenting cells and, 60, 61
Leukocytes
antigen-presenting cells and, 76
APC-T cell binding, 97
cell surface, 61, 63
tissue distribution, 48, 51, 53
CD5 B cell and, 145
HIV infection and, 400
natural killer cells and, 188, 189, 295
effector mechanisms, 243, 263
genetic control, 222
surface phenotype, 201, 208
spontaneous autoimmune thyroiditis and, 492
Ligands
antigen-presenting cells and, 64, 65, 68, 69, 87
antigen processing, 88, 89, 92
cell surface, 61
T cells, 94-96, 101
CD5 B cell and, 146
HIV infection and, 391
natural killer cells and, 221, 247, 265

Light microscopy, antigen-presenting cells and, 51, 52
Lipid
antigen-presenting cells and, 65
HIV infection and, 387
natural killer cells and, 217
spontaneous autoimmune thyroiditis and, 439, 491
Lipocortin, immunoglobulin E biosynthesis and, 24, 25, 38
Lipopolysaccharide
antigen-presenting cells and, 68, 70, 76, 80
antigen processing, 89, 90, 92
cell surface, 57, 59, 61-63
immunogeneity, 104
tissue distribution, 49
CD5 B cell and, 159
anatomic localization, 121
marker for activation, 126
physiology, 133-135, 142, 143
HIV infection and, 402
immunoglobulin E biosynthesis and, 6, 8, 9, 11
natural killer cells and, 289
spontaneous autoimmune thyroiditis and, 474
Liver
CD5 B cell and, 141, 158
natural killer cells and, 283, 296, 297
genetic control, 222
hematopoiesis, 276
tissue distribution, 220, 221
Long terminal repeats
HIV infection and
etiological agent, 380, 382, 385
immunopathogenic mechanism, 399-402
spontaneous autoimmune thyroiditis and, 464
Low-density lipoprotein, antigen-presenting cells and, 89
Lymph node cells, immunoglobulin E biosynthesis and
antibody response, 3-5
binding factors, 12, 14, 16, 17
Lymph nodes
antigen-presenting cells and, 65, 71-73, 76
immunogeneity, 102
T cells, 85, 94
tissue distribution, 50-52, 54, 55
HIV infection and, 410

natural killer cells and, 211, 219, 220, 228, 298
Lymphoblasts, *see also* B lymphoblasts; T lymphoblasts
  antigen-presenting cells and, 94, 96, 103
  natural killer cells and, 231
  spontaneous autoimmune thyroiditis and, 469
Lymphocyte choriomeningitis virus, natural killer cells and, 244, 245, 283, 284
Lymphocytes, *see also* specific lymphocyte
  antigen-presenting cells and, 65, 91, 95, 105
  CD5 B cell and, 117, 118, 149, 150, 153, 157, 161
    bone marrow transplantation, 130
    lineage, 128, 129
    malignancies, 123
    marker for activation, 125, 126
    ontogeny, 121, 122
    physiology, 135, 137-139
    surface antigen, 143-145
  HIV infection and
    immune response, 410, 411
    immunopathogenic mechanism, 390, 392, 393, 397, 398, 400
  immunoglobulin E biosynthesis and
    antibody response, 3-8, 11
    antibody response suppression, 33, 38
    binding factors, 13, 14, 19-22, 24, 25
  natural killer cells and, 187-189
    adaptive immunity, 291
    alterations, 302
    antimicrobial activity, 289
    antitumor activity, 297, 299
    cell-mediated cytotoxicity, 190, 194-196
    congenital defects, 224-226
    cytotoxicity, 252-255, 257, 258, 260, 261
    differentiation, 230, 231, 234
    effector mechanisms, 243, 246
    genetic control, 222, 223
    hematopoiesis, 272-274, 276, 280, 282
    identification, 197, 199
    malignant expansion, 226
    morphology, 214, 216
    reproduction, 270
    surface phenotype, 201, 205-207, 209-213
    tissue distribution, 219, 220
  spontaneous autoimmune thyroiditis and
    altered thyroid function, 456, 462

    cellular immune reactions, 451, 453, 455
    disturbed immunoregulation, 470-472, 474, 477, 481
    genetics, 487
    potential effector mechanisms, 466, 467, 469
Lymphoid cells
  CD5 B cell and, 125
  HIV infection and, 382, 388
  immunoglobulin E biosynthesis and, 11
  natural killer cells and, 188, 221
  spontaneous autoimmune thyroiditis and, 435, 491
    cellular immune reactions, 454
    disturbed immunoregulation, 475, 476, 481
    histopathology, 440, 442, 443
Lymphoid organs
  antigen-presenting cells and, 104
    APC-T cell binding, 95
    immunogeneity, 102, 103
    interaction with T cells, 82-84
    tissue distribution, 50-52
  CD5 B cell and, 122
  natural killer cells and, 211, 266
  spontaneous autoimmune thyroiditis and
    cellular immune reactions, 449, 450
    disturbed immunoregulation, 477
    histopathology, 444
    humoral immune reactions, 446, 447
    potential effector mechanisms, 469
Lymphokine-activated killer cells, 188, 259, 260, 296
Lymphokines
  antigen-presenting cells and, 75, 80, 87
    cell surface, 63
    immunogeneity, 103, 104
    T cells, 83, 84, 99-101
  immunoglobulin E biosynthesis and
    antibody response, 7-11
    antibody response suppression, 32, 33, 39
    binding factors, 12, 22-28
  natural killer cells and, 189, 289, 290, 293
    differentiation, 233
    effector mechanisms, 235, 262-266
    morphology, 216
    reproduction, 271
    tissue distribution, 220
  spontaneous autoimmune thyroiditis and, 472, 473, 477

Lymphoma
  CD5 B cell and, 123–125
    Ig gene expression, 150–152, 155, 156
    natural killer cells and, 190, 228
Lymphotoxin
  immunoglobulin E biosynthesis and, 10
  natural killer cells and, 278, 279
Lysosomes
  antigen-presenting cells and, 52
  natural killer cells and, 214, 218, 225, 238

M

Macrophages
  antigen-presenting cells and, 68, 80, 104
    antigen processing, 89, 90
    cell surface, 61, 62
    immunogeneity, 103, 104
    interaction with T cells, 93, 94
    T cell, 86, 95, 97, 99
    tissue distribution, 48, 51, 54, 55
  CD5 B cell and, 120–122, 132
  HIV infection and, 413
    activation, 400, 402
    immunopathogenic mechanism, 392–397
    neuropsychiatric manifestations, 404
  immunoglobulin E biosynthesis and
    antibody response suppression, 30, 33, 36, 37
    binding factors, 20, 21, 27
  natural killer cells and, 189, 288–290
    congenital defects, 224
    differentiation, 229
    effector mechanisms, 235, 237, 262, 263, 265, 266
    hematopoiesis, 274, 278
    identification, 296
    malignant expansion, 228
    reproduction, 270
    surface phenotype, 201, 202, 211–213
    tissue distribution, 220
  spontaneous autoimmune thyroiditis and, 492, 494
    disturbed immunoregulation, 475, 476
    genetics, 488
    histopathology, 440, 442
    potential effector mechanisms, 467, 468
Magnesium, natural killer cells and, 249, 250

Major histocompatibility complex
  antigen-presenting cells and, 45, 47, 87, 104, 105
    antigen presentation, 64, 66–69, 71–73, 75–80
    antigen processing, 87–89, 91, 92
    APC-T cell binding, 95–97, 99
    cell surface, 57–60
    immunogeneity, 103
    T cells, 82, 83, 85, 101
    tissue distribution, 51–54
  CD5 B cell and, 137, 142, 160
  HIV infection and, 380, 411
    immunopathogenic mechanism, 386, 389, 391, 392
  immunoglobulin E biosynthesis and
    antibody response, 2, 29, 33
    binding factors, 25, 27
  natural killer cells and, 187, 188, 292
    cytotoxicity, 190
    effector mechanisms, 239, 240, 242, 257, 259, 261
    surface phenotype, 201, 211
  spontaneous autoimmune thyroiditis and, 435, 491, 493, 494
    breeding, 436–438
    effector mechanisms, 467, 469
    function, 459, 461, 462, 464
    genetics, 481–491
    immune reactions, 450, 455
    immunoregulation, 470–472, 476, 477
Mesenteric lymph node cells, immunoglobulin E biosynthesis and
  antibody response, 3–5
  binding factors, 12, 14, 16, 17
Mitochondria
  natural killer cells and, 214
  spontaneous autoimmune thyroiditis and, 442, 448
Mitogens
  antigen-presenting cells and, 71, 73, 100
    tissue distribution, 54
  CD5 B cell and, 140, 142, 147
  HIV infection and, 390, 391, 398, 399
  natural killer cells and, 206, 261, 264
  spontaneous autoimmune thyroiditis and, 491, 493
    cellular immune reactions, 452, 456
    disturbed immunoregulation, 470–474, 476
    genetics, 488

potential effector mechanisms, 467
Mixed leukocyte cultures, natural killer cells and, 295
Mixed-leukocyte reaction, antigen-presenting cells and, 65, 71-73, 75, 76, 78-80
 APC-T cell binding, 95, 97, 99
 cell surface, 59, 61
 T cell, 83, 84, 99
 tissue distribution, 48, 49, 53, 54
Mls antigens, antigen-presenting cells and, 47
 antigen presentation, 64, 76-79
 APC-T cell binding, 95, 99
Monoclonal antibodies
 antigen-presenting cells and, 70, 76, 77, 96
  cell surface, 58, 60-62
  tissue distribution, 50, 51, 53
 CD5 B cell and, 117
  genetic influence, 143-147
  Ig gene expression, 153, 155
  physiology, 133, 134
  primordial immune network, 160
 HIV infection and, 386
 immunoglobulin E biosynthesis and
  antibody response, 8, 31, 33-35
  binding factors, 16, 18-22, 24, 27
 natural killer cells and, 198, 296
  congenital defects, 224, 225
  differentiation, 233
  effector mechanisms, 243, 258
  hematopoiesis, 278, 279
  surface phenotype, 200, 201, 205, 207, 208, 210, 211
  tissue distribution, 219, 220
 spontaneous autoimmune thyroiditis and, 435
  altered thyroid function, 460-462
  cellular immune reactions, 454, 455
  disturbed immunoregulation, 472, 479
  histopathology, 442
  potential effector mechanisms, 466
Monocytes
 CD5 B cell and, 142
 HIV infection and
  activation, 400, 402, 403
  immunopathogenic mechanism, 392-397
  neuropsychiatric manifestations, 404
 spontaneous autoimmune thyroiditis and, 475
Monocytoids, CD5 B cell and, 141-143

Morphine, natural killer cells and, 268
Morphology
 HIV infection and, 378
 natural killer cells and, 214-218, 292
  antimicrobial activity, 283, 290
  cytotoxicity, 249, 250, 253, 256, 258
  differentiation, 234
  hematopoiesis, 275, 281
  identification, 197, 198
  malignant expansion, 226, 227
  reproduction, 271
  surface phenotype, 210, 213
  tissue distribution, 219, 220
 spontaneous autoimmune thyroiditis and, 444, 467, 472
mRNA
 CD5 B cell and, 147
 HIV infection and, 380, 381, 392, 397
 immunoglobulin E biosynthesis and, 16
 natural killer cells and, 210, 246, 254, 263, 265, 266
Multiple sclerosis, natural killer cells and, 301, 302
Mutagenesis
 HIV infection and, 386
 spontaneous autoimmune thyroiditis and, 464
Mutation
 antigen-presenting cells and, 80, 103
 CD5 B cell and, 132, 146, 154, 155
 HIV infection and
  etiological agent, 381, 383
  immune response, 408
  immunopathogenic mechanism, 388, 400
 immunoglobulin E biosynthesis and, 16, 38
 natural killer cells and, 225

N

Natural cytotoxic cells, 213, 286
Natural killer cell cytotoxic factor, 241, 250, 251, 253, 262, 302
Natural killer cells, 187-189
 adaptive immunity
  B cell response, 291-294
  T cell response, 294, 295
 alterations, 300-303

antimicrobial activity
  antiviral activity, 282–288
  infection, 288–291
antitumor activity
  cancer patients, 297–300
  experimental animals, 295, 296
cell-mediated cytotoxicity, 189–196
CNS, 266–269
congenital defects, 224–226
differentiation, 229–234
effector mechanisms, 234, 235
  cytotoxicity, 248–254
  lymphocyte production, 262–266
  receptors, 242–248
  regulation, 254–262
  target cells, 235–242
genetic control, 222–224
hematopoiesis, 272, 273
  graft-versus-host reaction, 280–282
  inhibition, 276, 277
  regulation, 273–276
  soluble factors, 277–280
HIV infection and, 411
identification, 196–199
malignant expansion, 226–229
morphology, 214–218
reproduction, 269–272
surface phenotype, 199–201, 207, 208
  experimental animals, 210–214
  FcR antigen, 201–205
  HNK-1, 206, 207
  NKH-1 antigen, 205, 206
  T cell-associated antigens, 208–210
tissue distribution, 219–221
Negative regulatory element, HIV infection and, 381, 382
Neurological abnormalities, HIV infection and, 377, 413
Neuropsychiatric manifestations, HIV infection and, 395, 403–405
Neutralizing antibodies, HIV infection and, 407, 408, 410, 413
NKH-1, natural killer cells and, 188, 293, 294, 302
  CNS, 266, 267
  differentiation, 233, 234
  effector mechanisms, 261
  reproduction, 271
  surface phenotype, 205, 206
  tissue distribution, 219, 220
Nucleotides
  CD5 B cell and, 144
  HIV infection and, 383, 384
  immunoglobulin E biosynthesis and, 16, 20
  natural killer cells and, 202, 252

O

Obese strain chickens, spontaneous autoimmune thyroiditis in, see Spontaneous autoimmune thyroiditis
Oligosaccharides, immunoglobulin E biosynthesis and, 16, 18, 19, 23
Opiods, natural killer cells and, 268, 269
OVA, immunoglobulin E biosynthesis and
  antibody response, 8
  antibody response suppression, 29, 30, 32–37, 39
  binding factors, 27

P

Parallel tubular arrays, natural killer cells and, 216, 218, 256, 281
Peanut agglutinin
  antigen-presenting cells and, 86
  immunoglobulin E biosynthesis and, 15, 18
Peptides
  antigen-presenting cells and, 87, 104
  antigen presentation, 64, 66, 71, 74, 76, 77, 79, 81
  antigen processing, 87, 88, 90–92
  T cells, 82, 96, 97, 99, 101
HIV infection and
  immune response, 406, 410
  immunopathogenic mechanism, 389, 391, 392
  neuropsychiatric manifestations, 404
immunoglobulin E biosynthesis and
  antibody response, 39
  binding factors, 15–17, 20, 23, 25
natural killer cells and, 202, 204, 268, 303
Perforin, natural killer cells and, 251
Peripheral blood
  CD5 B cell and, 122, 131
  autoimmune diseases, 150
  marker for activation, 127
  surface antigen, 147

HIV infection and
  immune response, 411
  immunopathogenic mechanism, 394,
    397, 400, 402, 403
  natural killer cells and, 289, 293, 298,
    300, 303
    CNS, 266
    differentiation, 232-234
    effector mechanisms, 252, 254, 258, 264
    hematopoiesis, 275, 277, 279
    identification, 199
    malignant expansion, 226
    morphology, 216
    surface phenotype, 201, 205, 206
  spontaneous autoimmune thyroiditis
    and, 447
    cellular immune reactions, 449, 451
    disturbed immunoregulation, 471,
      473, 474
Peripheral blood lymphocytes
  CD5 B cell and, 144, 149
  HIV infection and, 388
  natural killer cells and, 187, 294, 297,
    301, 302
    antimicrobial activity, 286-289
    cell-mediated cytotoxicity, 195
    CNS, 267
    cytotoxicity, 254, 258-261
    differentiation, 234
    effector mechanisms, 234, 240, 243, 246
    genetic control, 222
    hematopoiesis, 275, 276
    lymphokines, 264, 265
    morphology, 214, 217, 218
    reproduction, 270
    surface phenotype, 205-209
    tissue distribution, 219
  spontaneous autoimmune thyroiditis
    and, 492
    cellular immune reactions, 452, 453, 456
    disturbed immunoregulation, 471, 472,
      475, 479
    effector mechanisms, 469
    genetics, 487, 488
    humoral immune reactions, 447, 449
Peripheral blood mononuclear cells
  HIV infection and
    activation, 398, 400, 403
    immune response, 411
    immunopathogenic mechanism,
      390-392

immunoglobulin E biosynthesis and
  antibody response, 6, 7, 9, 12, 38
  binding factors, 21, 22
Peripolesis, spontaneous autoimmune
  thyroiditis and, 442, 447, 469
pH
  antigen-presenting cells and, 88
  immunoglobulin E biosynthesis and
    antibody response, 8, 33, 34, 36
    binding factors, 12
  natural killer cells and, 263
  spontaneous autoimmune thyroiditis
    and, 446
Phenotype
  CD5 B cell and, 120, 122
    malignancies, 124
    physiology, 132, 135, 140, 142
  HIV infection and, 384
  immunoglobulin E biosynthesis and, 10, 12
  natural killer cells and, 292, 298, 302
    cell-mediated cytotoxicity, 195
    differentiation, 229, 231-233
    effector mechanisms, 246, 260, 264
    genetic control, 223
    hematopoiesis, 274-277
    identification, 197-199
    malignant expansion, 226-228
    reproduction, 271
    surface, 199-214
    tissue distribution, 220
  spontaneous autoimmune thyroiditis and,
    435-437
    disturbed immunoregulation, 470
    genetics, 484, 488
Phorbol myristic acetate, CD5 B cell and,
  125, 126, 141
Phospholipase
  immunoglobulin E biosynthesis and
    antibody response, 39
    binding factors, 18, 24-26, 28
  natural killer cells and, 249
Phospholipids, immunoglobulin E
  biosynthesis and, 26
Phosphorylation
  antigen-presenting cells and, 101
  immunoglobulin E biosynthesis and, 24
Phytohemagglutinin
  HIV infection and, 390, 398, 399, 401
  spontaneous autoimmune thyroiditis
    and, 492
    cellular immune reactions, 452, 455

disturbed immunoregulation, 470,
471, 473
genetics, 487
potential effector mechanisms, 467
Plaque-forming cells
CD5 B cell and
physiology, 130–132, 137, 139
surface antigen, 144
spontaneous autoimmune thyroiditis
and, 446
Plasma
antigen-presenting cells and, 45, 52, 53
CD5 B cell and, 132
HIV infection and, 408
immunoglobulin E biosynthesis and, 4–6,
9, 13
natural killer cells and, 267, 268
spontaneous autoimmune thyroiditis and
clinical symptoms, 440
disturbed immunoregulation, 476,
479–481
genetics, 488
humoral immune reactions, 446, 447
potential effector mechanisms, 467, 469
Plasma membrane
antigen-presenting cells and, 51, 68
HIV infection and, 393
natural killer cells and, 253
Plasminogen activator, natural killer cells
and, 254
Polymorphonucleated leukocytes, natural killer
cells and, 189, 190, 194, 201–204, 260
Polypeptides
antigen-presenting cells and, 82, 88
CD5 B cell and, 142
immunoglobulin E biosynthesis and,
17–19, 34
natural killer cells and, 202, 203, 208, 213
Pore-forming protein, natural killer cells
and, 251–254, 262, 291
Precursor cells, HIV infection and, 395–397
Priming
antigen-presenting cells and, 65, 68, 71–73,
75, 80
T cells, 82, 83, 85, 86, 94
tissue distribution, 56
CD5 B cell and, 137, 139
immunoglobulin E biosynthesis and
antibody response, 6, 29, 30, 32, 33,
36–39
binding factors, 14, 22–24, 26, 28

Prostaglandins, natural killer cells and,
250, 257
Protein
antigen-presenting cells and, 46, 64–73, 77
antigen processing, 87, 88, 90, 91
cell surface, 60
immunogeneity, 104
T cells, 86, 94, 99, 101
CD5 B cell and, 126
Ig gene expression, 150, 153, 154, 157
physiology, 131, 134
primordial immune network, 160
surface antigen, 146
HIV infection and
activation, 398–402
etiological agent, 378–382, 384, 385
immune response, 405–407, 409, 411
immunopathogenic mechanism, 387,
392, 395
immunoglobulin E biosynthesis and, 1
antibody response, 2, 3, 11
antibody response suppression, 31, 32,
34, 39
binding factors, 16–18, 20, 22, 24–27
natural killer cells and, 284, 287, 291
cytotoxicity, 252, 255
effector mechanisms, 241, 242, 244–246
lymphokines, 263, 265
surface phenotype, 203, 205
spontaneous autoimmune thyroiditis and,
462, 476, 479
Protein kinase
antigen-presenting cells and, 101
CD5 B cell and, 125
HIV infection and, 382
immunoglobulin E biosynthesis and, 26
natural killer cells and, 249, 271
Proteolysis
antigen-presenting cells and, 66, 87, 88
CD5 B cell and, 130, 161
immunoglobulin E biosynthesis and, 16,
17, 20
natural killer cells and, 203, 250, 254
spontaneous autoimmune thyroiditis
and, 461

R

Radioimmunoassay, immunoglobulin E
biosynthesis and, 1, 20

Reproduction, natural killer cells and, 269-272
Retrovirus
 HIV infection and, 377
  etiological agent, 378, 380, 383, 384
  immune response, 406, 407, 409
  immunopathogenic mechanism, 391
 immunoglobulin E biosynthesis and, 17
 natural killer cells and, 303
Rheumatoid arthritis
 CD5 B cell and, 136, 147, 148-150
 natural killer cells and, 300
RNA
 HIV infection and, 403
  etiological agent, 378, 380
  immunopathogenic mechanism, 387, 395
 immunoglobulin E biosynthesis and, 21
 natural killer cells and, 203, 241, 242, 284

S

Sex steroids, spontaneous autoimmune thyroiditis and, 480, 481
Simian immunodeficiency virus, HIV infection and, 378, 385, 404
Spleen
 antigen-presenting cells and, 69-72, 74-76, 78-81
  antigen processing, 92
  immunogeneity, 102
  T cells, 83, 85
  tissue distribution, 47, 50-52, 56
 CD5 B cell and, 120-123
  genetic influence, 147
  Ig gene expression, 152, 157
  lineage, 128
  physiology, 130, 132, 133
  primordial immune network, 159
 immunoglobulin E biosynthesis and
  antibody response, 5, 8, 11
  antibody response suppression, 29, 32-34, 36, 37
  binding factors, 13-15, 22-26, 28
 natural killer cells and, 187, 283, 289, 290, 292, 300
  CNS, 268
  congenital defects, 226
  differentiation, 229, 230
  effector mechanisms, 234, 260, 262
  genetic control, 223

hematopoiesis, 274, 276
identification, 199
malignant expansion, 228
surface phenotype, 210, 211, 213
tissue distribution, 220, 221
spontaneous autoimmune thyroiditis and
 cellular immune reactions, 450, 452, 454, 456
 disturbed immunoregulation, 471, 473-476, 481
 humoral immune reactions, 446, 447
Spontaneous autoimmune thyroiditis in obese strain chickens, 433-435, 491-494
 altered thyroid function, 456-465
 breeding, 435-438
 cellular immune reactions, 449-456
 clinical symptoms, 438-440
 genetics
  dysfunctions, 487-491
  MHC, 481-486
  target organ, 485, 487
 histopathology, 440-444
 humoral immune reactions, 444-449
 immunoregulation, 469
  extrinsic, 476-481
  intrinsic, 470-476
 potential effector mechanisms, 465-469
Spontaneous cellular cytotoxicty, 451, 452
Steroids, spontaneous autoimmune thyroiditis and, 480, 481
Systemic lupus erythematosus, natural killer cells and, 300, 301

T

T cells
 antigen-presenting cells and, 47, 64-74, 76, 77
  antibody responses, 81-86
  antigen presentation, 78-81
  antigen processing, 87, 90-92
  APC-T cell binding, 95-99
  cell surface, 57, 59, 61-63
  immunogeneity, 102-104
  T cell growth, 99-101
  tissue distribution, 49, 50, 52-57
 CD5 B cell and, 118, 162
  bone marrow transplantation, 130
  lineage, 129
  marker for activation, 125, 126

physiology, 137, 140-142
primordial immune network, 160, 161
surface antigen, 143-147
HIV infection and
  activation, 398-400, 402
  etiological agent, 378, 379, 382
  immune response, 405, 409, 410
  immunopathogenic mechanism, 385, 387-392, 394
  neuropsychiatric manifestations, 405
immunoglobulin E biosynthesis and, 1, 28-30, 32-39
  antibody response, 4-12
  binding factors, 12, 13, 15-24, 26-28
natural killer cells and, 188, 190
  adaptive immunity, 291-296
  antimicrobial activity, 289
  CNS, 266
  congenital defects, 225, 226
  cytotoxicity, 248, 255, 257-262
  effector mechanisms, 240, 244, 245, 247, 248
  genetic control, 222
  hematopoiesis, 272-275, 277-281
  identification, 196, 198, 199
  lymphokines, 264, 265
  malignant expansion, 227, 228
  morphology, 218
  reproduction, 271
  surface phenotype, 200, 204-213
  tissue distribution, 219-221
spontaneous autoimmune thyroiditis and, 434, 491, 492, 494
  altered thyroid function, 461, 462
  cellular immune reactions, 449-452, 454-456
  disturbed immunoregulation, 470-472, 475, 481
  genetics, 488-490
  histopathology, 442, 444
  humoral immune reactions, 445, 446
  potential effector mechanisms, 465-469
T lymphoblasts
  antigen-presenting cells and, 76, 84, 102
  spontaneous autoimmune thyroiditis and, 467, 473
T lymphocytes
  antigen-presenting cells and
    immunogeneity, 103
    T cells, 86, 96, 99
    tissue distribution, 48, 54

CD5 B cell and, 118, 126
  physiology, 131
  surface antigen, 143, 144, 147
HIV infection and, 379
  immunopathogenic mechanism, 385, 386, 388, 390, 391, 397
natural killer cells and, 188, 197, 294
  congenital defects, 225
  differentiation, 232
  effector mechanisms, 257, 265
spontaneous autoimmune thyroiditis and
  cellular immune reactions, 454, 455
  disturbed immunoregulation, 472-474, 477
  potential effector mechanisms, 466-469
Target-binding cells, natural killer cells and, 230, 269
Target cells
  HIV infection and
    etiological agent, 378, 384
    immune response, 409, 411
    immunopathogenic mechanism, 400
  natural killer cells and, 292, 294
    antimicrobial activity, 285-288
    cytotoxicity, 249-256, 259
    effector mechanisms, 234-242
    hematopoiesis, 280
    lymphokines, 262-264
    receptors, 242-248
  spontaneous autoimmune thyroiditis and, 451
Target organ, spontaneous autoimmune thyroiditis and
  defect, 456-465
  genetics, 482, 485, 487
Testosterone, spontaneous autoimmune thyroiditis and, 480, 481
Thymic nurse cells, spontaneous autoimmune thyroiditis and, 455, 456, 475, 491
Thymus
  antigen-presenting cells and, 47, 48, 81
  CD5 B cell and, 120, 121, 129
  natural killer cells and, 187, 188, 273, 276
    effector mechanisms, 239
    genetic control, 222
    malignant expansion, 228
  spontaneous autoimmune thyroiditis and, 492
    cellular immune reactions, 449-451, 454
    disturbed immunoregulation, 474-476
    histopathology, 434, 444

humoral immune reactions, 445, 447
  potential effector mechanisms, 466, 468
Thyroglobulin, 491
  altered thyroid function, 456, 459-461
  cellular immune reactions, 450, 451
  genetics, 485
  humoral immune reactions, 446, 447
  potential effector mechanisms, 466, 469
Thyroglobulin autoantibodies, 491, 492
  altered thyroid function, 457, 459, 460, 462
  cellular immune reactions, 449, 451
  disturbed immunoregulation, 481
  effector mechanisms, 466-469
  genetics, 482, 484-487
  humoral immune reactions, 444-448
Thyroid
  antigen-presenting cells and, 76
  spontaneous autoimmune thyroiditis and, see Spontaneous autoimmune thyroiditis
Thyroid epithelial cells, spontaneous autoimmune thyroiditis and, 493
  altered thyroid function, 458, 459, 461-463
  clinical symptoms, 440
  disturbed immunoregulation, 472
  effector mechanisms, 469
  genetics, 497
  histopathology, 442
Thyroid-infiltrating lymphocytes, 492
  effector mechanisms, 466, 467, 469
  immunoregulation, 473, 475
Thyroid-stimulating hormone, 457, 458, 461
Thyroiditis, see Spontaneous autoimmune thyroiditis
Thyroxine, 437, 439, 457, 470
Transcription
  HIV infection and, 380-382, 399, 401
  immunoglobulin E biosynthesis and, 21
  natural killer cells and, 265
  spontaneous autoimmune thyroiditis and, 477
Transferrin
  antigen-presenting cells and, 89
  natural killer cells and, 209, 240
Transplantation
  antigen-presenting cells and, 75, 76, 80
  CD5 B cell and, 128-130
  natural killer cells and, 187, 293, 302
    differentiation, 231, 232
    hematopoiesis, 273, 280-282

spontaneous autoimmune thyroiditis and, 457, 458
Trinitrophenyl
  antigen-presenting cells and, 68, 69, 79, 80
  T cells, 86, 97
  tissue distribution, 49
  CD5 B cell and, 160, 161
Trypsin, immunoglobulin E biosynthesis and, 25
Tubulin, natural killer cells and, 302
Tumor
  antigen-presenting cells and, 66, 67, 100
  CD5 B cell and, 118, 125
    Ig gene expression, 150, 151, 156
    marker for activation, 126
  natural killer cells and, 187-189, 295-300
    CNS, 267
    differentiation, 231, 234
    effector mechanisms, 235, 238, 257, 259, 262
  spontaneous autoimmune thyroiditis and, 450
Tumor necrosis factor
  HIV infection and, 394, 402-404
  natural killer cells and, 286, 289, 290
    differentiation, 233
    effector mechanisms, 251, 262, 265, 266
    hematopoiesis, 278, 279, 281
    reproduction, 271
    surface phenotype, 213
Tunicamycin, immunoglobulin E biosynthesis and, 18, 19
Turnover, antigen-presenting cells and, 49, 50, 52

U

Urea-denatured OVA, immunoglobulin E biosynthesis and, 29, 30, 33

V

Vaccination, HIV infection and, 408, 411, 413
Vesicles
  antigen-presenting cells and, 68, 87, 89
  HIV infection and, 393, 396
  natural killer cells and, 214, 216, 217, 221
Vesicular stomatitis virus, natural killer cells and, 286, 287

Viral antigens, antigen-presenting cells and, 47, 80, 81
Virus-dependent cellular cytotoxicity, natural killer cells and, 286

X

X chromosome-linked lymphoproliferative disorder, natural killer cells and, 224, 283, 299

CONTENTS OF RECENT VOLUMES

Volume 37

Structure, Function, and Genetics of Human Class II Molecules
  ROBERT C. GILES AND J. DONALD CAPRA

The Complexity of Virus–Cell Interactions in Abelson Virus Infection of Lymphoid and Other Hematopoietic Cells
  CHERYL A. WHITLOCK AND OWEN N. WITTE

Epstein–Barr Virus Infection and Immunoregulation in Man
  GIOVANNA TOSATO AND R. MICHAEL BLAESE

The Classical Complement Pathway: Activation and Regulation of the First Complement Component
  NEIL R. COOPER

Membrane Complement Receptors Specific for Bound Fragments of C3
  GORDON D. ROSS AND M. EDWARD MEDOFF

Murine Models of Systemic Lupus Erythematosus
  ARGYRIOS N. THEOFILOPOULOS AND FRANK J. DIXON

Immune Response (Ir) Genes of the Murine Major Histocompatibility Complex
  RONALD H. SCHWARTZ

The Molecular Genetics of Components of Complement
  R. D. CAMPBELL, M. C. CARROLL, AND R. R. PORTER

Molecular Genetics of Human B Cell Neoplasia
  CARLO M. CROCE AND PETER C. NOWELL

Human Lymphocyte Hybridomas and Monoclonal Antibodies
  DENNIS A. CARSON AND BRUCE D. FREIMARK

Maternally Transmitted Antigen
  JOHN R. RODGERS, ROGER SMITH III, MARILYN M. HUSTON, AND ROBERT R. RICH

Phagocytosis of Particulate Activators of the Alternative Complement Pathway: Effects of Fibronectin
  JOYCE K. CZOP

INDEX

INDEX

Volume 38

The Antigen-Specific, Major Histocompatibility Complex-Restricted Receptor on T Cells
  PHILIPPA MARRACK AND JOHN KAPPLER

Volume 39

Immunological Regulation of Hematopoietic/Lymphoid Stem Cell Differentiation by Interleukin 3
  JAMES N. IHLE AND YACOB WEINSTEIN

Antigen Presentation by B Cells and Its Significance in T–B Interactions
ROBERT W. CHESNUT AND HOWARD M. GREY

Ligand–Receptor Dynamics and Signal Amplification in the Neutrophil
LARRY A. SKLAR

Arachidonic Acid Metabolism by the 5-Lipoxygenase Pathway, and the Effects of Alternative Dietary Fatty Acids
TAK H. LEE AND K. FRANK AUSTEN

The Eosinophilic Leukocyte: Structure and Function
GERALD J. GLEICH AND CHERYL R. ADOLPHSON

Idiotypic Interactions in the Treatment of Human Diseases
RAIF S. GEHA

Neuroimmunology
DONALD G. PAYAN, JOSEPH P. MCGILLIS, AND EDWARD J. GOETZL

INDEX

Volume 40

Regulation of Human B Lymphocyte Activation, Proliferation, and Differentiation
DIANE F. JELINEK AND PETER E. LIPSKY

Biological Activities Residing in the Fc Region of Immunoglobulin
EDWARD L. MORGAN AND WILLIAM O. WEIGLE

Immunoglobulin-Specific Suppressor T Cells
RICHARD G. LYNCH

Immunoglobulin A (IgA): Molecular and Cellular Interactions Involved in IgA Biosynthesis and Immune Response
JIRI MESTECKY AND JERRY R. MCGHEE

The Arrangement of Immunoglobulin and T Cell Receptor Genes in Human Lymphoproliferative Disorders
THOMAS A. WALDMANN

Human Tumors Antigens
RALPH A. REISFELD AND DAVID A. CHERESH

Human Marrow Transplantation: An Immunological Perspective
PAUL J. MARTIN, JOHN A. HANSEN, RAINER STORB, AND E. DONNALL THOMAS

INDEX

Volume 41

Cell Surface Molecules and Early Events Involved in Human T Lymphocyte Activation
ARTHUR WEISS AND JOHN B. IMBODEN

Function and Specificity of T Cell Subsets in the Mouse
JONATHAN SPRENT AND SUSAN R. WEBB

Determinants on Major Histocompatibility Complex Class I Molecules Recognized by Cytotoxic T Lymphocytes
JAMES FORMAN

Experimental Models for Understanding B Lymphocyte Formation
PAUL W. KINCADE

Cellular and Humoral Mechanisms of Cytotoxicity: Structural and Functional Analogies
JOHN DING-E YOUNG AND ZANVIL A. COHN

Biology and Genetics of Hybrid Resistance
MICHAEL BENNETT

INDEX

Volume 42

The Clonotype Repertoire of B Cell Subpopulations
NORMAN R. KLINMAN AND PHYLLIS-JEAN LINTON

The Molecular Genetics of the Arsonate Idiotypic System of A/J Mice
GARY RATHBUN, INAKI SANZ, KATHERYN MEEK, PHILIP TUCKER, AND J. DONALD CAPRA

The Interleukin 2 Receptor
KENDALL A. SMITH

Characterization of Functional Surface Structures on Human Natural Killer Cells
JEROME RITZ, REINHOLD E. SCHMIDT, JEAN MICHON, THIERRY HERCEND, AND STUART F. SCHLOSSMAN

The Common Mediator of Shock, Cachexia, and Tumor Necrosis
B. BEUTLER AND A. CERAMI

Myasthenia Gravis
JON LINDSTROM, DIANE SHELTON, AND YOSHITAKA FUJII

Alterations of the Immune System in Ulcerative Colitis and Crohn's Disease
RICHARD P. MACDERMOTT AND WILLIAM F. STENSON

INDEX

Volume 43

The Chemistry and Mechanism of Antibody Binding to Protein Antigens
ELIZABETH D. GETZOFF, JOHN A. TAINER, RICHARD A. LERNER, AND H. MARIO GEYSEN

Structure of Antibody–Antigen Complexes: Implications for Immune Recognition
P. M. COLMAN

The $\gamma\delta$ T Cell Receptor
MICHAEL B. BRENNER, JACK L. STROMINGER, AND MICHAEL S. KRANGEL

Specificity of the T Cell Receptor for Antigen
STEPHEN M. HEDRICK

Transcriptional Controlling Elements in the Immunoglobulin and T Cell Receptor Loci
KATHRYN CALAME AND SUZANNE EATON

Molecular Aspects of Receptors and Binding Factors for IgE
HENRY METZGER

INDEX

Volume 44

Diversity of the Immunoglobulin Gene Superfamily
TIM HUNKAPILLER AND LEROY HOOD

Genetically Engineered Antibody Molecules
SHERIE L. MORRISON AND VERNON T. OI

Antinuclear Antibodies: Diagnostic Markers for Autoimmune Diseases and Probes for Cell Biology
ENG M. TAN

Interleukin-1 and Its Biologically Related Cytokines
CHARLES A. DINARELLO

Molecular and Cellular Events of T Cell Development
B. J. FOWLKES AND DREW M. PARDOLL

Molecular Biology and Function of CD4 and CD8
JANE R. PARNES

Lymphocyte Homing
 TED A. YEDNOCK AND STEVEN D. ROSEN

INDEX

Volume 45

Cellular Interactions in the Humoral Immune Response
 ELLEN S. VITETTA, RAFAEL FERNANDEZ-BOTRAN, CHRISTOPHER D. MYERS, AND VIRGINIA M. SANDERS

MHC–Antigen Interactions: What Does the T Cell Receptor See?
 PHILIPPE KOURILSKY AND JEAN-MICHEL CLAVERIE

Synthetic T and B Cell Recognition Sites: Implications for Vaccine Development
 DAVID R. MILICH

Rationale for the Development of an Engineered Sporozoite Malaria Vaccine
 VICTOR NUSSENZWEIG AND RUTH S. NUSSENZWEIG

Virus-Induced Immunosuppression: Infections with Measles Virus and Human Immunodeficiency Virus
 MICHAEL B. MCCHESNEY AND MICHAEL B. A. OLDSTONE

The Regulators of Complement Activation (RCA) Gene Cluster
 DENNIS HOURCADE, V. MICHAEL HOLERS, AND JOHN P. ATKINSON

Origin and Significance of Autoreactive T Cells
 MAURICE ZAUDERER

INDEX

Volume 46

Physical Maps of the Mouse and Human Immunoglobulin-like Loci
 ERIC LAI, RICHARD K. WILSON, AND LEROY E. HOOD

Molecular Genetics of Murine Lupus Models
 ARGYRIOS N. THEOFILOPOULOS, REINHARD KOFLER, PAUL A. SINGER, AND FRANK J. DIXON

Heterogeneity of Cytokine Secretion Patterns and Functions of Helper T Cells
 TIM R. MOSMANN AND ROBERT L. COFFMAN

The Leukocyte Integrins
 TAKASHI K. KISHIMOTO, RICHARD S. LARSON, ANGEL L. CORBI, MICHAEL L. DUSTIN, DONALD E. STAUNTON, AND TIMOTHY A. SPRINGER

Structure and Function of the Complement Receptors, CR1 (CD35) and CR2 (CD21)
 JOSEPH M. AHEARN AND DOUGLAS T. FEARON

The Cellular and Subcellular Bases of Immunosenescence
 MARILYN L. THOMAN AND WILLIAM O. WEIGLE

Immune Mechanisms in Autoimmune Thyroiditis
 JEANNINE CHARREIRE

IINDEX